SPRINGER PUBLISHING

AF716843

GET THE MOST FROM YOUR BOOK

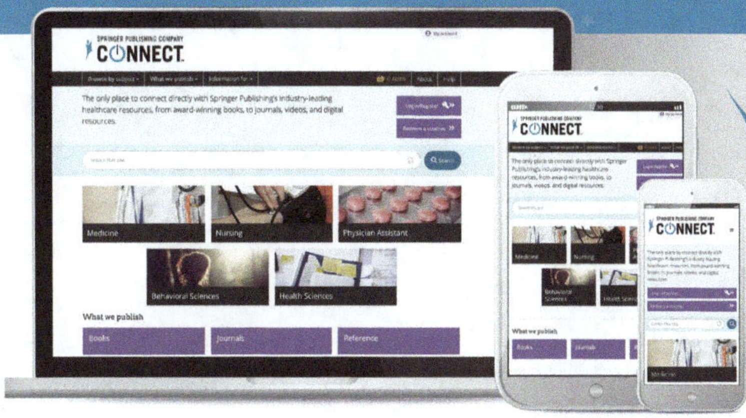

SPRINGER PUBLISHING
CONNECT™

VOUCHER CODE:

1T2LKXHN

Online Access

Your print purchase of *Life Cycle Nutrition for Public Health Professionals*, includes **online access via Springer Publishing Connect**™ to increase accessibility, portability, and searchability.

Insert the code at http://connect.springerpub.com/content/book/978-0-8261-8623-2 or scan the QR code and insert the voucher code today!

*Having trouble? Contact our customer service department at **cs@springerpub.com***

Instructor Resource Access for Adopters

Let us do some of the heavy lifting to create an engaging classroom experience with a variety of instructor resources included in most textbooks SUCH AS:

INSTRUCTOR MANUAL

POWERPOINTS

TEST BANK

Visit **https://connect.springerpub.com/** and look for the **"Show Supplementary"** button on your **book homepage** to see what is available to instructors! First time using Springer Publishing Connect?

Email **textbook@springerpub.com** to create an account and start unlocking valuable resources.

LIFE CYCLE NUTRITION FOR PUBLIC HEALTH PROFESSIONALS

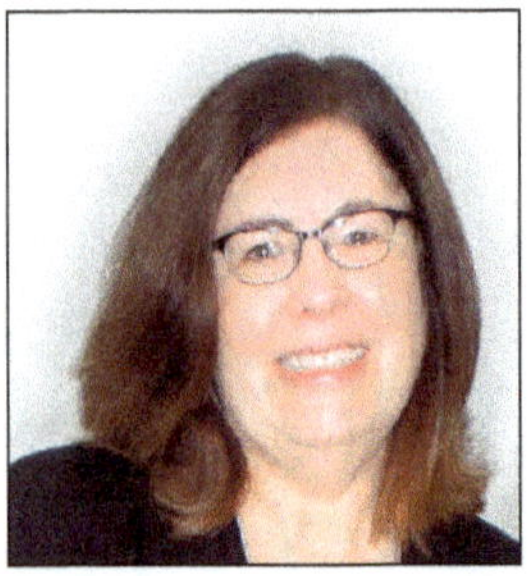

Dr. Kyle L. Thompson, DCN, RDN, is Associate Professor of Nutrition and Director of Graduate Programs in Public Health Nutrition at Appalachian State University. Dr. Thompson earned her Doctorate of Clinical Nutrition (DCN) from Rutgers, the State University of New Jersey, and her Master of Science in Nutrition from East Carolina University. From 2010 to 2017, she directed the Appalachian State Dietetic Internship Program. During her career, Dr. Thompson has received awards including a Teaching Award and a Service Award from Appalachian State's Beaver College of Health Sciences, an Outstanding Service Award from the Doctor of Clinical Nutrition Program, the Rutgers School of Health Professions, and the 2013 Outstanding Dietetic Educator: Dietetic Internship award from the North Carolina Dietetic Association and the Area 6 Nutrition and Dietetics Educators and Preceptors. She was named a Chancellor's Innovation Scholar for her proposal for developing rural-focused, interprofessional simulations for dietetics education. She has served with the Academy of Nutrition and Dietetics Evidence Analysis Library and Simulation Task Force. She has published a variety of scholarly papers, and has presented at meetings and webinars including the Food and Nutrition Conference and Expo (FNCE) 2013, 2014, 2015; the National Rural Health Association National Conference (2018, 2019), the American Public Health Association Annual Meeting (2019), Nutrition and Dietetics Educators and Preceptors (2019), and Nutrition Educators of Health Professionals (2020). Dr. Thompson is participating in a project with the World Public Health Nutrition Association focused on competencies for public health nutrition professionals, and is the Appalachian State University Liaison to the Association of State Public Health Nutritionists (ASPHN). She served as an Associate Editor for a textbook, *Public Health Nutrition: Rural, Urban, and Global Community*-Based Practice, published by Springer Publishing Company in spring 2020, and recently collaborated with the American Heart Association and the Aramark Corporation to publish the *Healthy for Life Educators' Guide.* Dr. Thompson's research agenda is focused on rural public health nutrition practice and nutrition and dietetics education. Dr. Thompson's passion is mentoring students to become compassionate, competent health and nutrition professionals who will make a positive difference for individuals, communities, the nation, and the world.

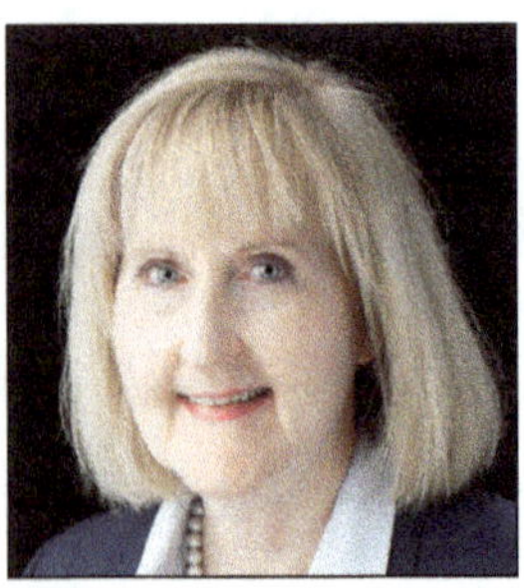

M. Margaret Barth, PhD, MPH, serves as Professor and Chair of Nutrition and Health Care Management at Appalachian State University. Dr. Barth received her PhD in Nutrition and Food Science from the University of Illinois, Urbana-Champaign; MPH from the University of Illinois, Chicago; MBA from the Kellogg School of Management, Northwestern University, and BS in Nutrition and Medical Dietetics from the University of Illinois, Chicago. Dr. Barth has served in leadership roles in academia and food organizations in areas of nutrition, food systems, and sustainability and developed research and service learning projects in the United States, Mexico, South America, the Philippines, and China. Publications include authorship of more than 50 scientific research papers along with invited review articles, book chapters, and government references on nutritional quality, public health nutrition, food safety, and community food systems. She was the recipient of the highest alumni award from the University of Illinois, College of Agriculture, Consumer, and Environmental Sciences in 2014. In addition to professional activities in the American Public Health Association (APHA), the World Public Health Nutrition Association (WPHNA), and the Association of State Public Health Nutritionists (ASPHN), she serves as an advisor to nonprofit corporations.

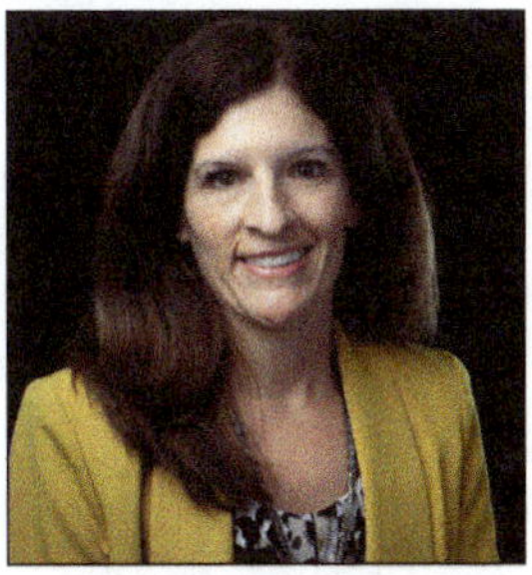

Dr. Melissa D. Gutschall, PhD, RD, is a Professor of Nutrition and Director of Graduate Programs in Nutrition in the Department of Nutrition and Healthcare Management at Appalachian State University, located in Boone, NC. She received her doctoral degree from The Pennsylvania State University in 2006 and has been a registered dietitian for 22 years. She has taught nutrition for 17 years at the undergraduate and graduate levels, served as the Director of the Didactic Program in Dietetics for 5 years, and served as a faculty internship coordinator for 8 years. She regularly serves as an advisor for graduate student research and capstone projects in the area of dietetics and public health nutrition. She has authored and coauthored over 40 publications and over 80 presentations related to nutrition education, rural nutrition, food insecurity, and chronic disease. She has authored *Nutrition and Health*, a supplementary text for introductory nutrition courses, published by Kendall Hunt Publishing in 2011; "Sports Nutrition for the Health Professional," a survey course offered by e-text, published by Caduceus International Publishing in 2018; and contributed to "Public Health Nutrition in the Rural United States: An Interprofessional Framework for Effective Nutrition Interventions" in *Public Health Nutrition: Rural, Urban, and Global Community*-Based Practice, published by Springer Publishing Company in 2020. Dr. Gutschall received the 2012 Inaugural College of Health Sciences Outstanding Teaching Award, the 2016 Beaver College of Health Sciences Research Award, and the 2020 Cratis D. Williams Graduate School 100 Scholars Award. She was selected as the Outstanding Dietetics Educator for 2014 by the North Carolina Dietetics Association, for the Chancellor's Inaugural Class of the Academic Leadership Development Program in 2015, and for the UNC-BRIDGES Academic Leadership Program for Women in 2021. Dr. Gutschall continues to practice clinically on an interdisciplinary team providing care for children with special needs in the Appalachian Region. She has served with the Academy of Nutrition and Dietetics Evidence Analysis Library and Simulation Task Force, and currently serves on the North Carolina Academy of Nutrition and Dietetics executive board in the role of President-Elect; she has earned the status of Fellow of the Academy of Nutrition and Dietetics. Her current research agenda is aimed at using her experience to bridge the gap between food insecurity and chronic illness in the rural population of Watauga County through a Food is Medicine initiative funded by the Blue Cross Blue Shield Foundation of NC, in collaboration with the Hunger and Health Coalition and Appalachian Regional Healthcare System.

LIFE CYCLE NUTRITION FOR PUBLIC HEALTH PROFESSIONALS

Kyle L. Thompson, DCN, RDN

M. Margaret Barth, PhD, MPH

Melissa D. Gutschall, PhD, RD

SPRINGER PUBLISHING

Springer Publishing Company, LLC
902 Carnegie Center, Suite 140, Princeton, NJ 08540
www.springerpub.com
connect.springerpub.com

Acquisitions Editor: David D'Addona
Compositor: Amnet
Production Editor: Dennis Troutman

ISBN: 978-0-8261-8622-5
ebook ISBN: 978-0-8261-8623-2
DOI: 10.1891/9780826186232

SUPPLEMENTS:

SPRINGER PUBLISHING CONNECT™ | A robust set of instructor resources designed to supplement this text is located at **http://connect.springerpub.com/content/book/978-0-8261-8623-2.** Qualifying instructors may request access by emailing **textbook@springerpub.com.**

Instructor Materials:
Instructor Manual: 978-0-8261-8624-9
PowerPoints: 978-0-8261-8626-3
Test Bank: 978-0-8261-8625-6
Sample Syllabus: 978-0-8261-8627-0

Printed by LSI

Library of Congress Cataloging-in-Publication Data
Names: Thompson, Kyle L., editor. | Barth, M. Margaret, editor. | Gutschall, Melissa D., editor.
Title: Life cycle nutrition for public health professionals / [edited by] Kyle L. Thompson, M. Margaret Barth, Melissa D. Gutschall.
Description: New York, NY : Springer Publishing Company, [2024] | Includes bibliographical references and index.
Identifiers: LCCN 2023039336 (print) | LCCN 2023039337 (ebook) | ISBN 9780826186225 (paperback) | ISBN 9780826186232 (ebook)
Subjects: MESH: Nutritional Physiological Phenomena | Public Health—methods | Population Health | Life Course Perspective
Classification: LCC RA425 (print) | LCC RA425 (ebook) | NLM QU 145 | DDC 362.1—dc23/eng/20230922
LC record available at https://lccn.loc.gov/2023039336
LC ebook record available at https://lccn.loc.gov/2023039337

Printed in the United States of America.

To the public health and public health nutrition leaders of the future,
that your training in community-focused nutrition across the life span
will strengthen your efforts in building health, wellness, and resilience—
and encourage and bless all those you serve locally and globally
in every life stage

CONTENTS

III. PUBLIC HEALTH AND NUTRITION: KEY TOPICS AND TRENDS

CONTRIBUTORS

Caroline Brantley, MS, RD, LDN Doctoral Candidate, Department of Human Nutrition and Hospitality Management, University of Alabama, Tuscaloosa, Alabama

David R. Buys, PhD, MSPH, CPH, FGSA Associate Professor, Department of Food Science, Nutrition, and Health Promotion, Mississippi State University, Mississippi

Amy B. Dailey, PhD, MPH Associate Professor and Chair, Health Sciences Department, Gettysburg College, Gettysburg, Pennsylvania

Onyedikachi Emmanuel Chike Department of Agricultural and Applied Economics, Texas Tech University, Lubbock

Melissa D. Gutschall, PhD, RD Professor and Director, Graduate Programs in Nutrition, Appalachian State University, Boone, North Carolina

Jennifer Noll Folliard, MPH, RDN Maternal Child Health Director, South Dakota Department of Health, Sioux Falls, South Dakota

Rosa K. Hand, PhD, RDN, LD, FAND Assistant Professor, Department of Nutrition, Case Western Reserve University, Cleveland, Ohio

Soghra Jarvandi, MD, MPH, PhD Associate Professor, Department of Family and Consumer Sciences, University of Tennessee, Knoxville, Tennessee

Natasha Johnson-Griffin NASA Capacity Building Program/Universities Space Research Association, MS with concentration in Public Health Nutrition, Appalachian State University, Boone, North Carolina

Linda L. Knol, PhD, RD Professor, Department of Human Nutrition and Hospitality Management, University of Alabama, Tuscaloosa, Alabama

Conrad Lyford, PhD Department of Agricultural and Applied Economics, Texas Tech University, Lubbock

Joshua D. Miller, BSc Doctoral Student, Department of Nutrition, University of North Carolina at Chapel Hill, Chapel Hill, North Carolina

Karen L. Probert, MS, RDN President, Mountain Valley Consulting, Inc., Executive Director, Association of State Public Health Nutritionists, Tuscon, Arizona

Janani Rajbhandari-Thapa, PhD Associate Professor, University of Georgia, Athens, Georgia

Jessica Soldavini, PhD, MPH, RD, LDN Assistant Professor, Department of Nutrition, University of North Carolina at Chapel Hill, Chapel Hill, North Carolina

Sonja Kassis Stetzler, MA, RDN Effective Connecting, Charlotte, North Carolina

Kyle L. Thompson, DCN, RDN, LDN Associate Professor and Director, Graduate Programs in Public Health Nutrition, Department of Nutrition and Health Care Management, Appalachian State University, Boone, North Carolina

PREFACE

Welcome to this textbook, *Life Cycle Nutrition for Public Health Professionals*. It was written as the result of interactions with other public health nutrition academicians, practitioners, and graduate students that indicated the need for such a text, developed from a public health and community-based focus. This text links to the expressed Public Health 3.0 strategy that supports the need for public health leaders to develop and embrace community-wide approaches to assuring conditions in which all people can be healthy. Thus, the text considers nutrition through the entire human life course as viewed through a population health lens. The text is designed for public health students who will benefit from enhanced knowledge of nutrition principles and nutrition students who will benefit from enhanced knowledge of public health principles, as well as public health nutrition practitioners. A distinguished group of authors have collaborated to develop the contents. The text's title is descriptive of the information it provides, and the content is described in detail here.

First, this text is about nutrition. Its specific focus is human nutrition. Human nutrition is the science of food and nutrients, and encompasses everything connected with how people obtain food and water, ingest nutrients from food, process nutrients in their bodies, and utilize nutrients to fuel their individual and collective human lives. Everything—yes, everything—in human life has some connection to nutrition because all human activity is supported in one way or another by food and nutrition. Through the power of nutrients to energize the body and provide substrates for its functions, human beings are able to work, play, create art, engage in science, build cities, grow and prepare food, go to school, raise families, laugh, sleep, nurture relationships, build meaningful lives, and so much more. Food and its nutrients are essential to life.

Second, this text is about life cycle nutrition. In this emphasis, the text is in alignment with the 2025 Dietary Guidelines for Americans, which for the first time provide life cycle–specific nutrition guidance. During each life cycle stage, human beings and communities require the same nutrients, but in varying amounts according to the physiologic needs of the particular stage. Every life cycle stage presents immense potential for growth, development, and maturation. Because the human life course is a continuum from one life cycle stage to the next, appropriate nutrition at earlier stages impacts health and quality of life at every subsequent stage up through older adulthood. This text focuses on recommendations for appropriate nutrition at each life cycle phase, and highlights key public health nutrition issues and social determinants throughout the life span.

Third, this text is written from a public health perspective. The first sentence of Chapter 1 states: "The health of the public is inseparably aligned with the nutrition of the public." Public health is concerned with the entire process of healthcare from policy to community health interventions to the quality of clinical care for individuals. However, public health's primary emphasis is on enacting and/or implementing the laws, regulations, policies, programs, and initiatives that impact population health and safety, such as those directed toward access to quality healthcare, social determinants of health, food safety, and community environments. All of these factors impact people's ability to achieve their maximum health potential. Laws, regulations, and policies that make adequate safe and healthful food available to all will improve the public's health. Effectively addressing community conditions and social determinants of health that present barriers to populations' ability to access adequate healthful food will improve the public's health. Thus, this nutrition textbook seeks to provide relevant knowledge points, expert insights, and practical strategies within the domain of public health. The purpose of the text is to provide education for current and future public health and nutrition practitioners that will result in an improved global health and nutrition environment and thus improvements in countless individual lives and their communities.

Finally, this text is written for public health professionals, including public health nutrition professionals. In support of Public Health 3.0, public health professionals seek to engage communities as partners in improving their nutrition environments and improving their health outcomes. Implementation of needs-based, evidence-based nutrition interventions that are collaborative, respectful, and culturally sensitive is a worthy goal, and one this textbook seeks to promote by contributing to the training of future and current professionals. The authors and editors hope that the knowledge, skills, and guidance obtained from this text will enhance professionals' ability to conduct effective public health nutrition interventions, inspire creativity and ingenuity in addressing public health nutrition problems, and contribute to the sense of meaning and purpose that comes from pursuing a vocation focused on improving the lives of others.

Sincerely,

Kyle L. Thompson, DCN, RDN

M. Margaret Barth, PhD, MPH

Melissa D. Gutschall, PhD, RD

ACKNOWLEDGMENTS

Chapter 12: The editors would like to thank Amanda Hege, MPH, RDN, Department of Nutrition and Healthcare Management, Appalachian State University, for assisting in the development of the Chapter 12 case study.

Chapter 14: The editors would like to thank Dr. Manan Roy, PhD, Department of Nutrition and Healthcare Management, Appalachian State University, for providing assistance in reviewing Chapter 14.

Appendix A: The editors would like to thank the following graduate nutrition students from the Department of Nutrition and Healthcare Management, Appalachian State University, for assisting in the development of Appendix A:

Emily Bowles

Benjamin O'Donnell

Cheyenne Westhoven

SPRINGER PUBLISHING RESOURCES

SPRINGER PUBLISHING CONNECT™

A robust set of instructor resources designed to supplement this text is located at **http://connect.springerpub.com/content/book/978-0-8261-8623-2.** Qualifying instructors may request access by emailing **textbook@springerpub.com.**

LMS Common Cartridge With All Instructor Resources

Instructor Manual

Test Bank with multiple-choice questions (including full rationales) of various types, including recall, higher level of reasoning, and application.

Instructor Chapter PowerPoints

I

LIFE CYCLE NUTRITION FROM THE PUBLIC HEALTH PERSPECTIVE: PRINCIPLES AND PRACTICE

1

LIFE CYCLE NUTRITION FROM A PUBLIC HEALTH PERSPECTIVE: AN INTRODUCTION TO FOUNDATIONAL CONCEPTS AND APPROACHES

Kyle L. Thompson

LEARNING OBJECTIVES

At the end of this chapter, students will be able to:

1. Define *public health, nutrition, public health nutrition, life cycle*, and the *public health approach to life cycle nutrition*.
2. List and describe at least five subdisciplines of nutrition science.
3. Explain six foundational understandings that inform public health and public health nutrition practice.
    - Describe and explain the functions of the six classes of nutrients and two non-nutritive components of foods (Appendix A).
    - Summarize the process of human **digestion** (Appendix A).
    - Explain the components of MyPlate (Appendix B) and the *Dietary Guidelines for Americans* (www.dietaryguidelines.gov/sites/default/files/2021-03/DGA_2020-2025_Infographic_MakeEveryBiteCount.pdf).
4. Explain five basic principles of life cycle nutrition.
5. For each life cycle stage, describe associated nutrition goals and public health nutrition concerns.
6. Explain possible harms of uninformed nutrition practice, four questions to use when evaluating nutrition information, and four sources of reliable nutrition information.

INTRODUCTION

The health of the public is inseparably aligned with the nutrition of the public. Whether or not populations have dependable access to adequate, wholesome, and nutritious **food** largely determines whether those populations will thrive and meet their potential for health and quality of life. Thus, the scope of public health practice includes ensuring good nutrition for populations, and public health nutrition as a specialty area of public health has come to the forefront in recent years. This chapter introduces the foundational concepts of public health and public health nutrition, as well as discussing approaches to nutrition science and its applications to population health through the human life cycle.

A PUBLIC HEALTH APPROACH TO LIFE CYCLE NUTRITION

According to the Centers for Disease Control and Prevention (CDC) of the U.S. Department of Health and Human Services (DHHS), the role of **public health** is to "protect and improve the health of communities through policy recommendations, health education and outreach, and research for disease detection and injury prevention."[1] Thus, public health nutrition can be considered the branch of public health that seeks to protect and improve community health through nutrition policy recommendations, nutrition education and outreach, and research focused on the prevention, detection, and management of nutrition-related diseases. As a branch of nutrition science, **life cycle nutrition in public health** applies the functions of public health nutrition to specific life cycle stages. The following pages provide an introduction and overview of the functions, foundations, and basic principles of public health, public health nutrition, and life cycle nutrition in public health.

Public Health

Dr. Charles E. Winslow was an eminent bacteriologist who was instrumental in founding the Yale School of Public Health in the early 20th century.[2] In a classic article published in 1920, *The Untilled Fields of Public Health,* Dr. Winslow penned a definition of public health that has been adapted over the years and could be considered a de facto mission statement for public health practice.[3,4] In fact, the CDC, in their online *Public Health 101 Series: Introduction to Public Health,* last updated in 2021, begins the course with this definition credited to Dr. Winslow:

> Public health is "the science and art of preventing disease, prolonging life, and promoting health through the organized efforts and informed choices of society, organizations, public and private communities, and individuals" (p. 30).[3,4]

In today's world of public health, each phrase of Dr. Winslow's definition has been expanded to encompass ever-widening circles including local, regional, national, and international settings; diverse groups and populations of people around the world; and myriad organizations, communities, and social structures. Echoing Dr. Winslow's realization of the importance of organized action and societal factors in promoting public health, current public health practitioners understand that disease prevention and health promotion in populations are crucially impacted by environments and **social determinants of health (SDOH).** Practitioners understand, too, that successful efforts to positively impact SDOHs rely on collaborations and cooperation among broad constituencies of organizations, communities, groups, and individuals. In fact, the principles and practice of public health are universal in scope, and apply to all people, all over the world.

10 Essential Public Health Services

What are the key functions carried out by public health professionals in their mission of preventing disease and promoting health in populations? In 1994, the Core Public Health Functions Steering Committee, comprising persons from the U.S. Public Health Service and other leading public health organizations, developed the original **10 Essential Public Health Services Framework.**[5] The original *Framework* served for over 25 years as guide for education and practice in the discipline of public health.

In 2020, the *Framework* was revised and updated to reflect current practice.[5] The 2020 revision was carried out by a task force consisting of public health experts and leaders, and key organizations including the CDC. Notably, in making recommendations for revisions to the framework, the task force actively sought and utilized input from the broader public health practitioner community. The 10 Essential Public Health Services (Revised, 2020) are stated as follows:

1. Assess and monitor population health status, factors that influence health, and community needs and assets.
2. Investigate, diagnose, and address health problems and hazards affecting the population.
3. Communicate effectively to inform and educate people about health, factors that influence it, and how to improve it.
4. Strengthen, support, and mobilize communities and partnerships to improve health.
5. Create, champion, and implement policies, plans, and laws that impact health.
6. Utilize legal and regulatory actions designed to improve and protect the public's health.
7. Assure an effective system that enables equitable access to the individual services and care needed to be healthy.
8. Build and support a diverse and skilled public health workforce.
9. Improve and innovate public health functions through ongoing evaluation, research, and continuous quality improvement.
10. Build and maintain a strong organizational infrastructure for public health.[5]

The scope of practice of public health professionals who practice in both general and specialty areas (such as public health nutrition) is defined by the *Framework.* Public health professionals may act generalists, working across the broad range of functions, or as specialists, focusing their efforts in one or a few defined areas.

Nutrition in Public Health

Like public health, the field of nutrition science is so vast it can literally be described as touching every area of life. **Nutrition** has been defined as the:

> science of food, the nutrients and other substances therein, their action, interaction and balance in relation to health and disease, and the process by which the organism ingests, absorbs, transports, utilizes and excretes food substances (p. 194).[6]

All living things require nutrients and continuously engage in the complex metabolic processes that facilitate the consumption, absorption, and utilization of nutrients.[7]

Nutrition as a physiologic process is, however, just the proverbial "tip of the iceberg": the relationship between food and human beings also involves deep and significant social, economic, historical, aesthetic, emotional, psychological, relational, and even spiritual meanings and implications.

In response to the breadth of the discipline of nutrition, a number of subdisciplines and/or specialty areas have emerged over the past century—most in recent decades. A few examples include but are not limited to public health nutrition, nutrition policy, dietetics and medical nutrition therapy, nutritional epidemiology, nutrient research, food science, culinary nutrition, environmental nutrition, sustainable agriculture, food safety and regulation, and food emergency management.

Some disciplines of nutrition science, such as dietetics and medical nutrition therapy, are primarily applicable to individuals. For example, nutrition and dietetics professionals (registered dietitians/registered dietitian nutritionists [RDs/RDNs]) in the United States are credentialed and qualified to design individualized meal plans and provide highly tailored medical nutrition therapy based on a patient's or client's specific health condition(s) and medical record. Other aspects of nutrition science are primarily applicable to populations. Public health nutrition practitioners including RDs and RDNs, public health professionals working to impact community health, food safety specialists, food distribution and supply chain specialists, and nutritional epidemiologists are examples of professionals whose focus is on nutrition issues that impact population groups and communities.

Public Health Nutrition as a Specialty Area of Public Health

Public health nutrition (PHN) is a specialty area of public health practice. The Academy of Nutrition and Dietetics has defined PHN as, "The application of nutrition and public health principles to improve or maintain optimal health of populations and targeted groups through enhancements in programs, systems, policies, and environments" (p. 5).[8] PHN practitioners apply the principles and services of public health within population nutrition settings. Table 1.1 lists the 10 Essential Public Health Services along with examples of associated PHN applications.

The Life Cycle: A Continuum of Human Development

Human development takes place on a continuum extending from the **prenatal** period through death. Unless interrupted by premature death, persons progress through the stages of infancy, young and older childhood, adolescence, young and middle adulthood, and older adulthood. The **hierarchy of needs** proposed by Maslow identifies nutrition as a foundational survival need.[9,10] A lack of nutrients ultimately results in the death of the organism.[10] But, beyond basic survival, the adequacy and quality of nutrients ingested by individuals plays a crucial role in physical and mental health at each life stage.

The human life cycle encompasses a lifelong process of continuous change and development that begins **in utero** during pregnancy, then progresses through the stages of infancy, young and older childhood, adolescence, young and middle adulthood, and older adulthood, ending at death. At each stage of the life span, humans develop by changing, adapting, and growing within their environments. Human development encompasses a multitude of areas, including but not limited to physical, cognitive, intellectual, creative,

Table 1.1. 10 Essential Public Health Services With Specific Examples of Public Health Nutrition Applications

Public Health Essential Functions	Public Health Nutrition Applications: Specific Examples
Assess and monitor population health status, factors that influence health, and community needs and assets.	*Participate in a comprehensive community health assessment to determine a community's nutrition environment, nutrition problems, and nutrition resources.*
Investigate, diagnose, and address health problems and hazards affecting the population.	*Based on appropriate data, implement collaborative obesity prevention initiatives for children and adults within localities, including components such as nutrition education; partnerships with local stakeholders such as the medical community, schools, and retailers; healthful cooking classes; social media messaging; and development of opportunities for safe physical activity such as walking paths and park prescription programs.*
Communicate effectively to inform and educate people about health, factors that influence it, and how to improve it.	*Work with local food retailers on a campaign to develop in-store messages and a social media campaign promoting fruit and vegetable consumption.*
Strengthen, support, and mobilize communities and partnerships to improve health.	*Partner with community organizations to develop mobile delivery options for residents.*
Create, champion, and implement policies, plans, and laws that impact health.	*Become a member of a public policy committee or task force within one's professional organization.*
Utilize legal and regulatory actions designed to improve and protect the public's health.	*Collaborate with food production industries to develop food safety quality assurance plans.*
Assure an effective system that enables equitable access to the individual services and care needed to be healthy.	*Promote local agriculture and local food networks to improve community access to fresh vegetables, including the development of shared processing facilities for small producers—and optimize utilization of SNAP and WIC Farmers Market benefits.*
Build and support a diverse and skilled public health workforce.	*Work in higher education or serve as a preceptor or mentor to develop and train future PHN professionals.*
Improve and innovate public health functions through ongoing evaluation, research, and continuous quality improvement.	*Conduct an epidemiologic study of the relationships among population eating patterns—including food insecure populations—and incidence of chronic diseases in a particular region.*
Build and maintain a strong organizational infrastructure for public health.	*Work with statewide food banks to develop a comprehensive disaster plan to ensure maintenance of basic functions and sharing of resources in the event of disasters.*

PHN, public health nutrition; SNAP, Supplemental Nutrition Assistance Program; WIC, Women, Infants, and Children.
Source: Adapted from Centers for Disease Control and Prevention. 10 essential public health services. Updated 2021. https://www.cdc.gov/publichealthgateway/publichealthservices/essentialhealthservices.html

functional, emotional, social, moral, and spiritual domains.[11] Adequate nutrition supports basic survival.[10] But, beyond survival, the adequacy and quality of nutrients ingested by individuals play a crucial role in physical, emotional, and mental health at each life stage.

Child Development

The words *human development* often bring to mind children and adolescents—and the fascination of watching them grow through childhood and adolescence into adulthood. Human development progresses rapidly throughout childhood and adolescence, and successful passage through each milestone sets the stage for a productive adult life. While there is some debate in the scientific literature regarding the nature of the prolonged effects of environmental deprivation in infancy and early childhood, it is generally agreed that there are periods when lack of desirable inputs results in severe and lifelong impacts.[12]

Critical periods of child development are thought to be specific time periods—with a well-defined beginning and ending—when the brain and body are ideally aligned for a crucial developmental advancement to occur. Once the time period ends, the window for normal development of the specific ability closes.[13] An example of a critical period is the development of binocular vision, or the ability to coordinate both eyes to achieve depth perception, in babies between 2 and 4 months of age, and at this stage, nutrients such as vitamin A must be available for optimal development of vision.[14]

Over the approximately 100 year history of the critical period theory of human development, there has been a growing general consensus that only a few periods are truly critical. The term sensitive period may be a better descriptor of many behavioral, linguistic, and even emotional developmental tasks.[12] A sensitive period of child development is a time when brain and body alignment are optimal for a particular developmental task; however, the time period during which the task can be accomplished remains somewhat malleable.[13,15] Thus, more or less extensive degrees of remediation and development remain possible. Examples of sensitive periods may include language learning, the acquisition of familial and cultural food preferences, and the development of human attachments and social behaviors, highlighting the importance of rich and loving environments for children, including at mealtimes.[16]

Nutrition and nutrient adequacy and quality play crucial roles in child development, and are essential for optimal progression through the critical and sensitive periods of the pediatric life cycle stages.[15] Thus, in public health settings, the task of ensuring access to adequate healthful, nutrient-rich foods for all children and adolescents is a key concern.

Adult Development

Human development is not limited to children. Adults, including older adults, learn, adapt, and change throughout life, most often in response to life experiences as well as the ongoing process of physical aging.[11,17] Once basic needs for survival are met, successful adult development is characterized by ongoing growth in qualities including but not limited to maturity, empathy, self-understanding, acceptance of self and others, the practice of kindness and compassion toward self and others, cultivation of positive relationships, a **growth mindset**, a sense of purpose and meaning, and the ability to handle life's inevitable highs and lows with resilience and strength. As adults progress through the life cycle, nutrition for disease prevention and management and the impacts of nutrition in previous life stages, take on greater importance.

At each human life stage, and during each developmental task, nutrition plays a critical role because nutrients fuel every human activity. Thus, a public health approach to nutrition seeks to address social determinants of health and environmental factors that present barriers to good nutrition for adults and children. **Nutrition security**, or access to adequate calories and nutrients to promote health and prevent chronic disease, is a primary goal of PH practice.[18] To this end, PH and PHN professionals encourage and promote access to healthful food for all persons at every life cycle stage. In relation to adults, promotion of access to healthful food can include addressing lack of access to full-service grocery stores, nutrition and cooking skills education, and promotion of governmental and nongovernmental resources and services available to fill nutrition gaps. PH and PHN professionals advocate for **food systems** and food environments that are just and equitable, and that support optimal human health, well-being, and quality of life for all, throughout the life span.

What Is a Public Health Approach to Life Cycle Nutrition?

For the purposes of this text, the *public health approach to life cycle nutrition* will be defined as the application of public health principles to population nutrition issues and problems at each stage of the human life cycle. The term *public health nutrition* (as a subdiscipline of public health) is used interchangeably in this text with the terms *nutrition in public health* and *a public health approach to life cycle nutrition.*

AN APPROACH TO THE PRACTICE OF NUTRITION IN PUBLIC HEALTH SETTINGS

A Foundation for Nutrition Practice in Public Health Settings

An important ethical imperative for all who work in health-associated fields is to develop an in-depth understanding of their disciplines so that professionals can address the often-delicate balance between benefits and possible risks and harms of interventions.[19] Nutrition information—and misinformation—is readily available and easily accessed. Thus, anyone who works in nutrition-related fields of public health should have a good basic knowledge of nutrition science, and understand the potential of nutrition interventions to help *and* harm.

Key Understandings to Inform Public Health Nutrition Approaches and Interventions

1. *Nutrition touches every aspect of life.*

Humans require a continual supply of nutrients throughout the entire life span. During thousands of years of human history, humans devoted the majority of their waking hours to the acquisition, preparation, and consumption of food and thus food's component nutrients. The *hierarchy of needs* proposed by Maslow identifies nutrition as a foundational survival need.[10] Food is basic to human existence. Every individual and collaborative human activity is fueled by food. On the population level, *food systems*—and their organizations, structures, and outcomes—inevitably lead to economic, political, ethical, cultural, physical and mental health, and social/emotional outcomes, whether good or ill.[20] Thus, it is crucial for PHN professionals to be aware of the plethora of contextual factors surrounding food and nutrition impacts and interventions. Effective professionals understand the broad spectrum of nutrition needs across the life span, and similarities and differences in nutrition needs among life stage groups.

2. Six major classes of nutrients, plus non-nutrient bioactive substances, are found in food. These substances are made available for use by the human body during the process of digestion.

All nutrition science begins with a discussion of the six kinds of nutrients found within solid and liquid foods: protein, fats, carbohydrates, vitamins, minerals, and water.[21] Humans obtain nearly all their nutrients from food consumption. Ingested nutrients support both the structural components and the functional processes of the human body, and provide the energy and the necessary substrates to carry out the chemical reactions of life.

Food also provides components that are not nutrients but play roles in human health, nutrition, and digestion. Two key examples are fiber and phytochemicals. Dietary fiber consists of carbohydrate structures of plants that are not digested or absorbed by the body.[22] Phytochemicals are bioactive, non-nutrient chemicals found in plants that may play roles in promoting health and preventing chronic disease.[23]

Digestion is the biologic process by which the nutrients in food become available to the human body. During digestion, food is ingested, broken down into its molecular components by both physical and chemical processes, and absorbed and utilized by the body. In the final stages of digestion, the waste products of nutrient breakdown are excreted. A concise review of basic human nutrition and digestion is found in **Appendix A.** It is highly recommended that students complete this self-guided review during their study of Chapter 1 of this text.

3. A myriad of attempts have been made throughout history to determine the ideal diet for humans. Current science-based dietary recommendations are reflected in the official dietary guidance tools provided to their citizens by the governments of many of the world's nations.

Although the statement often attributed to Hippocrates, "Let food by thy medicine and medicine by thy food" appears nowhere in the known works of Hippocrates and seems to be a modern misquotation, it is clear that from ancient times Hippocrates and many others noticed a connection between food and health.[24] In public health, dietary guidelines for large groups of healthy people are useful in formulating broad food and nutrition recommendations to promote health and the prevention of disease.

More than 100 countries have developed their own dietary guidance tools and graphics to deliver nutrition messages population-wide.[25,26] A few examples include Japan's Spinning Top visual aid, Bolivia's fan-shaped graphic, the Malaysian Food Pyramid, a color-coded representation of the Burj Khalifa to illustrate the United Arab Emirates' dietary guidelines, Finland's Food Triangle and Food Plate, China's Food Pagoda, Sierra Leone's Food Guide, and Kenya's Dietary Guidelines.[27–33] In the United States, three broad dietary guidance tools have been developed for applications in population health: the Dietary Reference Intakes (DRIs), the Dietary Guidelines for Americans (DGAs), and MyPlate.[34–36] Concise reviews of the DRIs, DGAs, and MyPlate are found in **Appendices C, D, and B**, respectively. It is highly recommended that students complete this self-guided review during their study of Chapter 1 of this text.

4. Nutrition and nutrition science are extremely complex.

A vast web of interconnected factors impacts all nutrition research and intervention. The study of nutrition encompasses complex relationships among food systems, people, specific foods and their properties, **bioavailability of nutrients**, genetics, state of physical health, the food environment, geographic location, economics, culture, and a plethora of other influences.[37] It is challenging, to say the least, to isolate the effects of specific nutrients in the body, to determine whether or not particular nutrition interventions are effective, and to accurately assess the influence of population-wide PHN interventions. When conducting nutrition research, the number of potential **confounders** can quickly become overwhelming, to the point that some experts have suggested the development of research methods unique to the complexity of nutrition science.[38,39]

Pharmaceutical research differs from nutrition research in several ways. In a randomized controlled trial designed to test a pharmaceutical, participants usually begin a study without any prior exposure to the drug of interest, and are provided with *one* intervention consisting of a standard dose of pharmaceutical *a*. Factors including but not limited to regimen compliance, disease state, the concurrent use of other pharmaceuticals, and even the ingestion of certain foods can confound results. However, in a given pharmaceutical study there may be fewer confounders to control, and in the end, it will be possible to compare differences in measured outcomes between the study group and a control group that differs appreciably in only one factor: *not* receiving the study drug.

People who participate in nutrition research usually live in normal human settings, creating formidable challenges to controlling confounding factors. Not the least of these challenges is that subjects have likely been consuming the nutrients of interest for years prior to the study, making establishment of baseline status for a particular nutrient difficult.[37] Participants in a nutrition study, or a nutrition intervention, may faithfully follow a prescribed regimen—whether for an individual food or nutrient or meal plan—during the entirety of a particular study. Concurrently, those participants are going about their unique lives and engaging in their usual habits. Nutrients are highly interactive, and are sensitive to the individual's genetic influences. Amount and intensity of physical activity, hours of sleep, the subject's usual environmental surroundings, and even the degree of stress experienced can impact the metabolism of nutrients. While valuable nutrition research can sometimes be conducted in specialized, isolated facilities such as metabolic research units, these are extremely expensive, require significant disruption of usual life activities on the part of subjects, and do not replicate normal life settings.[40]

In public health, research often takes place by necessity in real-world surroundings. Populations exist within geographic environments that can promote or hinder healthful nutrition. PHN research and interventions are influenced by a variety of SDOH such as access to wholesome and healthful food, socioeconomic status, housing, availability of cooking and refrigeration equipment, the number of retail food outlets nearby, nutrition education opportunities, education level, and more. For these and other reasons, public health professionals distinguish between **efficacy** (results of an intervention under ideal conditions) and **effectiveness** (results of an intervention in real-world settings).[41] The two are often not the same, and the truism "If it sounds good it must *be* good" should be approached with caution when implementing PHN studies.[41]

The PHN professional does well to maintain an attitude of humility in regard to the body of nutrition knowledge available to us. While much has been learned during the relatively short history of nutrition science, and the amount of nutrition knowledge grows with each passing year, the greatest breakthroughs in nutrition research likely still lie ahead. Methodologies designed for nutrition research will continue to develop, and the technology available to isolate the effects of specific nutrients will continue to improve. The practical application of genetics to nutrition science—so that the composition of a particular individual's ideal diet for optimizing health can be determined—is an exciting and advancing frontier still in its earlier stages of development. The complexity of nutrition science means that our understanding of the relationships among nutrients, human genetics, environmental factors, and human health will most likely develop gradually over many years.

5. Like all other health interventions, nutrition interventions require a careful assessment of possible harms.

Nutrition plays a tremendously important role across the entire spectrum of human health and well-being. Appropriate and adequate nutrition can support optimal physical, mental, and emotional well-being. Beyond those outcomes, medical nutrition therapy is a key component of effective treatment and management of both acute and chronic diseases and conditions. However, because of the complexity of nutrition, and the body of evidence that a variety of eating patterns and cultural foodways can support optimal human health, careful consideration should be given to the possible effects of nutrition interventions.

While supportive nutrition interventions can elicit many positive outcomes, they do not often cure disease (an exception is the correction of an identified nutrient deficiency before permanent physiologic damage has occurred). Professionals should maintain an attitude of skepticism regarding claims that one particular food /food group or one dietary plan is "ideal" for all persons, or that nutritional regimens can eliminate disease, or that in regard to supplements, "the more the better." As in most areas of life, the 20th-century saying, "if it sounds too good to be true, it probably is," is likely to hold true.[42]

Nutrition interventions should be based on the best knowledge and evidence available, and practitioners should utilize an evidence-based approach.[43] The possible impacts, both positive and negative, of nutrition interventions should be very carefully considered in the planning phases. In public health, harms may occur when interventions are implemented in the face of a lack of evidence—sometimes because the intervention "sounds like a good idea." In 1936, sociologist Robert K. Merton wrote a paper proposing what has come to be known popularly as **the law of unintended consequences.**[44] That is, actions—however well intentioned—may have results, either positive or negative, that are different from, or in addition to, expected outcomes.

As an example, consider the development of dietary messaging regarding fat. Beginning in 1984 with reports from the National Institutes of Health (NIH) and the National Cholesterol Education Program (NCEP), and continuing throughout the 1990s despite a lack of clear evidence, dietary fat came to be viewed unfavorably.[45] Public health messaging at the time led many to believe that dietary fat should be avoided and individuals' consumption should be as low as possible. The food industry responded by replacing much fat in food products with refined carbohydrates.[45] Products such as low-fat cookies and pastries were developed that contained only small amounts of fats but substantial amounts of added sugars and other carbohydrates, as well as additional sodium to compensate for flavor deficits resulting from lack of fat. Since that time, emerging evidence has suggested that consumption of excessive amounts of refined carbohydrates may have had unintended consequences, including possible associations with poor cardiac and metabolic outcomes.[45]

A knowledgeable approach to nutrition recognizes that in the history of man's scientific endeavors, nutrition science is a newcomer.[46] An understanding of diet as a factor in health has existed since ancient times, but nutrition as a branch of science has been recognized for considerably less than 200 years. Mozaffarian, Rosenberg, and Uauy have suggested that nutrition science was approached in a "reductionistic" manner during the late 19th and 20th centuries.[46] While a natural progression in the development of nutrition science, the reductionistic approach emphasized individual nutrients, their functions, and the impacts of their deficiencies in the diet.[47] In recent decades, there has been a growing recognition that a reductionistic approach is inadequate to explain the linkages among nutrients and health—and that an approach focusing on usual dietary patterns and foods is more explanatory when determining etiologies of chronic diseases.[46,47]

6. Know where to obtain reliable nutrition information.

Accurate nutrition information as well as misinformation are both readily available via the internet and social media. Nutrition misinformation can include claims of nutrition "cures" for serious and even terminal diseases, the presentation of certain foods as "good" or "bad," advertisements for "quick and easy" weight loss methods, promised benefits of supplementation along with the attitude that "more supplements are better," claims of "changing one's metabolism" with specific diets or supplements, diets based on extreme restriction of calories, diets promising benefits by eliminating entire food groups or combining certain food groups, claims that only organic foods are beneficial, and much more. Such claims can sound reasonable and feasible, and are often accompanied by testimonials or research studies of questionable quality.

When evaluating nutrition information and claims, public health and PHN professionals should keep in mind the complexity of nutrition science, the possible harms of nutrition interventions, and the imperative for practitioners to obtain nutrition information and guidance from reliable sources. Table 1.2 provides suggestions for evaluating nutrition information and claims. Table 1.3 provides a list of reliable sources of nutrition information.

Key Understandings to Inform Public Health Nutrition Approaches and Interventions Throughout the Life Cycle

Life cycle nutrition is a subspecialty of nutrition science. While the general principles of nutrition science apply to life cycle nutrition, several additional considerations are important to an understanding of nutrition throughout the life cycle.

1. Nutrition has important impacts in every stage of the life cycle.

Nutritional intake and status have sequential and cumulative effects on health outcomes from the beginning to the end of life.[48] As an example, consider the influence of a key PHN issue, **food insecurity**, on health and well-being throughout the life cycle.

Food insecurity during pregnancy has been associated with less-than-optimal pregnancy outcomes such as heightened risk of prematurity, a higher rate of infant hospitalizations in the months after birth, low birth weight, and small-for-gestational-age status.[49] The experience of food insecurity in childhood and adolescence is associated with **adverse childhood experiences (ACEs)** and is linked with poor physical and mental health outcomes.[50] Food-insecure young adults may suffer from higher rates of chronic disease and obesity.[51] The productivity and success of young adults may also be linked to food insecurity: in college student populations, food insecurity has been linked to worse academic performance and mental health problems, especially in students with diagnosed medical disorders.[52] A U.S. Department of Agriculture (USDA) Economic Research Service publication reported that in working-age adults with incomes at or below 200% of the federal poverty level, food insecurity is associated with a greater likelihood of 10 specific chronic diseases, and an overall increase in the risk of chronic disease in general.[53] Food insecurity increases the risk of adult depression, stress, and anxiety, and these sequelae may become more pronounced as age increases.[54] By older adulthood, cumulative impacts associated with poor

Table 1.2. Suggested Guidelines for Evaluating Nutrition Information and Claims

Suggested Evaluation Questions	Criteria for Evaluation	Best Sources	Use Caution; Check Further
1. What is the source of the nutrition information?	• Credentials and educational background of the information provider • Website domain • Reputability of agencies and organizations	• Sources with academic degrees from accredited universities • Sources with recognized practitioner credentials such as RDN, LDN, CHES • Websites with the domains .gov, .edu, .org; maintained by governmental agencies, accredited educational institutions, reputable nonprofit organizations	• Source lacks academic training in nutrition, or has degree from a non-accredited institution • Websites with .com or .net domains • Confirm qualifications of organizations providing nutrition information
2. What kind of information and/or evidence supports the nutrition claims?	• Method of obtaining information and/or evidence	• Evidence based on systematic reviews, meta-analyses, and/or research studies published in peer-reviewed academic journals • High-quality databases maintained by governmental agencies, accredited educational institutions, reputable nonprofit organizations	• Anecdotal evidence such as testimonials • Claims of clinical research studies not found in recognized academic journals, or using questionable methodology, or not published • Research studies funded by for-profit entities (*Note:* Research funding provided by a for-profit agency does not imply the research is poorly executed or invalid; however, it is a signal to use additional caution in evaluating potential conflicts of interest that could impact findings.)

3. Is the provider of nutrition information also selling products associated with the information?	• Potential conflicts of interest	• Qualified information providers who do not have a financial stake in the product • Neutral third-party evaluators such as governmental agencies, accredited educational institutions, reputable nonprofit organizations that disclose potential conflicts of interest	• Information source has a financial stake in the product being described • Third-party evaluators with a disclosed conflict of interest; evaluate on a case-by-case basis
4. Are the information and claims reasonable in light of the current state of nutrition science?	• Claims made for the results of applying the provided nutrition information	• Use all of the sources listed in this column to evaluate the reasonableness of nutrition claims (qualified professionals, reputable governmental, educational, and nongovernmental organizations, qualified evaluators without financial conflicts of interest in products touted, studies published in peer-reviewed academic journals)	• Nutrition claims touting spectacular results such as the cure of serious/terminal diseases, rapid and easy weight loss, major improvements in athletic performance • Claims promoting specific diets as the answer to attaining optimal health; claims that including or eliminating certain foods or food groups from the diet will promote optimal health • Claims that particular supplements are essential to achieving or maintaining health goals • CHES, certified health education specialist; LDN, licensed dietitian nutritionist; RDN, registered dietitian nutritionist.

Table 1.3. Examples of Agencies and Organizations Providing Reliable Nutrition Information for Public Health and Public Health Nutrition Professionals

Agency or Organization	Web Address
1. U.S. Department of Agriculture (USDA)	www.usda.gov
2. USDA Food and Nutrition Service	www.fns.usda.gov
3. USDA Food Safety and Inspection Service	www.fsis.usda.gov
4. U.S. Department of Health and Human Services (DHHS)	www.hhs.gov
5. Centers for Disease Control and Prevention (CDC)	www.cdc.gov
6. Dietary Guidelines for Americans	www.dietaryguidelines.gov
7. Tufts University, Friedman School of Nutrition Science and Policy	nutrition.tufts.edu
8. Academy of Nutrition and Dietetics	eatright.org
9. American Public Health Association	www.apha.org
10. Association of State Public Health Nutritionists (ASPHN)	asphn.org
11. American Diabetes Association	diabetes.org
12. American Heart Association	www.heart.org
13. Feeding America	www.feedingamerica.org

lifetime nutrition may include multiple chronic diseases, increased risk of infections and hospitalizations, reduced functional ability, suboptimal quality of life, and substantially reduced life span.[48,55]

2. There are key nutrition goals for each stage of the life cycle.

Adequate nutrition during pregnancy and lactation supports the appropriate growth of the fetus and infant. In infancy, nutrition goals include the provision of adequate calories and nutrients to promote optimal physical growth and development, successful completion of initial steps in establishing a positive relationship with food by respecting the infant's feeding cues and signals, and achieving appropriate social and emotional growth engendered by warm, responsive, and caring feeding experiences provided by parents and/or caregivers. Throughout childhood, adolescence, and adulthood, the achievement of desired nutrition goals enhances both human development and enjoyment of life.

In the culminating stages of the life cycle, adequate nutrition for older adults is essential for the prevention and management of chronic disease, optimization of functional ability, and maintenance of quality of life. Social and emotional aspects of nutrition remain important even in the older adult life stage; research indicates that commensality, or eating together, has a significant impact on older adult nutritional intake.[56] Table 1.4 provides examples of specific life cycle-related nutrition needs and goals.[57,58]

Table 1.4. Life Cycle Nutrition Goals for Each Life Stage

Life Cycle Stage	Nutrition Goals
Prenatal period	*Maternal*: Appropriate weight gain Reduced risk of pregnancy complications Reduced risk of preterm birth *Infant*: Healthy birth weight Appropriate weight for gestational age Reduced risk of neural tube defects
Infancy (Birth–1 year)	Appropriate growth and development Possible reduced risk of chronic disease in adulthood Successful initial development of feeding skills and attitudes toward food
Childhood (2–12 years)	Appropriate growth and development Reduced risk of childhood overweight and obesity Growth of independence in self-feeding including food preparation
Adolescence (13–19 years)	Achievement of optimal growth Reduced risk of adolescent overweight and obesity Transition to independence and adulthood in feeding and nourishing oneself Development of a positive relationship with food
Adulthood (young and middle adulthood: 20–44 years and 45–64 years, respectively; these ranges are approximate)	Prevention of chronic disease as adulthood progresses Reduced risk for a variety of physical and mental health problems Maintenance of a healthful weight
Older Adulthood (65+ years; young-old, middle-old, oldest-old: 65–74 years, 75–84 years, 85+ years, respectively)	Reduced risk for a variety of physical and mental health problems, including chronic diseases and infections Maintenance of functional ability and independence as long as possible Maintenance of ability to participate actively in all aspects of life, including food acquisition and meal preparation, as long as possible Maintenance of optimal quality of life

3. The six basic classes of nutrients remain constant throughout life; however, at different life stages, proportions and amounts of nutrients needed differ.

For example, in pregnancy, key nutrients such as iron and calcium are needed in significantly larger amounts than in other life stages. The required amounts are difficult to obtain from eating alone, hence the need for a special prenatal vitamin supplement to ensure adequate intake. Calorie needs—also called energy needs—are proportionately greater in infancy and adolescence than in other life stages. Differing life stage needs help guide nutrition interventions for specific population groups.

4. The nutritional practices of parents and caregivers have strong effects on their developing children's nutrition practices throughout life.

Food- and eating-related memories are established in infancy and early childhood, are some of our most persistent preferences, and are very difficult to change in later life.[59,60] Parents and caregivers have a profound impact not only on the adequacy of children's nutrition, but also on the development of the ability to nourish oneself competently throughout the life span. Ellyn Satter has described four components of her Satter Eating Competence Model that define eating competence: (1) an approach to food and eating that is healthful and positive; (2) the application of eating skills that promote exploration and acceptance of a wide variety of foods; (3) the ability to nourish oneself optimally, that is, to consume appropriate amounts and types of nutrients to support health, activity, and weight stability; and (4) appropriate skills for interacting with contextual factors surrounding food and managing family meals, including food acquisition, storage, preparation, and consumption.[61]

Parent and caregiver modeling profoundly impact children's behavior and growth in their ability to interact in positive ways with food and eating. Thus, PH and PHN professionals may wish to identify opportunities to educate parents and caregivers regarding healthful nutrition and eating strategies to promote their children's lifelong positive relationship with food.

5. Environmental factors, including social determinants of health, impact nutrition status at each stage of the life cycle.

SDOH are defined by the DHHS, Office of Disease Prevention and Health Promotion (ODPHP), as "the conditions in the environments where people are born, live, learn, work, play, worship, and age that affect a wide range of health, functioning, and quality-of-life outcomes and risks."[62] Nutrition status is strongly impacted by SDOH. For example, consider the associations among a household's location and its ability to access food. Factors including the location's urbanity or rurality, neighborhood characteristics such as safety, transportation infrastructure, and the surrounding food environment affect access to grocery stores, food assistance programs and facilities, farmers markets, gardening space and supplies, and more. Household-related resources, including a food budget and the availability of cooking and refrigeration equipment also impact food access.

While it is useful to categorize SDOH for purposes of education, monitoring, and research, it is important to remember that SDOH are interdependent. Challenging life circumstances in one area, such as housing, tend to have strong impacts on all the other SDOH affecting an individual. Conversely, an improvement in one SDOH area tends to have multiple positive effects in other areas. For example, acquisition of stable housing may result in substantial improvements for an entire multiple life-stage household economic well-being, health and nutrition status, educational opportunities, environmental factors, and quality of life in the community.

The DHHS ODPHP has suggested five major domains to categorize SDOH: (1) economic stability; (2) educational access and quality; (3) healthcare access and quality; (4) neighborhood and built environment; and (5) social and community context.[62] Table 1.5 provides a list of the five major SDOH domains and examples of associated potential nutrition impacts.

Table 1.5. Five Major Domains of the Social Determinants of Health and Associated Potential Nutrition Impacts of Suboptimal Factors

Five Major Domains of SDOH[62]	Potential Nutrition Impacts of Suboptimal SDOH Factors
1. Economic stability	• Inadequate financial resources to purchase adequate nutritious food • Unstable housing: impacts ability to obtain, store, and prepare food; increases difficulty of managing household meals
2. Educational access and quality	• Lack of nutrition knowledge to understand appropriate self- and household nourishment, including household food management and cooking skills • Lack of knowledge of available food resources, including food budgeting and nutrition assistance programs • Lack of knowledge of the relationships among nutrition and chronic diseases
3. Healthcare access and quality	• Higher rates of nutrition-related chronic diseases • Inadequate opportunities for medical nutrition therapy and disease-related nutrition education • Greater risk of malnutrition, including both under- and overnutrition
4. Neighborhood and built environment	• Lack of transportation infrastructure and/or safety considerations may impact ability to reach food centers such as full-service grocery stores, food resource facilities such as food pantries, farmers markets, food assistance programs • Locality/region may lack adequate numbers of full-service grocery stores and other food acquisition centers (food deserts), making access to food difficult
5. Social and community context	• Lack of social and community supports—which may promote feelings of negativity, isolation, loneliness, and/or being overwhelmed with problems—can contribute to a number of mental health sequelae (such as depression and anxiety), which may negatively impact nutrition status

WHAT WORKS: MYPLATE

MyPlate is the consumer-focused dietary guidance tool developed, updated, and maintained by the United States Department of Agriculture (USDA) Center for Nutrition Policy and Promotion (CNPP). MyPlate is designed to translate the recommendations of the Dietary Guidelines for Americans into clear, simple, and actionable messages that can be applied by consumers to make healthful dietary choices. As a visual aid, the MyPlate graphic conveys the concept of consuming a variety of healthful foods from the five food groups in recommended proportions.

The MyPlate website, available in English and Spanish, provides a wealth of resources for use in disseminating accurate nutrition information to individuals and populations. Among many others, these include:

- Personalized MyPlate Food Plans
- Dietary recommendations and targeted nutrition resources for each life cycle stage
- Detailed information, including suggested foods and portion sizes for each of the five food groups
- MyPlate Kitchen, a wide variety of consumer-friendly recipes, and cooking instruction
- Tips for healthy eating on a budget
- Written materials such as infographics, handouts and tip sheets, tools such as shopping lists, videos, and much more; some materials are available in multiple languages
- Availability of MyPlate as a computer application
- Resources for professionals, including toolkits on a variety of topics

Familiarity with the MyPlate website provides a rich resource for professionals to draw on when communicating nutrition knowledge and imparting nutrition skills in population health settings.

SUMMARY

The practice of nutrition in public health settings is primarily focused on nutrition-related disease prevention, detection, and management, as well as the implementation of supportive public policy to achieve these goals. A life cycle approach to public health nutrition applies the principles of public health nutrition practice to the needs of specific life-stage population groups.

Public health practitioners can prepare to implement population-focused nutrition interventions and policies by learning the basic principles of both public health and nutrition science. By disseminating approaches to nutrition that are aligned with best public health practices, the health and quality of life of populations can be greatly enhanced.

KEY CHAPTER CONCEPTS

1. According to the CDC of the DHHS, the role of *public health* is to "protect and improve the health of communities through policy recommendations, health education and outreach, and

research for disease detection and injury prevention."[1] The role of *public health nutrition*, therefore, is to protect and improve the health of communities through nutrition policy recommendations, nutrition and health education and outreach, and research into the associations among nutrition and the prevention and detection of disease.

2. The scope of practice of public health professionals who practice in both general and specialty areas (such as public health nutrition) is defined by the *10 Essential Public Health Services Framework*.[5] Public health nutrition is a specialty area of public health practice.

3. Human development takes place on a continuum extending from the prenatal period through death. Unless interrupted by premature death, persons progress through the stages of prenatal development, infancy, young and older childhood, adolescence, young and middle adulthood, and older adulthood. Human development encompasses a multitude of areas, including but not limited to physical, cognitive, intellectual, creative, functional, emotional, social, moral, and spiritual domains.[11] Adequate nutrition supports basic survival.[10] But, beyond survival, the adequacy and quality of nutrients ingested by individuals plays a crucial role in physical, emotional, and mental health at each life stage.

4. An important ethical imperative for all who work in health-associated fields is to develop a mature understanding of their disciplines so that professionals can address the often-delicate balance between benefits and possible risks and harms of interventions.[19]

5. This discussion covers six key understandings for public health and nutrition practice: (1) Nutrition touches every aspect of life. (2) Six major classes of nutrients, plus non-nutrient bioactive substances, are found in food. These substances are made available for use by the human body during the process of digestion. (3) A myriad of attempts has been made throughout history to determine the ideal diet for humans. Current science-based dietary recommendations are reflected in the official dietary guidance tools provided to their citizens by the governments of many of the world's nations. (4) Nutrition and nutrition science are extremely complex. (5) Like all other health interventions, nutrition interventions require a careful assessment of possible harms. (6) Know where to obtain reliable nutrition information.

6. Five key understandings for life cycle nutrition practice are discussed: (1) Nutrition has important impacts in every stage of the life cycle. (2) There are key nutrition goals for each stage of the life cycle. (3) The six basic types of nutrients remain constant throughout life; however, at different life stages, proportions and amounts of nutrients needed differ. (4) The nutritional practices of parents and caregivers have strong effects on their developing children's nutrition practices throughout life. (5) Environmental factors, including social determinants of health, impact nutrition status at each stage of the life cycle.

7. Public health practitioners can prepare to implement population-focused nutrition interventions and policies by learning the basic principles of both public health and nutrition science. By disseminating approaches to nutrition that are aligned with best public health practices, the health and quality of life of populations can be greatly enhanced.

CASE STUDY AND QUESTIONS

You are working in a county public health department, and are preparing educational materials for a community nutrition initiative. You've been asked to prepare one-page fact sheets on nutrition for several life cycle stages. Choose one life stage group (pregnancy, infancy, early childhood, later childhood, adolescence, young adulthood, middle adulthood, older adulthood) and prepare a one-page fact sheet describing basic nutrition needs of the life stage group. You may wish to consider using a table to format your information. Use a reliable source of information (such as your textbook) and include the following knowledge points:

- Definition of the life stage
- Calorie needs (kcal/kg/day)
- Protein needs (g/kg/day)
- Fluid needs (oz/day, or mL/day, or mL/kg)
- Micronutrients of concern, including recommended amounts of key micronutrients
- Fiber needs
- Key nutrition goals for your group
- How population nutrition status is assessed for your age group
- Recommended healthful diet for a healthy person in your chosen life stage group
- Key nutrition issues for this life stage group in regard to individual health
- Key public health nutrition issues for this life stage group

DISCUSSION QUESTIONS

1. Dr. Charles E. Winslow's 1920 definition of *public health* is still broadly used today. How is his definition still applicable to public health practice? What, if any, updates, additions or revisions to the definition might you suggest?
2. Discuss and explain the statement, "Every individual and collaborative human activity is fueled by food." Would you describe yourself as agreeing or disagreeing with this statement, and why?
3. How would you define *human development*?
4. Referring to Table 1.4, **Life Cycle Nutrition Goals for Each Life Stage,** describe how nutrition goals differ among the stages. What similarities and differences do you see among the stages? What broad similarities do you see between pediatric and adult life cycle stages?
5. How do developmental tasks differ between childhood and adulthood? How do developmental processes differ between children and adults?
6. What do you think are reasons that questionable/false nutrition claims are at times accepted by the public?
7. Review MyPlate.gov, one of the dietary guidance tools provided by the U.S. government to its citizens. Discuss both the MyPlate illustration and its associated website. What do you see as strengths of the tool? What do you see as weaknesses? What, if any, might be some suggestions for improvement?
8. Go to the MyPlate "Life Stages" web page at www.myplate.gov/life-stages. Explore and discuss several of the different life stage links. How do MyPlate recommendations shift for various life stages?
9. How would you describe "a knowledgeable approach to nutrition"? What are some characteristics of a public health nutrition practitioner who practices in a knowledgeable way?
10. While the six classes of primary nutrients don't change, the amounts and proportions of nutrients required can vary during different life stages. What are some examples of these variations, and how can they be addressed by public health practitioners?

SUGGESTED LEARNING ACTIVITIES

1. Choose two or three dietary guidance systems provided by national governments to their citizens (www.fao.org/nutrition/education/food-dietary-guidelines/regions/en). Compare and contrast the guidance systems. Describe and compare your chosen systems' strengths, and suggest areas for improvement.
2. Choose two life stage groups and write a 1.5- to 2-page paper contrasting and comparing nutritional similarities and differences for the two groups.
3. Select an advertisement for a nutritional supplement of some kind. Your product could be a supplement pill, a protein drink, or any variety of other items. You can obtain your advertisement from the internet, a magazine, or a brochure or pamphlet, or elsewhere. You may wish to refer to Table 1.2 for evaluation criteria. Review the advertisement and answer the following questions:
    - What is the source of the nutrition information?
    - What kind of information and/or evidence supports the nutrition claims?
    - Is the provider of nutrition information also selling products associated with the information?
    - For which life stage is this product being marketed? What are the safety implications of the use of this product?
    - After completing your review, how would you evaluate the reliability of the information provided about the nutrition product?
4. Review the history of trans fats and dietary advice in the United States (www.ncbi.nlm.nih.gov/pmc/articles/PMC8452362). Could the story of trans fats and dietary advice be utilized as an example of disseminating dietary advice prior to obtaining adequate research on short- and long-term effects of that advice? Why or why not? Summarize your response in a 1- to 2-page paper.
5. Choose one of the five major social determinants of health. Prepare a list of three to five public health nutrition issues related to your chosen social determinant. For each issue identified, provide a brief (one or two sentences) explanation of how the issue relates to the chosen social determinant of health.

RESOURCES FOR FURTHER LEARNING

- *The Association of State Public Health Nutritionists* (ASPHN): https://asphn.org
    - Information, resources, service opportunities, PHN-focused events and continuing education, and networking for public health nutrition and public health professionals
- *USDA Nutrition.gov*: www.nutrition.gov
    - Source of reliable/credible nutrition information to help make healthy eating choices; offers a variety of topic choices and links to resources
- *Evaluating Internet Health Information: A Tutorial From the National Library of Medicine*: https://medlineplus.gov/webeval/webeval.html
    - An interactive online tutorial focused on methods for evaluating health information websites and information
- *Nutrition Misinformation: How to Identify Fraud or Misleading Claims Fact Sheet*; Colorado State Extension: https://extension.colostate.edu/topic-areas/nutrition-food-safety

-health/nutrition-misinformation-how-to-identify-fraud-and-misleading-claims-9-350
  - A fact sheet describing common health and nutrition scams and how to identify them
- *Life Stage Nutrition*; USDA National Agricultural Library: www.nal.usda.gov/legacy/fnic/life-stage-nutrition
  - Provides food and nutrition resources for a variety of life cycle stages
- *Life Stages*: www.myplate.gov/life-stages
  - MyPlate website; provides life stage–specific nutrition tips, recipes, and resources including cooking skills strategies

SPRINGER PUBLISHING CONNECT™ | **A robust set of instructor resources designed to supplement this text is located at http://connect.springerpub.com/content/book/978-0-8261-8623-2. Qualifying instructors may request access by emailing textbook@springerpub.com.**

REFERENCES

1. One Health Initiative. News: U.S. Centers for Disease Control and Prevention (CDC). Population health training [One Health in Action]. Accessed October 22, 2023. https://onehealthinitiative.com/u-s-centers-for-disease-control-and-prevention-cdc-population-health-training-one-health-in-action.
2. Kemper S. C.E.A. Winslow, who launched public health at Yale a century ago, still influential today. *Yale News*. June 2, 2015. https://news.yale.edu/2015/06/02/public-health-giant-c-ea-winslow-who-launched-public-health-yale-century-ago-still-influe
3. Centers for Disease Control and Prevention. PH 101 series: introduction to public health. Accessed May 25, 2022. https://www.cdc.gov/training/publichealth101/public-health.html
4. Winslow C. The untilled fields of public health. *Science, New Series*. 1920;51(1306):23–33. https://doi.org/10.1126/science.51.1306.23
5. Centers for Disease Control and Prevention. 10 essential public health services. Updated 2021. https://www.cdc.gov/publichealthgateway/publichealthservices/essentialhealthservices.html
6. Lagua RT, Claudio VS. *Nutrition and Diet Therapy Reference Dictionary*. 5th ed. Blackwell Publishing; 2004.
7. Nutrition. In: *Dorland's Illustrated Medical Dictionary*. 33rd ed. Saunders; 2019.
8. Lehigh Valley Dietetic Association. House of Delegates Backgrounder: Public health nutrition: It's every member's business. Fall 2012. http://www.eatrightlehighvalley.org/wp-content/uploads/2016/07/hodpublichealthnutrition-1.pdf
9. Kenrick DT, Griskevicius V, Neuberg SL, Schaller M. Renovating the pyramid of needs: contemporary extensions built upon ancient foundations. *Perspect Psychol Sci*. 2010;5(3):292–314. https://doi.org/10.1177/1745691610369469
10. Taormina RJ, Gao JH. Maslow and the motivation hierarchy: measuring satisfaction of the needs. *Am J Psychol*. 2013;126(2):155–177. https://doi.org/10.5406/amerjpsyc.126.2.0155
11. Arnett JJ, Robinson O, Lachman ME. Rethinking adult development: introduction to the special issue. *Am Psychol*. 2020;75(4):425–430. https://doi.org/10.1037/amp0000633
12. Colombo J, Gustafson KM, Carlson SE. Critical and sensitive periods in development and nutrition. *Ann Nutr Metab*. 2019;75(suppl 1):34–42. https://doi.org/10.1159/000508053
13. Cisneros-Franco JM, Voss P, Thomas ME, de Villers-Sedani E. Critical periods of brain development. *Handb Clin Neurol*. 2020;173:75–88. https://doi.org/10.1016/B978-0-444-64150-2.00009-5
14. Horwood AM. Typical and atypical development of ocular alignment and binocular vision in infants—the background. American Academy of Opthamology; 2019. https://www.aao.org/disease-review/typical-atypical-development-of-ocular-alignment-b
15. Graf GH, Biroli P, Belsky DW. Critical periods in child development and the transition to adulthood. *JAMA Netw Open*. 2021;4(1):e2033359. https://doi.org/10.1001/jamanetworkopen.2020.33359
16. Fox NA. What do we know about sensitive periods in human development and how do we know it? *Hum Dev*. 2014;57(4):173–175. https://doi.org/10.1159/000363663
17. Staudinger UM. The positive plasticity of adult development: potential for the 21st century. *Am Psychol*. 2020;75(4):540–553. https://doi.org/10.1037/amp0000612

18. U.S. Department of Agriculture. Food and nutrition security. Accessed July 27, 2022. https://www.usda.gov/nutrition-security
19. Lorenc T, Oliver K. Adverse effects of public health interventions: a conceptual framework. *J Epidemiol Community Health.* 2014;68(3):288. https://doi.org/10.1136/jech-2013-203118
20. Food and Agriculture Organization of the United Nations. *In Brief to The State of Food and Agriculture 2021. Making Agrifood Systems More Resilient to Shocks and Stresses.* Food and Agriculture Organization of the United Nations; 2021. https://doi.org/10.4060/cb7351en
21. Jéquier E, Constant F. Water as an essential nutrient: the physiological basis of hydration. *Eur J Clin Nutr.* 2010;64(2):115–123. https://doi.org/10.1038/ejcn.2009.111
22. Guan ZW, Yu EZ, Feng Q. Soluble dietary fiber, one of the most important nutrients for the gut microbiota. *Molecules.* 2021;26(22):6802. https://doi.org/10.3390/molecules26226802
23. Liu RH. Potential synergy of phytochemicals in cancer prevention: mechanism of action. *J Nutr.* 2004;134(12 suppl):3479S–3485S. https://doi.org/10.1093/jn/134.12.3479S
24. Cardenas D. Let not thy food be confused with thy medicine: the Hippocratic misquotation. *e-SPEN J.* 2013;8(6):e260–e262. https://doi.org/10.1016/j.clnme.2013.10.002
25. Painter J, Rah J-H, Lee Y-K. Comparison of international food guide pictorial representations. *J Am Diet Assoc.* 2002;102(4):483–489. https://doi.org/10.1016/s0002-8223(02)90113-6
26. Food and Agriculture Organization of the United Nations. Food-based dietary guidelines. Accessed July 25, 2022. https://www.fao.org/nutrition/education/food-dietary-guidelines/background/en
27. Food and Agriculture Organization of the United Nations. Food-based dietary guidelines—Japan. Accessed July 26, 2022. https://www.fao.org/nutrition/education/food-dietary-guidelines/regions/countries/japan/en
28. Food and Agriculture Organization of the United Nations. Food-based dietary guidelines—Bolivia. Accessed July 26, 2022. https://www.fao.org/nutrition/education/food-dietary-guidelines/regions/countries/bolivia-plurinational-state-of/en
29. Food and Agriculture Organization of the United Nations. Food-based dietary guidelines—Malaysia. Accessed July 26, 2022. https://www.fao.org/nutrition/education/food-dietary-guidelines/regions/countries/malaysia/en
30. Food and Agriculture Organization of the United Nations. Food-based dietary guidelines—United Arab Emirates. Accessed July 26, 2022. https://www.fao.org/nutrition/education/food-dietary-guidelines/regions/countries/united-arab-emirates/en
31. Food and Agriculture Organization of the United Nations. Food-based dietary guidelines—Finland. Accessed July 26, 2022. https://www.fao.org/nutrition/education/food-dietary-guidelines/regions/countries/finland/en
32. Food and Agriculture Organization of the United Nations. Food-based dietary guidelines—China. Accessed July 26, 2022. https://www.fao.org/nutrition/education/food-dietary-guidelines/regions/countries/china/en
33. Food and Agriculture Organization of the United Nations. Food-based dietary guidelines—Sierra Leone. Accessed July 26, 2022. https://www.fao.org/nutrition/education/food-dietary-guidelines/regions/countries/sierra-leone/en
34. Office of Disease Prevention and Health Promotion. Dietary reference intakes. U.S. Department of Health and Human Services. Updated August 18, 2023. https://health.gov/our-work/nutrition-physical-activity/dietary-guidelines/dietary-reference-intakes
35. U.S. Department of Agriculture, U.S. Department of Health and Human Services. *Dietary Guidelines for Americans 2020–2025.* 9th ed. U.S. Department of Health and Human Services; December 2020. https://www.dietaryguidelines.gov/sites/default/files/2021-03/Dietary_Guidelines_for_Americans-2020-2025.pdf
36. U.S. Department of Agriculture. MyPlate. 2020. https://www.myplate.gov
37. Weaver CM, Miller JW. Challenges in conducting clinical nutrition research. *Nutr Rev.* 2017;75(7):491–499. https://doi.org/10.1093/nutrit/nux026
38. Santos S, Zugna D, Pizzi C, Richiardi L. Sources of confounding in life course epidemiology. *J Dev Orig Health Dis.* 2019;10(3):299–305. https://doi.org/10.1017/S2040174418000582
39. Vitolins MZ, Case TL. What makes nutrition research so difficult to conduct and interpret? *Diabetes Spectr.* 2020;33(2):113–117. https://doi.org/10.2337/ds19-0077
40. National Institute of Diabetes and Digestive and Kidney Diseases. Metabolic Clinical Research Unit. National Institutes of Health. Accessed July 7, 2022. https://www.niddk.nih.gov/research-funding/at-niddk/labs-branches/diabetes-endocrinology-obesity-branch/metabolic-clinical-research-unit

41. Secretary's Advisory Committee on National Health Promotion and Disease Prevention Objectives for 2020. *Evidence-Based Clinical and Public Health: Generating and Applying the Evidence*. U.S. Department of Health and Human Services; 2010. https://health.gov/sites/default/files/2021-11/Committee%27s%20Report%20on%20Evidence-Based%20Clinical%20and%20Public%20Health-%20Generating%20and%20Applying%20the%20Evidence.pdf
42. Oxford University Press. Something sounds too good to be true, it probably is. In: *The Oxford Dictionary of Phrase and Fable*. 2nd ed. Oxford University Press; 2006. https://doi.org/10.1093/acref/9780198609810.001.0001
43. Brannon PM, Taylor CL, Coates PM. Use and applications of systematic reviews in public health nutrition. *Annu Rev Nutr*. 2014;34:401–419. https://doi.org/10.1146/annurev-nutr-080508-141240
44. Merton RK. The unanticipated consequences of purposive social action. *Am Sociol Rev*. 1936;1(6): 894–904. https://doi.org/10.2307/2084615
45. Ebbeling CB, Young IS, Lichtenstein AH, et al. Dietary fat: friend or foe? *Clin Chem*. 2018;64(1):34–41. https://doi.org/10.1373/clinchem.2017.274084
46. Mozaffarian D, Rosenberg I, Uauy R. History of modern nutrition science—implications for current research, dietary guidelines, and food policy. *BMJ*. 2018;361:k2392. https://doi.org/10.1136/bmj.k2392
47. Nix E. Proposed changes to nutrition curricula in higher education. *J Nutr Educ Behav*. 2022;54(11): 1042–1046. https://doi.org/10.1016/j.jneb.2022.08.005
48. Wickramasinghe K, Mathers JC, Wopereis S, Marsman DS, Griffiths JC. From lifespan to healthspan: the role of nutrition in healthy ageing. *J Nutr Sci*. 2020;9:e33. https://doi.org/10.1017/jns.2020.26
49. Sandoval VS, Jackson A, Saleeby E, Smith L, Schickedanz A. Associations between prenatal food insecurity and prematurity, pediatric health care utilization, and postnatal social needs. *Acad Pediatr*. 2021;21(3):455–461. https://doi.org/10.1016/j.acap.2020.11.020
50. Testa A, Jackson DB. Adverse childhood experiences and food insecurity in adulthood: evidence from the national longitudinal study of adolescent to adult health. *J Adolesc Health*. 2020;67(2):218–224. https://doi.org/10.1016/j.jadohealth.2020.02.002
51. Nagata JM, Palar K, Gooding HC, Garber AK, Bibbins-Domingo K, Weiser SD. Food insecurity and chronic disease in U.S. young adults: findings from the national longitudinal study of adolescent to adult health. *J Gen Intern Med*. 2019;34(12):2756–2762. https://doi.org/10.1007/s11606-019-05317-8
52. McArthur LH, Gutschall M, Fasczewski KS, Jackson A. Food insecurity among college students with and without medical disorders at a university in Appalachia. *J Appalach Health*. 2020;2(2):36–48. https://doi.org/10.13023/jah.0202.04
53. Gregory CA, Coleman-Jensen A. *Food Insecurity, Chronic Disease, and Health Among Working-Age Adults*. Economic Research Report No. 235. U.S. Department of Agriculture, Economic Research Service; 2017.
54. Pourmotabbed A, Moradi S, Babaei A, et al. Food insecurity and mental health: a systematic review and meta-analysis. *Public Health Nutr*. 2020;23(10):1778–1790. https://doi.org/10.1017/S136898001900435X
55. Petersen CL, Brooks JM, Titus AJ, Vasquez E, Batsis JA. Relationship between food insecurity and functional limitations in older adults from 2005-2014 NHANES. *J Nutr Gerontol Geriatr*. 2019;38(3): 231–246. https://doi.org/10.1080/21551197.2019.1617219
56. Björnwall A, Mattsson Sydner Y, Koochek A, Neuman N. Eating alone or together among community-living older people—a scoping review. *Int J Environ Res Public Health*. 2021;18(7):3495. https://doi.org/10.3390/ijerph18073495
57. Holman DM, Grossman M, Henley SJ, Peipins LA, Tison L, White MC. Opportunities for cancer prevention during midlife. *Am J Prev Med*. 2014;46(3 0 1):S73–S80. https://stacks.cdc.gov/view/cdc/32862.
58. Lee SB, Oh JH, Park JH, Choi SP, Wee JH. Differences in youngest-old, middle-old, and oldest-old patients who visit the emergency department. *Clin Exp Emerg Med*. 2018;5(4):249–255. https://doi.org/10.15441/ceem.17.261
59. Koehler J, Leonhaeuser IU. Changes in food preferences during aging. *Ann Nutr Metab*. 2008;52 (suppl 1):15–19. https://doi.org/10.1159/000115342
60. Fostinelli S, De Amicis R, Leone A, et al. Eating behavior in aging and dementia: the need for a comprehensive assessment. *Front Nutr*. 2020;7:604488. https://doi.org/10.3389/fnut.2020.604488
61. Satter E. Eating competence: definition and evidence for the Satter Eating Competence model. *J Nutr Educ Behav*. 2007;39(5 suppl):S142–S153. https://doi.org/10.1016/j.jneb.2007.01.006
62. Office of Disease Prevention and Health Promotion. Healthy People 2030: social determinants of health. https://health.gov/healthypeople/priority-areas/social-determinants-health

2

PUBLIC HEALTH NUTRITION PRACTICE THROUGHOUT THE LIFE CYCLE

Jennifer Noll Folliard and Rosa K. Hand

LEARNING OBJECTIVES

At the end of this chapter, students will be able to:

1. Identify one domestic and one international public health nutrition program in each life course stage.
2. Define evidence-based practice and apply the principles of evidence-based practice to public health nutrition.
3. Name the 10 essential public health services and explain how equity underlies each one.
4. Connect ethical principles in public health to evidence-based practice and equity.
5. Format a PICO question and search for evidence to support implementation of a public health program.

INTRODUCTION

In order to deliver effective **population health** interventions, practitioners must understand the essential components of an evidence-based framework for public health and public health nutrition practice. This chapter provides an in-depth discussion of key public health concepts, including **health equity**, public health theoretical constructs and models, **social determinants of health**, and ethical practice, including scope of practice considerations. The chapter concludes with information on public health nutrition settings and programs.

LIFE CYCLE NUTRITION IN POPULATION HEALTH

Public health nutrition practitioners utilize a set of public health knowledge and skills as well as a strong foundational knowledge of nutrition to optimize human development, realization, and utilization and achieve health equity or reduce **health**

Table 2.1. Foundational Models and Theories for Public Health and Community Nutrition

Model/Theory	Brief Description
Socio-ecological model	Developed by McLeroy and colleagues, the socio-ecological model posits that there are interacting spheres of influence that impact a person's health behaviors and health. Those spheres include individual factors (e.g., knowledge, beliefs, attitudes, skills, preferences); intrapersonal factors (e.g., family and friends); institutional factors (e.g., schools, churches workplaces); community/environmental factors (e.g., neighborhoods); and societal factors (e.g., laws, policy, social norms).[23]
Social determinants of health	An explanation of the social conditions (economic stability, education, neighborhood, and built environment, health and healthcare, social and community context) and related underlying factors that influence people's disease.
Life course theory	A framework that describes how health outcomes in each life stage are influenced by the long-term effects of exposures during critical periods (e.g., pregnancy, infancy), by long-term health habits across the life course, and through the interaction of biologic, behavioral, psychological, social, economic, environmental, and equity factors.

Source: Table reprinted with permission from Bruening M, Udarbe AZ, Yakes Jimenez E, Stell Crowley P, Fredericks DC, Edwards Hall LA. Academy of Nutrition and Dietetics: Standards of Practice and Standards of Professional Performance for registered dietitian nutritionists (competent, proficient, and expert) in public health and community nutrition. *J Acad Nutr Diet.* 2015;115(10):1699–1709.e39, fig 4. https://doi.org/10.1016/j.jand.2015.06.374

inequities. Public health nutrition practice across the life cycle requires an understanding of the models and theories in public health and community nutrition, which are briefly reviewed in Table 2.1.

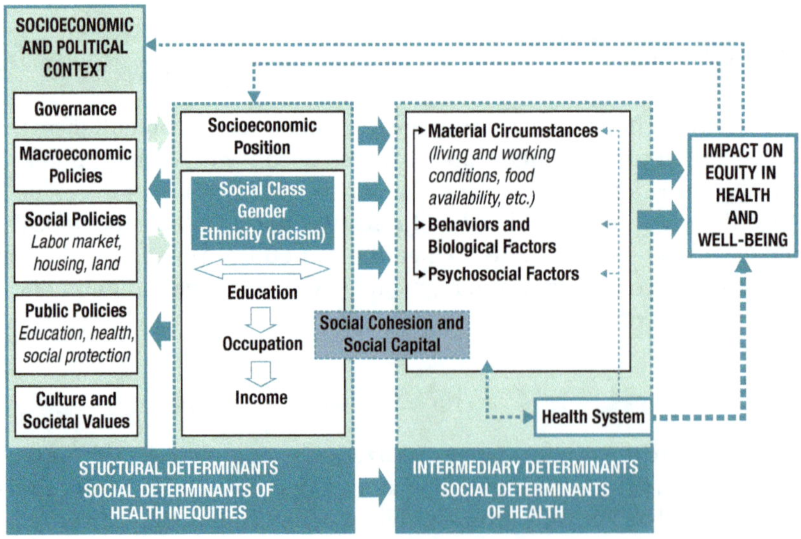

Figure 2.1. Framework for the social determinants of health.
Source: Solar O, Irwin A. *A Conceptual Framework for Action on the Social Determinants of Health.* World Health Organization; 2010: fig A. https://www.who.int/publications-detail-redirect/9789241500852

Optimal population health is shaped by social determinants of **health**, or the circumstances in which people are born, grow, live, work, and age (Figure 2.1).[1] These determinants shape the choices that are available for individual behavior. Identifying the social determinants of health helps to identify areas for program and policy intervention. For example, healthy food access is classified as a material circumstance, social determinant of health, which is perpetuated by structural socioeconomic inequities.

A final guiding framework is the 10 Essential Public Health Services[2] (Figure 2.2). This framework guides communities, and public health practitioners to achieve optimal health for all by organizing the 10 essential services into three core functions: (1) population assessment, (2) policy, law, and regulation development, and (3) enforcement and quality assurance and improvement.[2] At the center of the 10 Essential Public Health Services framework, touching all essential services, is equity.[2] Public health and public health nutrition practitioners who focus on life cycle nutrition can build adaptive and

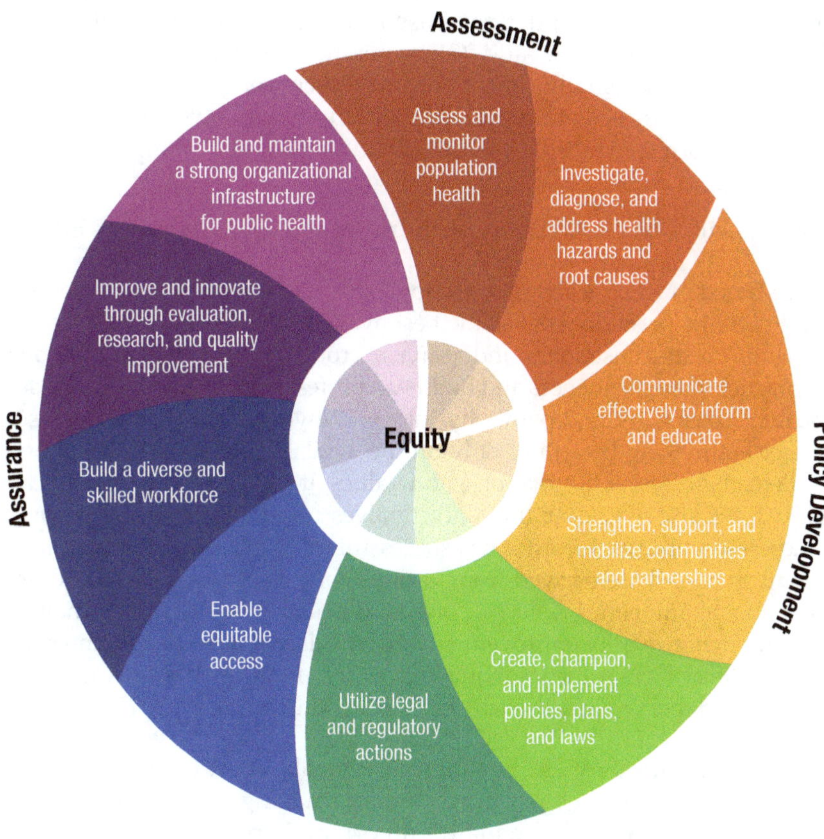

Figure 2.2. The 10 Essential Public Health Services Framework. ***To protect and promote the health of all people in all communities*** the 10 Essential Public Health Services provide a framework for public health to protect and promote the health of all people in all communities. To achieve optimal health for all, the essential public health services actively promote policies, systems, and services that enable good health and seek to remove obstacles and systemic and structural barriers, such as proverty, racism, gender discrimination, and other forms of oppression, that have resulted in health inequities. Everyone should have a fair and just opportunity to achieve good health and well-being.

Source: Centers for Disease Control and Prevention. *10 essential public health services*. Accessed August 30, 2023. https://www.cdc.gov/publichealthgateway/publichealthservices/essentialhealthservices.html

equitable systems, and have a responsibility to dismantle systems that perpetuate **structural inequities**. To understand systems level inequities the public health practitioner must understand how to identify population disparities in disease burden and diagnose the root cause using the social determinants of health.

Public health and public health nutrition practitioners work within programs, governing bodies, and research institutions to perform these essential public health services.[3] Specific examples include identifying population health problems; obtaining grant funding; creating, implementing, and evaluating intervention programs for individuals and groups; and creating policy and conducting research.[3]

PRINCIPLES OF EVIDENCE-BASED PUBLIC HEALTH NUTRITION PRACTICE

Evidence-based practice (EBP) is conceptualized as a three-legged stool. EBP involves making decisions and recommendations based on (1) the best available scientific evidence, (2) professional expertise, and (3) preferences of the impacted individual or group.[4] Criticisms of EBP usually center around the concept that it is a "cookie cutter" approach and utilizes only scientific evidence with no room for preferences or expertise.[4] However, this is incorrect. Multiple sources, including the CDC emphasize all three aspects of EBP.[4–6]

In nutrition specifically, the Academy of Nutrition and Dietetics defines EBP as follows:

> Evidence-based practice is an approach to health care wherein credentialed nutrition and dietetics practitioners use the best available evidence to make decisions for patients/clients, customers, individuals, groups, or populations. Evidence-based practice values, enhances and builds on professional expertise, a knowledge of disease mechanisms, and pathophysiology. It involves complex and conscientious decision making based not only on the available evidence but also on patient/client characteristics, situations, and values. It recognizes that health care is individualized and ever changing and involves uncertainties and probabilities. Evidence-based practice incorporates successful strategies that improve patient/client outcomes and are derived from various sources of evidence, including research, national guidelines, policies, consensus statements, systematic analysis of clinical experience, quality improvement data, specialized knowledge, and skills of experts. Evidence-based practice requires clear communication about the source(s) of evidence and their weight in each decision-making process (pp. 1569–1570).[4]

EBP emphasizes the need for clear communication about the quality of evidence and/or which "leg" of the stool is being relied upon in making a recommendation or decision.[4] This type of terminology is equally important in public health practice so that partner organizations and stakeholders are clear on the source and quality of evidence underpinning a recommendation.

In order to identify the best available scientific evidence for EBP, public health nutrition practitioners must first begin by framing a specific question that will be searchable. This is referred to as the "ask" step of EBP.[7] The formula for specific searchable questions is usually defined with the PICO acronym: Population, Intervention, Comparison, Outcome.[7] Framing a question in this manner helps focus the search process for the next step of EBP, also known as "acquire."[7] In the acquire step, a public health nutrition practitioner attempts to identify all possible sources of scientific evidence relevant to the PICO question. The third step of EBP is "appraise," during which a public health nutrition practitioner evaluates the quality of the science in the papers and reports they found.[7] One barrier to appraise is obtaining the full text of every article to be evaluated; it is essential to evaluate the full text and not just an abstract. In the appraise step, the focus is usually on the type of resource (guideline, systematic review/meta-analysis, randomized controlled trial, or observational study) and the validity, magnitude, and relevance of the finding. Finally, in the "apply" step of EBP, public health nutrition practitioners integrate the scientific evidence with their own expertise and the preferences of the group with whom they are working.[7] During this step, public health nutrition practitioners may find the frameworks and language around shared decision-making helpful in presenting the options to the group and in elucidating the group's values, desires, resources, and preferences. Some authors suggest there is a fifth step of EBP, "evaluate," in which the public health nutrition practitioner determines whether their recommendation/decision led to the desired outcomes and what they would do differently in the future.[7] The evaluate step is not a major focus of this chapter, but it does emphasize that EBP is a continual process that shares some elements with quality improvement. An evidence-based public health nutrition practitioner searches the literature with some frequency to determine whether any updated evidence exists that should change their typical practice. The steps of the EBP process are summarized in Table 2.2.

Public health and public health nutrition practitioners have a responsibility to engage in EBP/decision-making. Indeed, EBP is the 10th domain of the American Public Health Association Public Health Code of Ethics, and is highly relevant to considerations of proportionality and fair allocation of scarce resources.[8] Health professions in general have recognized a responsibility to practice in an evidence-based manner. As discussed in the next section, the training of **registered dietitian nutritionists (RDNs)** specifically prepares them to search and evaluate the literature as is necessary in the acquire and appraise steps of EBP, making them helpful participants or partners in this process.

PRINCIPLES OF ETHICAL PUBLIC HEALTH NUTRITION PRACTICE

Along with using EBP, other important ethical considerations in public health practice are the principle of harm reduction; issues around inclusion, diversity, equity, and access (IDEA); the need to evaluate outcomes; and scope of practice.

Harm Reduction

Although the exact phrasing is of some contention, the foundation of medical ethics is the balance of benefits and harms and ensuring that benefits are expected to outweigh harms.[9] This principle should also guide public health practice. In the 2002 Principles of Ethical Practice of Public Health, principle 9 provides the same concept but is worded positively: "Public health programs and policies should incorporate a variety of approaches that anticipate and respect diverse values, beliefs, and cultures in the community."[10] In 2019, the American Public Health Association provided a revised Public Health Code of Ethics, which weaves throughout the concept of harm reduction and proportionality to benefit.[8] All of the components of the Public Health Code of Ethics are relevant to public health nutrition but are too extensive for thorough review here.

Inclusion, Diversity, Equity, and Access

Another area of public health ethics that deserves special attention is IDEA. As it allocates scarce resources, public health has a responsibility to mitigate existing **health**

Table 2.2. Descriptions and Public Health Nutrition Examples of the Evidence-Based Practice Process

EBP Step	Brief Description/Key Terms	Example
Ask	Frame the question to be answered so that it is specific enough to be searchable. A frequent acronym for these questions is PICO—population, intervention, comparison, outcome. PICO questions will be less helpful if you are searching for the answer to a background question (e.g., about the rates or characteristics of a specific disease or condition). Background questions can be important in orienting yourself to a situation but don't require the steps of EBP outlined here in order to be answered.	Unsearchable question: How should my WIC program encourage breastfeeding? Comments: This question is unsearchable because the outcome or goal is unclear as are the potential options. A background question to be answered might be what the rates of breastfeeding are for the public health nutrition professional's state/community. PICO format helping to define the question for searching: Population: WIC mothers who have just given birth and expressed an interest in breastfeeding Intervention: Daily text messages supportive of breastfeeding in the first 6 weeks of life Comparison: Weekly, in-person breastfeeding support group sessions in the first 6 weeks of life Outcome: Percentage of women still breastfeeding at 6 months of life
Acquire	Search the literature for papers, reports, etc. that might answer the PICO question. PICO elements can be used in the search terms; usually the outcome is not part of the search in order to reduce bias.	Search pubmed for: breastfeeding support strategies and WIC 29 results are identified

Appraise	Evaluate the papers/reports that were found to identify the highest quality evidence. Guidelines and meta-analyses/systematic reviews are summative documents that include the results of multiple studies; therefore, these are the highest quality evidence because they incorporate the variation found in different studies. Guidelines and meta-analyses/systematic reviews should be used first, and if they are unavailable, then single studies should be evaluated. When evaluating single studies, the goal is to determine whether the study was well designed so that the conclusions are believable (validity), whether the results/conclusions are strong enough to matter (magnitude), and whether the results/conclusions are relevant to your PICO question (relevance).	Among the 29 results, a review is identified that has a promising title and abstract (Impact of Breastfeeding Interventions Among United States Minority Women on Breastfeeding Outcomes: A Systematic Review).[24] Review of that paper identifies that they summarized several WIC interventions that include phone or text messaging support and had promising results.[24] This paper is high quality because it is a systematic review. It discusses the quality of each included paper. The CDC has a guide to evaluating evidence in the context of violence prevention that may be helpful in other areas as well.[6]
Apply	Integrate the scientific evidence with professional expertise and the preferences/resources of the group being served to come to a decision/recommendation. Shared decision-making principles and language may be helpful in presenting the options and elucidating the desires of the group.	Based on the systematic review it appears that both in-person and text messaging breastfeeding support have potential. The public health nutrition practitioner now needs to use their own expertise about feasibility and their observations of what works in their community, as well as finding out what stakeholders prefer, in order to pick which program to implement first.
Evaluate	Determine whether the decision led to the expected outcomes; would the decision be the same in the future or is there more evidence that would change the decision?	After implementing the program monitor outcomes to determine if anticipated impact is achieved. Monitor the literature to determine if new evidence suggests a different approach should be investigated.

CDC, Centers for Disease Control and Prevention; EBP, evidence-based practice; WIC, Special Supplemental Nutrition Program for Women, Infants, and Children.

disparities and not create new ones, even for future generations.[8] Public health nutrition practitioners are well versed in incorporating community feedback into programming but should be particularly mindful of including all stakeholders and not excluding any previously marginalized groups in order to solicit diverse opinions.[8] IDEA principles connect closely with the public health commitment to improving social determinants of health[8] and the fact that equity is at the center of the 10 essential public health services.

Evaluate Outcomes

As part of EBP, and as a requirement of many granting agencies, public health nutrition practitioners have a responsibility to evaluate the outcomes of their programs. Outcome evaluation helps determine whether scarce resources were spent appropriately, and informs decision-making for future programs and initiatives. It aligns closely with the 9th Domain of the Public Health Code of Ethics (Evaluate and Continuously Improve Processes, Programs, and Interventions).[8] While program evaluation does not always require the full rigor of research, the Public Health Code of Ethics asks that public health practitioners invest "resources in collecting ethically and methodologically sound evidence."[9] Understanding research design and methods and/or collaborating with partners who do are important to resource-efficient data collection. Large federal agencies that support public health nutrition programs may also run centralized evaluation efforts; public health and public health nutrition practitioners should remain alert to new findings from these evaluations even if they do not conduct direct evaluation themselves.

Scope of Practice

Because public health is an interdisciplinary, collaborative field, public health practitioners may have a variety of backgrounds and levels of education, from community health workers or those bringing their own experience to the task at hand, through physicians and other doctorate holders. In public health nutrition in the United States, the RDN credential may be particularly relevant and beneficial. (Some other countries have dietitians or other titles with similar educational requirements; however, these are not reviewed in depth here.) RDNs complete coursework in basic, social, and nutritional sciences and at least 1,000 hours of practical experience before completing a national exam.[11] After initial exam-based credentialing, RDNs must complete 75 hours of continuing professional education every 5 years.[11] RDNs can be supported in their work by nutrition and dietetic technicians, registered (NDTRs), who complete truncated but similar requirements.[12] At the time of this writing, the minimum level of education for an RDN is a bachelor's degree and for the NDTR, an associate's degree, but beginning in 2024, the profession will require a master's degree for newly credentialed RDNs.[13]

The scope of practice for an individual RDN is defined by their own individual education both generally and in a specific area of practice, federal and state regulations, organizational policies and procedures, and practice area accreditation organizations (e.g., Public Health Accreditation Board).[11] Of particular importance is the role of state laws and regulations related to licensure or certification of RDNs. Both credentialing (national) and licensure or certification (state) seek to protect the public from the harm of incompetent or unqualified practitioners.[11,14] Licensure varies from state to state but usually includes qualifications that are either explicitly holding the RDN credential, or mirroring the RDN requirements exactly.[14] Licensure also establishes the scope of practice for RDNs in that state, meaning that only certain practitioners can provide the services established within the scope.[14] For example, in a particular state, only an RDN with licensure or a physician might be able to provide medical nutrition therapy to individual patients or clients.

Nonlicensed practitioners, including public health nutrition practitioners, can provide general nutrition information backed up by science (e.g., mirroring the Dietary Guidelines for Americans) but should not provide individualized, therapeutic nutrition advice. There are likely inadequate RDNs for all of the public health nutrition needs, so part of the ethical distribution of scarce resources is determining which activities require an RDN, and focusing their efforts, while delegating appropriate tasks that do not require a license to other types of public health nutrition practitioners. All practitioners, whether licensed or nonlicensed, are expected to consult and carefully comply with their statutory scope of practice and protected titles as set forth in their state licensure laws. Best use of resources might include having a RDN available for more complex or individualized questions, and/or responsible for creating or reviewing program materials related to nutrition, and training and/or supervising nonlicensed public health nutrition practitioners to provide appropriate programs.

In public health settings, the Certified Health Education Specialist (CHES) certification is a highly recognized credential. Persons with the CHES certification are specialists in health promotion and education in the health field which may include general, science-based nutrition education. Persons holding the CHES credential have met academic preparation qualifications, passed a national competency-based examination, and are required to comply with continuing education requirements. As with other professional certifications and credentials, careful adherence to any related statutory requirements is essential.[15]

SETTINGS FOR PUBLIC HEALTH NUTRITION PRACTICE THROUGHOUT THE LIFE CYCLE

The Academy of Nutrition and Dietetics defines public health nutrition as the "application of nutrition and public health principles to design programs, systems, policies and environments that aims to improve or maintain the optimal health of populations and targeted groups." In a 2015 paper from the Academy of Nutrition and Dietetics, the authors estimated that 11% of RDNs currently report that their primary practice area is community nutrition and that demand for this profession would significantly increase in the next decade. The authors noted that a workforce increase of 113% would be required to achieve a ratio of one public health nutrition practitioner per 50,000 people.

Public health nutrition practitioners work in a variety of settings that address nutrition needs across the life span. Federal, state, or local health, human, or social service agencies positions administer or deliver programs and services (see Table 2.3) to address populations in need of additional nutritional support and education. Public health nutrition practitioners also work in research institutions to test and develop the evidence base for public health and public health nutrition practice. Healthcare, hospital, or health insurance represent emerging settings for public health nutrition practitioners, providing an opportunity to link clinical practice to evidence-based population health initiatives.

Public health nutrition practitioners typically work as a part of an interdisciplinary team that may include different sectors of the community, including but not limited to community- and faith-based organizations, safety net healthcare providers, and health and hospital systems. **Systems thinking** or a systems approach is critical for a public health nutrition practitioner to adopt and requires the integration and consideration of multiple disciplines.[16]

Public Health Nutrition Policies and Programs

The life course theory states that there are certain points in life when rapid growth and development can occur or not, depending on the environment. The economic and societal costs of stunted growth and the management of nutrition-related disease can have devastating effects on a population. Societies and corresponding governments have a vested interest in preventing food and nutrition-related disease or stunted growth and development. According to the socio-ecological model, policy and systems provide the framework for health and health behavior. Thus, many policies and systems are targeted at times of high nutrition risk during the life course.

U.S. Domestic Public Health Nutrition Programs and Policies

Major U.S. domestic policies and programs that support human growth and development and thus a thriving society are presented in **Appendix D**, organized by life course stage (note this is not a comprehensive list; other programs may exist that touch public health nutrition). Many of these programs attempt to improve food access (a social determinant of health), including affordability and palatability/consumption and have generated improvements on health outcomes and overall healthcare costs.[17]

Table 2.3. Partial List of U.S.-Supported International Public Nutrition Programs, Organized by Life Course Stage

Life Course Stage	Program	Eligibility (Emergency or Nonemergency)	Major Provisions
Food insecure population, all ages	Food For Peace Title II	Qualifying international NGO or other organization Emergency and non emergency projects (vast majority emergency projects)	U.S.-sourced commodities Distributed directly to population At least 75% of nonemergency commodities must be value-added commodities (processed, fortified, or bagged commodities), and at least 50% of bagged, whole-grain commodities must be bagged in the United States.
	Bill Emerson Humanitarian Trust	Emergency reserve funds	Makes funds or commodities rapidly available for emergency food needs in humanitarian contexts
	Farmer to Farmer (Food for Peace Title V)	Potential volunteers apply directly to the coordinating NGOs and are selected based on the needs of the individual or organization in the developing country.	Finances short-term (typically 2- to 4-week) volunteer placements in developing countries to provide technical assistance to farmers Does not finance food distribution

Table 2.3. Partial List of U.S.-Supported International Public Nutrition Programs, Organized by Life Course Stage (*continued*)

Life Course Stage	Program	Eligibility (Emergency or Non-Emergency)	Major Provisions
Pregnant and nursing mothers; young children and school age children	McGovern-Dole International Food for Education and Child Nutrition	Priority countries identified through USDA based on criteria including per capita income, literacy, and malnutrition rates	Advance food security, nutrition, and education for children (with an emphasis on girls) in priority countries via in-kind aid that is distributed in school meals Provides encouragement and technical assistance to support the development of national school feeding programs in recipient countries
	Emergency Food Security Program	Four criteria to decide which market-based intervention is best suited to the recipient country context: market appropriateness, feasibility, project objectives, and cost	Market-based assistance program, aiding in the form of food vouchers, cash transfers, or the local or regional procurement of commodities
	Community Development Fund	Includes both short-term emergency food assistance programs and longer-term food security assistance (e.g., agricultural development and nutrition assistance programs)	Typically, 5-year programs aimed at addressing the root cause of food insecurity
School-age children	Local and Regional Food Aid Procurement Program	Priority countries identified through USDA based on criteria including per capita income, literacy, and malnutrition rates	Finances the provision of locally and regionally procured foods to beneficiaries USDA provides funding to partner organizations, which then procure eligible commodities in the area in which the commodities will be distributed. USDA determines nutritional, quality and labeling standards required of all procured commodities.

(*continued*)

Table 2.3. Partial List of U.S.-Supported International Public Nutrition Programs, Organized by Life Course Stage (*continued*)

Life Course Stage	Program	Eligibility (Emergency or Non-Emergency)	Major Provisions
School-age children *(cont.)*	Food for Progress	Statute directs USDA, when awarding projects, to consider a country's commitments to promote economic freedom and expand efficient domestic commodity markets.	USDA donates U.S. agricultural commodities to international organizations, NGOs, foreign governments, or private entities, which can then distribute the commodities to beneficiaries or raise funds for development projects by selling the commodities locally. Minimum annual provision from the program is 400,000 metric tons of commodities.
	Feed the Future	U.S. Agency for International Development (USAID); eligibility based on level of need, program potential to promote growth, partnership opportunities, host government commitment, and other factors.	Addresses both food/nutrition security AND poverty within the countries identified at greatest risk for stunting and wasting. Develops sustainable solutions, including agricultural production that impacts food and nutrition; and develops community and country economies GDP.

NGO, nongovernmental organization; USDA, U.S. Department of Agriculture.
Source: Casey AR, Morgenstern EM. *U.S. International Food Assistance: An Overview.* Congressional Research Service; 2021. https://crsreports.congress.gov/product/pdf/R/R45422

U.S.-Supported International Public Health Nutrition Programs and Policies

Although many U.S.-supported international nutrition programs are targeted at improving food security, defined by U.S. Agency for International Development (USAID) as "when all people at all times have both physical and economic access to sufficient food to meet their dietary needs for a productive and healthy life," different modalities are used to achieve this goal.[18] The first modality is in-kind, or commodities grown/packaged in the United States and shipped to other countries.[19] The second modality is market-based assistance, which can be in the form of direct cash, food voucher, or locally purchased food in country.[20] A partial list of U.S.-supported international policies and programs that promote human growth and development and thus a thriving society are presented in Table 2.3, organized by life course stage.

WHAT WORKS

U.S. Domestic Public Health Nutrition Program

The Special Supplemental Nutrition Assistance Program for Women, Infants, and Children (WIC) became a permanent program in 1975.[21] Since then, it has provided nutrition and nutrition education to millions of families during a window of rapid growth and development for the mother, fetus, infant, and child.[22] WIC provides this support for those families who are both at nutritional risk and meet the income threshold.[23] WIC is operated by each of the 50 states, Indian Tribal Organizations, and territories. Nearly half of the babies born in the United States are eligible for or enrolled in WIC.[24] WIC is delivered in a variety of settings, and partners with a variety of food retail establishments, but the program must adhere to national nutrition standards for products provided in the food package.

WIC has an extensive evaluation history. The most recent systematic review of the literature conducted by the Agency for Healthcare Research and Quality (AHRQ) found that maternal WIC participation associated with purchasing healthier foods and with improved diets for pregnant women and children resulted in improved birth outcomes, lower infant mortality, and better child cognitive development.[25] For every $1 invested in the WIC program, $2.48 is saved in other societal costs (e.g., education, safety net programs).[26] These measures of effectiveness provide policy makers the information needed to support the program and have contributed to its longevity.

U.S.-Supported International Public Health Nutrition Program

The use of micronutrient powders (MNP) to address high prevalence of iron deficiency anemia in childhood is an effective public health nutrition program. MNP are defined as “a mixture of vitamins and minerals, enclosed in single-dose sachets—which are stirred into a child’s portion of food immediately before consumption.”[27] A 2017 review identified that over 50 countries were implementing this intervention.[28] MNP can be delivered in a variety of formats, through different community based and facility-based settings. One U.S.-supported MNP intervention in Uganda is both market-based and in-kind.[29]

SUMMARY

Effective public health and public health nutrition practice are grounded within a framework that includes the goal of health equity for all people, a foundation of evidence-based public health theory and intervention models, an understanding of social determinants of health, the delivery of evidence-based interventions, competence within one’s practice scope, and a commitment to ethical practice. Building one’s career on these foundational components will foster and enhance practice across a broad range of settings and programs.

KEY CHAPTER CONCEPTS

- A variety of models including the socio-ecological model, social determinants of health, life course theory, and the 10 essential public health services help to guide and organize the work of public health nutrition practitioners in a variety of settings.
- Evidence-based practice combines scientific evidence with practice expertise and community preferences.

- Finding scientific evidence is a systematic process starting with clearly defining a question (ask), searching for evidence (acquire), and determining the quality of the evidence (appraise), before making, communicating, and implementing a decision or plan (apply).
- Ethical issues in public health nutrition practice include the principle of harm reduction, ensuring equitable distribution of resources, evaluating outcomes, and respecting scope of practice.
- Domestic and international public health nutrition programs exist to support food security and human development in each life course stage.

CASE STUDY AND QUESTIONS

The WIC program follows nutrition requirements, as set by the U.S. Department of Agriculture. These standards are implemented by state and tribal agencies, who design the food package for the state or tribe. These may include different packaging and brands for categories of foods. In the case of infant formula, each state contracts with a specific infant formula manufacturer. These food packages and infant formula contracts are required to administer the program.

1. Compare state WIC food and infant formula packages.
2. What are important considerations each state or tribal agency should consider when designing the food package?
3. What U.S. Department of Agriculture policies dictate nutrition standards for the food package and infant formula?
4. How can supplemental nutrition programs, like WIC, support local retail markets?
5. In 2022, one of the largest infant formulas manufacturers recalled infant formula and shut down operations for months. What impact did this have on the food and nutrition security of families who depended on WIC for their formula?

DISCUSSION QUESTIONS

1. What life course stage(s) are underserved by public health nutrition programs? Why might that be?
2. What are the challenges to implementing EBP in a public health setting? What resources could help overcome these challenges?
3. Compare and contrast the socio-ecological model, social determinants of health, life course theory, and the 10 essential public health services.
4. Compare and contrast the domestic and international programs for a life course stage of your choosing.

SUGGESTED LEARNING ACTIVITIES

1. Identify the stores in your area that accept the Supplemental Nutrition Assisstance Program (SNAP). Identify the stores in your area that accept WIC. Which is more commonly accepted? Is there overlap between the stores that accept each program?

2. Visit a store in your area that accepts WIC. How easy is it to identify the foods that are WIC approved?
3. Compare the approved WIC foods for your state to the WIC package of another state.
4. View the Thrifty Food Plan (https://fns-prod.azureedge.us/sites/default/files/resource-files/TFP2021.pdf), on which SNAP allotments are based. How many of the listed foods do you eat frequently? Do you think the Thrifty Food Plan is practical and reasonable?
5. Format a PICO question on the topic of healthy eating interventions for SNAP beneficiaries and search PubMed to identify a useful article.
6. Identify the educational requirements and titles for dietitians in a non-U.S. country of your choice. How might the presence or absence of this profession impact public health nutrition in that country?

RESOURCES FOR FURTHER LEARNING

- Association of State Public Health Nutritionists: https://asphn.org
    - Information, resources, service opportunities, PHN-focused events and continuing education, and networking for public health nutrition and public health professionals
- Academy of Nutrition and Dietetics Public Health Community Nutrition Dietetic Practice Group: www.phcnpg.org/home
    - Provides information, resources, networking, and practice information for registered dietitians in public health and community nutrition
- Association of Maternal and Child Health Professionals (AMCHP): https://amchp.org
    - Specializes in advocacy, dissemination of best practices, consultation, and support of state public health leaders working in maternal and child health
- *Healthy People 2030*: https://health.gov/healthypeople
    - An initiative of the U.S. Department of Health and Human Services; provides national objectives for health and wellness over the coming decade; provides data and evidence for public health objectives
- American Public Health Association Food and Nutrition Section: www.apha.org/apha-comunities/member-sections/food-and-nutrition
    - As a practice section of the American Public Health Association, the Food and Nutrition section advocates for public health nutrition education, policies, and programs.
- National Commission for Health Education Credentialing. Certified Health Education Specialist (CHES): www.nchec.org/
    - Provides information on the CHES certification for practitioners who wish to meet academic, testing, and continuing education requirements to earn and maintain this certification.

SPRINGER PUBLISHING CONNECT™

A robust set of instructor resources designed to supplement this text is located at http://connect.springerpub.com/content/book/978-0-8261-8623-2. Qualifying instructors may request access by emailing textbook@springerpub.com.

REFERENCES

1. Solar O, Irwin A. *A Conceptual Framework for Action on the Social Determinants of Health.* World Health Organization; 2010. https://www.who.int/publications-detail-redirect/9789241500852
2. Centers for Disease Control and Prevention. 10 essential public health services. Accessed August 30, 2023. https://www.cdc.gov/publichealthgateway/publichealthservices/essentialhealthservices.html
3. Bruening M, Udarbe AZ, Yakes Jimenez E, Stell Crowley P, Fredericks DC, Edwards Hall LA. Academy of Nutrition and Dietetics: Standards of Practice and Standards of Professional Performance for Registered Dietitian Nutritionists (Competent, Proficient, and Expert) in Public Health and Community Nutrition. *J Acad Nutr Diet.* 2015;115(10):1699–1709.e39. https://doi.org/10.1016/j.jand.2015.06.374
4. Hand RK, Davis AM, Thompson KL, Knol LL, Thomas A, Proaño GV. Updates to the definition of evidence-based (dietetics) practice: providing clarity for practice. *J Acad Nutr Diet.* 2021;121(8): 1565–1573.e4. https://doi.org/10.1016/j.jand.2020.05.014
5. Sackett DL, Rosenberg WMC, Gray JAM, Haynes RB, Richardson WS. Evidence based medicine: what it is and what it isn't. *BMJ.* 1996;312(7023):71–72. https://doi.org/10.1136/bmj.312.7023.71
6. Puddy RW, Wilkins N. *Understanding Evidence Part 1: Best Available Research Evidence. A Guide to the Continuum of Evidence of Effectiveness.* Centers for Disease Control and Prevention; 2011. https://www.cdc.gov/violenceprevention/pdf/understanding_evidence-a.pdf
7. Albarqouni L, Hoffmann T, Straus S, et al. Core competencies in evidence-based practice for health professionals: consensus statement based on a systematic review and Delphi survey. *JAMA Netw Open.* 2018;1(2):e180281. https://doi.org/10.1001/jamanetworkopen.2018.0281
8. American Public Health Association. *Public Health Code of Ethics: Issue Brief.* American Public Health Association; 2019. https://www.apha.org/-/media/files/pdf/membergroups/ethics/code_of_ethics.ashx
9. Retsas S. First do no harm: the impossible oath? (Rapid response). July 22, 2019. https://www.bmj.com/content/366/bmj.l4734/rr-2
10. Thomas JC, Sage M, Dillenberg J, Guillory VJ. A code of ethics for public health. *Am J Public Health.* 2002;92(7):1057–1059. https://doi.org/10.2105/AJPH.92.7.1057
11. Academy Quality Management Committee and Scope of Practice Subcommittee of Quality Management Committee. Academy of Nutrition and Dietetics: scope of practice for the registered dietitian. *J Acad Nutr Diet.* 2013;113(suppl 6):17–28. https://doi.org/10.1016/j.jand.2012.12.008
12. Academy Quality Management Committee and Scope of Practice Subcommittee of Quality Management Committee. Academy of Nutrition and Dietetics: scope of practice for the dietetic technician, registered. *J Acad Nutr Diet.* 2013;113(suppl 6):46–55. https://doi.org/10.1016/j.jand.2012.12.006
13. Commission on Dietetic Registration. 2024 graduate degree requirement—registration eligibility. 2023. https://www.cdrnet.org/graduatedegree
14. Phillips W, Tuma PA. Consumer protection through professional regulation. J Acad Nutr Diet. 2019;119(9):1561–1563. https://doi.org/10.1016/j.jand.2019.05.028
15. National Commission for Health Education Credentialing. Certified Health Education Specialist. Accessed November 13, 2023. https://www.nchec.org/
16. Leischow SJ, Milstein B. Systems thinking and modeling for public health practice. *Am J Public Health.* 2006;96(3):403–405. https://doi.org/10.2105/AJPH.2005.082842
17. Office of Disease Prevention and Health Promotion. Access to foods that support healthy dietary patterns. Accessed August 30, 2023. https://health.gov/healthypeople/priority-areas/social-determinants-health/literature-summaries/access-foods-support-healthy-dietary-patterns
18. Casey AR, Morgenstern EM. *U.S. International Food Assistance: An Overview.* Congressional Research Service; 2021. https://crsreports.congress.gov/product/pdf/R/R45422
19. U.S. Department of Agriculture Food and Nutrition Service. Special Supplemental Nutrition Program for Women, Infants, and Children (WIC). Accessed August 30, 2023. https://www.fns.usda.gov/wic
20. Agency for Healthcare Research and Quality. Maternal and childhood outcomes associated with the Special Supplemental Nutrition Program for Women, Infants and Children (WIC). Published December 1, 2020. https://effectivehealthcare.ahrq.gov/products/outcomes-nutrition/protocol
21. Nianogo RA, Wang MC, Basurto-Davila R, et al. Economic evaluation of California prenatal participation in the Special Supplemental Nutrition Program for Women, Infants and Children (WIC) to prevent preterm birth. *Prev Med.* 2019;124:42–49. https://doi.org/10.1016/j.ypmed.2019.04.011

22. Nyhus Dhillon C, Sarkar D, Klemm RD, et al. Executive summary for the micronutrient powders consultation: lessons learned for operational guidance. *Matern Child Nutr*. 2017;13(suppl 1):e12493. https://doi.org/10.1111/mcn.12493
23. SPRING. *SPRING's Contribution to Industrial Food Fortification in Uganda;* SPRING; 2017:1–20. https://www.spring-nutrition.org/sites/default/files/publications/briefs/spring_uganda_food_fortification.pdf

II

LIFE STAGE NUTRITION WITH A PUBLIC HEALTH FOCUS

3

NUTRITION IN PREGNANCY: POPULATION HEALTH PERSPECTIVES

Kyle L. Thompson

LEARNING OBJECTIVES

At the end of this chapter, students will be able to:

1. Summarize the overall process of a normal pregnancy by describing major developmental milestones that occur in each of the three stages.
2. Describe guidelines for normal nutrition in healthy pregnancy, including (a) recommendations for appropriate weight gain and (b) nutrition goals in pregnancy.
3. Explain how **social determinants of health (SDOH)** impact pregnancy outcomes.
4. Describe key **public health nutrition (PHN)** issues related to pregnancy and analyze various approaches to solutions.
5. Describe and explain pregnancy nutrition considerations for population health.
6. Analyze policy approaches to nutrition in pregnancy.
7. List and describe key U.S. and global programs for addressing nutrition in pregnancy.

INTRODUCTION

The **life course theory** posits that health and nutrition practices during each stage of the life cycle impact every subsequent stage, on a continuum from birth through death.[1,2] From the perspective of the life course theory, pregnancy is especially impactful since it is the first life cycle stage. Research continues to suggest robust connections among pregnancy nutrition, pregnancy outcomes, and health status throughout life.[3,4] The importance of adequate prenatal care, nutrition education, and nutrition resourcing during pregnancy—for example, ensuring access to healthful food and supplementation as indicated—is difficult to overemphasize. Population pregnancy outcomes have tremendous significance for a society's physical, mental, and economic well-being, as well as its overall quality of life.[5] This chapter discusses healthful nutrition in normal pregnancy as well as PHN approaches to ensuring good nutrition for all during pregnancy.

THE PROCESS OF PREGNANCY

Pregnancy is a remarkable life cycle stage, with its own unique physiology and even its own unique organ—the placenta. During pregnancy, a new human being develops from conception to birth. Nutritional status even before pregnancy is important to conception and a healthy pregnancy, and will be covered later in this chapter. The following is an overview of the process of pregnancy.

Overview of Pregnancy

A normal full-term pregnancy lasts about 39 weeks or a bit longer than 9 months, and the expected **length of pregnancy** and estimated due date are calculated from the first day of the last menstrual period.[6,7] Because conception typically takes place about 2 weeks following the first day of the last menstrual period, the actual time of gestation is closer to 38 weeks, or slightly more than 9 full months. Healthcare professionals usually describe the 9 months of pregnancy as occurring in three consecutive 3-month periods called the first, second, and third **trimesters**.

First Trimester (0 Through 12 Weeks)

Health behaviors and actions to prepare for pregnancy can positively impact the earliest developmental stages, and can reduce the risk of some congenital disorders. During the first trimester, initial differentiation and development of virtually all body systems and tissues takes place. By the end of this period, fetal development will focus primarily on growth and maturation of existing systems. Important milestones during the first trimester are discussed here.

Fetal Development

- Conception occurs when an egg cell is fertilized by a sperm cell.
- The fertilized egg, called a **zygote**, begins to grow as its cells reproduce. As the number of its cells increases, the zygote becomes a *blastocyst* that travels via a fallopian tube into the uterus, and implants into the uterine wall. The blastocyst is soon surrounded by a fluid-filled membrane that will become the amniotic sac.[7,8]
- By about 4 weeks, the blastocyst has developed into an **embryo**, and is about ¼ inch in length. During the embryonic period, the major systems of the body, including the nervous, digestive, and circulatory systems, are developing. The neural tube, which will become the brain and spinal cord, closes, and cardiac activity begins.[8,9]
- By about 8 weeks, the embryo has developed into a **fetus**, and is about 1¼ inches long. During the subsequent weeks of the first trimester, body systems including the kidneys and cardiovascular system continue to develop and begin to function. Arms and legs are forming from initial buds and are visible.[8]
- By about 12 weeks, the fetus's external genitalia and other primary body parts are formed. All organs, arms and legs, bones, and muscles are in place. The body's systems, including the brain and nervous system, digestive system including the liver, circulatory system, and urinary system are functioning.[7]

Maternal Changes

Many maternal physiologic changes occur in the first trimester that provide for the transfer of nutrients to the fetus, including development of the placenta, expansion of body fluids and increased blood volume, and increased absorption and decreased excretion of micronutrients in order to provide for both maternal and fetal needs. Because initial differentiation and development of the fetal body is complete by about 12 weeks, the risk of **early pregnancy loss** drops significantly at this time.[8] A majority of early pregnancy losses occur in the first trimester because of fetal genetic or developmental anomalies that are incompatible with life.[10,11] The first trimester of pregnancy often brings unfamiliar symptoms such as nausea—often called **morning sickness**—and fatigue. Typically, these symptoms resolve by the end of the first trimester.

Second Trimester (13 Through 27 Weeks)

During the second trimester of pregnancy, growth and development of organs, body systems, and other physical characteristics continue at a rapid pace. Important events during the second trimester are noted here.

Fetal Development

- By about 16 weeks, the fetus is about 5 inches long and is beginning to make purposeful movements such as sucking its thumb. The auditory system is functional and the fetus can hear sounds.[8]
- By about 20 weeks, fetal movement has probably been noticed. The skin is thickening, fingerprints have formed, and there may be an evident sleeping-waking schedule.[7,8] Sensory regions in the brain are maturing. The fetus is about 10 inches long and weighs about 1 lb. Notably, 20 weeks is halfway through pregnancy.
- By about 24 weeks, the fetus's bone marrow is producing its own blood cells. The developing fetus is growing stronger and its lungs have developed but are not yet ready for the outside world. Preterm infants born at 23 to 24 weeks are often able to survive with medical support provided within a hospital equipped with a neonatal intensive care unit (NICU). At this stage, the fetus is about 12 inches long and has reached a weight of about 2 lb.[7,8]
- By about 27 weeks, the nervous system continues developing rapidly. Eyelids are capable of blinking.[8] The fetus is about 14 inches long and weighs around 2 to 3 lb.

Maternal Changes

The second trimester is sometimes thought of as the easiest months of pregnancy, since symptoms such as nausea, morning sickness, and fatigue have typically resolved or lessened. Also, the at-times uncomfortable conditions of late pregnancy resulting from a larger, rapidly growing fetus have not yet developed.

Third Trimester (28 Through 40 Weeks)

During the third trimester of pregnancy, the fetus continues to grow larger, accumulate fat, and gain weight. Before 2013, babies born between 37 and 42 weeks' gestation were considered *term*. Based on new research indicating that key developments in the lungs, liver, and brain occur between 37 and 39 weeks' gestation, in 2013 the American College of Obstetricians and Gynecologists (ACOG) changed the definition of **full term** to 39 weeks' gestation.[12] Revised terminology describing the completion of pregnancy has been provided by the ACOG, including **early term** (37–38 weeks and 6 days), full term (39–40 weeks and 6 days), **late term** (41–41 weeks and 6 days), and **post term** (42 weeks and beyond).[6] Achieving a full-term pregnancy is a key goal for achieving optimal maternal and infant outcomes.

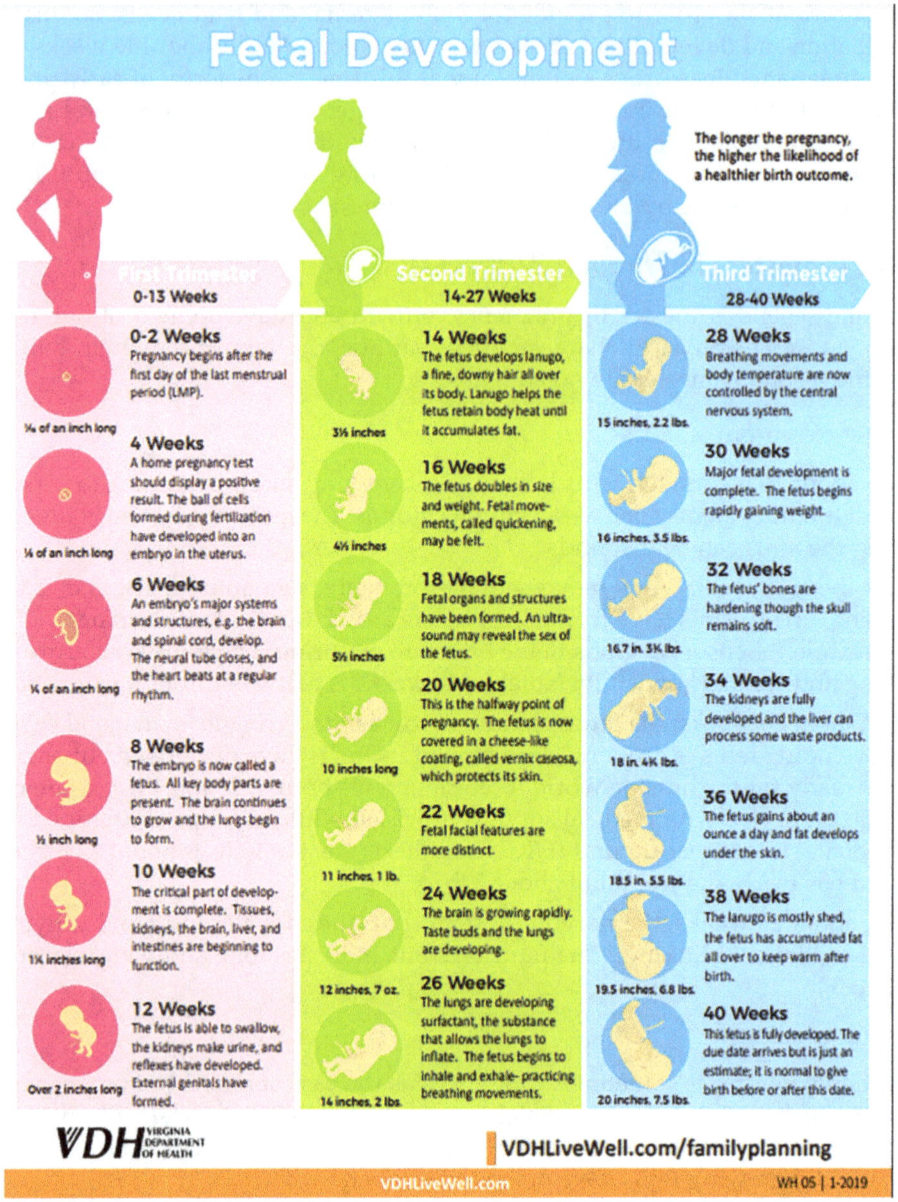

Figure 3.1. Fetal development milestones by trimester.
Source: Virginia Department of Health. Fetal development. 2019. https://www.vdh.virginia.gov/content/uploads/sites/65/2019/03/Fetal-Development-chart12-18-18-1.pdf

Fetal Development

- By about 30 weeks, metabolic systems such as control of body temperature have developed. Brain development continues with greater capabilities to process stimuli.[8] The fetus is about 17 inches in length and weighs up to 5 lb.
- By about 34 weeks—and now in the ninth month of pregnancy—all body systems continue to grow, mature, and develop in preparation for the upcoming first encounter with the outside world. Lung development is nearly complete.

The fetus is about 18 inches long and weighs 6 to 7 lb and is gaining about ½ lb per week.

- By weeks 37 to 38 (early term) the fetus is nearly ready for birth, but important additional lung, liver, and brain development is occurring at this time.
- By week 39, the fetus is full term and ready for birth, weighing about 7 to 9 lb and measuring about 18 to 20 inches long.[8]

Maternal Changes

During the third trimester, the growing fetus often presses on maternal organs, potentially causing discomforts such as frequent urination, shortness of breath, heartburn, hemorrhoids, and back and muscle aches.[13] The hormone **relaxin** promotes softening and stretching of the pelvic muscles and ligaments throughout pregnancy to promote and prepare for a safe delivery.[14] However, looser pelvic muscles and ligaments, the weight of nearly developed fetus, and the fetus's dropping lower into the pelvis in late pregnancy can result in awkwardness while walking. Adequate, effective prenatal care and good nutrition both contribute significantly to optimal pregnancy outcomes. Figure 3.1 illustrates fetal development milestones by pregnancy trimester.[9]

GENERAL NUTRITION GUIDELINES FOR A HEALTHFUL PREGNANCY

Goals for Nutrition in Pregnancy

Nutrition during pregnancy is a crucial factor in promoting optimal fetal and maternal outcomes. While humans require the same nutrients throughout the entire life cycle, albeit in differing amounts, pregnancy is a time during which needs for certain nutrients increase substantially. Working to ensure access to adequate food to support recommended weight gain and sufficient intake of key nutrients is an important function of public health and public health nutrition professionals.

Major goals for nutrition in pregnancy are listed here:

- Achieve appropriate and adequate consumption of calories and nutrients to support appropriate maternal weight gain and adequate and appropriate fetal growth (relates to good prenatal care, also a *Healthy People 2030* goal).[15–17]
- Reduce the risk of *preterm delivery* by maintaining good nutritional status (also a *Healthy People 2030* goal).[17–19]
- Reduce the risk of poor pregnancy and delivery outcomes by maintaining good nutritional status (relates to good prenatal care, also a *Healthy People 2030* goal).[20,21]
- Set the stage for the initiation and development of healthy feeding practices in infancy, as well as a return to prepregnancy maternal weight status.[17,22]

Preparing for a Healthy Pregnancy

Wherever possible, taking specific steps before becoming pregnant can reduce the risk of poor pregnancy outcomes. Nutrition plays an important role in preparation for pregnancy, and nutrition education prior to becoming pregnant is an important PHN function. The Centers for Disease Control and Prevention (CDC) provides a web page titled "Planning for Pregnancy"[23] that recommends helpful several actions to set the stage for a healthy pregnancy:

- See a health provider for a general checkup to assess criteria including but not limited to:
  - The status of any current health conditions, and concerns regarding their management
  - Preventive care updates needed, including vaccinations and health screenings
  - Medications currently used, in relation to pregnancy
  - Current health behaviors and lifestyle influences
- Consume 400 mcg of folic acid daily, either from a supplement or from fortified foods, to reduce the risk of congenital neural tube disorders such as anencephaly and spina bifida.[23,24] Consumption of folate-rich foods such as fruits and vegetables, especially green leafy vegetables, is recommended.
- Avoid environmental contaminants or potentially harmful substances. Stop smoking. Do not consume alcohol, and do not use drugs other than those medically prescribed.
- Consult with a health provider in regard to achieving and maintaining a healthy weight. Both obesity and underweight are associated with poor pregnancy outcomes.[25]
- Address mental health status. The CDC states that there are two major factors impacting mental health: (a) valuing oneself and (b) feeling positive about one's life.[23] If anxiety, depression, or other negative feelings persist and interfere with one's daily life, it is wise to seek help from a health provider.[23]

Official Nutrition Guidance for Healthy Pregnancy

The *Dietary Guidelines for Americans, 2020–2025*

For the first time in its history, the *Dietary Guidelines for Americans 2020–2025* (DGAs) provide dietary guidance for life stages, including pregnancy.[26] Prepared jointly by the U.S. Department of Agriculture (USDA) and the U.S. Department of Health and Human Services (DHHS), the DGAs are updated every 5 years and based on the most current scientific evidence.[26] Specific guidance for life cycle stages provides helpful tools for tailoring dietary recommendations to individual needs. Concerns addressed in the dietary guidelines for pregnancy include appropriate weight gain in pregnancy, healthy dietary patterns, and specific nutrient needs and concerns. Table 3.1 provides a healthy dietary pattern for pregnancy, at two calorie levels. Table 3.2 provides a sample ~2,220-calorie one-day meal plan for a normal pregnancy. An Executive Summary of the DGAs can be found at www.dietaryguidelines.gov/sites/default/files/2020-12/DGA_2020-2025_ExecutiveSummary_English.pdf

Table 3.1. Healthy Dietary Pattern for Women Who Are Pregnant or Lactating, at Two Daily Calorie Levels

Food Group	1,800 Calories per Day	2,200 Calories per Day
Vegetables (cups/day)	2.5	3
Fruits (cups/day)	1.5	2
Dairy (cups/day)	3	3

(continued)

Table 3.1. Healthy Dietary Pattern for Women Who Are Pregnant or Lactating, at Two Daily Calorie Levels (*continued*)

Food Group	1800 Calories per Day	2200 Calories per Day
Grains (oz/day)	6	7
Protein Foods (oz eq*/day)	5	6
Oils (g/day)	24	29
Upper limit on calories for other uses (kcal)	140	250

*One oz eq (ounce equivalent) is defined by the U.S. Department of Agriculture as 1 oz lean meat, poultry, or seafood, 1 egg, ¼ cup cooked beans or tofu, 1 tbsp peanut butter, ½ oz nuts or seeds.
Source: Adapted from U.S. Department of Agriculture, U.S. Department of Health and Human Services. *Dietary Guidelines for Americans, 2020-2025*. 9th ed. U.S. Department of Health and Human Services; 2020. https://www.dietaryguidelines.gov

Table 3.2. Sample Menu for Pregnancy*

Life Cycle Stage	Sample Meal†
Pregnancy (A daily prenatal vitamin may be prescribed by the healthcare provider; if prescribed, take as directed.)	**Breakfast:** ½ cup oatmeal with 1 tsp brown sugar and 1 tbsp walnuts; 2-egg omelet with ¼ cup mushroom/pepper mix and ½ oz shredded cheese, 1 cup fresh strawberries, 1 cup milk **Lunch**: Salad: 1 cup baby spinach, 2 oz cooked shredded chicken, ½ cup mandarin orange slices, 1 tbsp crushed pecans, 1 tbsp dried cranberries, 2 tbsp shredded carrots, 1 tbsp salad dressing of choice, 1 small roll with 1 tsp butter, 1 cup milk **Afternoon snack**: 1 cup fruit/green vegetable smoothie, 2 tbsp walnuts **Dinner:** 1 cup spaghetti (whole grain preferred), ½ cup tomato pasta sauce of choice, 2 oz ground beef, 2 tbsp grated parmesan cheese, ½ cup cooked broccoli tossed with tossed with 1 tsp olive oil, 1-oz slice garlic bread with 1 tsp butter/garlic spread **Evening snack:** ½ cup yogurt of choice mixed with ¼ cup granola

*Meal provides about 2,200 kcal (adjust number of servings/portion sizes to meet lower or higher calorie needs). Menu Assumes healthy pregnancy, for example, no conditions such as gestational diabetes or hypertensive disorders; adjust per food sensitivities and/or allergies; prenatal care should include physician management of any health conditions, and individualized medical nutrition therapy should be provided by a Registered Dietitian Nutritionist.
†Water to drink if not otherwise indicated.

Dietary Reference Intakes

The Dietary Reference Intakes (DRIs) are a set of values that describe recommended ranges of intake for nutrients, energy, and fiber in healthy persons.[27] The DRIs are provided for age and sex groupings, and are developed and periodically updated by the National Academies of Science, Engineering, and Medicine (NASEM). The work is funded jointly by the governments of the United States and Canada, which provide support but do not participate in the NASEM review process in order to maintain the scientific independence of the work.[28]

The DRI values include the following categories:

- Recommended Dietary Allowances (RDAs): The amount of a particular nutrient thought to be adequate to meet the needs of nearly all members of a population group. The RDA is calculated from the particular nutrient's EAR, and cannot be calculated if an EAR is not available.
- Estimated average requirement (EAR): The amount of a particular nutrient thought to meet the needs of half of the members of a population group. Based on research evidence, the EAR is used to calculate that particular nutrient's RDA.
- Adequate intake (AI): The amount of a particular nutrient thought to be adequate to meet the needs of a particular population group. An AI is an educated guess; it is used when research evidence to determine an EAR is not available.
- Estimated energy requirement (EER): The amount of energy, expressed as calories, thought to promote energy balance in given population groups.
- Tolerable upper intake level (UL): The highest amount of a nutrient that can be consumed by most persons without causing adverse effects.
- Chronic disease risk reduction intake (CDRR): The amount of a nutrient above or below which chronic disease risk is expected to decrease in healthy populations. A CDRR is currently available for sodium.
- Acceptable macronutrient distribution range (AMDR): Ranges of proportional intakes of macronutrients (protein, fat, and carbohydrate), expressed as percentages of total daily calorie intake, thought to be associated with reduced risk of chronic disease.[27]

DRI values specific to pregnancy should be used to guide dietary advice and meal planning interventions provided during pregnancy. Nutrients of special concern include folic acid (folate), iron, calcium, and vitamin D. For some nutrients, such as folate and iron, it may be difficult to consume adequate amounts through dietary intake alone.[15] Recommended intakes of nutrients during pregnancy may be found in the Dietary Guideline's Appendix 1 at the following link: www.dietaryguidelines.gov/sites/default/files/2021-03/Dietary_Guidelines_for_Americans-2020-2025.pdf.

MyPlate: Pregnancy and Lactation

MyPlate is the consumer-oriented dietary guidance plan provided by the USDA.[29] MyPlate was launched in 2011, and replaced the previous USDA Food Pyramid in providing consumers with information and resources to choose healthful foods and meals. MyPlate is administered by the USDA Center for Nutrition Policy and Promotion (CNPP), which has been providing consumer nutrition guidance to the public since 1994.[30] MyPlate is revised every 5 years based on revisions of the DGAs. Current MyPlate resources are based on the 2020–2025 DGAs, and provide general nutrition guidance as well as targeted information—for the first time—for life stages including pregnancy. The MyPlate resource is simple and flexible, and can accommodate a wide variety of personal likes and dislikes, cultural foodways, and budget needs.

The *MyPlate: Pregnancy and Lactation* resource includes a wealth of relevant and reliable dietary guidance, resources, and recommendations. Resources include general tips for a healthful diet during pregnancy as well as recommendations for issues specific to pregnancy, such as fish/seafood consumption, prenatal vitamins, food safety in pregnancy, and avoidance of alcohol consumption. The MyPlate plan provides personalized menu options, and the MyPlate Kitchen provides cooking instruction and a variety of recipes. MyPlate is available at myplate.gov. The MyPlate graphic is found in **Appendix B**.

World Health Organization Guidelines for Nutrition in Pregnancy

The World Health Organization (WHO) provides globally focused pregnancy care guidelines that are based on the following questions: "What are the evidence-based practices during antenatal care that improve outcomes and lead to a positive pregnancy experience?" and "How should these practices be delivered?"[31] Nutrition is one of the five major domains of care addressed by the guidelines. Examples of nutrition interventions recommended are as follows:

- Provision of nutrition education on healthful eating and physical activity during pregnancy; tailored education for undernourished populations on increasing daily calorie and protein intake
- Daily oral iron and folate supplementation (30 to 60 mg elemental iron and 400 mcg folate); daily calcium supplementation for populations with low calcium intake

WHO guidelines for nutrition during pregnancy are designed to improve maternal and infant outcomes globally, including low- and middle-income countries where dietary intake of healthful foods may be inadequate to meet needs. However, it is noted in the guidelines that availability of resources is a barrier to implementing the recommendations.[31]

Weight Gain Recommendations in Pregnancy

Weight status during pregnancy is an important indicator that can be used, in the context of an overall medical and nutritional assessment, as an indicator of possible maternal and fetal outcomes. Both inadequate and excessive weight gain in pregnancy are associated with an increased risk of poor outcomes, while weight gain within recommended parameters is associated with desirable pregnancy outcomes.

Inadequate Maternal Weight Gain, Small-for-Gestational-Age Births, and Preterm Birth

Inadequate maternal weight gain may increase the risk of giving birth to a **small-for-gestational-age (SGA)** infant. SGA is defined as a birth weight less than the 10th percentile for gestational age.[32] Infants with SGA status are at higher risk of death during the **neonatal period**, with about 22% of infant deaths worldwide during the neonatal period associated with SGA status.[18]

The incidence of **prematurity**, or **preterm birth,** is increased in SGA infants, as are breastfeeding difficulties, illness, and developmental challenges, delays, and disabilities that can persist throughout life.[33] Prematurity is categorized by gestational age: (1) extremely preterm—prior to 28 weeks' gestation; (2) very preterm—28 to 32 weeks' gestation; (3) moderate to late preterm—32 to 37 weeks.[34] Infants born before 37 weeks' gestation are at increased risk for a number of poor outcomes up to and including death, with the likelihood of complications increasing by the degree of prematurity.

Preterm birth is a major public health issue because it is the leading global cause of death in children under 5 years of age, and because nutrition is a key factor in its prevention. Death rates from prematurity are much higher in low-income countries due to a lack of availability and access to appropriate medical care. About 50% of infants born prior to 32 weeks' gestation in low-income countries die, a startling comparison with high-income countries in which most very preterm infants survive.[34]

Excessive Maternal Weight Gain, Macrosomia, and Large-for-Gestational-Age Births

Excessive maternal weight gain may increase the risk of **macrosomia** or a **large-for-gestational-age (LGA)** birth. Macrosomia is diagnosed at any gestational age if the fetus weighs more than 4,000 g (8 lb, 13 oz), and risk substantially increases once fetal weight reaches 4,500 g (9 lb, 15 oz).[35,36] LGA status is diagnosed when birth weight is above the 90th percentile for a given gestational age.[35]

Both macrosomia and LGA births are associated with heightened maternal risk for delivery injuries, postpartum hemorrhage, increased need for cesarean delivery, and extended labor. Infants with macrosomia or LGA may present with respiratory problems, low blood sugar, and increased risk of jaundice.[36] Additionally, large infants are at higher risk for **shoulder dystocia** during delivery, in which the infant's head is delivered but the shoulder become wedged against the mother's pubic bone. Considered an obstetric emergency, shoulder dystocia requires immediate intervention. The condition can result in broken bones and other complications including permanent nerve damage.[37]

Because there is are important relationships between pregnancy weight status and birth outcomes, chronic disease risk, and one's long-term health outlook, promotion of appropriate weight status in pregnancy is an important public health and public health nutrition initiative. The CDC reported a study that found only 32% of women gained weight within the recommended guidelines during pregnancy, with 21% gaining less weight than desired, and 48% gaining more weight than desired.[33] Regular prenatal care appointments that include weight monitoring are an essential component of appropriate weight management in pregnancy. Table 3.3 provides current desirable weight gain goals for pregnancy in singleton births. Table 3.4 provides desirable weight gain recommendations for twin births.

Table 3.3. Maternal Weight Gain Recommendations for Singleton Births

BMI Prior to Pregnancy	Desirable Weight Gain
Underweight: BMI <18.5	20–40 lb
Normal weight: BMI 18.5–24.9	25–35 lb
Overweight: BMI 25.0–29.9	15–25 lb
Obese: BMI ≥30.0	11–20 lb

BMI, body mass index.
Source: Adapted from Centers for Disease Control and Prevention. Weight gain during pregnancy. Updated June 13, 2022. https://www.cdc.gov/reproductivehealth/maternalinfanthealth/pregnancy-weight-gain.htm

Table 3.4. Maternal Weight Gain Recommendations for Twin Births

BMI Prior to Pregnancy	Desirable Weight Gain
Underweight: BMI <18.5	50–62 lb
Normal weight: BMI 18.5–24.9	37–54 lb
Overweight: BMI 25.0–29.9	31–50 lb
Obese: BMI ≥30.0	25–42 lb

BMI, body mass index.
Source: Adapted from Centers for Disease Control and Prevention. Weight gain during pregnancy. Updated June 13, 2022. https://www.cdc.gov/reproductivehealth/maternalinfanthealth/pregnancy-weight-gain.htm

The desirable rate of weight gain in pregnancy varies by trimester. For a healthy person beginning pregnancy at a normal BMI, a weight gain of 0–4.5 lb during the first trimester is adequate. During the second and third trimesters, a steady weight gain averaging about 1 lb to slightly more than 1 lb per week is desirable for persons beginning pregnancy at a normal BMI.[38]

To support appropriate weight gain, an average of about 300 additional calories per day over usual adequate intake is required.[39] Thus, over the length of an average pregnancy lasting about 280 days, an additional 80,000 calories must be consumed to support fetal growth and development. The distribution of these calories varies by trimester, with no additional calories being needed during the first trimester, and about 340 and 450 additional calories needed daily during the second and third trimesters, respectively.[39]

Recommendations for Education on Weight Gain in Pregnancy

PHN practitioners should be prepared to provide education to groups and populations on the importance of adequate weight gain in pregnancy. Concerns about excessive weight gain can lead to reluctance to consume adequate calories to support appropriate weight gain—a crucial key to achieving desirable birth outcomes. The U.S. Preventive Services Task Force has recommended that effective behavioral counseling be provided to promote adequate and to prevent excessive weight gain in pregnancy.[40]

Helpful information to provide to clients may include:

- The usual composition of pregnancy weight gain (see Table 3.5)
    - It is normal to accumulate some fat during pregnancy; note that fat stores are about 25% of total weight gain in normal pregnancy, with the remaining 75% of weight gain composed of lean tissue. While the purpose of this fat accumulation is poorly understood, in an evolutionary sense it may have been preparation for times of low food availability, or it could help to support lactation.[41]

  - By observing weight gain guidelines per prepregnancy BMI, and consuming a healthful diet following pregnancy, it is likely that most pregnancy weight will be lost within 6 to 12 months following pregnancy; about half of this weight loss will occur in the first 6 weeks after giving birth; lactation is helpful in promoting weight loss.[42]
- The wide variety of positive pregnancy outcomes associated with recommended weight gain; see previous sections of this chapter
- Recommendations for additional calorie intake per trimester, which may help dispel the myth that one should "eat for two (adults)" during pregnancy (see Table 3.6)
  - First trimester: No additional calories needed
  - Second trimester: About 340 additional calories per day needed (the equivalent of a substantial snack)
  - Third trimester: About 450 additional calories per day needed (the equivalent of an additional small meal)[38]
- The strong likelihood that pregnancy weight gain will be lost if one stays within desirable weight gain guidelines[42]
- Encourage lactation as an aid to losing pregnancy weight
- Practical instruction in nutrition self-management skills as needed, including resource availability and access (e.g., Supplemental Nutrition Assistance Program [SNAP], Special Supplemental Nutrition Program for Women, Infants, and Children [WIC]), meal planning, meal and snack preparation, and the like)

Table 3.5 provides a breakdown of the components of weight gain in normal pregnancy. Table 3.6 provides examples of snacks and small meals at appropriate calorie levels.

Table 3.5. Components of Weight Gain, by Average Weight of Component, in Normal Pregnancy With a 30-Pound Weight Gain

Component of Pregnancy Weight Gain	Average Weight
Fetus	7 lb (3.12 kg)
Growth of breasts and uterus	5 lb (2.27 kg)
Placenta	1.5 lb (0.68 kg)
Amniotic fluid	2 lb (0.91 kg)
Increased blood volume	3.5 lb (1.59 kg)
Increased fluid volume	3 lb (1.36 kg)
Fat stores	7 lb (3.12 kg)

Source: Adapted from Mayo Clinic. Pregnancy weight gain: what's healthy? February 9, 2022. https://www.mayoclinic.org/healthy-lifestyle/pregnancy-week-by-week/in-depth/pregnancy-weight-gain/art-20044360

Table 3.6. Sample Snacks and Small Meals for the Second and Third Trimesters of a Healthy Pregnancy*

Pregnancy Stage	Sample Snacks and Small Meals†	Tips and Hints
Second trimester: Sample snacks providing about 340 kcal	1. Sliced medium apple, 2 tbsp peanut butter, 1 tbsp shelled sunflower seeds 2. 6 whole-grain crackers, 1.5 oz cubed cheddar cheese, 1 small orange 3. ½ cup hummus, 10 baked tortilla chips, ½ cup baby carrots 4. 1 cup low-fat Greek plain yogurt mixed with 1 cup blueberries and 3 tbsp walnuts or pecans	Strive to include protein, carbohydrate, and fat in each snack to promote nutritional balance and satiety.
Third trimester: Sample small meals providing about 450 kcal	1. Sandwich made with 2 slices whole-grain bread, 3 oz sliced turkey, 1 tbsp mayonnaise, lettuce and tomato; ½ cup peaches canned in juice; 8 oz skim or 2% dairy milk or fortified almond milk 2. 1 scrambled egg, 2 whole-grain waffles, 1 tbsp maple syrup, 2 tsp butter, 1 small orange 3. Bean burrito made with one flour tortilla, ½ cup mashed beans, 1 oz grated cheese, 1 tbsp salsa, shredded lettuce; ½ sliced avocado	During pregnancy, it may be more comfortable to consume several mini-meals and snacks throughout the day rather than three larger meals.

*Assumes healthy pregnancy, with no conditions such as gestational diabetes or hypertensive disorders; adjust per food sensitivities and/or allergies; prenatal care should include physician management of any health conditions, and individualized medical nutrition therapy should be provided by a registered dietitian nutritionist.
†Water to drink if not otherwise indicated.

SPECIFIC NUTRIENT NEEDS IN PREGNANCY

Macronutrients

Macronutrients include the **energy-yielding nutrients** protein, carbohydrate, and fat. Proportions of macronutrients in relation to total caloric intake are important to overall health and pregnancy outcomes. The DRIs provide recommendations for macronutrient distribution in pregnancy, and these are found in Table 3.7.[26] Note that AMDRs remain the same throughout all three trimesters for all age groups.

Energy (Calorie) Needs

Energy (calorie) needs during pregnancy should support adequate but not excessive weight gain. Calorie needs are also impacted by prepregnancy BMI status and by the presence of special medical conditions, for which individualized nutrition assessment and therapy should be provided by a physician or registered dietitian nutritionist. Adequacy of energy consumption in pregnancy is evaluated by regular weight monitoring at prenatal visits, during which progression toward desired but not excessive weight gain is evaluated. Table 3.8 provides average calorie needs during pregnancy, based on EERs. Note that recommendations are based on a prepregnancy BMI in the normal range; calorie needs should be adjusted by a physician or registered dietitian nutritionist for prepregnancy BMIs in the underweight, overweight, and obese categories.

Table 3.7. Acceptable Macronutrient Distribution Ranges by Age in Pregnancy*

Stage of Pregnancy	Acceptable AMDRs in Percentage of Total Calories, Ages 14–18 Years	Acceptable AMDRs in Percentage of Total Calories, Ages 19–50 Years
First trimester	Protein: 10%–30% Carbohydrate: 45%–65% Fat: 25%–35%	Protein: 10%–35% Carbohydrate: 45%–65% Fat: 20%–35%
Second trimester	Protein: 10%–30% Carbohydrate: 45%–65% Fat: 25%–35%	Protein: 10%–35% Carbohydrate: 45%–65% Fat: 20%–35%
Third trimester	Protein: 10%–30% Carbohydrate: 45%–65% Fat: 25%–35%	Protein: 10%–35% Carbohydrate: 45%–65% Fat: 20%–35%

*Percentages are based on Dietary Reference Intake values. Needs may also be affected by activity levels or special conditions.
AMDR, acceptable macronutrient distribution range.
Source: U.S. Department of Agriculture, U.S. Department of Health and Human Services. *Dietary Guidelines for Americans, 2020-2025*. 9th ed. U.S. Department of Health and Human Services; 2020. https://www.dietaryguidelines.gov

Table 3.8. Calorie Needs by Age in Pregnancy for Those Beginning Pregnancy at BMI 18.5–24.9*

Stage	EER for Pregnancy in Calories: Ages 14–18 Years	EER for Pregnancy in Calories: Ages 19–30 Years	EER for Pregnancy in Calories: Ages 31–50 Years
First trimester	2,368 + 0	2,403 + 0	2,403 + 0
Second trimester	2,368 + ~340	2,403 + ~340	2,403 + ~340
Third trimester	2,368 + ~452	2,403 + ~452	2,403 + ~452

*Values are based on Dietary Reference Intake. Needs may also be affected by activity levels or special conditions.
Source: U.S. Department of Agriculture, U.S. Department of Health and Human Services. *Dietary Guidelines for Americans, 2020-2025*. 9th ed. U.S. Department of Health and Human Services; 2020. https://www.dietaryguidelines.gov

Protein Needs

Recent research based on the U.S. National Health and Nutrition Examination Survey (NHANES) indicates that about one in eight pregnant women do not consume adequate protein.[43] Sufficient protein intake is essential to support optimal fetal growth and development. The RDA for protein during pregnancy increases from 0.8 g/kg/day in the first trimester to 1.1 g/kg/day by the second and third trimester, to support healthful pregnancy, adequate fetal growth, and desired birth outcomes. During pregnancy, consumption of protein from a variety of sources should be encouraged. Protein foods include meats, poultry, fish, beans, and tofu, among others. Table 3.9 provides recommendations for protein during pregnancy by trimester.

Carbohydrate Needs

It is recommended that 45% to 65% of total calories come from carbohydrates during a normal pregnancy, with six to nine servings of whole grains per day.[39] Foods composed primarily of carbohydrates include grains, fruits, and some vegetables. The DGAs describe grain servings in ounce-equivalents; examples of ounce-equivalents are one slice whole-grain bread, ½ cup cooked brown rice, one 6-inch whole wheat or whole corn tortilla, 1 cup flaked whole-grain cereal, and ½ cup cooked whole-grain pasta.[44] Carbohydrate guidelines may require individualization for persons with preexisting or gestational diabetes.

While further high-quality research on the topic is needed, there is evidence that excessive added sugar consumption during pregnancy may contribute to excessive weight gain and subsequent poor outcomes including delivery and metabolic complications. Excessive added sugar consumption is defined as intake of added sugars that exceeds 10% of total calories; note that this is a whole-population recommendation for those 2 years of age and up, and there is no specific guideline for pregnancy.[45] Primary sources of added sugars include sugary beverages, highly sweetened foods such as cookies, snack cakes, and pastries, and processed foods such as sugary cereals.[46] It is recommended that during pregnancy, added sugar intake not exceed 10% of total calories. Note that carbohydrate recommendations are identical for all age groups. Table 3.10 provides recommendations for carbohydrate during pregnancy by trimester.

Fat Needs

Overall fat needs in pregnancy are described as a percentage of total calories. For a person consuming 2,000 calories per day, for example, keeping total fat intake within the recommended range of 20% to 35% of total calories would result in the consumption of 400 to

Table 3.9. Protein Requirements in Pregnancy by Trimester

Trimester	Daily Protein Requirement: Total Intake (g) and by Weight (g/kg), Ages 14–50 Years*
First trimester	71 (increases from 0.8 to 1.1)
Second trimester	71 (1.1)
Third trimester	71 (1.1)

*Needs also affected by activity levels or special conditions.
Source: Adapted from U.S. Department of Agriculture, U.S. Department of Health and Human Services. *Dietary Guidelines for Americans, 2020-2025*. 9th ed. U.S. Department of Health and Human Services; 2020. https://www.dietaryguidelines.gov

700 fat calories per day. It is recommended that saturated fat consumption be limited to no more than 10% of total calories, and about 75% of those who are pregnant exceed this amount.[26]

AI values have been developed for linolenic acid (an omega-3 fat), and linoleic acid (an omega-6 fat). Linolenic and linoleic acid are fats essential to humans that can only be obtained from the diet.[26] Because linoleic acid occurs in vegetable oil, it is found in many processed foods; thus, intake levels tend to be substantially higher than intakes of linolenic acid. The majority of fat calories consumed should come from healthful fat sources, including nuts such as walnuts, seeds such as flaxseed, oils such as olive and flaxseed oil, fatty fish such as salmon, and avocados, among other foods. Decosahexanoic acid (DHA) and eicosapentanoic acid (EPA) are omega-3 fats found primarily in fish. Because these fats are important in fetal brain and nervous system development, consumption of

Table 3.10. Carbohydrate Requirements in Pregnancy by Trimester

Trimester	Daily Carbohydrate Requirement for Pregnancy, Ages 14–50 Years
First trimester	175 g
Second trimester	175 g
Third trimester	175 g

*Needs also affected by activity levels or special conditions.
Source: Adapted from U.S. Department of Agriculture, U.S. Department of Health and Human Services. *Dietary Guidelines for Americans, 2020-2025*. 9th ed. U.S. Department of Health and Human Services; 2020. https://www.dietaryguidelines.gov

Table 3.11. Acceptable Macronutrient Distribution Range and Adequate Intakes for Fat During Pregnancy*

Trimester	Fat Needs, Ages 14–18 Years	Fat Needs, Ages 19–50 Years
First trimester	25%–35% of total calories α-Linolenic acid: 1.4 g/day Linoleic acid: 13 g/day	20%–35% of total calories (α-Linolenic acid: 1.4 g/day) (Linoleic acid: 13 g/day)
Second trimester	25%–35% of total calories α-Linolenic acid: 1.4 g/day Linoleic acid: 13 g/day	20%–35% of total calories α-Linolenic acid: 1.4 g/day Linoleic acid: 13 g/day
Third trimester	25%–35% of total calories α-Linolenic acid: 1.4 g/day Linoleic acid: 13 g/day	20%–35% of total calories α-Linolenic acid: 1.4 g/day Linoleic acid: 13 g/day

*Needs also affected by activity levels or special conditions.
Source: Adapted from U.S. Department of Agriculture, U.S. Department of Health and Human Services. *Dietary Guidelines for Americans, 2020-2025*. 9th ed. U.S. Department of Health and Human Services; 2020. https://www.dietaryguidelines.gov

two servings of fish per week (up to 12 oz) is recommended. Table 3.11 provides AMDRs and AIs for fat intake including essential fats during pregnancy by age groups. Note that recommendations vary only by age group.

Water Needs

Proper hydration is important in all life phases including pregnancy. Water intake includes the consumption of other beverages and all foods provide water in greater or lesser amounts—especially fruits, vegetables, and soups. It is recommended that water be consumed as the primary beverage during pregnancy. Table 3.12 provides water intake AIs during pregnancy.

Micronutrients of Special Concern During Pregnancy

Recommended amounts of certain micronutrients are substantially increased during pregnancy. DRI recommendations for micronutrient consumption during pregnancy are linked in Appendix C in this book and in Appendix 1 at the following link: www.dietaryguidelines.gov/sites/default/files/2021-03/Dietary_Guidelines_for_Americans-2020-2025.pdf.

Folate

Folate status prior to and during pregnancy is important in the prevention of congenital disorders including neural tube defects. The RDA for folate during all trimesters of pregnancy is 600 mcg/day.[26] The RDA is considered to be in addition to dietary folate consumed in dark green leafy vegetables, fruits, beans, and enriched grain products. Folate needs in pregnancy are at their highest level in the life span, compared with the RDA of 400 mcg/day for nonpregnant females ages 14 years and up.[26]

Iron

Iron needs in pregnancy are much higher than the iron needs of nonpregnant females, and because it can be difficult to obtain sufficient iron from food alone, there is usually a need for iron supplementation during pregnancy. Optimal maternal iron intake is vital for fetal growth and development. Additional iron is needed to oxygenate the larger amount of maternal blood volume required to supply the fetus and other pregnancy tissues with nutrients and oxygen. Good food sources of iron include meats and poultry, seafood, beans, dried fruits such as raisins, dark green leafy vegetables, and iron-fortified foods such as cereals and breads. It should be noted that iron sources can be classified

Table 3.12. Adequate Intake of Water During Pregnancy

Trimester	Water Needs (L/day),* Ages 14–50 Years
First trimester	3.0
Second trimester	3.0
Third trimester	3.0

*Needs also affected by activity levels or special conditions; 2.3 L as liquids including water.

Source: Adapted from National Academies Press. Dietary reference intakes for water, potassium, sodium chloride, and sulfate. 2005. https://nap.nationalacademies.org/read/10925/chapter/6

as heme (animal foods such as meat, poultry, eggs, and fish) and nonheme (plant foods such as beans and other legumes, dark green leafy vegetables such as spinach).[26] Heme iron is more easily absorbed by the body, but the absorption of nonheme iron can be improved by consuming it with sources of vitamin C. For example, consuming a meal of lentil soup with a fresh orange for dessert would enhance iron absorption. The RDA for iron during all trimesters of pregnancy is 27 mg/day.[26]

Iodine and Choline

The DGAs list two other nutrients for which needs increase during pregnancy. Iodine and choline are important in fetal neural development and may not be included in prenatal vitamins. The RDA for choline rises substantially during lactation to 550 mg. Foods providing iodine include dairy foods, seafood, iodized salt, and eggs. Foods providing choline include dairy products and most protein foods such as meats, seafood, eggs, and beans and legumes. The RDA for iodine during all trimesters of pregnancy is 220 mcg/day compared with 150 g/day for nonpregnant females ages 14 to 70+ years.[26] The RDA for choline during all trimesters of pregnancy is 450 mg/day compared with 425 mg/day for nonpregnant females ages 14 to 70+ years.[26] During lactation, the RDA for choline increases substantially to 550 mg/day.

Calcium

The need for calcium is not increased during pregnancy, but adequate intake is important to spare the mother's bone mass as the fetal bones grow and to reduce the risk of **hypertensive disorders of pregnancy**.[31,48] The RDA for calcium during all trimesters of pregnancy for persons 14 to 18 years of age is 1,300 mg/day. The RDA for calcium for all trimesters of pregnancy for persons 19 to 50 years of age is 1,000 mg/day.[26]

Prenatal Vitamins

Prenatal vitamins can be helpful in meeting the increased nutrient needs of pregnancy and in compensating for any nutritional gaps, and should be taken as directed by one's health provider. If it is determined by a health provider that additional folate is indicated per higher risk for fetal neural tube defects, additional prenatal vitamins should not be taken but the increased folate should be provided in a separate supplement.[48] In addition to a prenatal vitamin, the ACOG recommends consumption of 200 mg/day DHA to promote optimal fetal neurologic development.[48] It is important for healthcare providers to assess nutritional intake including all supplements currently used when recommending prenatal vitamins and supplements during pregnancy.

Fiber and Physical Activity in Pregnancy

Fiber

Dietary fiber consists of those components of plant foods that are not digested, and is provided by the consumption of fruits, vegetables, and whole grains. Dietary fiber provides many benefits for digestion, glucose metabolism, weight management, and more.[49] In pregnancy, adequate fiber intake reduces the risk of developing constipation and hemorrhoids, gestational diabetes, and hypertensive disorders.[50] Evidence indicates that a majority of pregnant women do not meet recommended guidelines for intake from various nutrient groups, including fruits and vegetables, which are rich sources of dietary

Table 3.13. Adequate Intake for Fiber During Pregnancy

Trimester	Fiber Needs (g/day),* Ages 14–50
First trimester	28
Second trimester	28
Third trimester	28

*Needs also affected by special conditions.
Source: Adapted from National Academies Press. Dietary reference intakes for energy, carbohydrate, fiber, fat, fatty acids, cholesterol, protein, and amino acids. 2005. https://nap.nationalacademies.org/catalog/10490/dietary-reference-intakes-for-energy-carbohydrate-fiber-fat-fatty-acids-cholesterol-protein-and-amino-acids

fiber.[26] PHN professionals should encourage adequate consumption of fruits, vegetables, and whole grains during pregnancy as a public health measure. Table 3.13 provides AI recommendations for fiber intake during pregnancy.

Physical Activity

Physical activity is very beneficial during pregnancy for promoting healthful weight management, optimal metabolic and digestive function, boosting mental health, and setting the stage for desired delivery outcomes. It is recommended that during pregnancy, *and after discussion with and approval from a healthcare provider,* healthy women should obtain about 150 minutes per week of aerobic exercise as able.[26] PH and PHN professionals should encourage appropriate physical activity during pregnancy, and should advocate for access and availability of safe physical activity venues in urban and rural settings.

Other Nutrition Concerns During Pregnancy

Avoidance of Alcohol

There is no known safe level of alcohol consumption during pregnancy; therefore, it is recommended that those planning to become pregnant or who are pregnant refrain from consuming any alcohol including wine, beer, hard liquor, or any other alcohol-containing beverage.[51] Alcohol is transmitted to the baby from the mother through the umbilical cord, and may lead to **fetal alcohol spectrum disorders** (FASDs) in the infant. Disabilities resulting from FASDs are lifelong and can be severe, including but not limited to facial abnormalities, shorter-than-expected height, problems with internal organs such as the heart and kidneys, poor coordination, learning problems, intellectual disabilities, behavioral problems such as poor concentration and hyperactivity, speech delays, and sensory issues such as poor hearing and/or vision.[51] Alcohol consumption during pregnancy is also associated with higher rates of miscarriage and stillbirths.[51]

Public health and public health nutrition professionals should be prepared to deliver education to populations on the importance of avoiding alcohol intake during pregnancy. The interdisciplinary healthcare team should help facilitate access to resources and treatment for persons planning to become pregnant or who are pregnant but may have difficulty in stopping their alcohol intake.

Table 3.14. Amounts of Caffeine in Selected Foods and Beverages

Food or Beverage	Amount of Caffeine (mg)*
Coffee, regular, 8 oz, brewed	137
Coffee, regular, 12 oz, brewed	206
Cola drink, 12 oz	46
Tea, 8 oz, steeped	48
Dark chocolate, 1 oz	12
Milk chocolate, 1 oz	6
Red Bull energy drink, 12 oz	67

*Amounts are approximate, but representative. Amounts of caffeine in brewed and steeped beverages may vary by brewing/steeping time, preparation method, and other factors.
Source: Adapted from Organization of Teratology Information Specialists. Caffeine.MotherToBaby. September 1, 2022. https://mothertobaby.org/fact-sheets/caffeine-pregnancy

Caffeine Intake

Caffeine is a chemical stimulant that occurs naturally in about 60 plant species, and thus is found in some food and beverages.[52] Common sources of caffeine in the diet include coffee, tea, colas, chocolate, energy drinks, and some medications. Amounts of caffeine in foods and beverages may not be clearly stated in labeling. In the United States, if caffeine is *added* to a food or beverage—for example, an energy drink—it must be included in the ingredient list, but there is no requirement that the *amount* of caffeine (usually in milligrams) be listed.[53] If caffeine occurs naturally in a food or beverage, as is the case with coffee, tea, or chocolate, there is no requirement that it be included in the ingredient list.[53]

Most health professional organizations recommend that caffeine intake during pregnancy be limited to 200 mg or less per day.[52,54] Intake levels at this amount have not been associated with infertility or increased risk of miscarriage, congenital disorders, growth restrictions, or other pregnancy problems.[52] While no final determination can be made at this time regarding the effects of high levels of caffeine intake on miscarriage (generally considered >300 mg/day), some studies have suggested higher rates of pregnancy loss with increasing amounts of caffeine intake; thus, if one consumes caffeine, adhering to consumption guidelines is prudent.[52] Research is ongoing. The public will benefit from education on caffeine consumption guidelines during pregnancy. Table 3.14 provides caffeine content of common foods and beverages.

Fish and Seafood Consumption

Fish and seafood are excellent sources of vital nutrients to support a healthy pregnancy and optimal fetal development. Evidence of moderate strength indicates that fish consumption as a component of an overall healthful diet during pregnancy is beneficial for fetal brain and nervous system development. Strong evidence indicates fish consumption promotes heart health.[55] Important nutrients provided by fish consumption include protein, omega-3 fatty acids, iron, choline, zinc, vitamin D, and iodine.[55] The DGAs recommend fish and seafood consumption up to a total of 12 oz per week as part of a healthful diet during pregnancy.

The element mercury occurs naturally in the environment, and also enters the environment as a result of human actions.[56] Mercury accumulates and is converted to methylmercury in bodies of water where fish live. Nearly all fish absorb methylmercury into their tissues from the food they consume, and nearly all human exposure to methylmercury comes through eating fish and seafood.[57] The highest levels of methylmercury tend to be found in larger fish that eat other fish as a major part of their food intake. Excessive consumption of methylmercury over time can damage the brain and nervous system of humans, and developing infants appear to be particularly vulnerable. Methylmercury may also be passed to infants through lactation.[56]

It is not necessary to avoid all seafood consumption during pregnancy and lactation, as recommended amounts of fish and seafood can be eaten without exceeding safety guidelines. Because the nutritional benefits of fish consumption are substantial for both maternal health and fetal development, the DGAs recommend consumption during pregnancy of 8 to 12 oz per week of a variety of fish and seafood *that are lower in mercury*.[26] All raw seafood should be avoided, and all seafood consumed should be cooked to an internal minimum temperature of 145°F (63°C).[58]

While the U.S. Food and Drug Administration (FDA) provides information on specific species that are lower in mercury, these recommendations are more global and national in nature. The Environmental Protection Agency (EPA) provides a list of links to state, territory, and tribal information on state, regional, and local fish advisories, and these agencies' advisory websites should be consulted prior to consuming locally caught fish (fishadvisoryonline.epa.gov/Contacts.aspx).[59]

Recommendations for Education on Fish and Seafood Consumption in Pregnancy

PHN practitioners should be prepared to educate and provide resources on safe fish and seafood consumption during pregnancy. The FDA provides several resources to assist in educating populations on the topic, including a consumer-friendly fact sheet, a frequently asked questions page, and a link to the EPA's list of links to local fish advisories.[55,56,59] Figure 3.2 provides a portion of the FDA's fact sheet on fish and seafood consumption during pregnancy.

Food Safety

Pregnancy is considered a time of increased maternal and fetal risk for foodborne illness due to the many changes that occur in body systems including the immune system. In addition to causing symptoms that can be severe, foodborne illness can result in hospitalization and pregnancy complications, miscarriage, injury to the infant, increased risk for premature birth, and even death.[58]

Foodborne illnesses of special concern during pregnancy include but are not limited to:

- Listeriosis, or infection with *Listeria monocytogenes*
    - This foodborne bacterium grows at refrigerated temperatures but is destroyed by heating food to recommended temperatures. In pregnancy, it usually causes mild maternal illness but can cause severe fetal illness that can lead to miscarriage or prematurity; it is estimated that miscarriage occurs in about 20% of *Listeria* cases. To avoid *Listeria* infection during pregnancy, follow general food safety guidelines, cook all foods to recommended temperatures, and refrain from consuming foods not recommended (see Figure 3.3).[60]

What is a serving? As a guide, use the palm of your hand.

Pregnancy and breastfeeding:
1 serving is 4 ounces

Eat 2 to 3 servings a week from the "Best Choices" list
(OR 1 serving from the "Good Choices" list).

Childhood:
On average, a serving is about:

1 ounce at age 1 to 3
2 ounces at age 4 to 7
3 ounces at age 8 to 10
4 ounces at age 11
Eat 2 servings a week from the "Best Choices" list.

Best Choices

Anchovy	Herring	Scallop
Atlantic croaker	Lobster. American and spiny	Shad
Atlantic mackerel	Mullet	Shrimp
Black sea bass	Oyster	Skate
Butterfish	Pacific chub mackerel	Smelt
Catfish	Perch, freshwater and ocean	Sole
Clam	Pickerel	Squid
Cod	Plaice	Tilapia
Crab	Pollock	Trout, freshwater
Crawfish	Salmon	Tuna, canned light (includes skipjack)
Flounder	Sardine	Whitefish
Haddock		Whiting
Hake		

Good Choices

Bluefish	Monkfish	Tilefish (Atlantic Ocean)
Buffalofish	Rockfish	Tuna, albacore/white tuna, canned and fresh/frozen
Carp	Sablefish	Tuna, yellow fin
Chilean sea bass/ Patagonian toothfish	Sheepshead	Weakfish/seatrout
Grouper	Snapper	White croaker/ Pacific croaker
Halibut	Spanish mackerel	
Mahi mahi/dolphinfish	Striped bass (ocean)	

Choices to Avoid HIGHEST MERCURY LEVELS

King mackerel	Shark	Tilefish (Gulf of Mexico)
Marlin	Swordfish	Tuna, bigeye
Orange roughy		

What about fish caught by family or friends? Check for fish and shellfish advisories to tell you how often you can safely eat those fish. If there is no advisory, eat only one serving and no other fish that week. Some fish caught by family and friends, such as larger carp. catfish, trout and perch, are more likely to have fish advisories due to mercury or other contaminants.

www.FDA.gov/fishadvice
www.EPA.gov/fishadvice

U.S. FOOD & DRUG ADMINISTRATION   EPA United States Environmental Protection Agency

Figure 3.2. U.S. Food and Drug Administration Partial Fact Sheet: Recommendations for Fish Consumption in Pregnancy.
Source: Reproduced from U.S. Food and Drug Administration. Advice about eating fish for those who might become or are pregnant or breastfeeding and children ages 1–11 years. Updated September 28, 2022. https://www.fda.gov/food/consumers/advice-about-eating-fish

- *Salmonella infection*, caused by *Salmonella enterica*
  - *Salmonella* is a foodborne bacterium most associated with eggs and poultry, although it can contaminate many types of foods and there are many pathways to becoming infected. For most individuals, salmonella infection means a few days of uncomfortable and unpleasant digestive symptoms. Although it is not common for salmonella infections to become severe, this can occur, especially in at-risk populations, and severe salmonella infection may increase the risk for poor pregnancy outcomes such as miscarriage, restricted fetal growth, and infection in the newborn. To avoid salmonella infection during pregnancy, follow general food safety guidelines, cook all foods (including poultry and eggs) to recommended temperatures, and refrain from consuming foods not recommended (see Figure 3.3).[61]
- Toxoplasmosis, caused by *Toxoplasma gondii*
  - *Toxoplasma* is a parasite that is highly associated with cats. Cats become infected after eating infected animals such as small rodents or birds; the parasite then reproduces in the cats' digestive systems. The parasite is not spread from person-to-person but by coming into direct or indirect contact with cat feces. Thus, litterboxes, sand, and soil (where cats may leave waste) are avenues of transmission. Since soil is at the base of our foodsystems, transmission is widespread in food and water, with about 50% of toxoplasmosis cases attributed to contaminated food.[62]
  - Maternal toxoplasmosis infection exposes the fetus to the infection. Miscarriage, stillbirth, or serious congenital disorders can result, including hearing loss, vision problems, and developmental delays.[63] To avoid toxoplasmosis during pregnancy, follow general food safety guidelines, cook all foods to recommended temperatures, and refrain from consuming foods not recommended. In addition, practice the following:
    - Wash hands thoroughly following contact with cats, soil, sand, cat litter, and unwashed vegetables.
    - Wash all fruits and vegetables thoroughly, and cook all meats, poultry, and fish to recommended temperatures.
    - Avoid changing litterboxes if possible, or wear gloves and thoroughly wash hands after completing the task. It is recommended to change litterboxes daily, since the parasite is not infectious for at least 1 to 5 days after feces is deposited.
    - Wear gloves while gardening or working in soil and sand; wash hands thoroughly after completing outdoor tasks (see Figure 3.3).[63]

Recommendations for Public Health Nutrition Practitioners: Education on Food Safety During Pregnancy

PHN practitioners should be prepared to provide education in food safety to pregnant women. The content of such education should include:[58]

- The importance of observing food safety best practices and precautions throughout pregnancy for maternal and infant health
- Specific foodborne illnesses of concern
- Basic food safety skills, including general food safety guidelines, instruction in handwashing; safely acquiring, storing, preparing, cooking, and cooling foods; proper washing of fruits and vegetables; using a food thermometer; avoiding cross-contamination; accessing food safety information, and the like

- Foods to avoid during pregnancy[58]
  - Unpasteurized juices and ciders
  - Unpasteurized or raw milk, and raw milk products including raw milk cheeses
  - Undercooked or raw eggs, or foods containing raw eggs (use a food thermometer)
  - Undercooked meats (use a food thermometer)
  - Raw fish, raw shellfish, or any type of raw seafood
  - Raw sprouts
  - Premade and/or prepackaged salads such as chicken and tuna salad, premade or prepackaged meat spreads or pâtés (commonly available in delis)
  - Raw cookie dough[58]
- Foods requiring special handling
  - Although the package may indicate that the item is ready to eat, heat all lunch meat, all styles of deli meat, hot dogs, and cold cuts to 165°F (74°C) to help prevent *Listeria* infection.
- Other measures
  - Toxoplasmosis prevention measures regarding contact with cats and litterboxes, gardening, and handling soil

Figure 3.3 provides an infographic from Foodsafety.gov on food safety basics during pregnancy, and may be useful in providing food safety education.

Special Nutrition and Dietary Needs in Pregnancy

During pregnancy, those with certain conditions or special dietary needs will require individualized nutrition assessment, recommendations, and ongoing monitoring from a physician or a registered dietitian nutritionist in order to provide the best opportunity for a safe pregnancy with good outcomes. Persons with the following conditions should be referred for further nutrition therapy:

- Diabetes diagnosed prior to pregnancy (type 1 or type 2)
- Gestational diabetes (diabetes diagnosed during pregnancy)
- Hypertensive disorders of pregnancy (chronic hypertension, gestational hypertension, preeclampsia/eclampsia)[64]
- **Hyperemesis gravidarum** (extreme, prolonged, and ongoing nausea and vomiting during pregnancy[65]
- Constipation and hemorrhoids
- Food allergies and/or intolerances
- Celiac disease
- Persons who have undergone bariatric surgery
- Vegan or vegetarian diets (these can result in excellent pregnancy outcomes, but special planning and client education are needed to ensure adequate intake of certain nutrients including iron, protein, vitamin B_{12}, and other nutrients as indicated by nutrition assessment)
- Any other health condition for which individualized nutrition advice would be beneficial

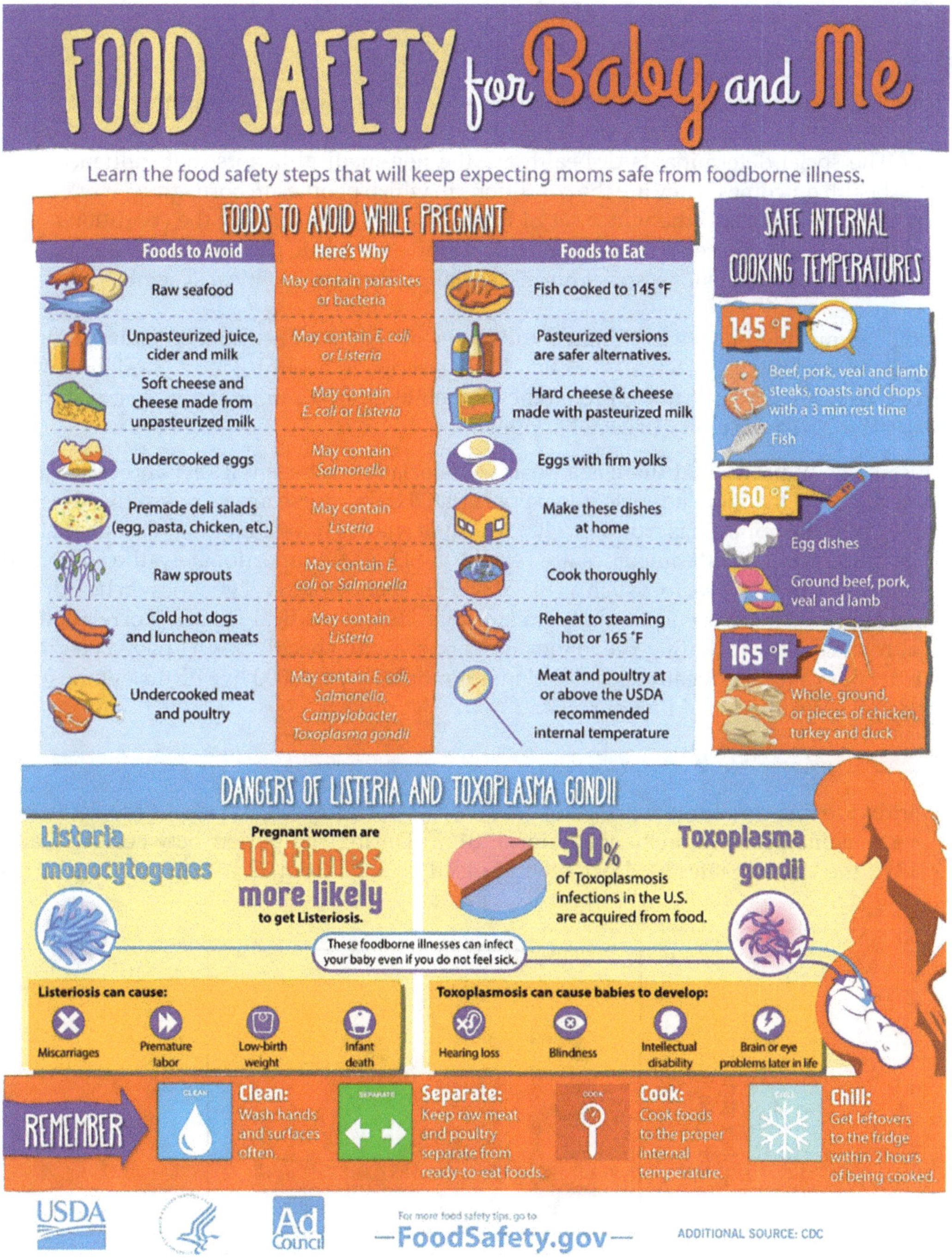
FOOD SAFETY for Baby and Me
Learn the food safety steps that will keep expecting moms safe from foodborne illness.
FOODS TO AVOID WHILE PREGNANT
Foods to Avoid
Here's Why
Foods to Eat
Raw seafood
May contain parasites or bacteria
Fish cooked to 145 °F
Unpasteurized juice, cider and milk
May contain E. coli or Listeria
Pasteurized versions are safer alternatives.
Soft cheese and cheese made from unpasteurized milk
May contain E. coli or Listeria
Hard cheese & cheese made with pasteurized milk
Undercooked eggs
May contain Salmonella
Eggs with firm yolks
Premade deli salads (egg, pasta, chicken, etc.)
May contain Listeria
Make these dishes at home
Raw sprouts
May contain E. coli or Salmonella
Cook thoroughly
Cold hot dogs and luncheon meats
May contain Listeria
Reheat to steaming hot or 165 °F
Undercooked meat and poultry
May contain E. coli, Salmonella, Campylobacter, Toxoplasma gondii
Meat and poultry at or above the USDA recommended internal temperature
SAFE INTERNAL COOKING TEMPERATURES
145 °F
Beef, pork, veal and lamb steaks, roasts and chops with a 3 min rest time
Fish
160 °F
Egg dishes
Ground beef, pork, veal and lamb
165 °F
Whole, ground, or pieces of chicken, turkey and duck
DANGERS OF LISTERIA AND TOXOPLASMA GONDII
Listeria monocytogenes
Pregnant women are 10 times more likely to get Listeriosis.
50% of Toxoplasmosis infections in the U.S. are acquired from food.
Toxoplasma gondii
These foodborne illnesses can infect your baby even if you do not feel sick.
Listeriosis can cause:
Miscarriages
Premature labor
Low-birth weight
Infant death
Toxoplasmosis can cause babies to develop:
Hearing loss
Blindness
Intellectual disability
Brain or eye problems later in life
REMEMBER
Clean: Wash hands and surfaces often.
Separate: Keep raw meat and poultry separate from ready-to-eat foods.
Cook: Cook foods to the proper internal temperature.
Chill: Get leftovers to the fridge within 2 hours of being cooked.
USDA
Ad Council
For more food safety tips, go to
—FoodSafety.gov—
ADDITIONAL SOURCE: CDC

Figure 3.3. Food safety education basics during pregnancy.
Source: Foodsafety.gov. Food safety for baby and me. 2020. https://www.foodsafety.gov/sites/default/files/2019-05/food-safety-infographic-pregnant-women.jpg

SOCIAL DETERMINANTS OF HEALTH: IMPACT ON PREGNANCY OUTCOMES

The CDC has adopted WHO's definition of social determinants of health[66]:

> The social determinants of health are the non-medical factors that influence health outcomes. They are the conditions in which people are born, grow, work, live, and age, and the wider set of forces and systems shaping the conditions of daily life. These forces and systems include economic policies and systems, development agendas, social norms, social policies and political systems.[67]

SDOH include but are not limited to factors such as income, housing status, education level, employment status, work conditions, access to healthful food, food insecurity, access to healthcare including prenatal care, neighborhood safety, access to community resources, and availability of social support.

Research indicates that there is a positive association between SDOH and health outcomes; that is, the more adverse a location's SDOH, the worse are its overall health outcomes, and the opposite is true as well.[68] Multiple studies have suggested that about 30% to 55% of overall health outcomes are related to SDOH.[69] Proportionately, the combined impact of nonmedical factors such as SDOH, health behaviors, and genetics on health and pregnancy outcomes is substantially greater than that of medical factors. Correlations of health outcomes—including pregnancy outcomes—with specific SDOH have been identified. For example, education level and infant mortality per 1,000 live births demonstrate a relationship, illustrated in Figure 3.4.[70,71]

Populations at Risk

Worldwide, maternal mortality rates (MMRs) have decreased by 34% since 2000, but have remained mostly unchanged since 2016.[72] During the period between 1990 and 2017 in the United States MMRs have increased by 58%, from 12 per 100,000 live births

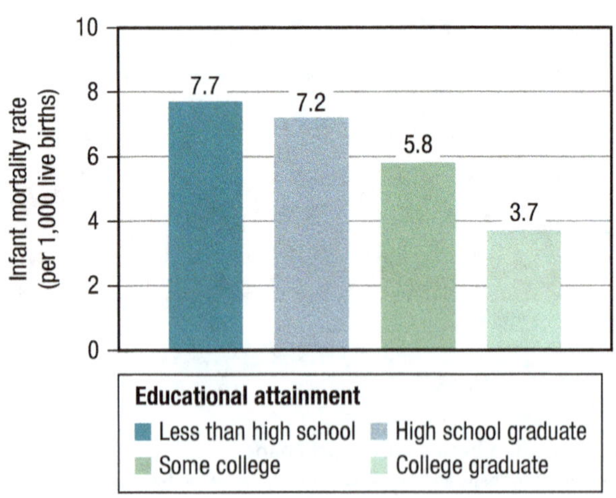

Figure 3.4. Infant mortality rate in the United States by mother's education, 2009.
Source: Mathews TJ, MacDorman MF. Infant statistics from the 2009 period linked birth/infant death dataset. *Natl Vital Stat Rep.* 2013;61:1–28.

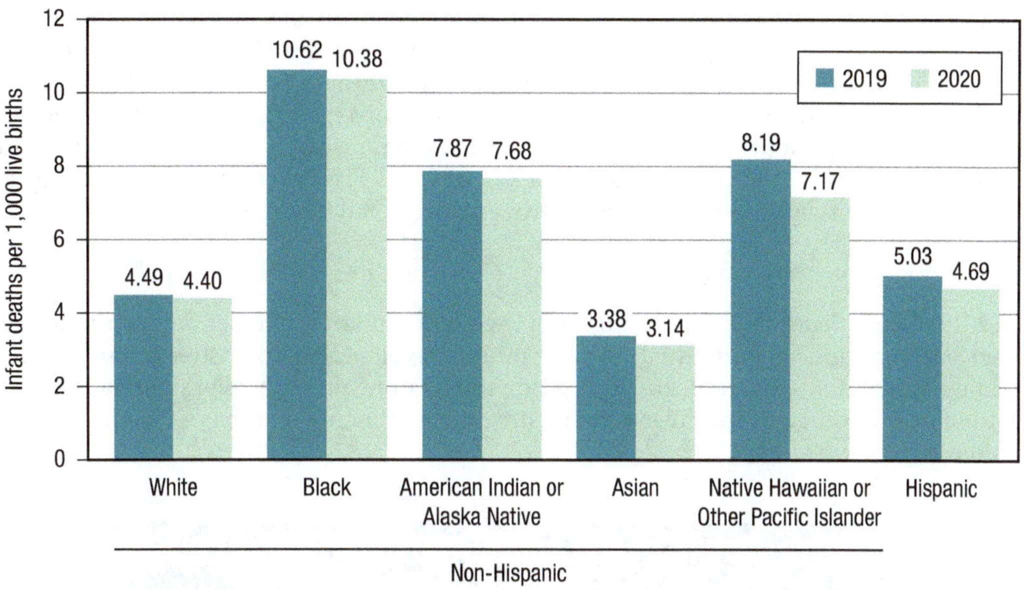

Figure 3.5. Infant mortality rate, by maternal race and hispanic origin: United States 2019 and 2020.

Source: Ely DM, Driscoll AK. *Infant mortality in the United States, 2020: data from the period linked birth/infant death file. Natl Vital Stat Rep. 2022;71(5):1–18. https://www.cdc.gov/nchs/data/nvsr/nvsr71/nvsr71-05*

in 1990 to 17 per 100,000 in 2017.[73] Infant mortality rates (IMRs) in the United States decreased between 2007 and 2017, falling from 6.75 to 5.79 deaths per 1,000 live births, a decrease of about 14%.[74] However, IMRs in the United States remain comparatively high. In 2022 Dagher and Linares pointed out that among the 36 countries participating in the Organisation for Economic Co-operation and Development (OECD), the United States ranks 33rd in IMR when compared with the OECD average rate of 3.31%.[73] Certain populations are at increased risk for poor pregnancy outcomes including maternal and infant deaths related to adverse SDOH. Figure 3.5 shows IMRs by maternal race and Hispanic origin; note the high rates of infant mortality among non-Hispanic Black, American Indian, Native Hawaiian and other Pacific Islander, and Hispanic populations.[75]

Dagher and Linares also point out three populations at substantially increased risk for *health disparities* leading to poor pregnancy outcomes: (1) persons of color; (2) underserved rural populations; and (3) persons with lower socioeconomic status.[73] Health disparities are defined by the CDC as "preventable differences in the burden of disease, injury, violence, or in opportunities to achieve optimal health experienced by socially disadvantaged racial, ethnic, and other population groups, and communities."[76] Disparities in pregnancy outcomes seem to persist even when specific SDOH are controlled for in data analysis, indicating that socioeconomic and other factors play a significant role in maternal and infant health.[77]

The effects of adverse impacts including racism, poverty, poor access to high-quality healthcare, lack of health insurance, food insecurity, lack of educational and/or economic opportunities, exposure to violence, and other negative factors appear to have a snowball effect on health throughout the life span.[73] The life course theory, which posits that each stage of the life cycle impacts all subsequent phases, supports this assertion.[1] Indeed,

SDOH have generational impacts since maternal health during pregnancy is reflected in the child's and thus the grandchildren's health throughout their life spans. Recent research has explored the concept of *weathering*, or biologic aging over time.[78,79] According to this theory, exposure to adverse SDOH results in worsening health over time and increases the risk of poor outcomes with maternal aging; research appears at this time to support this idea.[73] To improve maternal health, PH and PHN professionals should focus on effective interventions to promote improved nutritional (and other) SDOH.

A Framework for Impacting Social Determinants of Health in Pregnancy

In 2019, the de Beaumont Foundation proposed a model for strategies and tactics to impact SDOH at clinical, individual, and community levels called downstream, midstream, and upstream domains, respectively.[80] If one thinks of health as a river or stream, it follows that the source of the river—the upstream component—will have a major impact on downstream results.

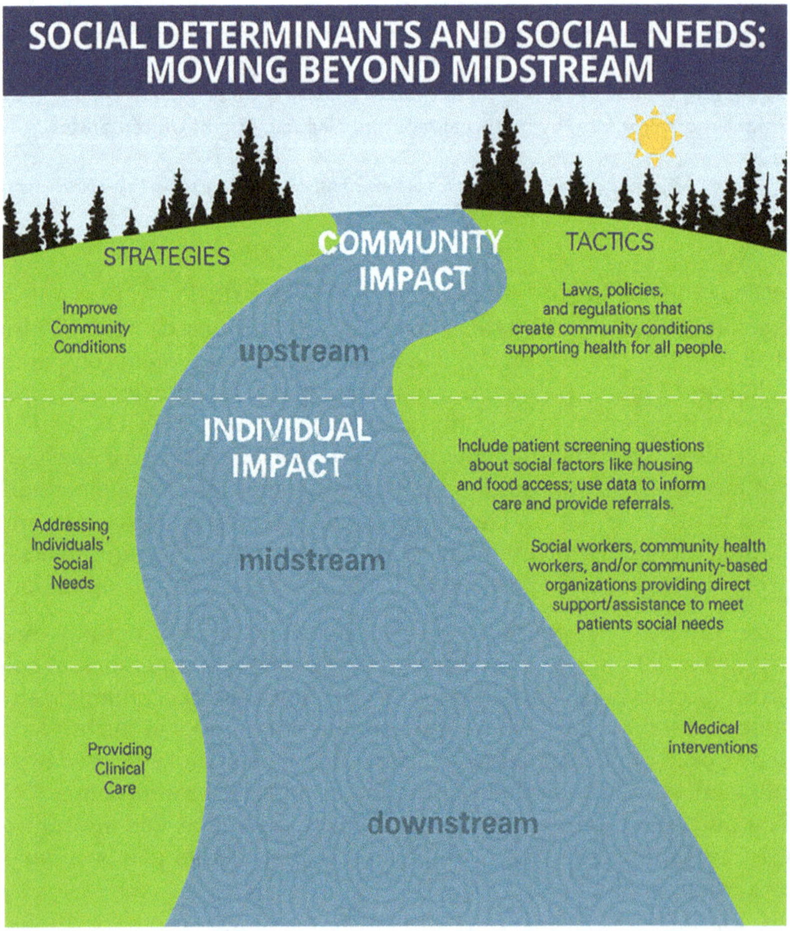

Figure 3.6. Strategies and tactics for impacting social determinants of health at upstream, midstream, and downstream levels.

Source: de Beaumont Foundation, Trust for America's Health. *Social determinants and social needs: moving beyond midstream. de Beaumont Foundation; 2019. https://debeaumont.org/wp-content/uploads/2019/04/social-determinants-and-social-needs.pdf*

Table 3.15. Examples: Upstream, Midstream, and Downstream Potential Impacts via Public Health Nutrition Interventions During Pregnancy

Level of Potential Benefits	Nutrition Interventions During Pregnancy	Potential Impacts Likely to Result in Better Pregnancy Outcomes
Upstream: benefits to the community	1. SNAP established by law (encourage and promote access) 2. WIC program, established by law (encourage and promote access) 3. Cultural foods available through WIC electronic benefit card, by WIC policy	1. Reduced food insecurity during pregnancy 2. Reduced food insecurity during pregnancy, access to prenatal care and monitoring 3. Improved food intake during pregnancy through provision of culturally appropriate nutritious foods
Midstream: benefits to the individual by addressing social needs	1. Screen prenatal patients for food insecurity at clinical visits or community venues as appropriate 2. Develop a food pantry at a local clinic where pregnant patients receive care	1. Referral to social services as needed to connect individuals with food assistance resources to reduce food insecurity (governmental and nongovernmental) 2. Point-of-service access to nutritious food to reduce food insecurity; opportunity for referrals to programs such as SNAP and WIC
Downstream (clinical): benefits to the individual by addressing individual healthcare needs in the clinic	1. Weight monitoring at regular prenatal visits 2. Provision of appropriate nutrient supplementation at regular prenatal visits as needed (usually a prenatal vitamin)	1. Fewer SGA births, fewer premature births 2. Fewer congenital disorders, optimal fetal growth and development, improved maternal nutrition status

SGA, small-for-gestational-age; SNAP, Supplemental Nutrition Assistance Program; WIC, Special Supplemental Nutrition Program for Women, Infants, and Children.

According to the model illustrated in Figure 3.6, clinical health encounters are downstream from SDOH that affect individuals, and individual impacts are downstream from societal conditions that affect SDOH. Thus, the greatest health and nutrition impacts will result from strategies and tactics that impact upstream factors in ways that promote health for everyone.

Table 3.15 illustrates examples of the **upstream, midstream,** and **downstream model** of SDOH applied to PHN issues impacting pregnancy outcomes.

Public Health Nutrition Issues Related to the Pregnancy Life Cycle Stage

Prenatal Care

Because nutrition is a crucial factor in promoting optimal pregnancy outcomes, PH and PHN professionals should work at all levels of influence to improve access to high-quality prenatal care, including nutrition care, for all. High-quality prenatal care at the downstream influence level (clinical care) includes ongoing weight monitoring, nutrition education and counseling on healthful dietary practices during pregnancy, and referrals for individualized nutrition care provided by a physician or registered dietitian nutritionist as needed. At the midstream level, interventions that can have major positive impacts include those that screen for pregnancy-related conditions including impacts of SDOH, develop resources and processes to support care and referral pathways, and develop interprofessional networks to address specific pregnancy-related SDOH from many different viewpoints in a coordinated way. At the upstream level, appropriate laws, policies, and regulations can provide the framework and scaffolding needed to promote the best possible pregnancy outcomes for all in order to benefit individuals and communities.

Rural Concerns

PH and PHN professionals should be aware of an ongoing crisis in rural pregnancy care related to the closure of many small rural hospitals in recent years. Between 2005 and 2017 approximately 125 rural hospitals closed, largely for financial reasons.[81] When a rural hospital closes, the effects on its surrounding communities and their SDOH can be profound, and these effects often include the loss of obstetric services. Other rural hospitals have remained open but have discontinued obstetric services due to low birth volumes, the cost of retaining staff and necessary equipment, liability concerns, and other financial issues.[81] The loss of access to rural obstetric services is demonstrated in increased rates of undesirable pregnancy outcomes, and these impacts are worse for rural residents who are people of color or who have low income levels.[81] Obstetric service closures have led to the definition of **maternity care deserts** by the March of Dimes as any county lacking a hospital or birthing center providing obstetric services or lacking a provider of obstetric care. PHN professionals should advocate for innovative solutions to making pregnancy care, including nutrition care, available regardless of location.

Food Security

The inability to access adequate amounts of nutritious food is of increasing concern during pregnancy. PHN professionals should work to promote food and nutrition programs and resources to pregnant clients/patients experiencing food insecurity. Federal programs include SNAP, WIC, and hands-on educational programs such as Supplemental Nutrition Assistance Program Education (SNAP-Ed). The Extended Food and Nutrition Education Program (EFNEP) is offered on the state/county level and partially funded by the federal government. PH and PHN professionals should familiarize themselves with local resources such as food pantries and farmers markets in order to make appropriate referrals. In addition, it is important to develop relationships and networks with local and regional social service professionals in order to maximize the effectiveness of recommendations.

Policy: Global Issues and Challenges

WHO reports that about 287,000 women died in 2020 from complications resulting from pregnancy and childbirth.[82] While this number represents a decrease from 2015's maternal mortality total of 303,000 women, it remains unacceptably high. In 2019, 900,000 infants across the globe died as a result of preterm birth.[34] Most maternal deaths are preventable; crucial to reducing maternal mortality numbers is the availability of adequate prenatal care and skilled professional care during and after birth to all.[82] It is thought that with appropriate care utilizing widely available, cost-effective interventions, three quarters of deaths resulting from preterm birth could also be prevented.[34]

The United Nations Children's Fund (UNICEF) provides interventions focused on improving access to nutritious food for women and adolescent girls, food fortification programs, nutrition education, vitamin/mineral supplementation during pregnancy, and weight gain monitoring, among others.[83] UNICEF engages in research with the purpose of improving maternal nutrition. The organization also encourages research and interventions focused on upstream/meta interventions to improve the nutritional environment for all life cycle stages including pregnancy: food systems development, expanded access to food and nutrition services, optimal nutrition communications, and economic empowerment and leadership development among women and adolescent girls.[83]

Public Health Nutrition Programs for the Pregnancy Life Stage

Appendix C provides a table of PHN programs by life stage.

WHAT WORKS : A CLOSER LOOK AT MYPLATE RESOURCES FOR PREGNANCY AND LACTATION

This chapter mentions that the Dietary Guidelines for Americans—for the first time—provide dietary information by life cycle stage. *MyPlate: Pregnancy and Lactation* provides many useful, consumer-focused tools for promoting good nutrition during pregnancy.[84] The resource provides an accurate, reliable, and client-friendly source of nutrition information for healthy pregnancies.

The *MyPlate: Pregnancy and Lactation* web page organizes information into five major categories:

- Eat Healthy: Provides tips on recommended foods to support a healthful diet; links to the Food and Drug Administration's recommendations for seafood consumption during pregnancy.
- Get Your Plan: Explains that calorie needs may change when one is pregnant or lactating; links to the "MyPlate Plan" tool to provide further information on a healthy meal plan during pregnancy.
- Ask About Supplements: Recommends adhering to physician recommendations for taking a prenatal vitamin/mineral supplement, or other supplements, when pregnant or lactating.
- Make Safe Choices: Provides recommendation that all alcohol consumption should be avoided during pregnancy; provides food safety guidelines and information on caffeine consumption and food allergy prevention.
- Resources: Links are provided to a wide variety of tip sheets and informational resources in English and Spanish; links are also provided to further information about three *MyPlate* technology tools:
    - *Shop Simple with MyPlate*: An app, accessible through a provided QR code, that focuses on budget-friendly healthy eating; provides location-specific information on healthy food sources such as farmers markets.

- o *MyPlate on Alexa*: MyPlate is available as an Alexa skill; provides nutrition information via the Amazon Alexa smart speaker; available through the free Amazon Alexa app found at Google Play or the App Store.
- o *Start Simple with MyPlate*: This app uses MyPlate as a guide for implementing healthier habits and monitoring progress; available through Google Play or the App Store.

MyPlate: Pregnancy and Lactation is a useful, regularly updated resource that can be recommended to consumers and clients to promote improved nutritional intake and thus contribute to optimal pregnancy outcomes.

SUMMARY

Population pregnancy outcomes have tremendous significance for a society's physical, mental, and economic well-being as well as its overall quality of life.[5] Proper prenatal nutrition is a crucial component in achieving optimal pregnancy outcomes. Good nutrition in pregnancy supports appropriate maternal weight gain, reduces adequate and appropriate fetal growth, reduces the risk of preterm delivery, reduces the risk of labor and delivery problems, and sets the stage for the development of healthy feeding practices in infancy. SDOH affect the outcomes of pregnancy, and PHN professionals should advocate for optimal nutritional SDOH such as the availability of healthful food for all. From the perspective of the life course theory, pregnancy is especially impactful since it is the first life cycle stage. Research continues to suggest robust connections among pregnancy nutrition, pregnancy outcomes, and health status throughout life.[3,4]

KEY CHAPTER CONCEPTS

1. The life course theory posits that health behaviors including nutrition practices during a given life cycle stage impact health during each subsequent life cycle stage, on a continuum from birth to death, and contextualized within environments consisting of social, economic, educational, and physical determinants. From a life course theory perspective, pregnancy is especially impactful since it is the first life cycle stage for each new human being.
2. A normal full-term pregnancy lasts about 39 weeks or slightly longer than 9 months, and the expected length of pregnancy and estimated due date are calculated from the first day of the last menstrual period.[6,7] Because conception typically takes place about 2 weeks following the first day of the last menstrual period, the actual time of gestation is closer to 38 weeks, or slightly more than 9 full months. Healthcare professionals usually describe the 9 months of pregnancy as occurring in three consecutive 3-month periods called the first, second, and third *trimesters*.
3. Before becoming pregnant, several actions are recommended to reduce the risk of poor pregnancy outcomes: Obtain a medical checkup; consume 400 mcg folate daily through supplementation, fortified foods, and/or folate-rich foods; avoid environmental contaminants and potentially harmful substances, quit smoking, stop alcohol intake, and do not use drugs other than those medically prescribed; if needed, obtain medical consultation in regard to achieving and maintaining a healthy weight; address any mental health concerns.

4. Goals for healthful nutrition in pregnancy can be generally described as adequate and appropriate maternal intake to promote optimal pregnancy outcomes such as maintenance of good maternal nutritional status, a safe delivery, reduced risk of congenital disorders, and a healthy birth weight for the infant.
5. Official dietary guidance for pregnancy includes the *Dietary Guidelines for Americans, 2020–2025* (DGAs), which for the first time provide dietary recommendations by life stage; the Dietary Reference Intakes, which provide reference values for nutrient intake during pregnancy; MyPlate, the U.S. consumer-focused dietary guidance tool, which is aligned with the DGAs and provides guidance for life stage groups; and the United Nations WHO guidelines for nutrition during pregnancy.
6. Appropriate weight gain in pregnancy is a key component of promoting healthful pregnancy outcomes. Prenatal care, monitoring, and education should be provided prior to and during pregnancy to promote the achievement of recommended weight gain goals per prepregnancy BMI.
7. Key nutrients of concern in pregnancy due to increased needs include protein, folate, iron, choline, and iodine. While needs do not increase during pregnancy, adequate calcium intake and vitamin D intake are important to maintain bone health.
8. Nutrition education in pregnancy should include information on food safety, fish and seafood consumption, alcohol consumption, caffeine consumption, and other topics as needed. PHN professionals should be aware of special conditions in pregnancy that require individualized nutrition therapy, and should refer such clients to a physician or RDN as indicated. Access to prenatal care including nutrition care, location-related concerns such as rurality, and food insecurity are concerns that may need to be addressed by PH and PHN professionals.
9. Populations at higher risk for health disparities associated with SDOH, leading to poor pregnancy outcomes, include persons of color, some rural populations, and persons with lower socioeconomic resources. To impact the underlying SDOH, upstream and midstream interventions are most effective, and lead to better downstream outcomes.

CASE STUDY AND QUESTIONS

You work in a public health department and have been asked to prepare a client handout, no longer than two pages (front and back), on pregnancy nutrition resources available in your locality. Your handout will be provided to clients in both a print version and as a downloadable PDF. Complete a search of available resources, then answer the following questions related to your project:

1. Which publicly funded resources will you include?
2. Which privately funded resources will you include?
3. What contact information will you provide for each resource?
4. For each resource, prepare a brief phrase/sentence that you can include as part of the handout to describe the resource's role in enhancing nutrition during pregnancy.
5. Arrange and format your handout. Consider readability, appearance, and accessibility. If possible, conduct a peer review with your classmates to receive and incorporate suggestions for your handout.

DISCUSSION QUESTIONS

1. This chapter posits that fetal development during pregnancy is the most important life cycle phase for each human being. Discuss the evidence underpinning this statement. Are there reasons you might disagree with or modify the statement?
2. Discuss: How can public health nutrition professionals best promote and educate groups and populations on the importance of taking specific actions to prepare for pregnancy?
3. In regard to nutrition-related prenatal care, which components do you see as being of key importance? What do you think are effective strategies for providing prenatal nutrition care?
4. Select three nutrients of concern during pregnancy. How might you educate a client on the importance of the chosen nutrients? What points would you include in your education? What sources of the nutrient would you recommend?
5. Discuss and describe the concept of upstream, midstream, and downstream impacts in public health. How can you apply this model to public health nutrition during pregnancy? What strategies and tactics would you suggest to reduce health disparities in pregnancy? What are the impact levels of your suggested strategies, and how could they best be implemented (e.g., laws, policies, regulations)?
6. Read the webpage "Barriers to Improving Rural Maternal Health" at www.ruralhealthinfo.org/toolkits/maternal-health/1/barriers. Which barriers seem most significant to you? Which barriers do you see as being nutrition-related? What role do you see for public health nutrition professionals in rural maternal health?
7. How could remote patient monitoring (RPM), often called telehealth, be utilized regionally, nationally, and globally to improve pregnancy outcomes? What barriers might exist to implementing RPM interventions in various settings?

SUGGESTED LEARNING ACTIVITIES

1. Prepare a presentation for your class or for a community group on recommendations, including nutrition recommendations, to prepare for a healthy pregnancy.
2. Review the *MyPlate: Pregnancy and Lactation* website. Choose a calorie level and a trimester, and prepare a 3-day healthy meal plan for pregnancy utilizing the *MyPlate* resources. You may wish to present your meal plan in a print or digital booklet form, and include several appropriate recipe suggestions, perhaps referring to the *MyPlate Kitchen* resource.
3. Design an educational tool, such as a fact sheet or brief presentation, addressing the importance of appropriate weight gain in pregnancy, and addressing possible client concerns about the need to gain weight.
4. Prepare a nutrition education presentation on food safety in pregnancy for a group of clients participating in the WIC program. Include a pre- and post-test in your materials. Present to an actual WIC client group, if possible, or simulate the experience with fellow students. Administer your pre- and post-tests and solicit feedback for presentation improvement; incorporate gathered suggestions.
5. Research laws, policies, and regulations in your locale that might have an impact on nutrition during pregnancy. Prepare a one- to two-page written brief on your findings.
6. Make arrangements to visit a WIC facility and speak with a staff member (director or nutritionist) on operations and functions of the facility, especially as related to interventions provided during

pregnancy, or invite a WIC staff member to visit your class as a speaker. Following the activity, write a brief reflection on your learnings.

RESOURCES FOR FURTHER LEARNING

- *MyPlate: Pregnancy and Breastfeeding*: www.myplate.gov/life-stages/pregnancy-and-breastfeeding
  - Information and many practical MyPlate resources including the MyPlate Planner, advice on pregnancy-focused nutrition topics such as fish consumption, and recipes/cooking tips for supporting good nutritional status during pregnancy
- *Special Supplemental Nutrition Program for Women, Infants, and Children:* www.fns.usda.gov/wic
  - Gateway to WIC programs, with many resources for applicants, agencies, and partners
- *Healthy Weight Gain During Pregnancy:* https://webassets.nationalacademies.org/whattogain
  - An interactive, engaging tool to obtain personalized weight gain recommendations for a healthy pregnancy; provides answers to a number of Frequently Asked Questions (FAQs) regarding pregnancy weight gain
- *Food and Drug Administration: Advice About Eating Fish for Those Who Might Become or Are Pregnant and Children Ages 1–11 Years:* www.fda.gov/media/102331/download
  - Consumer-friendly fact sheet with information on fish and seafood consumption during pregnancy, including a current list of recommended fish and seafood types, as well a list of fish and seafood to avoid
- *Morning sickness:* https://medlineplus.gov/ency/patientinstructions/000604.htm
  - Medical encyclopedia entry from the National Library of Medicine that provides information and evidence-based strategies on managing morning sickness
- *CDC Info-on-Demand: Fetal Alcohol Spectrum Disorders (FASDs):* (1) wwwn.cdc.gov/pubs/CDCInfoOnDemand.aspx?ProgramID=234; (2) www.cdc.gov/ncbddd/fasd/alcohol-use.html
  - Access to resources for health professionals to use in providing education on refraining from alcohol use during pregnancy; includes posters, brochures, and a Surgeon General's advisory card
  - Information on FASDs, including links to resources for finding treatment for problem drinking
- *Food Safety Booklet for Pregnant Women, Their Unborn Babies, and Children Under Five (2022):* www.fda.gov/media/83740/download
  - A printable PDF booklet providing detailed, consumer-friendly information on food safety during pregnancy
- *Rural Health Information Hub:* www.ruralhealthinfo.org
  - Comprehensive information and practical resources for addressing rural health issues, including health during pregnancy
- *March of Dimes Maternity Care Desert Dashboard:* www2.deloitte.com/us/en/pages/life-sciences-and-health-care/articles/march-of-dimes-maternity-care-deserts-dashboard.html
  - Interactive tool to evaluate availability of obstetric care and hospitals/birth centers, by county, in the United States

- *WHO Antenatal Care Guidelines 2016:* www.who.int/publications/i/item/9789241549912
  - Official WHO recommendations for antenatal care to support a positive pregnancy experience
- *SNAP-Ed and the EFNEP:* https://snaped.fns.usda.gov and www.nifa.usda.gov/grants/programs/capacity-grants/efnep/expanded-food-nutrition-education-program, respectively
  - SNAP-Ed: Effective hands-on nutrition education programs for participants in SNAP
  - EFNEP: Effective hands-on nutrition education programs provided for low-income populations by federal extension as a community outreach program

REFERENCES

1. Florida Department of Health. The life course theory. Florida Health: Maternal and Child Health Section. Updated June 8, 2022. https://www.floridahealth.gov/programs-and-services/womens-health/florida-life-course-indicator-report/life-course-theory-1.html
2. Wickramasinghe K, Mathers JC, Wopereis S, Marsman DS, Griffiths JC. From lifespan to healthspan: the role of nutrition in healthy ageing. *J Nutr Sci.* 2020;9:e33. https://doi.org/10.1017/jns.2020.26
3. Cho GJ, Kim J, Kim JY, et al. Adverse pregnancy outcomes and maternal chronic diseases in the future: a cross-sectional study using KoGES-HEXA data. *J Clin Med.* 2022;11(5):1457. https://doi.org/10.3390/jcm11051457
4. Likhar A, Patil MS. Importance of maternal nutrition in the first 1,000 days of life and its effects on child development: a narrative review. *Cureus.* 2022;14(10):e30083. https://doi.org/10.7759/cureus.30083
5. National Academies of Sciences Engineering and Medicine. *Birth Settings in America: Outcomes, Quality, Access, and Choice.* National Academies Press; 2020.
6. The American College of Obstetricians and Gynecologists. ACOG committee opinion no. 579: definition of term pregnancy. *Obstet Gynecol.* 2013;122(5):1139–1140. https://doi.org/10.1097/01.AOG.0000437385.88715.4a
7. Eunice Kennedy Shriver National Institute of Child Health and Human Development. About pregnancy. Updated January 31, 2017. https://www.nichd.nih.gov/health/topics/pregnancy/conditioninfo
8. Cleveland Clinic. Fetal development. Updated March 3, 2023. https://my.clevelandclinic.org/health/articles/7247-fetal-development-stages-of-growth
9. Virginia Department of Health. Fetal development. 2019. https://www.vdh.virginia.gov/content/uploads/sites/65/2019/03/Fetal-Development-chart12-18-18-1.pdf
10. Hardy K, Hardy PJ. 1(st) trimester miscarriage: four decades of study. *Transl Pediatr.* 2015;4(2): 189–200. https://doi.org/10.3978/j.issn.2224-4336.2015.03.05
11. Mayo Clinic. Miscarriage. October 16, 2021. https://www.mayoclinic.org/diseases-conditions/pregnancy-loss-miscarriage/symptoms-causes/syc-20354298
12. Eunice Kennedy Shriver National Institute of Child Health and Human Development. Know your terms: full term pregnancy. Updated June 2, 2022. https://www.nichd.nih.gov/ncmhep/initiatives/know-your-terms/moms
13. Mayo Clinic. 3rd trimester pregnancy: what to expect. March 9, 2022. https://www.mayoclinic.org/healthy-lifestyle/pregnancy-week-by-week/in-depth/pregnancy/art-20046767
14. Cleveland Clinic. Relaxin. October 17, 2022. https://my.clevelandclinic.org/health/body/24305-relaxin

15. Medline Plus. Pregnancy and nutrition. National Library of Medicine. Updated January 12, 2021. https://medlineplus.gov/pregnancyandnutrition.html
16. Đaković I, Soljačić-Vraneš H, Kuna K. Weight gain in pregnancy and weight retention after birth. *Open Access Maced J Med Sci.* 2019;7(4):614–616. https://doi.org/10.3889/oamjms.2019.141
17. Office of Disease Prevention and Health Promotion. Healthy People 2030: pregnancy and childbirth. U.S. Department of Health and Human Services. https://health.gov/healthypeople/objectives-and-data/browse-objectives/pregnancy-and-childbirth
18. Gillespie B. Nutritional status and the risk of preterm birth. In: Anumba DOC, Jayasooriya SM, eds. *Evidence Based Global Health Manual for Preterm Birth Risk Assessment.* Springer; 2022:41–51.
19. Best KP, Gomersall J, Makrides M. Prenatal nutritional strategies to reduce the risk of preterm birth. *Ann Nutr Metab.* 2020;76(suppl 3):31–39. https://doi.org/10.1159/000509901
20. Paknahad Z, Fallah A, Moravejolahkami AR. Maternal dietary patterns and their association with pregnancy outcomes. *Clin Nutr Res.* 2019;8(1):64–73. https://doi.org/10.7762/cnr.2019.8.1.64
21. Lassi ZS, Padhani ZA, Rabbani A, et al. Impact of dietary interventions during pregnancy on maternal, neonatal, and child outcomes in low- and middle-income countries. *Nutrients.* 2020;12(2):531. https://doi.org/10.3390/nu12020531.
22. Siega-Riz AM, Bodnar LM, Stotland NE, Stang J. The current understanding of gestational weight gain among women with obesity and the need for future research. *NAM Perspect.* 2020;2020:10.31478/202001a. https://doi.org/10.31478/202001a
23. Centers for Disease Control and Prevention. Planning for pregnancy. Updated February 15, 2023. https://www.cdc.gov/preconception/planning.html
24. Ami N, Bernstein M, Boucher F, Rieder M, Parker L. Folate and neural tube defects: the role of supplements and food fortification. *Paediatr Child Health.* 2016;21(3):145–154. https://doi.org/10.1093/pch/21.3.145
25. Office on Women's Health. Weight, fertility, and pregnancy. U.S. Department of Health and Human Services. Updated February 17, 2021. https://www.womenshealth.gov/healthy-weight/weight-fertility-and-pregnancy
26. U.S. Department of Agriculture, U.S. Department of Health and Human Services. *Dietary Guidelines for Americans, 2020–2025.* 9th ed. U.S. Department of Health and Human Services; 2020. https://www.dietaryguidelines.gov
27. Office of Disease Prevention and Health Promotion. Dietary reference intakes. U.S. Department of Health and Human Services. Updated January 18, 2023. https://health.gov/our-work/nutrition-physical-activity/dietary-guidelines/dietary-reference-intakes
28. Office of Disease Prevention and Health Promotion. Dietary reference intakes development. U.S. Department of Health and Human Services. Updated January 18, 2023. https://health.gov/our-work/nutrition-physical-activity/dietary-guidelines/dietary-reference-intakes/dietary-reference-intakes-development
29. U.S. Department of Agriculture. MyPlate. Accessed April 27, 2023. https://www.myplate.gov
30. U.S. Department of Agriculture Food and Nutrition Service. Center for Nutrition Policy and Promotion (CNPP). https://www.fns.usda.gov/cnpp
31. World Health Organization. *WHO Recommendations on Antenatal Care for a Positive Pregnancy Experience*. World Health Organization; 2016.
32. Osuchukwu OO, Reed DJ. Small for gestational age. In: *StatPearls*. StatPearls Publishing; 2022. https://www.ncbi.nlm.nih.gov/books/NBK563247
33. Centers for Disease Control and Prevention. Weight gain during pregnancy. Updated June 13, 2022. https://www.cdc.gov/reproductivehealth/maternalinfanthealth/pregnancy-weight-gain.htm
34. World Health Organization. Preterm birth; key facts. May 10, 2023. https://www.who.int/news-room/fact-sheets/detail/preterm-birth
35. Akanmode AM, Mahdy H. Macrosomia. In: *StatPearls*. StatPearls Publishing; 2023. https://www.ncbi.nlm.nih.gov/books/NBK557577
36. Cleveland Clinic. Fetal macrosomia. Updated May 13, 2022. https://my.clevelandclinic.org/health/diseases/17795-fetal-macrosomia
37. Davis DD, Roshan A, Canela CD, Varacallo M. Shoulder dystocia. In: *StatPearls.* StatPearls Publishing; 2022. https://www.ncbi.nlm.nih.gov/books/NBK470427
38. Institute of Medicine, National Research Council of the National Academies. Healthy weight gain during pregnancy. https://webassets.nationalacademies.org/whattogain

39. Kominiarek MA, Rajan P. Nutrition recommendations in pregnancy and lactation. *Med Clin North Am.* 2016;100(6):1199–1215. https://doi.org/10.1016/j.mcna.2016.06.004
40. U.S. Preventive Services Task Force. Final recommendation statement: healthy weight and weight gain in pregnancy: behavioral counseling interventions. May 25, 2021. https://www.uspreventiveservicestaskforce.org/uspstf/recommendation/healthy-weight-and-weight-gain-during-pregnancy-behavioral-counseling-interventions
41. Mayo Clinic Staff. Pregnancy Weight gain: what's healthy? February 9, 2022. https://www.mayoclinic.org/healthy-lifestyle/pregnancy-week-by-week/in-depth/pregnancy-weight-gain/art-20044360
42. Dugdale DC. Losing weight after pregnancy. Medline Plus. Updated October 17, 2021. https://medlineplus.gov/ency/patientinstructions/000586.htm
43. Murphy MM, Higgins KA, Bi X, Barraj LM. Adequacy and sources of protein intake among pregnant women in the United States, NHANES 2003–2012. *Nutrients.* 2021;13(3):795. https://doi.org/10.3390/nu13030795
44. U.S. Department of Agriculture. Grains: what foods are in the grains group? MyPlate. https://www.myplate.gov/eat-healthy/grains
45. Cioffi CE, Figueroa J, Welsh JA. Added sugar intake among pregnant women in the United States: national health and nutrition examination survey 2003–2012. *J Acad Nutr Diet.* 2018;118(5):886–895.e1. https://doi.org/10.1016/j.jand.2017.10.021
46. Goran MI, Plows JF, Ventura EE. Effects of consuming sugars and alternative sweeteners during pregnancy on maternal and child health: evidence for a secondhand sugar effect. *Proc Nutr Soc.* 2019;78(3):262–271. https://doi.org/10.1017/S002966511800263X.
47. Cleveland Clinic. Pregnancy: prenatal vitamins. January 1, 2018. https://my.clevelandclinic.org/health/drugs/9754-pregnancy-prenatal-vitamins
48. Anderson JW, Baird P, Davis RH Jr, et al. Health benefits of dietary fiber. *Nutr Rev.* 2009;67(4):188–205. https://doi.org/10.1111/j.1753-4887.2009.00189.x
49. Zerfu TA, Mekuria A. Pregnant women have inadequate fiber intake while consuming fiber-rich diets in low-income rural setting: evidences from analysis of common "ready-to-eat" stable foods. *Food Sci Nutr.* 2019;7(10):3286–3292. https://doi.org/10.1002/fsn3.1188
50. Centers for Disease Control and Prevention. Fetal alcohol spectrum disorders: alcohol use in pregnancy. Updated November 4, 2022. https://www.cdc.gov/ncbddd/fasd/alcohol-use.html
51. Organization of Teratology Information Specialists. Caffeine. MotherToBaby. September 1, 2022. https://mothertobaby.org/fact-sheets/caffeine-pregnancy
52. Kole J, Barnhill A. Caffeine content labeling: a missed opportunity for promoting personal and public health. *J Caffeine Res.* 2013;3(3):108–113. https://doi.org/10.1089/jcr.2013.0017
53. American College of Obstetricians and Gynecologists. ACOG committee opinion no. 462: moderate caffeine consumption during pregnancy. Obstet Gynecol. 2010;116(2 pt 1):467–468. https://doi.org/10.1097/AOG.0b013e3181eeb2a1
54. U.S. Food and Drug Administration. Advice about eating fish for those who might become or are pregnant or breastfeeding and children ages 1–11 years. Updated September 28, 2022.https://www.fda.gov/food/consumers/advice-about-eating-fish
55. U.S. Food and Drug Administration. Questions & answers from the FDA/EPA: advice about eating fish for those who might become or are pregnant or breastfeeding and children ages 1 to 11 years. Updated February 17, 2022. https://www.fda.gov/food/consumers/questions-answers-fdaepa-advice-about-eating-fish-those-who-might-become-or-are-pregnant-or#V
56. U.S. Environmental Protection Agency. How people are exposed to mercury. U.S. Department of the Interior. Updated March 28, 2023. https://www.epa.gov/mercury/how-people-are-exposed-mercury
57. Foodsafety.gov. People at risk: pregnant women. U.S. Department of Health and Human Services. Updated September 25, 2020. https://www.foodsafety.gov/people-at-risk/pregnant-women
58. U.S. Environmental Protection Agency. National listing of fish advisories: state, territory and tribe fish advisory contacts. U.S. Department of the Interior. March 21, 2018. https://fishadvisoryonline.epa.gov/Contacts.aspx
59. Centers for Disease Control and Prevention. Questions and answers: what are *Listeria*? U.S. Department of Health and Human Services. Updated August 23, 2023. https://www.cdc.gov/listeria/faq.html
60. Organization of Teratology Information Specialists. *Mother to Baby Fact Sheets: Salmonella.* National Library of Medicine; 2020. https://www.ncbi.nlm.nih.gov/books/NBK582942

61. Centers for Disease Control and Prevention. Toxoplasmosis: epidemiology and risk factors. Updated September 4, 2018. https://www.cdc.gov/parasites/toxoplasmosis/epi.html
62. U.S. Food and Drug Administration. *Toxoplasma*—food safety for moms to be. September 27, 2018. https://www.fda.gov/food/people-risk-foodborne-illness/toxoplasma-food-safety-moms-be
63. Khedagi AM, Bello NA. Hypertensive disorders of pregnancy. *Cardiol Clin.* 2021;39(1):77–90. https://doi.org/10.1016/j.ccl.2020.09.005
64. Medline Plus. Hyperemesis gravidarum. National Library of Medicine. Medline. Updated January 1, 2023. https://medlineplus.gov/ency/article/001499.htm
65. Centers for Disease Control and Prevention. Social determinants of health at CDC. Updated December 8, 2022. https://www.cdc.gov/about/sdoh/index.html
66. World Health Organization. Social determinants of health. 2023. https://www.who.int/health-topics/social-determinants-of-health#tab=tab_1
67. Solar O, Irwin A. *A Conceptual Framework for Action on the Social Determinants of Health*. World Health Organization; 2010.
68. Braveman P, Gottlieb L. The social determinants of health: it's time to consider the causes of the causes. *Public Health Rep.* 2014;129(suppl 2):19–31. https://doi.org/10.1177/00333549141291S206
69. Mathews TJ, MacDorman MF. Infant statistics from the 2009 period linked birth/infant death dataset. *Natl Vital Stat Rep.* 2013;61(8):1–28.
70. Green T, Hamilton T. Maternal educational attainment and infant mortality in the United States: does the gradient vary by race/ethnicity and nativity? *Demogr Res.* 2019;41(25):713–752. https://doi.org/10.4054/DemRes.2019.41.25
71. Suzuki E, Kouame C, Mills S. Progress in reducing maternal mortality has stagnated and we are not on track to achieve the SDG target: new UN report. World Bank Blogs; February 22, 2023. https://blogs.worldbank.org/opendata/progress-reducing-maternal-mortality-has-stagnated-and-we-are-not-track-achieve-sdg-target
72. Dagher RK, Linares DE. A critical review on the complex interplay between social determinants of health and maternal and infant mortality. *Children.* 2022;9(3):394. https://doi.org/10.3390/children9030394
73. Kamal R, Hudman J, McDermott D. What Do We Know about Infant Mortality in the U.S. and Comparable Countries? Peterson-KFF Health System Tracker. October 18, 2019. https://www.healthsystemtracker.org/chart-collection/infant-mortality-u-s-compare-countries
74. Ely DM, Driscoll AK. Infant mortality in the United States, 2020: data from the period linked birth/infant death file. *Natl Vital Stat Rep.* 2022;71(5):1–18. https://www.cdc.gov/nchs/data/nvsr/nvsr71/nvsr71-05
75. Centers for Disease Control and Prevention. Alzheimer's disease and healthy aging: health disparities. Updated January 31, 2017. https://www.cdc.gov/aging/disparities/index.htm
76. Hill L, Artiga S, Ranji U. Policy issue brief: racial disparities in maternal and infant health: current status and efforts to address them. KFF. Published November 1, 2022. https://www.kff.org/racial-equity-and-health-policy/issue-brief/racial-disparities-in-maternal-and-infant-health-current-status-and-efforts-to-address-them
77. Fishman S. An extended evaluation of the weathering hypothesis for birthweight. *Demogr Res.* 2020;43(31):929–968. https://doi.org/10.4054/DemRes.2020.43.31
78. Cohen PN. Maternal age and infant mortality for white, black, and Mexican mothers in the United States. *Sociol Sci.* 2016;3(2):32–38. https://doi.org/10.15195/v3.a2
79. de Beaumont Foundation, Trust for America's Health. Social determinants and social needs: moving beyond midstream. de Beaumont Foundation; 2019. https://debeaumont.org/wp-content/uploads/2019/04/social-determinants-and-social-needs.pdf
80. Rural Health Information Hub. Barriers to improving rural maternal health. Health Resources and Services Administration. May 17, 2021. https://www.ruralhealthinfo.org/toolkits/maternal-health/1/barriers
81. World Health Organization. Maternal mortality. February 22, 2023. https://www.who.int/news-room/fact-sheets/detail/maternal-mortality
82. UNICEF. Maternal nutrition: preventing malnutrition in pregnant and breastfeeding women. https://www.unicef.org/nutrition/maternal
83. Food and Nutrition Service. WIC frequently asked questions. U.S. Department of Agriculture. Updated April 4, 2023. https://www.fns.usda.gov/wic/frequently-asked-questions
84. U.S. Department of Agriculture. MyPlate: pregnancy and lactation. Accessed April 27, 2023. https://www.myplate.gov/life-stages/pregnancy-and-breastfeeding

4

INFANT NUTRITION

Melissa D. Gutschall

LEARNING OBJECTIVES

At the end of this chapter, students will be able to:

1. Describe the growth and developmental patterns of infants during the first year of life and how they relate to nutritional needs and feeding skills.
2. Identify key principles in promoting optimal nutrition intake for infants.
3. Compare and contrast breastfeeding versus bottle feeding methods, nutrition, trends, and challenges.
4. Describe the benefits of breastfeeding and why it is a major public health nutrition focus area.
5. Detail the recommendations for introducing complementary foods from 6 to 12 months.
6. Name key nutrients and feeding practices of public health concern for infants.
7. Identify needs for nutrition intervention and referral for common nutrition and feeding concerns among infants.
8. Explain how social determinants of health affect the feeding practices and health outcomes for infants.
9. Describe global efforts to improve breastfeeding rates as a method for improving infant mortality rates.
10. Recognize national public health nutrition programs available to assist families with infants in meeting nutrition recommendations.

INTRODUCTION

This chapter describes the nutritional needs for **infants**. The infant stage refers to the period of time from birth to 1 year of age, which includes a dynamic transition from total dependence on breast milk or formula to a diet inclusive of all solid foods (some in modified forms). The chapter also explores the **social determinants of health (SDOH)**, public health nutrition issues, population issues, and global challenges related to infant nutrition, as well as an example of an effective program to support optimal nutrition for early life. Overall, this stage demands a balance among meeting nutritional needs for rapid growth while promoting independence in feeding. The overarching nutritional goals during infancy include nutritional adequacy, growth, and the development of competence with self-feeding.

NORMAL NUTRITION SUMMARY

Nutritional adequacy is crucial to optimal growth and development during the infancy stage when body systems are continuing to develop following the birth of the child. *Healthy People 2030* goals related specifically to infants are aimed at increasing the number of infants who are breastfed at 6 months and 1 year of age.[1] The **Dietary Guidelines** have provided evidence-based recommendations on eating to promote health and prevent disease since 1980 and are strategically oriented toward public health nutrition as opposed to clinical care.[2] These guidelines are updated every 5 years, and the current version is the first set of guidelines to address infants as a distinct life stage. Specifically, and in line with the *Healthy People 2030* goals, the Dietary Guidelines recommend exclusive breastfeeding through 6 months of age and continued breastfeeding along with the introduction of solid foods until 1 year of age. When breastfeeding is contraindicated, iron-fortified infant formula is an appropriate substitution. Throughout this chapter, the term *infant formula* is used interchangeably with human milk substitute.

The Dietary Guidelines for infants introduce us to potentially problematic nutrients such as iron and vitamin D, recommending iron-fortified formula and foods during the first year of life as well as a vitamin D supplement for all infants being exclusively breastfed. Ultimately, the goal at 1 year is to promote a diet with variety, adequacy, and nutrient density, limiting added sugars and sodium. The **Dietary Reference Intakes (DRIs)** offer a set of more specific values that can be used to assess and plan nutrient intakes for healthy people and vary by sex and age,[3] and are classified by infants 0 to 6 months of age and 6 to 12 months of age. The DRIs are provided in **Appendix C**, and specific nutrients of concern for this age group are considered later in this chapter.

NUTRITIONAL GOALS FOR INFANTS

The overarching nutritional goals for childhood include (1) optimal growth and development, (2) nutritional adequacy, and (3) progression of feeding skills. At birth, infants are completely dependent on breast milk or **human milk substitutes** (infant formula) for all nutritional needs. Nutritional needs are primarily indicated by adequate calories and protein to achieve optimal growth. By 1 year of age human milk or formula is no longer the major source of calories and protein, and the child should now be consuming a variety of nutrient-dense **complementary foods** in manageable forms. Parents and caregivers act as the primary source of providing feeding and establishing the feeding environment.

Growth and Development

Infant birth weight is one of the best indicators of infant health. Full-term infants are born at 37 to 42 weeks of gestation with an ideal birth weight between 5.5 and 8.5 lb. Aside from the gestation period, infancy, particularly 0 to 6 months, is the most rapid period of growth among all the life stages.[4] Infant growth patterns generally show a doubling of birth weight by 4 to 6 months of age and tripling of birth weight by 1 year.[5] Birth length should double at the end of the first year, and head circumference, an indicator of brain growth, should also double by that time.[5] With this rapid growth comes a time for the greatest nutritional need relative to body size.

Growth is one of the best indicators of infant nutritional status. Regular monitoring of a child's growth is important to establish the individual growth pattern and identify any deviations from it. The three most regularly assessed infant growth measures are weight, length, and head circumference. Methods for assessing growth of infants include a calibrated infant scale, recumbent length board, and a nonstretch head circumference tape. Standardized methods, including trained staff with practice for consistency, are also important for growth assessment in infants.

The Centers for Disease Control and Prevention (CDC) Growth Charts are the recommended tool for monitoring a child's growth.[6] This resource provides sex-specific charts for infants from birth to 24 months to plot weight-for-age, length-for-age, and head circumference. Measuring and charting growth are subject to many potential sources of error (from measurement technique to incorrect plotting) that can be misinterpreted in the evaluation of growth. When measuring and interpreting growth in infants, the following situations warrant further evaluation: (1) a plateau in weight at several consecutive assessments, (2) a pattern of weight gain followed by weight loss, (3) not regaining weight lost during illness, and (4) a pattern of unexplained and unintentional weight gain.[7] Signs that an infant may not be eating enough include a weight loss of >7% birth weight, sleepiness or unresponsiveness, dry mucous membranes around the nose and mouth, and few wet diapers. Continued weight loss or plateau that is not resolved with increasing intake or breastfeeding competency should be evaluated by a medical professional for the risk of failure to thrive.

In addition to growth, nutrition is paramount to brain development, and thus cognitive, motor, and socioemotional skills development. This is evident by the fact that the very young infant feeds based on reflexes such as **rooting**, **suckling**, and the coordination of sucking, swallowing, and breathing.[8,9] In the older infant, the feeding environment interacts with the development of food preferences and language skills. Thus, the psychosocial stimulation offered by mealtimes plays a role in cognitive development. Organs and organ systems continue to develop following the birth of the infant. For example, while the gastrointestinal (GI) tract is functional at birth and sufficient to digest fats, protein, and simple sugars, GI muscle coordination and digestive enzyme levels continue to improve through 6 months of age.[10]

An infant's developmental skills parallel the progression in feeding skills as well as nutritional needs. For example, when the infant achieves head and trunk control, they can sit for feeding. With more crawling or walking, they are expending more energy. **Critical periods of childhood development** refer to particular time periods when a skill emerges and must be in place for subsequent learning to take place.[9] Critical periods in the development of oral feeding skills, a time that is typically a source of pleasure and exploring, may explain later feeding problems.[11] For example, a **premature** infant receiving respiratory support may associate oral sensations with discomfort and become a reluctant feeder.

Nutritional Adequacy

As stated previously, nutritional needs during the first 6 months are met entirely by breast milk or formula. The American Academy of Pediatrics (AAP) recommends breastfeeding for at least 12 months while the World Health Organization (WHO) recommends a continuation of breastfeeding for up to 2 years.[12] Ultimately, the decision to breastfeed and the duration of breastfeeding are up to the mother within the family dynamic. The Academy of Nutrition and Dietetics posits that exclusive breastfeeding provides optimal nutrition and health protection for the first 6 months of life and that breastfeeding with complementary foods from 6 months until at least 12 months of age is the ideal feeding pattern for infants.[13] The Academy of Nutrition and Dietetics (AND) further recognizes that breastfeeding as a public health strategy is implicated in reducing infant and child mortality, maternal morbidity, and overall healthcare costs. The role of the public health nutrition professional is to support the family's decision while providing evidence-based information about both sources of feeding, accurate feeding recommendations, and strategies to overcome any barriers to successful breastfeeding.

The benefits of breastfeeding are numerous and include those for the infant, mother, family, environment and society. For the infant, breastfeeding provides an easy-to-digest form of food that is nutritionally customized for their needs. It also provides superior immune protection and reduces the incidence of childhood illness[13] as well as chronic disease. Breast milk offers nutrients that are more **bioavailable** for the infant, for example, many minerals are attached to protein to promote absorption. For the mother, breastfeeding promotes bonding with the infant, protection from chronic disease, and potential benefits for weight management.[13] For the family, breastfeeding can save money, contributing to overall improvements in economic status, and for the environment, breastfeeding eliminates the need for manufacturing, packaging, and waste.

The role of the public health nutrition professional is to educate expectant mothers and families about these benefits, but understand that the decision is ultimately that of the family. The public health nutrition professional can also provide resources and referrals to support a mother who is initiating breastfeeding or having trouble breastfeeding. If a mother has chosen not to breastfeed or breastfeeding is not possible, human milk substitutes can offer a nutritionally complete and safe alternative. While breast milk and all its components can never be completely manufactured, some key differences between breast milk and human milk substitutes include the proportion of macronutrients, presence of immune protection factors and essential fatty acids, and the ideal ratio of nutrients to fluid for ideal hydration. Cow's milk should not be used in infancy due to the risk of GI bleeding, development of allergies, and lack of iron content.[14,15] The macronutrient and key micronutrient needs of infants are discussed next.

Energy and Macronutrient Needs

The DRIs provide specific recommendations for energy and nutrients for infants from 0 to 6 months and 7 to 12 months.[16] The AAP and the AND provide guidelines related to infant health, nutrition, and feeding. Energy needs for infants are higher relative to body weight than at any other life stage, ranging from 80 to 120 kcal/kg of body weight.[16] The large range in caloric needs varies with weight, growth rate, sleep/wake cycle, temperature/climate, physical activity, metabolic response to food, and health status of the infant. From 6 to 12 months of age, energy needs decrease to 98 kcal/kg. The DRI for protein intake for infants from birth to 6 months of age is 1.52 g/kg body weight and from 7 to 12 months is 1.2 g/kg body weight. Breast milk or formula provides an adequate amount of protein for the infant prior to the introduction of complementary foods. It is important that carbohydrate and fat content in the diet are sufficient to provide energy, sparing protein for the major purpose of growth. Fat is a critical source of essential fatty acids for infants, supplying a concentrated source of energy as well as supporting neurologic and brain development.[17] Infants, especially if premature, have limited stores of body fat such that fat should never be restricted during infancy.[18] The recommendation for fat in infants 0 to 6 months is 31 g, and 30 g for infants 7 to 12 months, also obtainable from an adequate amount of breast milk or infant formula in which fat makes up 40% to 50% of the calories.[16,19,20] In particular, the essential fatty acids include linoleic acid (LA), alpha-linolenic acid (ALA), and the polyunsaturated fats that are derived from them, docohexanoic acid (DHA) and arachidonic acid (ARA), are present in breast milk and included in infant formulas.

The first milk, **colostrum**, is particularly higher in protein than mature milk and contains several immune factors and nutrients.[21] While infants only take 1.5 to 2 tsp of colostrum during the first feedings, this thick yellow fluid is highly beneficial. Mature breast milk provides about 22 kcal/oz while infant formulas provide about 20 kcal/oz. Overall, infants take less volume of breast milk due to the self-regulation, composition, and nutrient density. Preterm infant formulas can contain 22 to 24 kcal/oz.

With the exception of premature infants, most nutrient needs are met through breast milk or human milk substitutes. There are a few cases, however, when micronutrient supplementation for infants is recommended, and supplementation is more fully described later in the chapter. There are also several specialty formulas on the market targeting the specific needs of premature infants and infants with food allergies or intolerances. The role of the public health nutrition practitioner is to assess the risk of nutrient deficiency or special feeding needs and refer families to a registered dietitian/nutritionist to guide them to the appropriate supplemental recommendations, particularly in the case of prematurity and special conditions.

Iron

Iron is the number one micronutrient deficiency worldwide, affecting about 2 billion people, mostly pregnant women and children.[22] **Iron deficiency** more likely shows up in toddlers and young children who are no longer receiving a major source of iron from breast milk or iron-fortified formulas and foods, but is critical for the rapid rate of growth occurring during infancy. Because iron plays a role in carrying oxygen in the blood, it is necessary for the expansion of blood cells that accompanies growth. Iron deficiency in infancy is also associated with neurodevelopment and behavior, manifesting as learning delays and poor cognitive, motor, and socioemotional development.[23,24] This provides further rationale for not introducing cow's milk, a source lacking in iron, during the first year of life. Additional risk factors for iron deficiency in infants include **low birth weight**, low socioeconomic status, and low intake of iron-rich complementary foods.[23] When infants transition to less breast milk and formula intake and more complementary foods from 6 to 12 months, iron-rich infant foods should include iron-fortified cereal/grains, meat, fish, poultry, eggs, beans, nut butters, and green leafy vegetables. The public health nutrition professional plays a key role in identifying these risk factors for iron deficiency in infants. Further information on iron deficiency screening and dietary measures to promote adequate iron intake are provided in the subsequent chapters on toddlers and young children. Referral to a healthcare provider or registered dietitian is appropriate in the case of suspected iron deficiency and recommendations for supplementation during infancy.

Vitamin D

Vitamin D intake is critical for optimal bone development and many other critical functions in the body. While breast milk is the optimal source of infant nutrition, it is not adequate in vitamin D. Infants should also spend limited time in direct sunlight or wear sunscreen, so they are unable to synthesize enough vitamin D in the body. The AAP recommends 400 IU of supplemental vitamin D each day for infants who are breastfed or even partially breastfed, as well as infants taking less than 1 L of infant formula per day.[25,26] Vitamin D supplements are available in liquid form administered by a dropper for infants. Most infant formulas include vitamin D in the recommended amount. Additional questions or concerns regarding vitamin D supplementation should be referred to a registered dietitian/nutritionist.

Vitamin K

Vitamin K plays a critical role in blood clotting, and newborn levels of the vitamin are low, which could lead to dangerous bleeding, referred to as **vitamin K deficiency bleeding (VKDB).**[27] Low levels of vitamin K are related to limited stores at birth and limited amounts in breast milk. Vitamin K is also synthesized by gut bacteria, and the intestinal flora is not composed of its full diversity until 6 months of age. VKDB affects up to 1 in 250 newborns and can occur up to 6 months after birth, involving bleeding from the umbilical cord, or bleeding in the brain. For these reasons, the AAP has recommended supplementing newborns with vitamin K since 1961.[27] This supplementation is received by injection within 6 hours of birth. While there has been some historical controversy over vitamin K injections, several studies have supported their safety and the value of the benefits over any minimal risks.[27]

Fluids

Breast milk or formula provides ample amounts of fluid for the infant from 0 to 6 months of age. The DRIs for water are 700 mL/day for 0- to 6-month-old infants and 800 mL for 7- to 12-month-old infants.[28] A safe source of water can be introduced in very small amounts once the infant reaches 6 months of age.[29] Water should only be provided in amounts of 2 to 3 oz to start so as not to cause satiety and replace nutrient-rich breast milk or formula. Too much water can also disrupt the sodium balance in bodily fluids, leading to severe consequences of seizure and even death. Juice is not needed to meet the fluid needs of infants, and it is more important during this time to help them develop a preference for milk and water. Sugar-containing beverages may fill the infant and limit their desire for nutrient-dense foods and liquids, as well as promote dental caries.[28] If juice is offered, it should not be introduced until at least 6 months of age, and from a cup. Rehydration products may be used temporarily following illness but, like juice, will result in energy or nutrient deficits if used longer term.

INFANT FEEDING

Hunger and Satiety Cues: The Role of Parents

Infant reflexes enable breastfeeding or bottle feeding soon after birth. A young infant may signal hunger by waking, crying, or sucking on their fist, and satiety by sealing their lips, turning their head away, or falling asleep while feeding. As development advances throughout the first year, an infant may point or reach for food to signal hunger and push food away and shake their head or even say "no" when they are full.[30] Parents are learning these cues and the appropriate responses to them while also gaining a sense of the child's temperament toward feeding. Parents may misinterpret discomfort as a sign of hunger as the infant is learning to self-calm and adapt to its environment. Parents can support a healthy feeding environment for infants by responding early and appropriately to these cues, recognizing the infant's abilities with feeding skills, balancing the infant's need for assistance while encouraging age-appropriate feeding skills, and allowing the infant to initiate and guide feeding interactions.[12] **Responsive feeding** recognizes and responds to the child's hunger and fullness cues in effort to help them learn to self-regulate their intake. The public health nutrition professional can help educate and support parents as they navigate these early steps in the feeding relationship.

Feeding Patterns

While feeding should be based on infant cuing, a breastfed newborn infant will typically eat every 1.5 to 2 hours due to the small stomach volume and rate of stomach emptying, totaling 10 to 12 feedings per day. A formula-fed infant may feed less frequently due to more complex digestion needed for formula. Various feeding patterns can evolve to meet these needs as the infant grows in the first few months of life, for example, providing more volume during the day to extend sleep time overnight.[31] A newborn infant may start by taking just 1 or 2 oz per feeding and progress over the first year to taking a total volume of 28 to 32 oz with less overall feeding occasions and a greater volume (6–8 oz) at each.[32] The total volume of formula/breast milk will decrease once complementary foods are offered from 6 months to 1 year of age. Parents should encourage their child to drink from an open cup as they approach 1 year of age, and completely wean from the bottle between 12 and 18 months.[33] Healthy infants are developmentally ready to begin drinking from a cup at 6 to 8 months, but are not yet skilled enough to meet all fluid needs.[11]

Parents may use a variety of feeding methods during the first year for various reasons and situations. If a mother chooses to stop breastfeeding prior to 1 year of age, the infant should be transitioned to iron-fortified infant formula for the remainder of the year.[34] When the child is *weaned* from breast milk or formula at 1 year, they should be provided with whole milk. Further discussion on the use of whole milk for toddlers is provided in Chapter 5.

Development of Feeding Skills and Relationships With Food

Introduction of Complementary Foods

Key developmental and feeding milestones parallel the growing and expanding nutritional needs of children to facilitate optimal growth and development (Table 4.1). Infants will transition from a diet of primarily breast milk or formula to a diet of all modified solid foods by 1 year of age. From birth to 6 months, infants can effectively suck and swallow, but have poor lip closure and head and neck control and push most solid foods out of the mouth, indicative of the liquid-based diet necessary during this time frame. At 4 to 6 months, infants begin to gain the ability to control the head and neck, sit with support, and move food from the front to the back of the mouth for swallowing. These are all signs that the infant is ready to begin eating complementary foods, meaning solid foods and fluids other than breast milk or formula. These first foods are pureed or strained, such as infant cereals and pureed fruits and vegetables. Commercial baby foods are labeled as stages 1 (from about 6 months), 2 (from about 8 months), and 3 (from about 10 months). With the increase in stages come increasing textures, food variety, and food mixtures as well as an increased packaging size. It is important to remember that these are not necessarily the serving sizes the infant needs, and parents should base feeding duration on satiety cues rather than finishing the predetermined serving. Complementary foods serve to provide the additional energy and nutrient needs no longer met by breast milk or formula.[35] Beginning to eat complementary foods offers the experience of new tastes and textures but also the oral stimulation of feeding from a spoon. The following list summarizes considerations for introducing solid foods to an infant:

Table 4.1. Infant Feeding Guidelines by Age and Developmental Skills

Age	Developmental Skills	Hunger Cues	Satiety Cues	Example Intake
Birth to 3 months	• Tongue thrust, rooting, gag reflex • Coordinates suck-swallow-breathe • Brings hands to mouth • Needs head support	• Opens and closes mouth • Brings hands to mouth • Uses rooting motions to search for feeding • Makes sucking noises and sucks on fingers, hands, or objects	• Slows or decreases sucking • Relaxes arms, legs, fingers • Pushes away or turns head away from nipple • Falls asleep	Breastfeeding 10–12 times per day OR 2–3 oz formula every 3–4 hours
4–7 months	• Transfers food from front to back of mouth with tongue • Uses up and down munching movement • Has head and neck control • Sits with support • Begins to grasp foods and bring to mouth • Takes spoonfuls of pureed foods; begins to eat mashed foods • Begins to drink small amounts from a cup held by feeder	• Smiles or coos during feeding to indicate wanting more • Moves head toward spoon or tries to swipe food toward mouth	• Releases nipple • Seals lips together • Shows distraction/ greater interest in surroundings • Turns head away from food	• Breastfeeding on demand OR 24–32 oz formula total Beginning at 6 months: • 1–2 oz iron-fortified infant cereals, breads • 2–4 oz each of cooked, plain, strained or pureed vegetables and fruits • 1–2 oz plain/ strained/ pureed meat, fish, poultry, eggs, cheese, yogurt, or legumes

(continued)

Table 4.1. Infant Feeding Guidelines by Age and Developmental Skills

Age	Developmental Skills	Hunger Cues	Satiety Cues	Example Intake
8–12 months	• Uses the jaw and tongue to mash foods • Uses rotary chewing motion • Sits unaided • Holds cup with two hands • Develops eye-hand-mouth coordination • Begins to eat soft, chopped table foods and desires to self-feed • Capable of eating a variety of textures	• Reaches for food or spoon • Points to food • Gets excited when food is presented • Expresses desire for food with words or sounds	• Slows pace of eating • Clenches mouth closed • Pushes food away • Verbally expresses "no" or "done"	• Breastfeeding on demand OR about 24 oz formula • 2–4 oz iron-fortified infant cereals and grains (breads, crackers, tortilla, noodles) • 4–6 oz each of chopped or diced fruits and vegetables • 2–4 oz chopped or diced meat, poultry, fish, eggs, cheese, yogurt, or mashed legumes

Source: U.S. Department of Agriculture Food and Nutrition Service. WIC infant nutrition and feeding guide. April 2019. https://wicworks.fns.usda.gov/resources/infant-nutrition-and-feeding-guide

1. Time the first feeding experience for when the baby is active and alert.
2. Use a small spoon with a shallow bowl and neutral temperature.
3. The baby should be able to open the mouth and extend the tongue toward the food.
4. Place the bowl of the spoon on the tongue with slight downward pressure, keeping the spoon level.
5. Pace the feeding on the infant's ability to swallow.
6. First meals will be only 5 or 6 baby spoons each.
7. Parent or caregiver should sit directly in front of the infant, making eye contact.
8. Infant should be in a seated position with hips and legs at 90 degrees.

From 6 months on, the variety of foods and textures will expand. At 5 to 9 months, the infant begins to position food between the jaws for chewing and can use up and down munching movements. They are able to sit more independently and grasp foods to bring them to the mouth (e.g., finger foods). Food variety will increase to more lumpy or mashed textures and expand to more fruits and vegetables, grains, and even soft/mashed meats. At 8 to 11 months, the infant is more competent with side-to-side tongue movements and begins to form lips around the rim of a cup. Ground or chopped foods, drinking from a cup, and self-feeding with fingers are the next feeding steps at this stage.

Finally, from 10 to 12 months, the infant can perform rotary chewing (grinding), feed with utensils, hold their own cup, and eat chopped foods or pieces of soft, cooked foods. It is important to note that a child does not develop mature chewing skills until toddler age and **weaning** is not complete until the calories from breast milk or formula are replaced by foods and other fluids. The following recommendations should be considered as the infant expands food variety:

1. The addition of infant cereals or foods to baby bottles to promote longer sleep is unfounded and not recommended; this practice inhibits development of skills to eat from a spoon and results in unnecessary calories.
2. When introducing new foods, introduce single-ingredient foods first (e.g, applesauce, bananas) before mixed foods (e.g., apples and bananas), and introduce foods one at a time with a few days in between to identify food allergies or intolerances.
3. Baby food desserts and snacks are not necessary, nor are they recommended.
4. Many regular household foods are appropriate for older infants such as yogurt, unsweetened applesauce, mashed potatoes, and oatmeal.
5. Perceptions of healthy infant foods and feeding methods will differ by cultural and ethnic background.[36]

Baby-Led Weaning

A newer feeding philosophy among infants is the idea of **baby-led weaning**, which as it sounds, promotes the infant's independence and lead in advancing to greater textures and solid foods.[37] While this idea is still based on developmental readiness, it may result in expediting the traditional progression of solid foods based on age timelines as indicated previously. Rather than continued spoon-feeding of puree textures, for example, this method promotes more self-feeding. For example, rather than a pureed banana, parents may provide slices of banana, and rather than pureed meats, soft ground beef may be provided for finger feeding. Safety and appropriateness of foods are still paramount, but this gives some flexibility to the family by allowing the infant to join in on the foods the entire family is eating, yet in smaller portions and modified forms as necessary. Similar to making homemade baby foods, this method may save time and money, promote cohesive family mealtimes, increase exposure to a greater variety of foods, and hone developmental skills such as oral-motor ability and self-regulation of hunger and fullness. It is important to note that baby-led weaning should still be guided by the signs of developmental readiness previously described and not begun prior to 6 months of age. Foods that pose a choking risk should also be avoided and are discussed later in the Food Safety section of this chapter. The public health professional can work with families interested in this feeding approach by guiding them to the appropriate resource for doing so.

SOCIAL DETERMINANTS OF HEALTH FOR INFANTS

SDOH refer to the social, economic, and physical conditions that may affect an individual's health[38] and are very important for explaining disparities in health status. According to the World Health Organization (WHO), SDOH can be described as "the conditions in which people are born, grow, work, live, and age, and the wide set of forces and systems shaping the conditions of daily life,"[1] thus playing a role in creating and sustaining health disparities across multiple levels including individual, interpersonal, community, and societal).[39]

This text describes the interplay between SDOH and health outcomes across the life course. For infants specifically, many health indicators overlap with maternal health status. Low education levels, limited access to healthcare, race, and discrimination can all contribute to disparities in **infant mortality** and birth outcomes. Discrepancies in healthcare can exist by race, residence, and socioeconomic status. Health outcomes are also affected by environmental exposures related to housing situation and type of employment. Much literature in the area of SDOH points to a substantial disparity in health outcomes for Black infants, supported by the higher **infant mortality rates** among Black infants previously discussed, and contributed to by structural racism across the life course.[39]

Interestingly, several SDOH also track along with the choice of infant feeding method.[13] Breastfeeding initiation rates are lower among younger women, obese women, those without a high school education, and those of lower income as is the continuation rate among those who do initiate breastfeeding. In turn, those mothers are also more likely to suffer the health consequences of not breastfeeding. The literature presents many influences on a mother's choice to breastfeed, leading *The Surgeon General's Call to Action to Support Breastfeeding* using a socioecological approach that considers strategies for overcoming barriers to breastfeeding from the family level (e.g., support) to the manufacturer level (e.g., marketing to minimize the effects on exclusive breastfeeding).[40] Table 4.2 highlights the role of the Public Health Nutrition Professional in Supporting Breastfeeding.

Table 4.2. Role of the Public Health Nutrition Professional in Supporting Breastfeeding
1. Demonstrate an understanding of the importance of exclusive breastfeeding for the first 6 months, continued breastfeeding until at least 12 months of age, and the role of breastfeeding and human milk in maintaining health and disease prevention.
2. Provide families with evidence-based information on breastfeeding in order to make the most informed choice on infant feeding method.
3. Offer general guidance for normal infant nutrition, recognizing early infant feeding cues, progression of feeding behaviors, and maternal nutrition.
4. Assess and recognize the need for additional nutrition information and support, and refer to the appropriate healthcare professional for complex breastfeeding problems.
5. Provide education in a culturally competent manner.
6. Evaluate challenges to breastfeeding and develop strategies for improvement.
7. Plan and implement nutrition education and interventions to support the breastfeeding family.
8. Participate in professional organizations that support breastfeeding.
9. Collaborate with other healthcare professionals to support breastfeeding.
10. Demonstrate ethical behavior when dealing with manufacturers of human milk substitutes.

Source: Office of the Surgeon General. *The Surgeon General's Call to Action to Support Breastfeeding.* U.S. Department of Health and Human Services; 2011. https://www.hhs.gov/surgeongeneral/reports-and-publications/breastfeeding/factsheet/index.html; Lessen R, Kavanagh K. Position of the Academy of Nutrition and Dietetics: promoting and supporting breastfeeding. *J Acad Nutr Diet.* 2015;115(3):444–449. https://doi.org/10.1016/j.jand.2014.12.014

PUBLIC HEALTH NUTRITION ISSUES FOR INFANTS

Poverty and Food Insecurity

Poverty is the leading public health issue related to nutritional status in children and is considered a primary SDOH. In 2015, it was reported that one in five children, or 15 million children, in the United States are living in poverty and 9 million are not covered by health insurance.[41] Poverty is a major driver in **food insecurity** in young children along with other SDOH that affect food access. In 2020, 14.8% of households with children were affected by food insecurity,[42] resulting in 9 million children facing hunger. Food insecurity rates were higher in single mother households, Black and Hispanic households, and those with incomes below the poverty line. Children who have experienced food insecurity suffer from delayed development, risk of chronic diseases like asthma and anemia, and behavioral problems.[43]

Lack of healthy food has implications for a child's physical and mental health, academic achievement, and future economic prosperity. In infants specifically, families may attempt to water down infant formula to make it last longer. This practice limits energy and nutrients needed to support adequate growth and development and can be dangerous, leading to other health problems resulting from electrolyte imbalances. Likewise, homemade formulas can increase risk for contamination leading to illness or infection. These practices may be common among food insecure families, but also came to light during recent manufacturer formula shortages and supply chain issues as a result of a global pandemic.[44] The U.S. Department of Health and Human Services and the CDC can provide families with guidance on locating formula during future shortages.[44,45] Food insecurity effects on the various lifecycle stages is discussed further in Chapter 9.

Prematurity and Special Conditions

Infants may experience a multitude of **special healthcare needs** related to premature birth and low birth weight, congenital anomalies, or genetic conditions. **Preterm** infants are born before 37 weeks of gestation and are classified by their gestational age and birth weight, the most important predictors of survival and health.[46] *Low birth weight* infants weigh less than 2,500 g; **very low birth weight** infants weigh less than 1,500 g, and **extremely low birth weight** infants weigh less than 1,000 g. An increase in the number of infants with ongoing special healthcare needs is growing due to advances in medical care for preterm deliveries. These infants may have increased energy and nutrient needs related to infections, fever, difficulty breathing, temperature regulation, and recovery from surgeries, and may rely on **parenteral** or **enteral feedings** depending on the maturity of the gut and other body systems at birth. Breast milk is the preferred infant feeding choice for preterm infants and its therapeutic benefits are only amplified by these situations.[47–49] Breast milk is still produced with an early delivery and is higher in protein to meet the unique needs of prematurity. New mothers are encouraged to pump their breast milk frequently to establish their supply.[50] Premature breast milk is fortified with micronutrients and can be provided orally or enterally, depending on the extent of prematurity, complications, and gut function of the infant.[51] If a mother cannot provide breast milk for the premature infant, and prefers to use human milk, donor milk from a milk bank can be considered. The Human Milk Banking Association of North America (HMBANA) offers a network of 31 nonprofit human milk banks across North America, providing pasteurized donor milk for use by fragile infants.[52] HMBANA believes in mobilizing the healing powers of donor milk and also sets guidelines for human milk safety.

Premature birth or low birth weight may or may not cause long-lasting disability depending on the gestational age at birth, birth weight, and available medical care. Regardless, these infants are at higher risk for a chronic physical, developmental, behavioral, or emotional condition and require health and related services of a type or amount beyond that required by children more generally. Often, these conditions are not diagnosed until later in childhood but there may be some common characteristics that appear during infancy to support a diagnosis, such as difficulty coordinating eating and breathing, failure to thrive, lack of hunger and satiety cues, and oral-motor feeding difficulties that affect the coordination of chewing and swallowing or acceptance of textures. More information about nutrition care and public health programs for special conditions are provided in Chapter 5.

Food Allergies and Intolerances

Although food allergies can begin in infancy, they are typically not confirmed until later in childhood[53] due to an array of reactions that build over time. More commonly, infants may experience food intolerances, causing symptoms like skin rashes, respiratory congestion, and gastrointestinal disturbances. Up to 3% of infants have a true cow milk allergy.[54] If protein or lactose intolerance is suspected, specialty infant formulas are available. Current recommendations do not indicate a need for a breastfeeding mother to restrict her diet, nor should she delay the introduction of specific allergenic foods during infant feeding, because these restrictions may in fact increase the baby's risk of developing allergies.[55,56] Avoiding foods may decrease nutritional adequacy, and lead to limited variety or rejection of foods later in childhood. It may be helpful to note the top eight allergenic foods are cow's milk, eggs, peanuts, tree nuts, fish, shellfish, soy, and wheat, in the case of identifying associations with specific symptoms.[55] Consultation with the healthcare provider or a registered dietitian should be sought in the case of a suspected **food allergy** for the most current recommendations for infant feeding.

Foodborne Illness and Food Safety

Foodborne illness is more common among children than adults given their lower immune capacity for handling an exposure to microorganisms, making infants a particularly vulnerable population with an immune system that is still developing. Common causes of foodborne illness include raw and undercooked meats, poultry, and eggs, and unpasteurized food and drink, particularly milk and soft cheeses.[57] Raw or cooked honey should also not be provided to infants under 1 year of age as it could contain the harmful *Clostridium botulinum* organism causing serious illness or death. Further information regarding food safety for children is provided in Chapter 5, and these same principles apply to infants approaching toddler age and eating a greater variety of these solid foods. More specific to infants are concerns with formula preparation and storage.[58] Formula should be prepared with a safe water source, refrigerated if not used within 2 hours of preparation, and discarded after 24 hours of refrigeration. Hands should be washed prior to preparation, and infant feeding items should be properly cleaned and sanitized. If the safety of the water supply is unknown, parents can contact their local health department for testing. Directions for mixing powdered formula should be followed carefully to ensure the proper concentration of energy and nutrients. Pumped breast milk should be used within 2 hours or frozen. Breast milk can be refrigerated for up to 4 days and breast milk that is frozen at 0°F or colder can be used for up to 12 months. Food safety practices are important in the home, child care centers, and food retail locations.

State cooperative extension agencies offer excellent food safety resources for families and organizations. If foodborne illness is suspected in a child, parents should seek immediate medical attention. The Child and Adult Care Food Program, a part of the U.S. Department of Agriculture Food and Nutrition Services provides guidelines and training tools for infant feeding in child care settings, including infant meal patterns, developmental readiness, and handling and storing breast milk, formula, and solid foods.[59] In addition to foodborne illness, several foods should be avoided in infancy and up to 4 years of age due to the risk of choking. These include popcorn, nuts and seeds, large chunks of meat or poultry or cheese, candy, hard raw fruits and vegetables unless finely chopped less than ½ inch, whole grapes or cherry tomatoes unless quartered, hot dogs, and thick layers of sticky foods like peanut butter.[60]

Immature Gastrointestinal Tract

Since it takes up to 6 months for the infant GI tract to mature,[10] bowel movements can be variable from diarrhea to constipation during this time. An infant that is breastfed also has typically soft or loose stools that could be mistaken for diarrhea by parents. **Colic** and **gastroesophageal reflux (GER)** are also common conditions during infancy that may be related to the immaturity of the gut. These conditions have not been found to affect nutrient absorption nor to hinder growth.[61]

Neonatal jaundice is another condition affecting up to 60% of full-term and 80% of preterm infants, relating to the ability to eliminate **bilirubin**, a yellow pigment that is a by-product of the fetal hemoglobin destruction after birth. This condition has some interconnections to metabolism, intestinal function, and volume of feedings to stimulate its removal from the body as well as potential factors in a mother's milk that inhibit the processing of bilirubin.[62] Consequences of elevated bilirubin in the body can be detrimental if it crosses the blood–brain barrier. If jaundice is suspected through visible signs of yellowing skin or whites of the eyes, the family should seek medical attention immediately.

Early Childhood Caries

Feeding practices established during infancy can contribute to the development of *early childhood dental caries,* often referred to as baby bottle tooth decay. The American Academy of Pediatric Dentistry and the AAP make several recommendations regarding the prevention of **early childhood caries.**[33,63] With the exception of a limited amount of juice after 6 months of age (4–6 oz), sugar-sweetened beverages should be avoided for infants. Small amounts of juice should only be offered in an open cup. Infants should not be put to bed with a bottle of formula, milk, or liquids containing sugars and should be weaned from the bottle by 12 to 18 months of age. Baby teeth should be wiped or brushed as soon as they emerge and infants should be seen by a dentist by 12 months of age.[64]

POPULATION CONSIDERATIONS

Population considerations related to infant health range from an increase in infant mortality rates to mounting evidence relating early nutrition exposures to disease processes later in life. Infant mortality is the death of an infant before 1 year of age[65] and is an important indicator of the health of a society. In the United States, in 2020, the infant mortality rate was 5.4 deaths per 1,000 live births, higher than the rate in several other developed countries. The infant mortality rate is double among African Americans.[65] The five leading causes of infant death are congenital disorders, preterm birth/low birth weight, sudden infant death syndrome, injuries, and pregnancy complications.[65]

The **first 1,000 days** refers to the time period from conception to age 2, a time that is most critical for the development of the body, brain, metabolism, and immune system, and setting the foundations for long-term health.[66] Nutritional status during the first 1,000 days lays a foundation for health for life and determines a child's ability to develop, learn, and thrive.[67] Additionally, nutrition exposures during the infancy period are being related to longer-term chronic disease risk such as type 2 diabetes and obesity. In fact, the Barker hypothesis, or **fetal origins of disease hypothesis**, states that the origins of chronic disease are programmed in the fetus as a response to the intrauterine environment.[68] Thus, nutrition exposures during fetal life and infancy are crucial to the long-term health of the individual, and infancy is the ideal time to begin setting the stage for lifelong health through infant feeding choice and diversity of nutrient-dense foods.

POLICY: GLOBAL ISSUES AND CHALLENGES

Worldwide, infant feeding is not only associated with optimal growth and development, but with childhood survival. Breastfeeding is predicted to save over 820,000 child lives each year, yet only 44% of infants 0 to 6 months old are breastfed.[69] Breastfeeding remains the best feeding method and is often therapeutic in difficult situations like prematurity, low birth weight, and HIV infection. WHO also reports that in many countries, infants do not meet the criteria of diet diversity and feeding frequency appropriate for their age. WHO recommends policies and practices in support of breastfeeding, such as longer duration of maternity leave, Baby-Friendly Hospital Initiatives, and community support services, put forth in the *Comprehensive* Implementation Plan on Maternal, Infant, and Young Child Nutrition.[70] A target of this plan is to increase the rate of exclusive breastfeeding among 0- to 6-month-old infants to 50%, and specific methods for doing so are outlined in the WHO/UNICEF Global Strategy for Infant and Young Child Feeding.[71] Baby-Friendly Hospitals are guided by the "Ten Steps to Successful Breastfeeding," which includes key clinical practices and management procedures such as ensuring that all staff are trained to support breastfeeding, that breastfeeding is initiated as soon after birth as possible, and that mothers have access to ongoing support and care upon discharge.[72]

Ultimately, WHO posits breastfeeding as a solution to improving infant mortality rates, child development, longer-term health outcomes, healthcare costs, and the economic status of families and nations.[70] This position is more fully detailed in the World Health Organization International Code of Marketing Breastmilk Substitutes, adopted in 1981 by the World Health Assembly.[73] The Code aims to protect and promote breastfeeding and ensure the proper use of human milk substitutes when necessary. Likewise, many other health organizations have shifted their efforts to quantifying not only the benefits of breastfeeding, but the risk of *not* breastfeeding.[13]

Despite several barriers to breastfeeding among new mothers, there are very few true medical contraindications to choosing this feeding method. More common reasons for discontinuing breastfeeding include perceived insufficient milk supply, painful breasts, and returning to work,[74] all of which can be targeted through the appropriate education and support for new mothers. This further supports the need for a socioecological approach, as previously mentioned, to promote breastfeeding from the individual to societal level.[13] Figure 4.1 and Table 4.3 provide additional examples and resources for promoting and supporting breastfeeding.

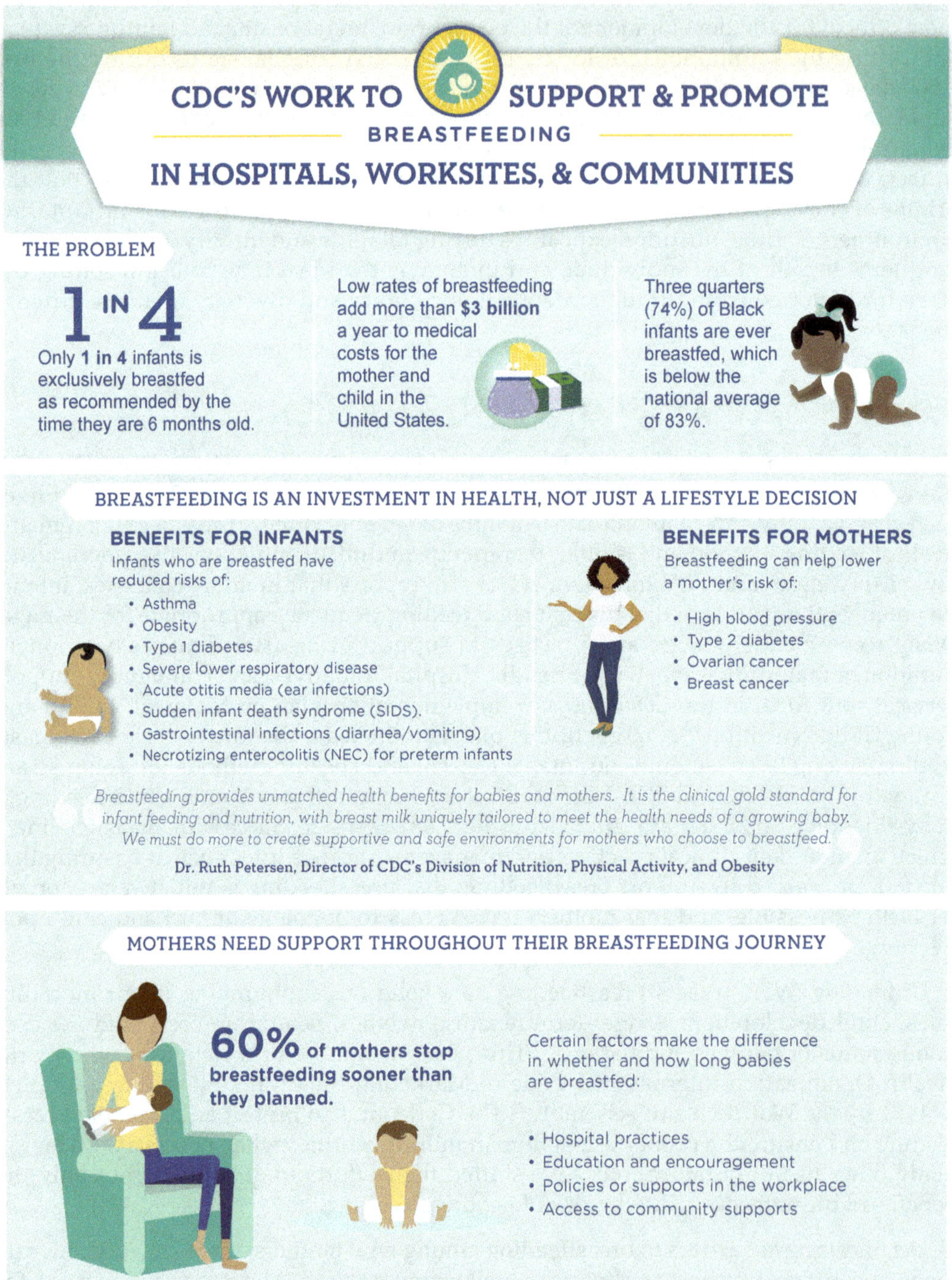

Figure 4.1. Breastfeeding infographic from the Centers for Disease Control and Prevention.
Source: Centers For Disease Control and Prevention. Fact sheets and infographics, CDC's work to promote and support breastfeeding in hospitals, worksites, and communities. Accessed October 18, 2023. https://www.cdc.gov/breastfeeding/pdf/breastfeeding-cdcs-work-508.pdf

(*continued*)

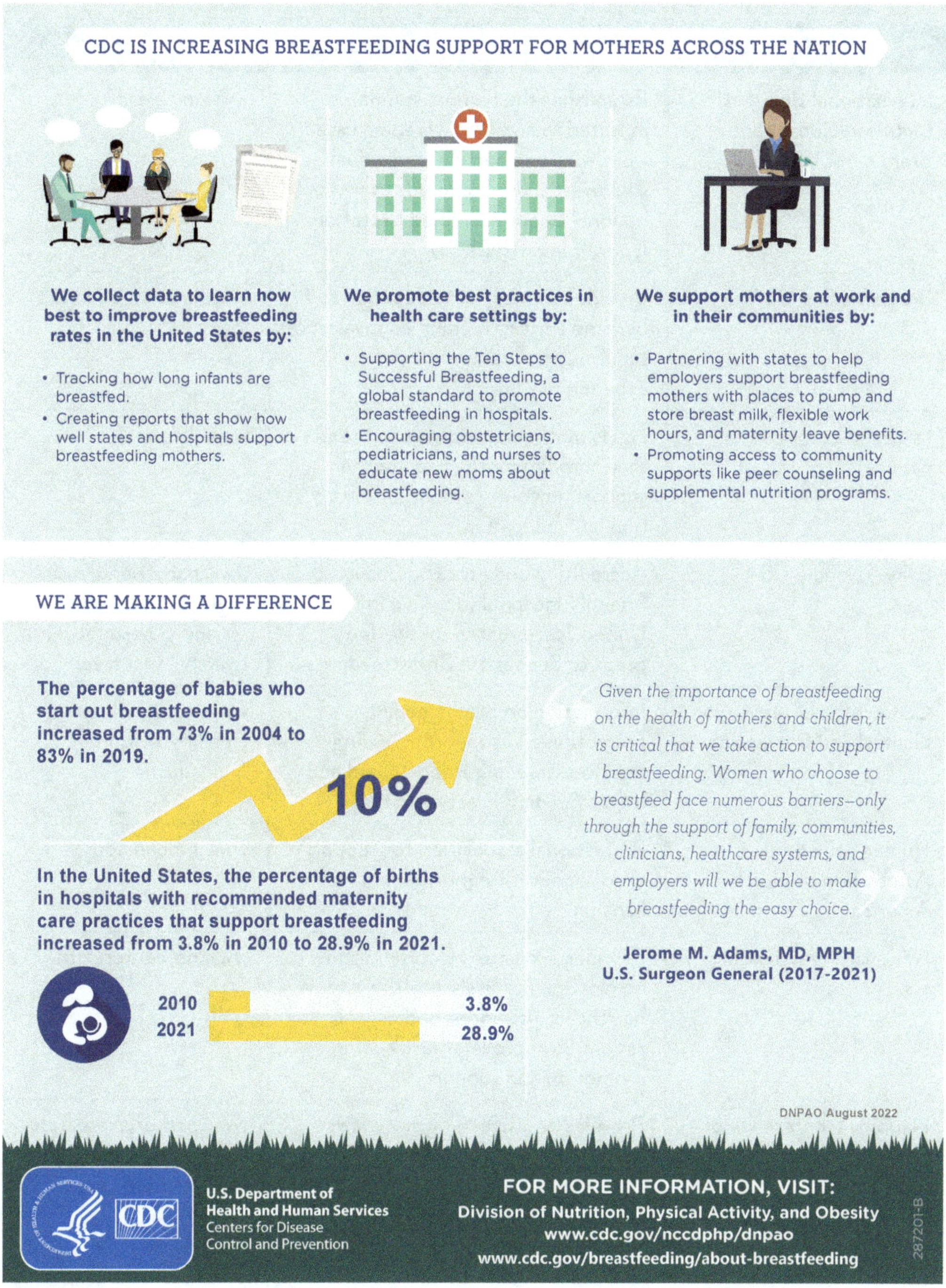
CDC IS INCREASING BREASTFEEDING SUPPORT FOR MOTHERS ACROSS THE NATION
We collect data to learn how best to improve breastfeeding rates in the United States by:
• Tracking how long infants are breastfed.
• Creating reports that show how well states and hospitals support breastfeeding mothers.
We promote best practices in health care settings by:
• Supporting the Ten Steps to Successful Breastfeeding, a global standard to promote breastfeeding in hospitals.
• Encouraging obstetricians, pediatricians, and nurses to educate new moms about breastfeeding.
We support mothers at work and in their communities by:
• Partnering with states to help employers support breastfeeding mothers with places to pump and store breast milk, flexible work hours, and maternity leave benefits.
• Promoting access to community supports like peer counseling and supplemental nutrition programs.
WE ARE MAKING A DIFFERENCE
The percentage of babies who start out breastfeeding increased from 73% in 2004 to 83% in 2019.
10%
In the United States, the percentage of births in hospitals with recommended maternity care practices that support breastfeeding increased from 3.8% in 2010 to 28.9% in 2021.
2010 3.8%
2021 28.9%
"Given the importance of breastfeeding on the health of mothers and children, it is critical that we take action to support breastfeeding. Women who choose to breastfeed face numerous barriers—only through the support of family, communities, clinicians, healthcare systems, and employers will we be able to make breastfeeding the easy choice."
Jerome M. Adams, MD, MPH
U.S. Surgeon General (2017-2021)
DNPAO August 2022
CDC
U.S. Department of Health and Human Services
Centers for Disease Control and Prevention
FOR MORE INFORMATION, VISIT:
Division of Nutrition, Physical Activity, and Obesity
www.cdc.gov/nccdphp/dnpao
www.cdc.gov/breastfeeding/about-breastfeeding
287201-B

Figure 4.1. (*continued*)

Table 4.3. Resources for Promoting and Supporting Breastfeeding

Organization	Description	Website
International Board of Lactation Consultant Examiners (IBLCE)	Establishes the highest standards in lactation and breastfeeding care worldwide and certifies individuals who meet these standards as International Board-Certified Lactation Consultants (IBCLCs)	www.iblce.org
Breastfeeding USA	Provides training and education to become a breastfeeding counselor; requires personal breastfeeding experience	www.breastfeedingusa.org
La Leche League International	Helps mothers worldwide to breastfeed through mother-to-mother support, encouragement, information, and education	www.llli.org
Baby-Friendly USA	Accrediting body for the Baby Friendly Hospital Initiative in the United States based on the Ten Steps to Successful Breastfeeding	www.babyfriendlyusa.org/about-us/baby-friendly-hospital-initiative/the-ten-steps
Centers for Disease Control and Prevention	Information on breastfeeding promotion and support including the Breastfeeding Report Card and Infant Feeding Practices Study	www.cdc.gov/breastfeeding/resources/guide.htm
Human Milk Banking Association of North America	Professional association for supporters of nonprofit donor human milk banking	www.hmbana.org
National Breastfeeding Center	Provides expertise to corporations/employers, hospitals/health systems, healthcare providers, and organizations to improve breastfeeding promotion and support	www.nbfcenter.com
National Conference of State Legislatures	Provides breastfeeding state laws	www.ncsl.org/research/health/breastfeeding-state-laws.aspx
National Institute of Child Health and Human Development, National Institutes of Health	Breastfeeding and breast milk resources and publications for patients and consumers	www.nichd.nih.gov/health/topics/breastfeeding/resources/Pages/patients-consumers.aspx#information

Table 4.3. Resources for Promoting and Supporting Breastfeeding (*continued*)

Organization	Description	Website
Office on Women's Health, U.S. Department of Health and Human Services (DHHS)	Tips, suggestions, information, and resources for breastfeeding women including Breastfeeding Fact Sheet and Your Guide to Breastfeeding	www.womenshealth.gov/breastfeeding
United States Breast-feeding Committee	Independent, nonprofit coalition of professional, educational and governmental organizations working collaboratively to protect, promote, and support breastfeeding	www.usbreastfeeding.org
U.S. Department of Agriculture (USDA)	Information and resources about nutrition during lactation	www.fnic.nal.usda.gov/lifecyclenutrition
USDA, Food and Nutrition Service	Breastfeeding promotion and support in the Special Supplemental Nutrition Program for Women, Infants, and Children	www.fns.usda.gov/wic/breastfeeding-promotion-and-support-wic
Health Resources Services Agency, Maternal and Child Health Board	Information, support services, and initiatives that support pregnant and lactating mothers	https://mchb.hrsa.gov/programs-impact/focus-areas/perinatal-infant-health/understanding-breastfeeding-benefits
U.S. National Library of Medicine, National Institutes of Health	Breastfeeding handouts in multiple languages	www.nlm.nih.gov/medlineplus/languages/breastfeeding.html

Source: Lessen R, Kavanagh K. Position of the Academy of Nutrition and Dietetics: promoting and supporting breastfeeding. *J Acad Nutr Diet.* 2015;115(3):444–449. https://doi.org/10.1016/j.jand.2014.12.014

PUBLIC HEALTH NUTRITION PROGRAMS FOR INFANTS

Federal child nutrition programs in the United States aim to ameliorate the effects of poverty, food insecurity, and poor nutrition described in this chapter. In fact, there is a great deal of evidence demonstrating the profound impacts of these programs on healthy growth and development during the infant and childhood years.[75] More specifically, these programs help lift families out of poverty and food insecurity, improve the intake of nutrient-dense foods, and reduce the risk of obesity and other health conditions. Table 4.4 provides a summary of federal nutrition programs that support the dietary needs of families with infants, with one specific program, the Special Supplemental Nutrition Program for Women, Infants, and Children (WIC) highlighted in the next section. See Table 4.5 for a snapshot of WIC food packages for infants.

In addition to these federally supported programs, a variety of nongovernmental and nonprofit organizations from the local to global level also exist to support the nutrition

Table 4.4. Summary of Federal Nutrition Programs Supporting Infants

Program Name	Description	Reach of Services	Eligibility	Website
WIC: Special Supplemental Nutrition Program for Women, Infants, and Children	Provides nutritional support to low-income women, infants, and children by providing foods, formula, and nutrition education	Provides farmers market vouchers Provides benefits to over 1.59 million participants	Children 0–5 years Pregnant, breastfeeding, and postpartum women	www.fns.usda.gov/wic
SNAP: Supplemental Nutrition Assistance Program	Provides supplemental income for the purchase of food for low-income families	The average SNAP benefit is $104 per month. Over 248,000 participating food retailers	All ages Must be at or below 130% of the poverty line to qualify	www.fns.usda.gov/snap/supplemental-nutrition-assistance-program
TEFAP: The Emergency Food Assistance Program	Provides food items to food banks, food pantries, and soup kitchens to be given out to the community. Most participants who enroll are elderly and have an income high enough to not qualify for SNAP.	In 2020, TEFAP provided over 2.4 billion meals.	All ages	www.fns.usda.gov/tefap/emergency-food-assistance-program
CACFP: Child and Adult Care Food Program	Reimburses child care and adult care facilities for meals and snacks that are served	Children participating in CACFP programs improved their intake of fruits and whole grains	0–18 years and 60+ years	www.fns.usda.gov/cacfp

needs of families with infants and young children. Examples include community food pantries, mobile food pantries and food lockers, and the United Nations Children's Fund (UNICEF) supporting the nutrition needs of infants and children in developing countries (www.feedingamerica.org, www.unicef.org).

Table 4.5. Snapshot of the WIC Food Packages for Infants*

Maximum Monthly Allowances (MMA) of Supplemental Foods for Infants†						
Foods	**Fully Formula Fed (FF)**		**Partially (Mostly) Breastfed (BF/FF)**		**Fully Breastfed (BF)**	
Food packages	Food Packages I-FF & III-FF A: 0–3 months B: 4–5 months	Food Packages II-FF & III-FF 6–11 months	Food Packages I-BF/FF & III-BF/FF A: 0–1 month B: 1–3 months C: 4–5 months	Food Packages II-BF/FF & III- BF/FF 6–11 months	Food Package I- BF 0–5 months	Food Package II-BF 6–11 months
WIC formula	A: 823 fl oz reconstituted liquid concentrate B: 896 fl oz reconstituted liquid concentrate	630 fl oz reconstituted liquid concentrate	A: 104 fl oz reconstituted powder B: 388 fl oz reconstituted liquid concentrate C: 460 fl oz reconstituted liquid concentrate	315 fl oz reconstituted liquid concentrate		
Infant cereal		24 oz		24 oz		24 oz
Infant food fruits and vegetables‡		128 oz		128 oz		256 oz
Infant food meat						77.5 oz

*Refer to the full regulation at *www.fns.usda.gov/wic* for the complete provisions and requirements for infant formula and infant foods in the WIC food packages.
†State agencies must provide at least the full nutrition benefit, as defined in §246.2, to non-breastfed infants.
‡At state agency option, older infants may be issued a cash-value voucher for fresh fruits and vegetables in lieu of a portion of jarred infant foods.
WIC, Special Supplemental Nutrition Program for Women, Infants, and Children.
Source: U.S. Department of Agriculture. WIC breastfeeding support. Accessed October 18, 2023. https://wicbreastfeeding.fns.usda.gov

WHAT WORKS: SPECIAL SUPPLEMENTAL NUTRITION PROGRAM FOR WOMEN, INFANTS, AND CHILDREN BREASTFEEDING PROMOTION AND SUPPORT

In addition to the food packages that support the nutritional needs of new mothers and infants, the WIC program offers a comprehensive breastfeeding promotion and support program. The goal of this program is to equip new mothers with the information, support, and resources they need to successfully breastfeed.[76] The program provides breastfeeding information and resources, peer counselors, a buddy program, and access to designated breastfeeding experts for more complex problems related to infant latching or milk supply. In the peer counselor program, WIC identifies and trains peer counselors from the community, ideally from WIC's target population and supporting the same racial and ethnic background as the mothers they support. Peer counselors are available outside of WIC's operational hours and clinic environment, and they have breastfed at least one baby. Peer counselors mentor and coach new breastfeeding mothers in a variety of areas such as comfortably breastfeeding in public, returning to work while breastfeeding, and helping with breastfeeding concerns. The Buddy Program offers a more informal network of new mothers who can share experiences and offer encouragement. Ultimately, WIC offers training and education through established curricula for all levels of breastfeeding support, from staff and volunteers to designated breastfeeding experts. For more complex questions or concerns around breastfeeding conditions (e.g., engorgement or mastitis), use of medications or alcohol while breastfeeding, or breastfeeding multiples, the WIC support system can also refer new mothers to the appropriate medical professional, registered dietitian/nutritionist, or board-certified lactation consultant. While historically, breastfeeding rates among WIC participants have been lower than those for nonparticipants, rates have increased by nearly 6% nationwide over the last decade from approximately 65% to 72%,[77] which may be attributable to this program.

SUMMARY

This chapter highlights the importance of infant feeding choice and the introduction of new foods in meeting the needs for rapid development, and establishing a foundation for lifelong dietary patterns that optimize health. Overarching nutritional goals during this stage include supporting growth and development, nutritional adequacy, and building feeding competency. Understanding the public health nutrition issues that affect families with infants can help identify the appropriate public resources and supports. Ultimately, the chapter provides convincing evidence of the need to promote breastfeeding as a public health nutrition strategy implicated in infant mortality and quality of life.

KEY CHAPTER CONCEPTS

1. Infancy is the most rapid period of growth and development of all life stages, and nutritional adequacy is paramount to optimizing the infant's potential.
2. Feeding behaviors are intricately related to physical, social, and emotional development and thus are shaped by the infant's environment and cognitive stimulation.

3. Breastfeeding is the optimal feeding method for infants, with numerous benefits for the infant, family, and society.
4. Infants progress from complete dependence on breast milk or human milk substitutes at birth to a diet including all modified solid foods at 1 year of age.
5. Social determinants of health are highly correlated with infant feeding choice.
6. Public health nutrition issues that require special consideration for infants and involvement of appropriate healthcare professionals include poverty and food insecurity, special conditions and prematurity, food allergies, food safety, maturation of the GI tract, and early childhood caries.
7. The infant mortality rate in the United States is higher than in several other developed countries; breastfeeding is proposed to be a comprehensive global solution to infant mortality rates.
8. The public health nutrition professional should build awareness for the benefits of and risks of not breastfeeding and offer resources and support through available community, state, federal, or international programs, particularly the WIC Breastfeeding Promotion and Support program.

CASE STUDY

You are a WIC nutritionist, and you've been asked to prepare a presentation for a small group education session of expecting parents on infant feeding during the first year of life. Consider the following in your presentation:

1. What information might you include about the decision between breastfeeding and formula feeding, that is, a comparison of each method and pros and cons of each?
2. What information could you include about hunger and satiety cues in infants for these new parents learning about the feeding relationship?
3. Are there particular nutrients or supplements of which parents should be made aware?
4. What additional resources could you provide to parents to help inform or support their feeding choice?
5. What questions do you think parents may have about feeding during the first year?
6. Describe the introduction of complementary foods considering the timeline from 6 to 12 months. Include the following:
    a. What foods can be introduced at various ages and what are the signs of developmental readiness for these foods?
    b. Compare the typical introduction of complementary foods to the idea of baby-led weaning.
    c. What other particular milestones or recommendations would you want to share with parents (i.e., dos and don'ts)?
    d. What foods should be avoided during the first year?
    e. Describe the ideal feeding environment for providing solid foods.
    f. Consider liquids as well as solid foods, for example, introducing water and juice.

7. Are there any resources besides WIC available for families struggling to meet the infant's first foods?
8. Use the following lesson plan template to prepare the lesson plan and any learning materials you would use.

LESSON PLAN TEMPLATE

Topic:	
Lesson Title:	
Location:	
Number of Participants:	Lesson Duration:

Lesson Objectives:

Summary of Tasks/Actions:

Materials/Equipment:

References:

Activities/Take-Home Tasks:

DISCUSSION QUESTIONS

1. Name the three overarching nutritional goals for infancy.
2. Consider how you would debate the promotion of breastfeeding as a public health nutrition focus area.
3. Review the national and international goals and objectives related to breastfeeding in the context of the socioecological model. Describe a strategy to help meet these goals at the individual, family, community, environmental, and policy level.
4. Describe the pattern of growth during the first year of life. How do growth and key developmental milestones parallel the nutrition recommendations during infancy?
5. Identify common nutritional areas for public health concern among infants. For which of these should further intervention be referred to other health professionals?
6. Describe the supplemental requirements of key nutrients during the first year of life?
7. Provide a basic timeline for the introduction of complementary foods from 6 to 12 months of age? What foods should be avoided during this time?
8. Describe the role of the parent in establishing the feeding relationship with their infant.
9. Explain three areas of public health concern related to infant feeding.
10. What social determinants of health impact feeding choice and health outcomes among infants?
11. Identify and discuss two public health nutrition support programs designed to improve nutritional intake for infants.

SUGGESTED LEARNING ACTIVITIES

1. Research or seek experience with a federal or nonprofit program that serves to meet the nutritional needs of infants. Note how your findings, experience, or observations relate to the information presented in this chapter.
2. Review the provisions of WIC food packages for infants. How do these foods support or refute the nutritional recommendations presented in this chapter?
3. Discuss the decision to breast or bottle feed with a friend or family member (this could be your mother, your child, or even your own decision). What were the major factors in this decision? If breastfeeding, were there any barriers and how did this mother overcome them? Were these barriers related to the individual, family, community, environment/society, or policy? How do your findings impact the way you might work with families to promote breastfeeding?
4. Identify local resources to help parents of infants in your area seek food and nutrition information and support. Create a flyer or brochure to share this information with the community.
5. Walk down the baby food aisle at your local grocery store and note your observations. What do you notice now that you've completed this chapter? Consider the types of foods available for infants. Do they seem to match the nutritional information included in this chapter? Are there particular promotional items or slogans that catch your eye? Which of these foods are necessary or not based on what you've learned from the chapter? Compare these items to the idea of baby-led weaning and consider the pros and cons of each.

6. Conduct further research on the nutritional content of breast milk as compared to a commercial formula. What are the major differences to note? What are the components of breast milk that are not available in infant formula?
7. Visit the website for the Human Milk Banking Association of North America to learn more about the donation and use of human milk. What situations might warrant use of a human milk bank and why is it beneficial? Who donates to a human milk bank? How is milk safety ensured? Does the milk maintain nutritive qualities? What is the cost of purchasing donated milk? Are there costs for donators?

RESOURCES FOR FURTHER LEARNING

- American Academy of Pediatrics Newborn and Infant Nutrition: www.aap.org/en/patient-care/newborn-and-infant-nutrition
  - Information, recommendations, and resources to optimize nutrition for newborns and infants
- Academy of Nutrition and Dietetics: www.eatright.org/for-baby
  - Provides resources related to breastfeeding and infant feeding with links to find a nutrition expert
- Baby-Friendly USA, Ten Steps to Successful Breastfeeding and International Code of Marketing Breastmilk Substitutes: www.babyfriendlyusa.org/for-facilities/practice-guidelines/10-steps-and-international-code
  - Outlines key clinical practices, management procedures, and restrictions on marketing breast milk substitutes for hospitals and birthing centers wishing to attain and retain the Baby-Friendly designation
- Centers for Disease Control and Prevention, National Center for Health Services, CDC Growth Charts: /www.cdc.gov/growthcharts
  - Provides up-to-date percentile curves showing the distribution of selected body measurements in infants from birth to 24 months
- Centers for Disease Control and Prevention, Infant and Toddler Nutrition: www.cdc.gov/nutrition/infantandtoddlernutrition/index.html
  - Provides information on infant feeding as well as food assistance and food systems resources such as during a national pandemic
- Centers for Disease Control and Prevention, Surgeon General's Call to Action to Support Breastfeeding: www.cdc.gov/breastfeeding/resources/calltoaction.htm
  - Provides key findings and action steps from the Surgeon General's Report
- Human Milk Banking Association of North America: www.hmbana.org/welcome2.html
  - Provides information about the Human Milk Bank Network in North America; assists in the location of a milk bank, and provides guidelines for donating and receiving milk
- Special Supplemental Nutrition Assistance Program for WIC: www.fns.usda.gov/wic
  - Provides comprehensive information about eligibility, programs, data, and additional resources

- U.S. Department of Agriculture, Feeding Infants in the Child and Adult Care Food Program: www.fns.usda.gov/cacfp
  - Provides training tools for CAFCP operators with infants enrolled at their child-care site
- U.S. Department of Agriculture, MyPlate: www.myplate.gov
  - Provides parent-friendly guidelines for infant feeding from birth to 6 months and 6 to 12 months and additional resources for new parents, including the safe preparation and storage of breast milk or formula
- World Health Organization Breastfeeding: www.who.int/health-topics/breastfeeding
  - Provides breastfeeding recommendations and resources including access to fact sheets and databases

SPRINGER PUBLISHING CONNECT™ | **A robust set of instructor resources designed to supplement this text is located at http://connect.springerpub.com/content/book/978-0-8261-8623-2. Qualifying instructors may request access by emailing textbook@springerpub.com.**

REFERENCES

1. *Office of Disease Prevention and Health Promotion. Healthy People 2030.* U.S. Department of Health and Human Services; 2021. www.health.gov/healthypeople
2. U.S. Department of Agriculture, U.S. Department of Health and Human Services. *Dietary Guidelines for Americans, 2020–2025.* 9th ed. U.S. Department of Health and Human Services; 2020. https://dietaryguidelines.gov
3. Office of Disease Prevention and Health Promotion. Dietary reference intakes. U.S. Department of Health and Human Services. Updated January 18, 2023. https://health.gov/our-work/nutrition-physical-activity/dietary-guidelines/dietary-reference-intakes
4. Zlotkin S. Neonatal nutrition. In: Linder MC, ed. *Nutritional Biochemistry and Metabolism With Clinical Applications.* 2nd ed. Elsevier; 1991:349–371.
5. Chumlea WD, LaMonte M. Physical growth and maturation. In: Samour PQ, King K, eds. *Pediatric Nutrition.* Jones & Bartlett Learning; 2013:15–20.
6. National Center for Health Statistics. CDC growth charts. Centers for Disease Control and Prevention. December 15, 2022. Accessed February 25, 2023. http://www.cdc.gov/growthcharts/cdc_charts.htm
7. Brown JE. *Nutrition Through the Life Cycle.* 7th ed. Cengage Learning; 2019.
8. Kail RV, Cavanaugh JC. *Human Development: A Lifespan View.* 2nd ed. Wadsworth Thomson Learning; 2000.
9. Santrock J. *Life-Span Development.* 7th ed. McGraw Hill; 1999.
10. American Academy of Pediatrics. Development of gastrointestinal function. In: Kleinman RE, Greer FR, eds. *Pediatric Nutrition.* 7th ed. American Academy of Pediatrics; 2014:15–40.
11. Shelton TL. Principles of child development and developmental assessment. In: Osborne L, ed. *Pediatrics.* Mosby; 2005:41–57.
12. Holt K, Woolridge NH, Storuy M, Sofka D, eds. *Bright Futures Nutrition.* American Academy of Pediatrics; 2011.
13. Lessen R, Kavanagh K. Position of the Academy of Nutrition and Dietetics: promoting and supporting breastfeeding. *J Acad Nutr Diet.* 2015;115(3):444–449. https://doi.org/10.1016/j.jand.2014.12.014
14. American Academy of Pediatrics. Formula feeding of term infants. In: Kleinman RE, Greer FR, eds. *Pediatric Nutrition.* 7th ed. American Academy of Pediatrics; 2014:61–81.
15. Nevin-Folino NL. *Pediatric Manual of Clinical Dietetics.* American Dietetic Association; 2008.
16. Institute of Medicine. *Dietary Reference Intakes for Energy, Carbohydrate, Fiber, Fat, Fatty Acids, Cholesterol, Protein, and Amino Acids.* National Academies Press; 2005.

17. Milner JA, Allison RG. The role of dietary fat in child nutrition and development: summary of an ASNS workshop. *J Nutr*. 1999;129:2094–2105. https://doi.org/10.1093/jn/129.11.2094
18. Krohn K, Demmelmair H, Koletzko B, Duggan C, Watkins J, Walker W. Macronutrient requirements for growth: fats and fatty acids. In: Duggan C, Watkins JB, Walker WA, eds. *Nutrition in Pediatrics*. 4th ed. BC Decker; 2008:59–65.
19. Lawrence RA, Lawrence RM. *Breastfeeding: A Guide for the Medical Profession*. 7th ed. Elsevier Mosby; 2011.
20. American Academy of Pediatrics. Fats and fatty acids. In: Kleinman RE, Greer FR, eds. *Pediatric Nutrition*. 7th ed. American Academy of Pediatrics; 2014:407–434.
21. Lima MS, Dimenstein R, Ribeiro KDS. Vitamin E concentration in human milk and associated factors: a literature review. *J Pediatr*. 2014;90(5):440–448. https://doi.org/10.1016/j.jped.2014.04.006
22. Gedfie S, Getawa S, Melku M. Prevalence and associated factors of iron deficiency and iron deficiency anemia among under-5 children: a systematic review and meta-analysis. *Glob Pediatr Health*. 2022;9. https://doi.org/10.1177/2333794X221110860
23. Prado EL, Dewey KG. Nutrition and brain development in early life. *Nutr Rev*. 2014;72(4):267–284. https://doi.org/10.1111/nure.12102
24. Lozoff B, Beard J, Connor J, Barbara F, Georgieff M, Schallert T. Long-lasting neural and behavioral effects of iron deficiency in infancy. *Nutr Rev*. 2006;64:S34–S91. https://doi.org/10.1301/nr.2006.may.s34-s43
25. Wagner CL, Greer FR. Prevention of rickets and vitamin D deficiency in infants, children, and adolescents. *Pediatrics*. 2008;122(5):1142–1152. https://doi.org/10.1542/peds.2008-1862
26. Kleinman RE, ed. *Pediatric Nutrition Handbook*. 6th ed. American Academy of Pediatrics; 2009.
27. Centers for Disease Control and Prevention. Frequently asked questions (FAQ's): vitamin K and the vitamin K shot given at birth. Accessed October 18, 2023. https://www.cdc.gov/ncbddd/vitamink/faqs.html
28. Institute of Medicine. *Dietary Reference Intakes for Water, Potassium, Sodium, Chloride, and Sulfate*. National Academies Press; 2005. https://doi.org/10.17226/10925
29. WebMD. What you need to know about water for infants. November 27, 2021. https://www.webmd.com/parenting/baby/what-you-need-to-know-water-infants
30. U.S. Department of Agriculture Food and Nutrition Service. *WIC Infant Nutrition and Feeding Guide*. U.S. Department of Agriculture; 2019. https://wicworks.fns.usda.gov/resources/infant-nutrition-and-feeding-guide
31. Butte NF, Wills C, Jean CA, Smith EO, Garza C. Feeding patterns of exclusively breastfed infants during the first four months of life. *Early Hum Dev*. 1985;12(3):291–300. https://doi.org/10.1016/0378-3782(85)90151-3
32. Centers for Disease Control and Prevention. How much and how often to feed infant formula. Accessed October 18, 2023. https://www.cdc.gov/nutrition/infantandtoddlernutrition/formula-feeding/how-much-how-often.html
33. American Academy of Pediatric Dentistry. Policy on early childhood caries (ECC): classifications, consequences, and preventive strategies. In: *Reference Manual of Pediatric Dentistry*. American Academy of Pediatric Dentistry; 2020:79–81.
34. American Academy of Pediatrics. Infant food and feeding. Updated July 6, 2021. https://www.aap.org/en/patient-care/healthy-active-living-for-families/infant-food-and-feeding
35. Brown KH. Complementary feeding. In: Duggan C, Watkins JB, Walker WA, eds. *Nutrition in Pediatrics*. 4th ed. BC Decker; 2008:411–416.
36. American Academy of Pediatrics. Cultural differences in infant feeding. Updated May 31, 2022. https://www.aap.org/en/patient-care/newborn-and-infant-nutrition/cultural-differences-in-infant-feeding
37. Cleveland Clinic. Baby-led weaning: what you need to know. October 27, 2021. https://health.clevelandclinic.org/baby-led-weaning
38. Francis L, DePriest K, Wilson M, Gross D. Child poverty, toxic stress, and social determinants of health: screening and care coordination. *Online J Issues Nurs*. 2018;23(3):2. https://doi.org/10.3912/OJIN.Vol23No03Man02
39. Dagher RK, Linares DE. A critical review on the complex interplay between social determinants of health and maternal and infant mortality. *Children*. 2022;9(3):394. https://doi.org/10.3390/children9030394

40. Office of the Surgeon General. *The Surgeon General's Call to Action to Support Breastfeeding*. U.S. Department of Health and Human Services; 2011. https://www.hhs.gov/surgeongeneral/reports-and-publications/breastfeeding/factsheet/index.html
41. Annie E. Casey Foundation. Demographics. Kids Count Data Center. Accessed October 18, 2023. https://datacenter.aecf.org
42. Coleman-Jensen A, Rabbitt MP, Gregory CA, Singha A. *Household Food Security in the United States in 2017*. ERR-256. U.S. Department of Agriculture, Economic Research Service; 2018. https://www.ers.usda.gov/webdocs/publications/90023/err-256.pdf
43. Feeding America. Hunger in America. https://www.feedingamerica.org/hunger-in-america/impact-of-hunger
44. U.S. Department of Health and Human Services. Information for families during the formula shortage. Accessed October 18, 2023. https://www.hhs.gov/formula/index.html
45. Centers for Disease Control and Prevention. Information for families during the infant formula shortage. Accessed October 18, 2023. https://www.cdc.gov/nutrition/infantandtoddlernutrition/formula-feeding/infant-formula-shortage.html
46. MacDorman MF, Matthews TJ. The challenge of infant mortality: have we reached a plateau? *Public Health Rep*. 2009;124(5):670–681. https://doi.org/10.1177/003335490912400509
47. Bankhead R, Boullata J, Brantley S, et al. Enteral nutrition practice recommendations. *J Parenter Enteral Nutr*. 2009;33(2):122–167. https://doi.org/10.1177/0148607108330314
48. Bhatia J. Human milk and the premature infant. *Ann Nutr Metab*. 2013;62(suppl 3):8–14. https://doi.org/10.1159/000351537
49. Schanler RJ, Lau C, Hurst NM, Smith E. Randomized trial of donor human milk versus preterm formula as substitutes for mothers' own milk in the feeding of extremely premature infants. *Pediatrics*. 2005;116:400–406. https://doi.org/10.1542/peds.2004-1974
50. Jones F. *Best Practice for Expressing, Storing, and Handling Human Milk*. 3rd ed. Human Milk Banking Association of North America; 2011.
51. American Academy of Pediatrics. Nutritional needs of the preterm infant. In: Kleinman RE, Greer FR, eds. *Pediatric Nutrition*. 7th ed. American Academy of Pediatrics; 2014:83–122.
52. Human Milk Banking Association of North America. Home page. Accessed September 19, 2023. https://www.hmbana.org/welcome2.html
53. Sicherer SH, Wood RA. Allergy testing in childhood: using allergen-specific IgE tests. *Pediatrics*. 2012;129:193–197. https://doi.org/10.1542/peds.2011-2382
54. American Academy of Pediatrics. Food allergy. In: Kleinman RE, Greer FR, eds. *Pediatric Nutrition*. 7th ed. American Academy of Pediatrics; 2014:845–862.
55. American Academy of Allergy, Asthma, & Immunology. Prevention of allergies and asthma in children. Accessed October 18, 2023. https://www.aaaai.org/tools-for-the-public/conditions-library/allergies/prevention-of-allergies-and-asthma-in-children
56. American Academy of Pediatrics. Food allergies and intolerances in newborns and infants. Updated May 31, 2022. https://www.aap.org/en/patient-care/newborn-and-infant-nutrition/food-allergies-and-intolerances-in-newborns-and-infants
57. Partnership for Food Safety Education. Common foodborne pathogens. Accessed October 18, 2023. https://www.fightbac.org/food-poisoning/foodborne-pathogens/
58. Centers for Disease Control and Prevention. Infant formula preparation and storage. Accessed October 18, 2023. https://www.cdc.gov/nutrition/infantandtoddlernutrition/formula-feeding/infant-formula-preparation-and-storage.html
59. Child and Adult Care Food Program. *Feeding Infants in the Child and Adult Care Food Program*. U.S. Department of Agriculture; July 2021. https://www.fns.usda.gov/tn/feeding-infants-child-and-adult-care-food-program
60. Academy of Nutrition and Dietetics. Do's and don'ts for baby's first foods. Published December 6, 2019. https://www.eatright.org/health/pregnancy/babys-first-foods/dos-and-donts-for-babys-first-foods
61. Thomas DW, Greer FR. Clinical report: probiotics and prebiotics in pediatrics. *Pediatrics*. 2010;126:1217–1231. https://doi.org/10.1542/peds.2010-2548
62. Centers for Disease Control and Prevention. Jaundice. Accessed October 18, 2023. https://www.cdc.gov/breastfeeding/breastfeeding-special-circumstances/maternal-or-infant-illnesses/jaundice.html
63. American Academy of Pediatrics. American Academy of Pediatrics updates recommendations on maintaining, improving children's oral health. December 19, 2022. https://www.aap.org/en/news

-room/news-releases/aap/2022/american-academy-of-pediatrics-updates-recommendations-on-maintaining-improving-childrens-oral-health
64. American Academy of Pediatrics. Nutrition and oral health. In: Kleinman RE, Greer FR, eds. *Pediatric Nutrition*. 7th ed. American Academy of Pediatrics; 2014:1167–1186.
65. Centers for Disease Control and Prevention. Infant mortality. Accessed October 18, 2023. https://www.cdc.gov/reproductivehealth/maternalinfanthealth/infantmortality.htm
66. Likhar A, Patil MS. Importance of maternal nutrition in the first 1,000 days of life and its effects on child development: a narrative review. *Cureus*. 2022;14(10):e30083. https://doi.org/10.7759/cureus.30083
67. Zero to Three: National Center for Infants, Toddlers and Families. *Nutrition in the first 1,000 days: A Foundation for Brain Development and Learning*. ThinkBabies; 2022. https://thousanddays.org/wp-content/uploads/1000Days-Nutrition_Brief_Brain-Think_Babies_FINAL.pdf
68. Almond D, Currie J. Killing me softly: the fetal origins hypothesis. *J Econ Perspect*. 2011;25(3):153–172. https://doi.org/10.1257/jep.25.3.153
69. World Health Organization. Infant and young child feeding. June 9, 2021. https://www.who.int/news-room/fact-sheets/detail/infant-and-young-child-feeding
70. World Health Organization. *Comprehensive Implementation Plan on Maternal, Infant, and Young Child Nutrition*. World Health Organization; 2014. http://apps.who.int/iris/bitstream/handle/10665/113048/WHO_NMH_NHD_14.1_eng.pdf
71. World Health Organization, UNICEF. *Global Strategy for Infant and Young Child Feeding*. World Health Organization; 2003. https://www.who.int/publications/i/item/9241562218
72. Baby-Friendly USA. The ten steps to successful breastfeeding. Updated 2018. https://www.babyfriendlyusa.org/for-facilities/practice-guidelines/10-steps-and-international-code
73. World Health Organization. *International Code of Marketing of Breast-*Milk Substitutes: Frequently Asked Questions. World Health Organization; 2017. https://apps.who.int/iris/bitstream/handle/10665/254911/WHO-NMH-NHD-17.1-eng.pdf
74. Brand E, Kothari C, Stark MA. Factors related to breastfeeding discontinuation between hospital discharge and 2 weeks postpartum. *J Perinat Educ*. 2011;20(1):36–44. https://doi.org/10.1891/1058-1243.20.1.36
75. Food Research & Action Center. *Child Nutrition Programs and Public Health: The Role of the Federal Child Nutrition Programs in Improving Health and Well-Being*. Food Research & Action Center; December 2017. https://frac.org/wp-content/uploads/hunger-health-role-federal-child-nutrition-programs-improving-health-well-being.pdf
76. U.S. Department of Agriculture. WIC breastfeeding support. Accessed October 18, 2023. https://wicbreastfeeding.fns.usda.gov
77. Kline N, Zvavitch P, Wroblewska K, Worden M, Mwombela B, Thorn B. *WIC Participant and Program Characteristics 2020*. U.S. Department of Agriculture Food and Nutrition Service; 2021.

5

TODDLER, PRESCHOOLER, AND SCHOOL-AGE CHILD NUTRITION

Melissa D. Gutschall

LEARNING OBJECTIVES

At the end of this chapter, students will be able to:

1. Describe the growth and developmental patterns of young children and how they relate to nutritional needs and feeding skills.
2. Identify key principles in promoting optimal nutrition intake for young children.
3. Name key nutrients and dietary patterns of public health concern for young children.
4. Identify needs for nutrition intervention and referral for common dietary concerns among young children.
5. Describe how the feeding environment of young children influences future dietary intake and disease risk.
6. Explain how social determinants of health affect the dietary intake of young children.
7. Recognize public health nutrition programs available to assist families with young children in meeting nutrition recommendations.

INTRODUCTION

This chapter describes the nutritional needs specific to **toddlers**, **preschoolers,** and **school-age children**. The toddler stage refers to children between the ages of 1 and 3 years, and the preschool stage between 3 and 5 years of age. The school-age stage is inclusive of middle childhood, or ages 5 to 10 years, and preadolescence, ages 9 to 11 years for girls and 10 to 12 years for boys. The chapter also explores the social determinants of health, public health nutrition issues, population issues, and global challenges related to children, as well as an example of an effective program solution. Overall, these stages demand a balance among meeting nutritional needs, addressing common nutrition problems, and preventing nutrition-related disorders while also building healthy eating and lifestyle habits. The overarching nutritional goals during childhood include dietary adequacy, physical growth, and the development of appropriate feeding skills and relationships with food.

NORMAL NUTRITION SUMMARY

Nutritional adequacy is crucial to optimal growth and development during these life stages. Toddlers and preschoolers, specifically, are being set up for their full growth and developmental potential, but nutrition is also important for cognitive development and exploration of their environment.[1] For the school-age child, nutrition goals should continue to focus on steady growth; cognitive, social, and emotional development; and the promotion of healthy eating patterns. The school-age classification includes both middle childhood (ages 5–10) and preadolescence (ages 9–11 for girls and 10–12 for boys). *Healthy People 2030* goals related specifically to nutrition for children include increasing the proportion of children who participate in the School Breakfast and Summer School Food Service programs, reducing **iron deficiency** in children 1 to 2 years of age, and reducing the proportion of children with obesity.[2]

The **Dietary Guidelines** have provided evidence-based recommendations on eating to promote health and prevent disease since 1980 and are strategically oriented toward public health nutrition as opposed to clinical care.[3] These guidelines are updated every 5 years. The current version focuses on the prevalence of chronic disease among Americans, dietary patterns as opposed to isolated foods or food groups, and the importance of a life-span approach. With respect to children, this is the first set of guidelines to address infants and toddlers and the distinct needs of every life stage. Table 5.1 provides a summary of food group recommendations based on the Dietary Guidelines for children.

The four major Dietary Guidelines for all Americans are as follows:

1. Follow a healthy dietary pattern at every life stage.
2. Customize and enjoy nutrient-dense food and beverage choices to reflect personal preferences, cultural traditions, and budgetary considerations.
3. Focus on meeting food group needs with **nutrient-dense** foods and beverages, and stay within calorie limits.
4. Limit foods and beverages higher in added sugars, saturated fat, and sodium, and limit alcoholic beverages.

Table 5.1. Food Group Intake Goals Amounts by Childhood Stage

Food Group	Toddler (12–23 Months)*	Preschooler/Middle Childhood (Ages 2–8 Years)*	Preadolescent (Ages 9–13 Years)*
Vegetables (cups/day)	⅔–1	1–2½	1½–3½
Fruits (cups/day)	½–1	1–2	1½–2
Dairy (cups/day)	1⅔–2	2–2½	3
Grains (oz/day)	1¾–3	3–6	5–9
Protein foods (oz/day)	2	2–5½	4–6½
Oils (g/day)	9–13	15–24	17–34

*Ranges vary by calorie needs and age.
Source: Adapted from U.S. Department of Agriculture, U.S. Department of Health and Human Services. *Dietary Guidelines for Americans, 2020-2025*. 9th ed. U.S. Department of Health and Human Services; 2020. https://www.dietaryguidelines.gov

Perhaps most paramount with regard to the dietary guidelines is promoting dietary variety, which ensures that children will obtain all necessary nutrients and develop an appreciation for all foods that will carry into adulthood. The Dietary Guidelines for Americans and MyPlate,[4] outlined by the U.S. Department of Agriculture (USDA), provide guidance and tools for healthy diets during various life stages, including childhood. MyPlate provides a visual for implementing the Dietary Guidelines in a practical way. Key messages promoted by MyPlate are making half the plate from fruits and vegetables, making half of all grain servings from whole grains, using fat-free or low-fat milk, choosing foods lower in added sodium and sugars, drinking water, and promoting physical activity.[4]

The **Dietary Reference Intakes (DRIs)** offer a set of more specific values that can be used to assess and plan nutrient intakes for health people and vary by sex and age.[5] The DRIs include the Recommended Dietary Allowance (RDA), or average daily intake level necessary to meet the needs of 98% of the population; adequate intakes (AIs) established when there is not enough evidence to set an RDA but a level probable to ensure nutritional adequacy; and the tolerable upper intake Level (UL), the maximum intake level that is unlikely to cause adverse health effects. A link to the DRIs for toddler through preschool age is provided in Appendix C, and specific nutrients of concern for this age group are considered later in this chapter.

NUTRITIONAL GOALS FOR CHILDREN

The overarching nutritional goals for childhood include (a) optimal growth, (b) nutritional adequacy, and (c) development and progression of feeding skills. All children should consume a varied and balanced diet appropriate for their age and ability and focused on nutrient density. Nutritional needs are typically dictated by adequate calories and protein to achieve optimal growth. Toddlers are no longer consuming human milk or formula as the major source of calories and protein, and should be consuming a variety of nutrient-dense complementary foods in manageable forms. Parents and caregivers act as the primary source of foods and mealtime routines. Preschoolers and young children have transitioned to the full diet of the family and continue to form dietary habits and patterns that set the foundations for prevention of chronic disease later in life. The eating environment expands to institutions and social influences on food choices with a growing autonomy for making food selections. The importance of social supports and healthy marketing and community policies[3] are evident throughout this chapter.

Growth

Children have diverse nutritional needs dependent on individual growth and development, but overall there is a decreased growth rate from the infancy stage. The average growth of toddlers is 8 oz (0.23 kg) and 0.4 inch (1 cm) of height per month.[6] Preschool growth slows to 4.4 lb (2 kg) per year and 2.75 inches (7 cm) per year.[6] A simultaneous decrease in appetite and interest in food accompanies this decreased growth velocity and increased developmental ability to explore and learn. Growth velocity slows further during the school-age years, but remains steady at an average of 7 lb (3–3.5 kg) and 2.5 inches (6 cm) annually.[6] It is not uncommon to see variability in appetite based on the timing of growth spurts in school-age children.

Regular monitoring of a child's growth is important to establish the individual growth pattern and identify any deviations from it. The Centers for Disease Control and Prevention (CDC) Growth Charts are the recommended tool for monitoring a child's growth.[7] This resource provides sex-specific charts for children ages 2 to 20 to plot weight-for-age, height-for-age, and body mass index (BMI) for age. For toddlers between 1 and 2 years of age, the birth to 36 months growth chart is used. It is important to evaluate the pattern of growth over time rather than one single measurement. Measuring and charting growth are subject to many potential sources of error (from measurement technique to incorrect plotting), which can be misinterpreted in the evaluation of growth. When measuring and interpreting growth in children, the following situations warrant further evaluation: (a) a plateau in weight, (b) a pattern of weight gain followed by weight loss, (c) not regaining weight lost during illness, and (d) a pattern of unexplained and unintentional weight gain.[8]

Nutritional Adequacy

A balanced diet from all food groups ensures that all **macronutrient** and **micronutrient** needs are met. This includes enough energy from carbohydrates, protein, and fat to fuel the rapid rates of growth previously described, along with key vitamins and minerals, such as iron for the expanding blood supply that accompanies growth and calcium for the developing bones. The Dietary Guidelines support a diet that includes whole grains, plenty of fruits and vegetables, lean protein sources, and low-fat dairy products. Nutrition problems can span from deficiencies to excesses. More information about specific nutrients of public health concern among young children is discussed later in this chapter.

A review of children's diets compared to the Dietary Guideline recommendations reveals that all age groups, from toddlers to preadolescents, consume lower than recommended amounts of vegetables, lean proteins, whole grains, and low-fat dairy products.[3] Dairy intake drops off after the age of 2 and fruit intake declines among 5- to 8-year-olds and thereafter. Among children 9 to 13 years of age, only grain intake meets the recommendations, but the majority of grains are from refined sources. The dietary pattern currently consumed by children nationwide is high in sodium, saturated fat, and added sugars with over half of children exceeding the suggested limits for these nutrients. In fact, data show that sugar-sweetened beverages make up 11% of total daily energy intake for young children and contribute up to a quarter (25%) of daily added sugar intake. Consequently, milk intake has declined as it is displaced by these beverage sources, which do not offer the same nutrient density. Thus, it is not surprising that calcium and vitamin D intake are of concern for public health nutrition. These dietary habits increase risk for chronic disease. Micronutrients of public health concern for all ages include calcium and vitamin D, potassium, and fiber. Requirements for them, as well as for iron and zinc, of specific concern to young children, are covered in the next section. Table 5.2 presents a 1-day sample meal plan for the toddler, preschooler, and school-age child that meets the food group recommendations within the Dietary Guidelines.

Energy Needs

Consideration of age, gender, height, weight, and physical activity is used to determine energy needs for children (DRIs).[9] A summary of estimated calorie needs by age group is presented in Table 5.3. Energy needs during the toddler phase are indicative of a slowing growth pattern compared to infancy and the needs for school-age children continue to be reflective of the slower, but steady growth during these years. With energy needs, it is

Table 5.2. One-Day Sample Meal Plans for Toddler, Preschooler, and School-Age Child Based on the Dietary Guidelines

Age	Sample Meals*
Toddler	**Breakfast**: 2 scrambled eggs and ¼ cup oatmeal, ½ sliced banana, with ½ cup of milk. **Morning snack**: ¼ cup Greek yogurt with ¼ cup blueberries **Lunch:** ½ grilled cheese sandwich on whole wheat bread and ½ cup bell peppers **Afternoon snack:** 1 cup veggie straws **Dinner:** 2 baked chicken tenders with ¼ cup roasted potatoes and ¼ cup broccoli **Evening snack**: 2 cookies, 1 cup milk
Preschool	**Breakfast**: 1 cheese and spinach omelet (2 eggs), 1 slice whole wheat toast, 1 cup milk. ½ cup fresh berries **Snack**: 1 cup apple slices with 1 tbsp peanut butter **Lunch**: ½ chicken quesadilla with 1 cup of corn and beans **Afternoon snack**: 2 tbsp hummus with veggie sticks **Dinner:** 2 oz BBQ baked chicken, ½ cup mashed potatoes, ½ cup asparagus, 1 cup milk **Evening snack**: 1 cup Greek yogurt with strawberries and ¼ cup granola
School-age	**Breakfast:** breakfast burrito (2 eggs, ¼ cup cheese, bell peppers, onions, and mushrooms), ½ cup fruit, 1 cup milk **Snack**: 1 banana and 1 tbsp peanut butter **Lunch**: 1 whole turkey avocado sandwich, ½ cup cucumber and 1 tbsp ranch dressing **Afternoon snack**: 1 cheese stick and ½ cup applesauce **Dinner:** 4 oz teriyaki salmon stir fry with veggies and ½ cup brown rice, 1 cup milk **Evening snack:** ½ cup chocolate pudding

*Water to drink if not otherwise indicated.

Table 5.3. Average Calorie Needs by Age and Sex for Children

Age	Calorie Needs, Female*	Calorie Needs, Male*
2–4 years	1,000–1,400	1,000–1,600
5–8 years	1,200–1,800	1,200–2,000
9–13 years	1,400–2,200	1,600–2,260

*Needs also affected by activity levels or special conditions.
Source: Adapted from U.S. Department of Agriculture, U.S. Department of Health and Human Services. *Dietary Guidelines for Americans, 2020-2025*. 9th ed. U.S. Department of Health and Human Services; 2020. https://www.dietaryguidelines.gov

important that calories come from nutrient-dense foods to ensure all *micronutrient* needs are met by the overall diet. Food consumption surveys show that children are exceeding the recommended intakes for fat and saturated fat, but not meeting the recommendations for dietary fiber nor key vitamins and minerals, discussed in the next section. Toddler to preschooler surveys show variability in dietary intakes among age groups with preschoolers more likely to fall short on recommended micronutrients.[10] Children's diets are commonly characterized by a lack of dietary diversity and irregular meal patterns.[11]

Protein Needs

The DRIs for protein can be found at the link provided in Appendix C. Needs are easily met by the American diet, but may be lower among children due to limited preference for protein-containing foods, development of competence with chewing and swallowing, and diets higher in refined carbohydrates. Because protein is an energy-contributing nutrient, it is important that overall energy needs are met in order to spare protein for its essential functions in growth and tissue development. A balance of high-quality proteins ensures that the needs for all essential amino acids are met. These proteins include lean meats, eggs, beans and legumes, nuts and seeds, and low-fat dairy products. Vegetarian diets can be appropriate and adequate if they meet energy needs and contain a variety of foods. A registered dietitian nutritionist should be consulted for assistance in assuring a vegetarian diet meets a child's protein needs.

Carbohydrates

The DRIs for carbohydrate can be found by accessing the link provided in Appendix C. The role of carbohydrates in the diet of young children are primarily to meet energy needs, sparing protein for its high demands in growth. As previously stated, the dietary patterns for carbohydrates include primarily highly refined sources such as sugars and processed grains, and low in fiber. The Dietary Guidelines promote half of carbohydrate intake from whole grain foods, which offer fiber and several micronutrients in addition to energy. Examples include whole grain cereals, breads, pastas, and rice. Parents of young children may need to be educated about how to identify sources of whole grains.

Fats

While fats offer a concentrated source of energy at 9 kcal/g, which also spares protein for the growth of new tissues, they are critical for brain and nervous system development in young children. In addition to these functions, fats offer a source of fat-soluble vitamins such as vitamin D. In fact, the recommendation to limit saturated fat to less than 10% of calories does not apply to children until the age of 2 for these reasons. Children are meeting the recommended level of intake of fats, but not from preferable sources. Children's diets are high in saturated fats that come primarily from animal sources and processed foods as opposed to unsaturated fats from plant-based sources like oil, nuts, and seeds. Fatty fish, like salmon, also provide omega-3 fatty acids that help support brain development and heart health. Omega-3 fatty acid intake is low in most Americans' diet, especially when compared to intake of omega-6 fatty acids present in oils and processed foods. Fish high in mercury content, however, should be avoided in the young child's diet.[12] These fish include shark, swordfish, and mackerel.

Vitamins and Minerals

The DRIs for micronutrients for children by age range are linked in Appendix C.[13,14] Children are consuming adequate amounts of most micronutrients with the exception of iron, calcium and vitamin D, zinc, and potassium.[10,15]

Iron

Iron is the number one micronutrient deficiency worldwide and iron deficiency is no stranger to young children in the United States. As toddlers transition from formula fortified with iron to regular milk, they are missing a major source of iron in the diet that may not be replaced with foods. Iron deficiency affects toddlers at a rate of 7%, but just 4% to 6% in school-age children.[16] Toddlers are at highest risk due to a combination of rapid growth and limited intake of iron-rich foods such as meat, fish, poultry, eggs, beans, nuts/nut butters, and green leafy vegetables. These foods are often not preferable to toddlers with a developing palate or difficult to consume based on chewing and swallowing ability. Meats should be cut into fine pieces so children can manipulate them successfully. They can also be prepared in different ways or offered as part of mixed dishes. Meats are also more expensive than other sources of iron. Alternative sources of iron such as eggs, beans and legumes, and nuts/nut butters should be promoted if meat intake is limited. Finally, high intakes of milk and juice may displace more nutrient-rich foods for young children. Recommendations are to limit drinking caloric beverages to mealtimes with only water offered in between. Interestingly, fortified grains are a major contributor of iron to the American diet, and vitamin C can assist with the absorption of iron from other foods. For example, consuming orange juice with an iron-fortified cereal will increase the absorption of that iron and thus its availability for use by the body.

Iron deficiency is more common among African American and Mexican American children.[17] The impacts are profound in the areas of cognitive and behavioral development.[18–19] In cases of iron deficiency, regular consumption of the high iron sources previously mentioned should be encouraged for the child, along with limiting milk intake to <24 oz per day and juice intake to <6 oz per day.[20] The American Academy of Pediatrics (AAP) recommends routine screening for iron deficiency at 12 months of age and additional screening at any age for children at increased risk (low-iron diet, high milk consumption, limited food access, strict vegetarian diets, chronic illness or genetic conditions, and children with special healthcare needs).[18,19,21] Referral to a healthcare provider or registered dietitian is appropriate in the case of iron deficiency to develop an intervention that includes iron-rich foods and/or supplementation according to the most current treatment guidelines. With iron deficiency comes an increased risk for lead toxicity due to a higher absorption capacity for lead. Other risk factors for lead toxicity are discussed in a later section.

Zinc

Mean intakes of zinc in toddlers and preschoolers have been documented as low.[22,23] The major sources of zinc are lean proteins such as seafood, poultry, eggs, nuts, beans, and legumes. Zinc is important in cell division, and thus growth and differentiation of new tissues, as well as immune function. As described previously, children's diets are low in lean protein sources, and consumption of these foods offers zinc as well as several other micronutrients required for children to grow and develop.

Calcium/Vitamin D

Calcium and vitamin D intake are critical for optimal bone development in young children. Upon weaning from breast milk or bottle feeding, continued provision of milk and other dairy foods is recommended in young children. As described previously, dairy intake is shown to decline after weaning, and remains one of the highest and most **bioavailable** sources of calcium and vitamin D in the diet. A common recommendation is for children to aim for three servings of dairy foods each day to meet this need. An increased amount of calcium and vitamin D are needed as children approach adolescence as puberty is the time in which peak bone mass is achieved. While low-fat dairy products are the optimal source, calcium-fortified foods, such as orange juice and almond or soy milk, may be useful in a vegetarian diet that excludes dairy. In addition to fortified foods, vitamin D is also made in the body with ample sunlight exposure. Assessment and recommendations for calcium and vitamin D supplementation should be sought from a registered dietitian/nutritionist if dairy foods or sunlight exposure are limited for any reason.

Other Nutritional Concerns for Young Children

Fluid Intake

Fluid needs for children vary depending on age, weight, sex, humidity, and activity level, but the DRIs include 4 cups per day for ages 1 to 3, 5 cups per day for ages 4 to 8, and 7 to 8 cups per day for ages 9 to 13.[9] Children should consume plain water as the primary source of hydration. Sugar-sweetened beverages (SSBs), including juice, fruit drinks, soda, and sports drinks, are not necessary in the diet of young children and are not recommended at all for children under the age of 2 as they could fill the child and displace more nutrient-dense foods in the diet.[24] SSBs do not contribute to any food group intake nor the dietary guidelines, containing a high calorie load with no other nutrient value. Fluid intake for children should come from water or low-fat dairy products. Juice can be included as part of a healthy diet if 100% juice is selected and in the recommended amounts of 4 to 6 oz for young children after 1 year of age.[24] Whole fruit intake is preferred over juice because of its fiber content. Juice should not be confused with the many juice and fruit drinks on the market that contain minimal juice. Appropriate juice sources should be identifiable on the package labeling as "100% fruit juice" or by looking for 0 added sugars on the Nutrition Facts label. Along with this, specialty toddler drinks and milks, promoted for additional nutrition content, are not necessary in the diets of young children and often contain added sugars and a higher price tag. Diets with a variety of nutrient-dense foods and low-fat milk (or alternative) should be promoted. As children approach preadolescence and may be participating more heavily in sports activities, the use of sports drinks may be considered by families. Sports drinks are included in the category of SSBs. A basic sports drink with a low amount of added sugar may be appropriate for longer bouts of activity, particularly in hot temperatures, but are not necessary for drinking on a regular basis or during play-based activities. These beverages may also contain caffeine. Safety limits for caffeine intake have not been established for young children, and thus, caffeine should be avoided in this population.

Fiber

Fiber is important for bowel regularity and chronic disease prevention. A delicate balance with fiber may be necessary in young children as they may alternate from constipation with too little fiber to diarrhea with too much fiber. Too many high-fiber foods can also replace other foods in the diet and inhibit the absorption of micronutrients such as calcium and iron.[20] Promoting a variety of whole grains and fruits and vegetables at the recommended amounts for age and with adequate fluids helps to establish bowel regularity. The DRIs have established AIs for fiber intake in children with 19 g/day in 1- to 3-year-olds, and 25 g in 4- to 8-year-olds. Fiber recommendations differ for boys and girls in the preadolescent stages of life with 26 g/day recommended for girls ages 9 to 13 and 31 g/day recommended for boys ages 9 to 13.[5]

Lead

While lead is not of dietary concern for children, it is worth mentioning from an environmental health standpoint. Blood levels of lead have been of concern historically in young children related to sources of lead as an external contaminant. Lead levels among young children are declining[2] due to a reduction in airborne sources of lead from gasoline and industrial emissions. Of particular risk are children living in older homes (built prior to 1978) where lead-based paint chips or dust remain from deteriorating lead paint.[25] Children are busy exploring their surroundings and do so by putting things in their mouth. Lead could also be introduced through contaminated water or parental occupations. High lead levels have been shown to disproportionately affect children living in poverty and minority groups.[25,26] Reduction of lead levels remains a Healthy People 2030 objective; there is no safe blood level of lead as it can affect the brain, liver, and kidneys, and lead to seizures, coma, and death at high levels.[25,27,28] The CDC uses a blood lead reference value of 3.5 mcg/dl to identify children with blood lead levels that are higher than most, based on the NHANES (National Health and Nutrition Examination Survey) 97.5th percentile of data among children 1 to 5 years of age from 2015–2018.[29] This is not health-based nor a regulatory standard, but may help identify more children as having lead exposure and seeking appropriate follow-up measures. The AAP recommendations are focused more on prevention than identification.[25,30] Mean lead levels in children ages 1 to 5 from 2013–2016 were 3.31 mcg/dL. The CDC recommends screening at age 9 to 12 months and again at 2 years; local and state health departments set screening protocols based on these recommendations and risk factors in their respective communities. Federal policy also requires lead screening for all children enrolled in Medicaid who are at higher risk.[25,30,31] Nutritionally, adequate intakes of iron and calcium may help prevent elevated lead levels by competing for absorption.[28] Therefore, monitoring risk factors for lead in the child's environment and ensuring an adequate diet can help reduce the occurrence of elevated lead levels in young children.

Development of Feeding Skills and Relationships With Food

Key developmental and feeding milestones typically parallel the growing and expanding nutritional needs of children to facilitate optimal growth and development. Toddlers will transition from a diet of primarily breast milk or formula to a diet of all modified solid foods between 1 and 2 years of age. Weaning from the breast or bottle is initiated between 12 and 14 months with a transition to whole milk. The AAP recommends breastfeeding for at least 12 months while the World Health Organization (WHO) recommends a continuation of breastfeeding for up to 2 years.[30] Ultimately, the decision to breastfeed, and the duration of breastfeeding is up to the mother within the family dynamic. The role of the public health nutrition professional is to support the family's decision while providing evidence-based information about both sources of feeding, accurate feeding recommendations, and strategies to overcome any barriers to successful breastfeeding.

Whole milk is provided during the second year of life to provide the fat necessary for rapid growth and brain development. At this point, the child is also transitioning to an open cup for drinking. *Gross and fine motor development* occurs from 12 to 18 months and provides the ability for children to chew foods of different textures with rotary tongue and jaw motions, as well as to become more competent in their self-feeding ability. These skills are refined by 18 to 24 months such that the toddler can handle more complex textures like meats and raw fruits and vegetables. An accompanying increase in visual/motor coordination helps the child use a cup and spoon more effectively, although they do prefer to eat with their hands first as an important developmental step. The **pincer grasp**, the ability to hold something between the thumb and first finger, facilitates picking up foods and bringing them to the mouth at around 12 months of age. In addition to physical development, children are growing in communication skills and independence. They desire and gain pleasure from self-feeding and exploring new tastes and textures. At this stage, children still need very close feeding supervision and appropriately modified foods due to the risk of choking. Feeding should take place in a seated position with parental interaction and established mealtimes.

Refinement of **gross** and **fine motor skills** continue into the preschool years and children at this age are competent with the use of utensils and a cup. Children can even be encouraged to take part in simple meal preparation tasks. The preschool age child is capable of activities such as tearing lettuce, rinsing fruits and vegetables, stirring, mashing potatoes, and peeling or cracking eggs. Regular mealtimes should occur seated at the table with adult supervision. The importance of parental role modeling remains highly influential during the preschool years. The rate of growth remains slow with fairly small intakes paralleling those needs. Fluctuations in appetite at this stage are normal as growth occurs in spurts and appetite is likewise variable. It is common for appetite to increase in advance of a growth spurt and then drop off again.

A child's **temperament** can affect their willingness to try and accept new foods[32] as well as the feeding dynamics at mealtime. Three temperamental categories have been identified: easy, difficult, and slow-to-warm-up. The easy child is willing to try new foods and accepts them with regularity. The difficult child is slow to adapt to new foods and can display negativity about them. The slow-to-warm-up child is also slow to adapt to new foods, but often does with repeated exposures to them, and with less difficulty. It is important not to rush or pressure a child to accept new foods, and if the temperament of the parent is mismatched to that of the child, the result may be more conflict over eating. Research shows that it may take eight to 10 exposures to a new food before it is accepted by a child,[33] that is, a child may refuse a food initially but learn to accept it with repeated exposure to it. Exposures can be any interaction with the food that involves multiple senses, even playing with the food before tasting it. Parent/caregiver modeling of trying new foods and enjoying mealtimes can also be helpful in promoting children's acceptance of a variety of foods.

The relationship between preferred foods and emotions has also been described in the literature. For example, children may have a preference for high fat or high sugar foods associated with social events or may desire foods that are used on a limited basis as a reward. Likewise, forcing children to eat foods can negatively affect their acceptance of these foods.[33–35] Young children display strong food likes and dislikes, and a fear of unfamiliar foods, **neophobia**, is common. **Food jags**, the repetitive intake of one or very few food items, are common with the preference for the foods described earlier but also the comfort that is brought by familiar foods. Suggestions to promote new foods include offering new foods with familiar foods, offering new foods in a similar form or texture to preferred foods (e.g., mashed, baked, or steamed), offering new foods in a form that will intrigue the child (e.g., shapes or with dipping sauces), starting with small portions, and offering praise even if the child only tastes the food. Large portion sizes can also be overwhelming for young children and parents often overestimate the amount of food needed. For example, the portion size recommendation for a toddler is 1 tbsp per year of age. Snacks are important to meet all nutrient needs given these small portion sizes, although

Table 5.4. Summary of Child Feeding Strategies
Respond appropriately to child hunger and satiety cues to promote self-regulation.
Avoid restrictive and forceful feeding practices to prevent desirability associated with particular foods.
Avoid food as reward to prevent emotional attachment to foods.
Promote a variety of foods through parental modeling.
Provide repeated exposures in different forms to increase acceptability of new foods.
Serve appropriate child-size portions to avoid overwhelming the child.
Serve foods in a positive environment with adult supervision and interaction; maintain family mealtimes as much as possible.
Include children in mealtime tasks such as preparation and cleanup to promote ownership of the foods being offered.
Provide acceptable choices to allow children to exert independence in the foods consumed.

Source: Adapted from Brown EJ. *Nutrition Through the Life Cycle.* Cengage Learning; 2019.

grazing, the continual ingestion of calories throughout the day, is advised against so that children come to mealtime with a healthy appetite. The amount eaten should be controlled by the child's hunger cues rather than the parents' pressure to eat more. Table 5.4 summarizes child feeding strategies based on the content of this chapter.

Young children have an **innate** (inborn, natural) ability to regulate their intake based on individual needs, but this ability is lost as children are exposed to more external cues to eating. That is, without external interference, children know when to eat and how much to eat.[36,37] While intake may vary from day to day, intake remains stable over a week's time.[38] However, children do not have the ability to self-select a balanced diet and that remains the responsibility of the parent. Ellyn Satter is a well-known authority on child feeding and developed the concept known as **division of responsibility** *in feeding*, considered a gold standard for feeding children (www.ellynsatterinstitute.org). Using the division of responsibility in child feeding sets the roles of the parent and child to promote a positive feeding environment without conflict or struggle. Using this principle, the child decides if they will eat and how much and the parent is responsible for establishing when (meal and snack schedule) and what the child will eat (offering a balanced diet with a variety of foods). By preventing grazing throughout the day, the child comes to the meal hungry and exercises independence with what they eat based on the internal hunger and fullness cues. The parent is not exerting any force that overrides the child's ability to self-regulate based on satiety. The child maintains some independence and choice as food habits are established. The role of parents helping children self-regulate becomes more important as they grow and expand on the number of stimuli that provide cues for eating.[39–45]

Responsive feeding refers to recognizing and responding to the child's hunger and fullness cues in an effort to help them learn to self-regulate. Signs that a child is hungry, particularly for toddlers who may not express hunger with words, include pointing to food, showing excitement at the sight of food, and using hand motions or sounds to indicate hunger. Likewise, a child may indicate they are full by turning away from food, turning the head away from food, or using hand motions or sound to indicate they are full. Parents are the largest influence on child feeding habits through determination of foods brought into the home, the way they are offered to the child, establishment of a positive feeding environment, and through their own modeling of foods eaten. Children thrive on routine mealtimes and imitating others in the home. Thus, parental nutritional knowledge, cooking ability, time constraints, and preference for convenience foods all affect the nutritional intake of children. The role of the public health nutrition professional is to offer information, support, and creative strategies to overcome these barriers to optimize the nutritional value of the child's diet.

Body image concerns may become apparent in school-age children as body fat increases to prepare for the adolescent growth spurt. BMI rebound, or **adiposity rebound,** which is an increase in BMI after infancy, typically occurring between ages 3 and 7 years, occurs earlier in females than males and may be associated with fears of overweight. Parental awareness of this stage of growth can be reassuring to children who are concerned with body weight or building more muscle at this stage. BMI rebound has only been associated with overweight and obesity when it occurs before the age of 5 years.[30,46,47] During this stage, physical development and motor coordination increase, leading to greater ability to participate in physical activity. Cognitive gains include the development of **self-efficacy** or confidence for performing a specific behavior, concrete operations, and cause-and-effect reasoning, leading to the formation of a sense of self and independence. With this growing independence comes the ability to determine activities and food choices with more external influences, such as peer pressure. Many outside influences in the school and social environment, including media, compete with desired food behaviors. Continued role-modeling by parents, setting family mealtimes, and involvement in food preparation are all associated with a higher quality diet in children.[48,49] Additionally, frequent eating outside the home is associated with higher calorie, fat, carbohydrate, and added sugar intake and lower fiber, milk, fruit, and vegetable intake among children.[50] Table 5.5 provides a summary of child feeding recommendations by age and stage covered in this section.

SOCIAL DETERMINANTS OF HEALTH FOR CHILDREN

Social determinants of health (SDOH) refer to the social, economic, and physical conditions that may affect an individual's health[51] and are very important for explaining disparities in health status. According to WHO, SDOH can be described as "the conditions in which people are born, grow, work, live, and age, and the wide set of forces and systems shaping the conditions of daily life."[2,52] SDOH include child maltreatment, child care and education, family financial support, physical environment, family social support, intimate partner violence, maternal depression and family mental illness, household substance abuse, firearm exposure, and parental health literacy. It is important to consider the effects of these factors on the availability of and access to food; for example, costs of medication may lead to trade-offs in food versus medicine within a family budget. SDOH also commonly affect the ability to obtain, cook, and store foods depending on available resources.

Healthy People 2030 takes a more focused approach on SDOH as critical to one's health, well-being, and quality of life, categorizing SDOH into five domains: economic stability, education access and quality, healthcare access and quality, neighborhood and built environment, and social and community context. Some examples specific to nutrition are

Table 5.5. Child Feeding Recommendations by Age and Stage	
12 to 36 months: Feeding toddlers	**Make food fun** • Offer different shapes and colors **Healthy snacks:** • Have healthy snacks available: - Fresh fruit - Yogurt - Vegetable sticks w/dip - Whole grain snacks: crackers, bread - Milk **Foods to avoid or limit:** - Junk food - Soft drinks - Sweets - Chips **Food refusal:**[a,b] • Try to stay calm. • Don't force a child to eat. • Offer new foods with familiar ones. • Start with a small serving and give more if hungry. • Encourage parents to be a positive role model for their child. **Mealtimes:** • At meals and snacks let children decide how much and even whether they eat from foods put on the table.[a,b] • Have three meals a day at set times with parent/caregiver involvement. • Offer sit-down snacks every 2 to 3 hours between times. • Let them eat their way: fingers or utensils, fast or slow, much or little, one or two foods, and in any order.[a,b] • Always supervise meals and snacks.
3 to 5 years: Feeding Preschoolers	**Foods:** • Meals can be simple: - 1 protein source—chicken - 1 whole grain—brown rice - 1 fruit—strawberries - 1 vegetable—green beans - 1 dairy—milk • Limit: processed foods and sugary drinks

(continued)

Table 5.5. Child Feeding Recommendations by Age and Stage (*continued*)

	Picky eaters:[c] • Continue to offer refused foods on multiple occasions. • Offer new foods with foods the child already likes. • Offer new foods at the beginning of the meal when the child is more hungry. **Mealtime:** • Have set mealtimes and limit snacking. • Involve children in simple meal prep tasks: pouring or stirring. It is okay if they make a mess! • Let children serve themselves.[c] • Do not force a child to finish everything on their plate.[c] • Turn off the TV and have a conversation instead. • Teach table manners. • Supervise meals and snacks. • Do not use food as a reward. • Do not use food to stop tantrums.

5 to 12 years: Feeding school-age children	**Foods:**
	• Provide a balanced diet including all food groups.
	• Avoid sugary drinks and snacks.
	• Offer healthy afterschool snack options:
	  - Fruit
	  - Vegetable and dip
	  - Yogurt
	  - Turkey sandwich
	Mealtime:
	• Always serve breakfast, even if it is "on the run."[d,e]
	• Allow the child to help with meal planning and preparation.[d,e]
	• Serve meals at the table, not in front of the TV.
	• Demonstrate healthy eating habits as a role model.

[a]HealthyChildren.org. Feeding & nutrition tips: your 3-year-old. Accessed September 28, 2022. https://www.healthychildren.org/English/ages-stages/toddler/nutrition/Pages/Feeding-and-Nutrition-Your-Three-Year-Old.aspx
[b]Better Health Channel. Eating tips for children (3)—older toddlers. Accessed September 28, 2022. https://www.betterhealth.vic.gov.au/health/healthyliving/eating-tips-for-older-toddlers
[c]Johns Hopkins Medicine. School-aged child nutrition. Published August 8, 2021. Accessed October 1, 2022. https://www.hopkinsmedicine.org/health/wellness-and-prevention/schoolaged-child-nutrition
[d]National Institute of Diabetes and Digestive and Kidney Diseases. Take charge of your health: a guide for teenagers. Accessed October 1, 2022. https://www.niddk.nih.gov/health-information/weight-management/take-charge-health-guide-teenagers
[e]MyPlate.gov. Healthy eating for teens. Accessed October 1, 2022. https://www.myplate.gov/tip-sheet/healthy-eating-teens

access to grocery stores or the financial ability to buy a variety of foods. These factors directly affect nutritional quality of the diet, nutritional status, and risk for chronic disease. Thus, improvement takes more than just promoting healthy foods, but making access to them possible by shifting the conditions in one's environment.

Child health outcomes in particular have been related to socioeconomic status, race, education, employment status, mental health, and family structure.[53] While some determinants may differ in relation to health outcomes, others, such as parental mental health and number of children in the household, are more universally associated with poor health outcomes. Poverty is a major SDOH affecting future health outcomes. Children of color, from single-parent households, and from immigrant families are most likely to live below the poverty line.[54] Living in impoverished conditions can lead to chronic stress, or toxic stress, affecting all areas of development from physical to cognitive health as well as risk for chronic disease in adulthood.[51,55] **Adverse childhood experiences (ACEs)** is a term used to refer to specific instances of child maltreatment, neglect, or exposure to parental substance abuse. ACEs have been linked to increased risk of chronic disease and costs of healthcare later in life.[52] For nutrition specifically, unmet social needs are related to **food insecurity** most directly, but also to indirect influences on nutritional status such as substance abuse, neglect, social isolation, and access to housing and utilities.

The AAP has called for greater attention to SDOH in clinical settings, through screening for social needs, familial risk factors, and ACEs that could predispose a child to unfavorable health outcomes.[52] Given the significant interplay between social factors and health outcomes, addressing SDOH from a young age has been suggested as a possible way to achieve the Triple Aim of healthcare: improving health quality and experiences, and reducing the cost of healthcare.[56] While the AAP supports SDOH screening within clinical settings in order to identify unmet social needs and adverse social circumstances, there is currently no standardized procedure or tool in existence and it may not be possible due to the many considerations of individual clinical practices. Screening is important for all clinicians and should be appropriate for the SDOH that affect each unique age and life stage as well as the most salient issues in a community. Screening practices could include multiple SDOH or specific areas such as food insecurity. Ultimately, effective practices for screening should include a team-based approach, incorporation into the electronic health record, and universal use to avoid any associated stigma. Many validated tools and associated resources exist for identifying SDOH[53] but point to the need for a more collaborative care model. Ideally, screening should identify a child/family's needs and connect them to the appropriate community support services, bridging the gap between healthcare and community health.[52] The role of the public health nutrition professional is crucial to care coordination and resource referrals with appropriate community agencies.

PUBLIC HEALTH NUTRITION ISSUES FOR CHILDREN

Poverty and Food Insecurity

Poverty is the leading public health issue related to nutritional status in children and falls within the domains of SDOH. In 2015, one in five children, or 15 million children, in the United States are living in poverty and 9 million are not covered by health insurance.[57] Some of the following issues are interrelated with poverty but are highlighted separately.

Food insecurity in young children aligns heavily with poverty and other SDOH that affect food access. In 2020, 14.8% of households with children were affected by food insecurity,[58] which means they struggled to provide enough food for their family due to limited resources at a given point during the year. Food insecurity rates were higher in single mother households, Black and Hispanic households, and those with incomes below the poverty line. Children accounted for 44% of SNAP (Supplemental Nutrition Assistance Program) participants in 2018. This is particularly concerning for young children with a high need for nutrients to support growth and development. Food insufficiency among children has been reported to manifest in behavioral, emotional, or academic problems.[59] Food insecurity effects on the various life cycle stages are discussed further in Chapter 8.

Overweight and Obesity

Overweight and obesity among young children is recognized as a major public health issue. The importance of developing healthy food habits, preferences, and behaviors early cannot be understated as they are highly indicative of dietary habits and consequential health outcomes later in life. Overweight and obesity disproportionately affect those from low-income and minority families.[60,61] While prevention is the preferred treatment for obesity, an expert committee formed from the American Medical Association and U.S. Department of Health and Human Services has published specific recommendations for the assessment, prevention, and treatment of child overweight and obesity.[62-65] Specific risk factors for overweight and obesity in young children include sedentary behaviors, SSB intake, screen time, skipping breakfast, eating outside the home, limited fruits and vegetables, and excessive portion sizes.[62,63] Overweight and obesity are more fully discussed in Chapter 10.

Eating Disorders

On the other hand, as children approach adolescence the potential development of **eating disorders** is also concerning. At this stage of development, body image and self-esteem take on increasing importance, coupled with social pressures from peers and social media that emphasize thinness for acceptance. Additional risk factors for eating disorders include underlying mental health issues such as depression, anxiety, or emotional trauma, as well as unhealthy family relationships that may include abuse or chaotic lifestyles. Common eating disorder categories include anorexia nervosa, associated with dietary restriction; bulimia nervosa, associated with purging; and binge eating disorder, accompanied by a cycle of binging and purging. An additional category, other specified feeding and eating disorders (OSFED), has been established to capture feeding and eating disorders that cause clinically significant distress but do not fully meet the criteria for one of the other disorders.[66] It is also important to mention orthorexia, an obsession with healthy eating, that currently has no formal diagnostic criteria. Early identification of risks and disordered eating behaviors for referral to the appropriate nutrition and mental health professionals are crucial for treatment and support as extreme behaviors can lead to nutritional deficiencies or even death. Treatment involves a team approach with potential interventions including a focus on making healthy lifestyle changes, body positivity, nutrition education, psychological therapy to treat the underlying emotional cause, restoration of body weight, and normalization of eating patterns.[67]

Special Conditions

Children may experience a multitude of special conditions related to premature birth, congenital anomalies, or genetic causes. Examples include cerebral palsy, disorders of nutrient metabolism, cleft lip and palate, physical defects, and Down syndrome, to name a few, as well as any accompanying developmental delays. **Special healthcare needs (SHCN)** is a generalized term used to capture this array of conditions as many are not diagnosed until the toddler or childhood age.[68] More specifically defined, children with special healthcare needs have or are at a high risk for a chronic physical, developmental, behavioral, or emotional condition and require health and related services of a type or amount beyond that required by children more generally. The special needs classification helps children receive support services without an official diagnosis. Of special needs children, 70% to 90% may have a nutrition-related problem.[69] Special conditions are associated with feeding difficulties such as oral-motor skills and swallowing, altered growth (short stature, failure to thrive, or obesity), drug-nutrient interactions, and the need for enteral or parenteral feeding support. Ultimately, a team of nutritional, medical, and developmental services are involved in the child's care. Public health programs to support families of special needs children include Early Intervention Programs, Early Head Start, WIC (Special Supplemental Nutrition Program for Women, Infants, and Children), state SHCN programs, and a variety of specialty clinics, formulas, and medical foods supported by the Maternal-Child Health Bureau of the U.S. Department of Health and Human Services.

Oral Health

Dental caries and compromised oral health are also related to continual drinking of SSBs throughout the day, another public health concern for children. Dental caries affect 37% of children in the United States, with rates increasing by age group (23% ages 2–5 and 56% ages 6–8). By adolescence, 58% of children have experienced some level of tooth decay.[70] Caution should be taken to limit food and beverage sources with added sugars. Recommendations for juice intake and added sugar intake were previously discussed. The American Academy of Pediatric Dentistry (AAPD) encourages healthcare providers and caregivers to implement preventive practices that can decrease a child's risks of developing tooth decay, including avoiding sugar-sweetened foods and beverages as well as maintaining oral hygiene measures and regular dental care.[71] The public health nutrition professional should include information about sugar intake and dental care in their work with children and families.

A confounding factor related to oral health is lack of fluoride intake, which depends on living situations and access to fluoridated water. For example, cities may provide fluoridated water, but rural areas depend on well water. A child's water consumption may vary between home and day care or school environments depending on these locations as well. Water used to prepare other beverages in the home should be considered a source if water is fluoridated, and fluoridated toothpaste is also a source once children begin brushing their teeth. Parents should consult with a child's physician for the most current recommendations on fluoride supplementation if there is a concern about these sources in the home. The American Dental Association, AAP, and AAPD make recommendations based on the water supply and age of the child.[72] Recommendations should be followed to prevent consumption of too much fluoride which leads to **fluorosis**, white or brown staining of the teeth caused by excessive ingestion of fluoride before the teeth have erupted.[72]

Food Allergies

Food allergies now affect 5% to 10% of preschool children.[73] **Food allergy** prevalence may be increasing due to better detection, sterile environments, timing of complementary foods, secondhand smoke, and low vitamin D in infants.[74] The most common allergens, referred to as the Big 8, account for 90% of allergic reactions: eggs, dairy, peanuts, tree nuts, fish, shellfish, wheat, and soy (but rarer cases can include any foods). Of these, milk, egg, and peanut allergies are most common among young children, affecting up to 5%.[75] Many children will outgrow allergies to milk, egg, and wheat, but not nuts.[75] If an allergy is suspected, it is important to direct families to their pediatrician for appropriate testing. Methods of testing include skin pricks, blood tests, skin patches, and oral food challenges.[76,77] Upon diagnosis, the nutrition professional can assist families with label reading to identify potential allergenic ingredients, locating affordable alternatives to preferred foods, coordinating with school meal staff, and navigating the effects of the allergy on the diet of the entire family.

Foodborne Illness

Foodborne illness is more common among children than adults given their lower immune capacity for handling an exposure to microorganisms. Common causes of foodborne illness include raw and undercooked meats, poultry, and eggs and unpasteurized food and drink, particularly milk and soft cheeses.[78] The Dietary Guidelines include food safety recommendations, and the FightBAC program developed by the Partnership for Food Safety Education provides food safety messaging in four areas: washing hands and surfaces often (Clean); avoiding cross-contamination (Separate); cooking to proper temperatures (Cook); and refrigerating promptly (Chill).[3] Put another way, most food safety behaviors can be classified under personal hygiene, cross-contamination, and temperature control. Food safety practices are important in the home, child care centers, and food retail locations. State cooperative extension agencies offer high-quality food safety resources for families and organizations. If foodborne illness is suspected in a child, parents should seek immediate medical attention.

Social Influences

School-age children are exposed to a growing number of external influences to food intake as they transition to greater time outside the home environment. Peers take on an increasing role in shaping food preferences and attitudes, as well as exposure to new foods. Children are making independent choices in school meal selections, afterschool snacks, and vending options. With increased screen time also comes greater exposure to food advertising. There is strong evidence that media impacts the amount and type of food consumed by children, including a preference for brand-name foods.[79] Advertised foods are often high in fat, sodium, and added sugars, and low in nutrients.[80,81] Many advertisements are for sugar-sweetened cereals or fast foods. Advertising for these foods is also fun, colorful, and exciting to entice young children. The average reported screen time for older children is 7.5 hours per day[82] and up to 2.5 hours per day for toddlers and preschool children.[83] Increased screen time is associated with increased risk for overweight and obesity due to the displacement of physical activity habits.[84] A confounding concern is the consumption of snacks, often in uncontrolled portions, while watching television or using the internet. Snacking makes up about 25% of daily calorie consumption for children ages 4 to 13, a significant amount when considering the low nutrient value of common snack foods.[85] In fact, most snack calories have been documented as coming from desserts and sweetened beverages.[86,87] Children take in 10% to 15% of total calories from SSBs and 50% of children ages 2 to 5 consume soft drinks).[21,88,89] Nutrition education efforts within schools and for families should equip children for making their own nutrient-dense food selections in these situations.

Physical Activity

The Dietary Guidelines and the AAP support recommendations for regular physical activity among children of all ages.[3,90] Physical activity patterns are considered here as a complementary aspect of healthy lifestyle behaviors in children, their role in supporting growth and development, and as a means of healthy weight management. Specific recommendations include promoting active play of a variety of activities and intensity levels among toddlers and preschoolers for 3 hours each day. For school-age children, 60 minutes per day of moderate to vigorous activity is encouraged, and should include a mixture of aerobic and strength-building activities for muscles and bones.[3] Likewise, it is recommended that screen time be eliminated for toddlers and limited to 2 hours per day or less for all other children. The most recent data suggest that only about 25% of children ages 6 to 13 are meeting the daily recommendations for physical activity, and this is a target for improvement in the *Healthy People 2030* objectives.[2]

Supplementation

All nutrient needs can be met by consuming a varied diet, and that is the preferred way to get nutrients due to the other health benefits offered by whole foods. In some cases, however, a child may need *supplementation* to ensure basic needs are met. First and foremost, if a child has a documented nutrient deficiency or is at high risk of developing a nutrient deficiency, the AAP recommends supplementation. Examples of children at risk for nutrient deficiency include those with inadequate appetite or following fad diets, those suffering from parental abuse or neglect, those with chronic disease, those who participate in a dietary program for weight management, those who consume a vegetarian diet without dairy products, and those who follow a vegan diet.[30] Despite these recommendations, young children have been documented to be major users of supplementation[91] and are typically the children least likely to benefit from supplementation, that is, those with adequate household incomes who already consume an adequate and varied diet. Caution should also be raised regarding the intake of multiple supplements that may risk exceeding the tolerable upper intake levels of nutrients. The role of the public health nutrition practitioner is to assess the risk of nutrient deficiency and refer families to a registered dietitian/nutritionist to guide them to appropriate supplemental products and amounts if there is a concern. The use of supplements other than vitamin/mineral supplements (e.g., herbal products) in young children should also be assessed by a registered dietitian/nutritionist or physician so that families can be guided to appropriate information on their use, safety, and monitoring (www.nccih.nih.gov).[92-94]

POPULATION CONSIDERATIONS

Several considerations are important from a population health perspective related to nutrition intake and behaviors established in childhood. First and foremost, dietary patterns established in childhood have been shown to carry into adulthood and thus affect health outcomes.[15,95,96] Nutrition behaviors in young children are strongly influenced by their external environment including parents, families, caregivers, peers, and media exposures. Nutrition messaging should promote healthy dietary patterns in line with the dietary guidelines and including a variety of nutrient-dense foods, prevention of excess weight gain, and inclusion of regular physical activity. Children are experiencing various stages of growth and development, and these rates and patterns vary from child to child. Thus, the overarching nutritional recommendations from this chapter should be promoted, but strategies for more focused assessment and intervention may need an individualized approach. In these cases, referral to the appropriate health professional, such as the registered dietitian, is essential. Examples from this chapter include vegetarian diets, iron deficiency, and childhood obesity. Children need adequate nutrients to prevent deficiencies, but also to support optimal growth, development, and health for a lifetime. Finally, all children need to learn self-feeding skills and develop a healthful relationship with food. Promotion of a positive feeding environment in the home including family mealtimes and avoiding the use of force, punishment, or reward associated with eating are critical because the home and family are the number one influence on a child's eating habits; family mealtimes play a significant role in improving nutritional quality of the diet as well as weight status in children.[48,49] Establishing these foundations will help to maintain a healthy dietary intake even in the midst of the multiple competing external influences described in this chapter.

POLICY: GLOBAL ISSUES AND CHALLENGES

Successful child feeding is associated not only with optimal growth and development but also with childhood survival. Nutrition challenges range from the extremes of malnutrition to obesity, with various nutrient deficiencies in between. Globally, undernutrition is associated with 2.7 million childhood deaths per year, accounting for 45% of overall childhood deaths.[97] In 2020, 149 million children worldwide under the age of 5 were classified as *stunted* (too short for age), 45 million were estimated to be *wasted* (too thin for age), and nearly 40 million were overweight or obese. Iron and vitamin A deficiencies are the most common micronutrient deficiencies affecting nearly 42% and 30%, respectively, of young children worldwide.[98] Vitamin A deficiency is attributable to significant numbers of blindness and death each year.[97] The Global Burden of Disease study[99] documents the significant public health impact of these deficiencies. Along with breastfeeding recommendations, discussed in Chapter 4, WHO's global strategy for infant and young child feeding promotes targeted policies and interventions to improve child growth, development, health, and survival. Specific objectives include raising awareness of the issues, building government and organizational commitment to solutions, and creating an environment where all families can make informed decisions about feeding practices for their children.[100] The global nutrition targets for 2025, specific to young children, include reducing the number of children under 5 who are **stunted** by 40%, ensuring that there is no increase in childhood overweight prevalence, and reducing childhood **wasting** to less than 5%.[101]

PUBLIC HEALTH NUTRITION PROGRAMS FOR CHILDREN

Federal child nutrition programs in the United States aim to ameliorate the effects of poverty, food insecurity, and poor nutrition described in this chapter. In fact, there is a great deal of evidence demonstrating that these programs are effective for reducing food insecurity, alleviating poverty, supporting economic stability, improving dietary intake and the nutrition environment, protecting against obesity, improving health outcomes, and boosting learning and development.[102] Table 5.6 provides a summary of federal nutrition programs that support children and families with children.

Table 5.6. Summary of Federal Child Nutrition Programs

Program Name	Description	Reach of Services	Eligibility	Website
WIC: Special Supplemental Nutrition Program for Women, Infants, and Children	Provides nutritional support to low-income women, infants, and children by providing foods, formula, and nutrition education	Provides farmers market vouchers Provides benefits to over 1.59 million participants	Children 0–5 years Pregnant, breast-feeding, and post-partum women	www.fns.usda.gov/wic
SNAP: Supplemental Nutrition Assistance Program	Provides supplemental income for the purchase of food for low-income families	The average SNAP benefit is $104 per month Over 248,000 participating food retailers	All ages; must be at or below 130% of the poverty line to qualify	www.fns.usda.gov/snap/supplemental-nutrition-assistance-program
TEFAP: The Emergency Food Assistance Program	Provides food items to food banks, food pantries, and soup kitchens to be given out to the community. Most participants who enroll are older adults who have an income high enough to disqualify them for SNAP benefits.	In 2020, TEFAP provided over 2.4 billion meals.	All ages	www.fns.usda.gov/tefap/emergency-food-assistance-program
School Meals: Breakfast, Lunch, Summer	Assists low-income families by providing reduced or free school lunches in public schools, nonprofit private schools, and child care facilities. During the summer children also qualify for the Summer Food Service Program that provides nutritious meals and snacks.	About 7.1 million children participate in the school lunch program.	PreK–12 students	www.fns.usda.gov/nslp
CACFP: Child and Adult Care Food Program	Reimburses child care and adult care facilities for meals and snacks that are served	Children participating in CACFP programs improved their intake of fruits and whole grains.	0–18 years and 60+ years	www.fns.usda.gov/cacfp

In addition to these federally supported programs, a variety of nongovernmental and nonprofit organizations from the local to global level also exist to support child nutrition needs. Examples include community food pantries, mobile food pantries and food lockers, school backpack programs, and the United Nations Children's Fund (UNICEF) supporting the nutrition needs of children in developing countries (www.feedingamerica.org, www.unicef.org).

WHAT WORKS: CHILD AND ADULT CARE FOOD PROGRAM

The Child and Adult Care Food Program (CACFP) is a federal program that provides reimbursements for nutritious meals and snacks to eligible children and adults who are enrolled for care at participating child care centers, day care homes, and adult day care centers. CACFP also provides reimbursements for meals served to children and youth participating in after-school care programs, children residing in emergency shelters, and adults over the age of 60 or living with a disability and enrolled in day care facilities (fns.usda.gov/cacfp). To qualify for reimbursement through CACFP, meals and snacks must meet specific meal component requirements and be served in minimum portion size amounts. The four meal component requirements at the time of this study were milk, fruit or vegetable, grains or bread, and meat or meat alternative (such as cheese, eggs, peanut butter, or tofu). A recent study of nutrition and activity in child care settings was conducted by the USDA.[103] Findings revealed that the majority of meals were meeting these requirements (88% of lunches and 97% of breakfasts and snacks). In fact, the meal level benchmarks for food groups exceeded those established by the USDA and the nutritional quality of CACFP meals offered was determined to be better than the average child's diet. While there is room for improvement to align with the Dietary Guidelines, and despite food waste of about one quarter of calories served, children ages 3 to 5 consumed three fifths or more of the minimum required components, contributing significantly to children's nutrient intake on child care days. Additionally, CAFCP meal participation was reported to improve diet quality specific to fruit and whole grain consumption among racially and ethnically diverse children in participating programs.[104] With CACFP reimbursement rates of 20% to 50% in food and labor costs, more early child care programs could benefit from increased reimbursement rates. Interestingly, almost all early child care programs offered at least one daily opportunity for physical activity with an average of 96 minutes/day.

SUMMARY

This chapter highlights the importance of dietary pattern formation during childhood on food intake habits that will influence health over the life span. Overarching nutritional goals during this stage include growth, nutrient density, and the development of a healthy relationship with food. Understanding the many factors that affect dietary choices can help identify the appropriate public health nutrition resources and supports needed by families with young children.

KEY CHAPTER CONCEPTS

1. The foundations for dietary patterns and health outcomes are established during childhood.
2. Nutrition behaviors are shaped by multiple factors, positive and negative, in the child's environment, but ultimately by the family and home environment.

3. Children's diets are lacking in key micronutrients and abundant in less nutrient-dense options such as added fats and sugars.
4. Nutrition messaging should aim to promote nutrient-dense food options, regular physical activity, and healthful food behaviors, and prevent excess weight gain.
5. Respect individual growth patterns of children and intervene appropriately upon significant deviations.
6. Identification of influences on children's dietary habits can offer areas for support or improvement.
7. Referrals to the appropriate nutrition and healthcare professionals are necessary for key childhood nutritional concerns such as nutrient deficiency, foodborne illness, eating disorders, and food allergies.
8. Build awareness for SDOH that impact food intake of children and offer support through available community, state, federal, or international programs.

CASE STUDY

J is a 6-year-old boy who lives with his father, Mr. W, and his 3-year-old sister in a farmhouse located on some acreage in a rural county. They live about 6 miles outside the nearest small town, population 3,000, where you are working at a community health clinic. J attends first grade at the county elementary school, and his sister attends all-day preschool in the same building. J's father has stable employment in a lower income job, but it does provide state workers' health insurance.

J's height and weight were recently measured by his general practice physician at J's 6-year well-child visit. His BMI exceeded the 95th percentile, placing him in the obese category. You receive a referral from J's physician to speak with Mr. W, and Mr. W schedules an appointment with you. Upon speaking with Mr. W, you learn the following:

Mr. W's job is demanding, and he finds himself returning home tired and stressed after picking up his children from their afterschool program. The last thing he feels like doing is preparing a home-cooked dinner, so often he purchases take-out from a local fast-food restaurant or grocery store deli. Otherwise, he makes sandwiches, scrambles eggs, or microwaves frozen meals. Other than apples, bananas, canned corn, and frozen peas, the family doesn't consume many fresh fruits and vegetables. Meals are often eaten in front of the TV. Breakfast is usually consumed in a hurry, and often consists of Pop-Tarts or granola bars eaten in the car while the children are being driven to school. The children often have a sugary juice drink for breakfast, which is less expensive than real orange juice. Mr. W knows he should cut back on J's screen time, but he hasn't prioritized this task. There is always so much to do at home once he picks up the children from school.

Mr. W is concerned that the doctor told him that J was too heavy. He has participated in the employee wellness program at his job, and has learned that childhood obesity is a major problem in the United States. He knows that J's diet is not ideal, and he wants to help his son avoid weight-related health problems in the future.

1. What are some considerations about J's weight status and growth chart percentile based on the content of this chapter?
2. Given what you know about J's living situation, what SDOH might be affecting his nutritional and weight status?
3. Identify at least three nutrition themes discussed in this chapter that are reflected by the presented case study.

4. What nutrients may be lacking in J's diet based on the reported intake? What nutrients might he be consuming in excess?
5. In your discussion, Mr. W tells you, "I do my best, but I just don't know how to cook, and I don't have time, anyway. Is there anything I can do to help J without needing to cook fancy meals?" How would you address his concern?
6. Based on the content of the chapter, what are three suggestions you would make for this family regarding food intake/behaviors?
7. Which community programs (federal, local, nonprofit) would be the most helpful for this family and why?
8. While the focus is on J, are there additional concerns for his 3-year-old sister based on the information in this chapter? Are there any additional resources that may be helpful to the food and nutrition needs of a younger child?

DISCUSSION QUESTIONS

1. Name the three overarching nutritional goals for childhood.
2. Review the *Healthy People 2030* objectives related to young children. Select two goals and consider interventions that may help us reach these goals.
3. Describe the pattern of growth from toddler through middle childhood. How does this growth parallel differences in eating skills and nutritional needs among childhood stages?
4. Discuss some common themes regarding feeding recommendations that support optimal intake for children across ages and stages (feeding skills and nutritional value).
5. Identify common nutritional areas for public health concern among children. For which of these should further intervention be referred to other health professionals?
6. Name some influences on children's dietary preferences and habits. What is the most important influence and why?
7. Think about the influences from childhood that shaped your eating habits. Describe one eating preference or habit you still hold from that time.
8. What are some tips you could recommend to parents struggling with a picky eater?
9. What SDOH impact dietary adequacy and intake among children?
10. Identify three common public health nutrition support programs designed to improve the nutritional quality of children's diets.

SUGGESTED LEARNING ACTIVITIES

1. Seek experience with a federal or nonprofit program that serves to meet the nutritional needs of children. Note how your experience and observations related to the information presented in this chapter.
2. Conduct an assessment of a child's intake for your own child, a friend, family member, community member, or client. Collect a dietary record for 1 to 3 days. Comparing the diet to the Dietary Guidelines, what food groups are lacking? What micronutrients might be of concern? Are there any other consumption or mealtime behavior patterns that may not be ideal based on the information presented in the chapter? What recommendations might you provide to improve the child's intake?

3. A female child is measured at 6-month intervals with the measurements and percentiles noted in Table 5.7. Are there any red flags based on this information? What could be reasons for the percentile increase in weight from 2.5 to 3 years of age? How might you intervene further based on this pattern?

Table 5.7. Weight and Height Measurements for a Female Child From 2 to 4 Years of Age

Age	Weight/Percentile	Height/Percentile
2 years	23.5 lb/10th	81 cm/10th
2.5 years	25 lb/10th	86 cm/10th
3 years	28 lb/25th	89 cm/10th
3.5 years	30 lb/25th	95 cm/25th
4 years	30 lb/10th	98 cm/25th

4. Identify local resources to help parents of young children in your area seek food and nutrition information and support. Create a flyer or brochure to share this information with the community.
5. Picky eating is very common among young children. Conduct an internet search for strategies to encourage new foods for picky eaters. What can you find to add to the information provided in this chapter? Consider creating a one-page infographic with the most successful strategies parents can use to promote new foods. What would you include? What strategies do you see repeatedly in the resources you review, and based on the chapter, which strategies do you think might work best?
6. Consider the implementation of SDOH screening at your facility. What would be important to include on the screening tool? Review some established screening tools to compare and contrast items included. Would one of these tools work effectively for your organization or community? Why or why not? What adaptations would you suggest?

RESOURCES FOR FURTHER LEARNING

- American Academy of Pediatrics: www.aap.org
  - Provides evidence-based information on optimal physical, mental, and social health and well-being for all children
- Centers for Disease Control and Prevention, National Center for Health Services, CDC Growth Charts: www.cdc.gov/growthcharts
  - Provides up-to-date percentile curves showing the distribution of selected body measurements in children, used to track childhood growth
- School Nutrition Association: https://schoolnutrition.org
  - Provides resources for advancing the accessibility, quality, and integrity of school meal programs
- Bright Futures: www.brightfutures.org
  - Includes education center and information about the components of the Bright Futures Project, a national health promotion project aimed at achieving optimal health for every child

- Child Nutrition Programs (National School Lunch, School Breakfast, Special Milk, Summer Food Service, and Child and Adult Care Food Programs): www.fns.usda.gov/child-nutrition-programs
  - Describes federally funded programs to support child nutrition through schools and child care facilities
- Team Nutrition: www.fns.usda.gov/tn/team-nutrition
  - An initiative of the USDA Food and Nutrition Service that provides resources for child nutrition programs
- The Center for Health and Health Care in Schools: www.healthinschools.org
  - Provides school-connected strategies for better health and school outcomes for children
- Model School Wellness Policies: www.schoolwellnesspolicies.org
  - Provides resources to assist school districts and stakeholders in updating and implementing school wellness policies
- Ellyn Satter Institute: www.ellynsatterinstitute.org
  - Evidence-based child feeding guidance for professionals, the public, and organizations
- United Nations Children's Fund: www.unicef.org
  - Information about international work to support child health
- Kids Count Data Center: www.datacenter.kidscount.org
  - Data about child health indicators, searchable by location.

SPRINGER PUBLISHING CONNECT™

A robust set of instructor resources designed to supplement this text is located at http://connect.springerpub.com/content/book/978-0-8261-8623-2. Qualifying instructors may request access by emailing textbook@springerpub.com.

REFERENCES

1. Center on Hunger, Poverty and Nutrition Policy. *Statement on the Link between Nutrition and Cognitive Development in Children*. Tufts University, School of Nutrition Science and Policy; 1994.
2. Office of Disease Prevention and Health Promotion. Child and adolescent development. *Healthy People 2030*. U.S. Department of Health and Human Services. Accessed October 19, 2023. https://health.gov/healthypeople/objectives-and-data/browse-objectives/child-and-adolescent-development
3. U.S. Department of Agriculture, U.S. Department of Health and Human Services. *Dietary Guidelines for Americans, 2020–2025*. 9th ed. U.S. Department of Health and Human Services; 2020. https://www.dietaryguidelines.gov
4. U.S. Department of Agriculture. ChooseMyPlate. Accessed October 19, 2023. https://www.myplate.gov
5. National Institutes of Health. Nutrient recommendations and databases. Accessed October 19, 2023. https://ods.od.nih.gov/HealthInformation/Dietary_Reference_Intakes.aspx
6. Kliegman RM, Stanton BF, St. Geme JW III, Schor NF, Behrman RE, eds. *Nelson's Textbook of Pediatrics*. 20th ed. Elsevier; 2016.
7. Centers for Disease Control and Prevention. CDC growth charts. National Center for Health Statistics. Updated December 15, 2022. http://www.cdc.gov/growthcharts/cdc_charts.htm
8. Brown JE. *Nutrition Through the Life Cycle*. 7th ed. Cengage Learning; 2019.
9. Institute of Medicine. *Dietary Reference Intakes for Energy, Carbohydrate, Fiber, Fat, Fatty Acids, Cholesterol, Protein, and Amino Acids*. National Academies Press; 2005.
10. Skinner JD, Carruth BR, Houck KS, et al. Longitudinal study of nutrient and food intakes of white preschool children aged 24 to 60 months. *J Am Diet Assoc*. 1999;99(12):1514–1521. https://doi.org/10.1016/S0002-8223(99)00371-5

11. Academy of Nutrition and Dietetics. Position of the Academy of Nutrition and Dietetics: nutrition guidance for healthy children ages 2-11 Years. *J Acad Nutr Diet*. 2014;114:1257–1276.
12. U.S. Food and Drug Administration. Advice about eating fish for those who might become or are pregnant or breastfeeding and children ages 1–11 years. Updated October 2021. https://www.fda.gov/food/consumers/advice-about-eating-fish
13. Institute of Medicine. *Dietary Reference Intakes for Calcium and Vitamin D*. National Academies Press; 2011. https://www.ncbi.nlm.nih.gov/books/NBK56070
14. Institute of Medicine. *Dietary Reference Intakes for Vitamin A, Vitamin K, Arsenic, Boron, Chromium, Copper, Iodine, Iron, Manganese, Molybdenum, Nickel, Silicon, Vanadium, and Zinc*. National Academies Press; 2001. https://www.ncbi.nlm.nih.gov/books/NBK222310
15. Nicklas TA, Hayes D. Position of the American Dietetic Association: nutrition guidance for healthy children ages 2 to 11 years. *J Am Diet Assoc*. 2008;108(6):1038–1047. https://doi.org/10.1016/j.jada.2008.04.005
16. Centers for Disease Control and Prevention. Iron deficiency—United States, 1999–2000. *MMWR Morb Mortal Wkly Rep*. 2002;51(40):897–899. https://doi.org/10.1001/jama.288.17.2114-jwr1106-2-1
17. Jiang Y, Ekono M, Skinner C. *Basic Facts About Low-Income Children: Children Under 6 Years, 2013*. National Center for Children in Poverty; 2015. https://www.nccp.org/wp-content/uploads/2015/01/text_1097.pdf
18. Centers for Disease Control and Prevention. Recommendations to prevent and control iron deficiency in the United States. *MMWR Recomm Rep*. 1998;47(RR-3):1–29. https://www.cdc.gov/mmwr/preview/mmwrhtml/00051880.htm
19. Baker RD, Greer FR, American Academy of Pediatrics Committee on Nutrition. Diagnosis and prevention of iron deficiency and iron deficiency anemia in infants and young children (0 to 3 years of age). *Pediatrics*. 2010;126(5):1040–1050. https://doi.org/10.1542/peds.2010-2576
20. Centers for Disease Control and Prevention. *Foods and Drinks to Avoid or Limit*. Accessed October 19, 2023. https://www.cdc.gov/nutrition/infantandtoddlernutrition/foods-and-drinks/foods-and-drinks-to-limit.html
21. American Academy of Pediatrics, Kleinman RE, eds. *Pediatric Nutrition Handbook*. 6th ed. American Academy of Pediatrics; 2009.
22. Picciano MF, Smiciklas-Wright H, Birch LL, Mitchell DC, Murray-Kolb L, McConahy KL. Nutritional guidance is needed during dietary transition in early childhood. *Pediatrics*. 2000;106:109–114. https://doi.org/10.1542/peds.106.1.109
23. Bowman SA, Gortmaker SL, Ebbeling CB, Pereira MA, Ludwig DS. Effects of fast-food consumption on energy intake and diet quality among children in a national household survey. *Pediatrics*. 2004;113:112–118. https://doi.org/10.1542/peds.113.1.112
24. American Academy of Pediatrics, Committee on Nutrition. The use and misuse of fruit juice in pediatrics. *Pediatrics*. 2001;107(5):1210–1213. https://doi.org/10.1542/peds.107.5.1210
25. American Academy of Pediatrics, Committee on Environmental Health. Lead exposure in children: prevention, detection, and management. *Pediatrics*. 2005;116:1036–1046. https://doi.org/10.1542/peds.2005-1947
26. U.S. Preventive Services Task Force. *Recommendation Statement: Elevated Blood Lead Levels in Children and Pregnant Women: Screening*. Agency for Healthcare Research and Quality; 2019. https://www.uspreventiveservicestaskforce.org/uspstf/recommendation/elevated-blood-lead-levels-in-childhood-and-pregnancy-screening
27. Centers for Disease Control and Prevention Advisory Committee on Childhood Lead Poisoning Prevention. Interpreting and managing blood lead levels <10 μg/dL in children and reducing childhood exposures to lead: recommendations of CDC's Advisory Committee on Childhood Lead Poisoning Prevention. *MMWR Recomm Rep*. 2007;56(RR-8):1–16. https://www.cdc.gov/mmwr/preview/mmwrhtml/rr5608a1.htm
28. Binns HJ, Campbell C, Brown MJ. Interpreting and managing blood lead levels of less than 10 mcg/dL in children and reducing childhood exposure to lead: recommendations of the Centers for Disease Control and Prevention Advisory Committee on Childhood Lead Poisoning Prevention. *Pediatrics*. 2007;120:e1285–e1298. https://doi.org/10.1542/peds.2005-1770
29. Centers for Disease Control and Prevention. Blood lead reference value. https://www.cdc.gov/nceh/lead/data/blood-lead-reference-value.htm
30. Advisory Committee on Childhood Lead Poisoning Prevention. *Low Level Lead Exposure Harms Children: A Renewed Call for Primary Prevention*. Centers for Disease Control and Prevention; 2012. https://www.cdc.gov/nceh/lead/acclpp/final_document_030712.pdf

31. Holt K, Woolridge NH, Story M, Sofka D, eds. *Bright Futures Nutrition*. American Academy of Pediatrics; 2011.
32. Chess S, Thomas A. Dynamics of individual behavioral development. In: Levine MD, Carey WB, Crocker AC, eds. *Developmental-Behavioral Pediatrics*. WB Saunders; 1992:84–94.
33. Fisher JO, Mitchell DC, Smiciklas-Wright H, Birch LL. Parental influences on young girls' fruit and vegetable, micronutrient, and fat intakes. *J Am Diet Assoc*. 2002;102:58–64. https://doi.org/10.1016/s0002-8223(02)90017-9
34. Birch LL, Fisher JO. Development of eating behaviors among children and adolescents. *Pediatrics*. 1998;101(3 pt 2):539–549. https://doi.org/10.1542/peds.101.S2.539
35. Birch LL, Fisher JO. Appetite and eating behavior in children. *Pediatr Clin North Am*. 1995;42:931–953. https://doi.org/10.1016/s0031-3955(16)40023-4
36. Satter E. The feeding relationship: problems and interventions. *J Pediatr*. 1990;117:181–189. https://doi.org/10.1016/s0022-3476(05)80017-4
37. Birch LL. Children's food acceptance patterns. *Nutr Today*. 1996;31:234–240. https://doi.org/10.1097/00017285-199611000-00003
38. Birch LL, Johnson SL, Andresen G, Peters JC, Schulte MC. The variability of young children's energy intake. *N Engl J Med*. 1991;324:232–235. https://doi.org/10.1056/NEJM199101243240405
39. Birch LL, Fisher JO. Food intake regulation in children, fat and sugar substitutes and intake. *Ann N Y Acad Sci*. 1997;819:194–220. https://doi.org/10.1111/j.1749-6632.1997.tb51809.x
40. Rolls BJ, Engell D, Birch LL. Serving portion size influences 5-year-old but not 3-year-old children's food intake. *J Am Diet Assoc*. 2000;100:232–234. https://doi.org/10.1016/S0002-8223(00)00070-5
41. Fisher JO, Rolls BJ, Birch LL. Children's bite size and intake of an entrée are greater with large portions than with age-appropriate or self-selected portions. *Am J Clin Nutr*. 2003;77:1164–1170. https://doi.org/10.1093/ajcn/77.5.1164
42. Fisher JO, Birch LL. Parents' restrictive feeding practices are associated with young girls' negative self-evaluation of eating. *J Am Diet Assoc*. 2000;100:1341–1346. https://doi.org/10.1016/S0002-8223(00)00378-3
43. Davison KK, Birch LL. Weight status, parent reaction, and self-concept in five-year-old girls. *Pediatrics*. 2001;107:46–53. https://doi.org/10.1542/peds.107.1.46
44. Abramovitz BA, Birch LL. Five-year-old girls' ideas about dieting are predicted by their mothers' dieting. *J Am Diet Assoc*. 2000;100:1157–1163. https://doi.org/10.1016/S0002-8223(00)00339-4
45. Satter E. Feeding dynamics: helping children to eat well. *J Pediatr Health Care*. 1995;9:178–184. https://doi.org/10.1016/s0891-5245(05)80033-1
46. Dietz WH. Critical periods in childhood for the development of obesity. *Am J Clin Nutr*. 1994;59:955–959. https://doi.org/10.1093/ajcn/59.5.955
47. Hughes AR, Sherriff A, Ness AR, Reilly JJ. Timing of adiposity rebound and adiposity in adolescence. *Pediatrics*. 2014;134:e1354–e1361. https://doi.org/10.1542/peds.2014-1908
48. Hammons AJ, Fiese BH. Is frequency of shared family meals related to the nutrition health of children and adolescents? *Pediatrics*. 2001;127(6):e1565–e1574. https://doi.org/10.1542/peds.2010-1440
49. Scaglioni S, Arrizza C, Vecchi F, Tedeschi S. Determinants of children's eating behavior. *Am J Clin Nutr*. 2011;94(6 suppl):2006S–2011S. https://doi.org/10.3945/ajcn.110.001685
50. Kranz S, Smiciklas-Wright H, Siega-Riz AM, Mitchell D. Adverse effect of high added sugar consumption on dietary intake in American preschoolers. *J Pediatr*. 2005;146:105–111. https://doi.org/10.1016/j.jpeds.2004.08.077
51. Francis L, DePriest K, Wilson M, Gross D. Child poverty, toxic stress, and social determinants of health: screening and care coordination. *Online J Issues Nurs*. 2018;23(3):2. https://doi.org/10.3912/OJIN.Vol23No03Man02
52. Narayan A, Raphael J, Rattler T, Bocchini C. Social determinants of health: screening in the clinical setting. Center for Child Health Policy and Advocacy at Texas Children's Hospital. May 14, 2018. https://www.texaschildrens.org/sites/default/files/uploads/documents/83176%20BRIEF%20Social%20Determinants%20of%20Health%20Policy%20Digital.pdf
53. Victorino CC, Gauthier AH. The social determinants of child health: variations across health outcomes—a population-based cross-sectional analysis. *BMC Pediatr*. 2009;9:53. https://doi.org/10.1186/1471-2431-9-53
54. Chung EK, Siegel BS, Garg A, et al. Screening for social determinants of health among children and families living in poverty: a guide for clinicians. *Curr Probl Pediatr Adolesc Health Care*. 2016;46(5):135–153. https://doi.org/10.1016/j.cppeds.2016.02.004
55. Shonkoff JP, Garner AS, Committee on Psychosocial Aspects of Child and Family Health, Committee on Early Childhood, Adoption, and Dependent Care, Section on Developmental and Behavioral

Pediatrics. The lifelong effects of early childhood adversity and toxic stress. *Pediatrics*. 2012;129(1):e232–e246. https://doi.org/10.1542/peds.2011-2663

56. Institute for Healthcare Improvement. *The IHI Triple Aim*. Accessed October 19, 2023. http://www.ihi.org/Engage/Initiatives/TripleAim/Pages/default.aspx
57. Annie E. Casey Foundation. Demographics. Kids Count Data Center. Accessed October 18, 2023. https://datacenter.aecf.org/
58. Coleman-Jensen A, Rabbitt MP, Gregory CA, Singh A. *Household Food Security in the United States in 2017*. ERR-256. U.S. Department of Agriculture, Economic Research Service; 2018. https://www.ers.usda.gov/webdocs/publications/90023/err-256.pdf
59. Shankar P, Chung R, Frank DA. Association of food insecurity with children's behavioral, emotional, and academic outcomes: a systematic review. *J Dev Behav Pediatr*. 2017 Feb/Mar;38(2):135–150. https://doi.org/10.1097/DBP.0000000000000383
60. Min J, Xue H, Wang Y. Association between household poverty dynamics and childhood overweight risk and health behaviours in the United States: a 8-year nationally representative longitudinal study of 16 800 children. *Pediatr Obes*. 2018;13(10):590–597. https://doi.org/10.1111/ijpo.12292
61. Skinner AC, Ravanbakht SN, Skelton JA, Perrin EM, Armstrong SC. Prevalence of obesity and severe obesity in U.S. children, 1999–2016. *Pediatrics*. 2018;141(3):e20173459. https://doi.org/10.1542/peds.2017-3459
62. Barlow SE, Expert Committee. Expert Committee Recommendations regarding the prevention, assessment, and treatment of child and adolescent overweight and obesity: summary report. *Pediatrics*. 2007;120(suppl 4):S164–S192. https://doi.org/10.1542/peds.2007-2329C
63. Davis MM, Gance-Cleveland B, Hassink S, Johnson R, Paradis G, Resnicow K. Recommendations for prevention of childhood obesity. *Pediatrics*. 2007;120(suppl 4):S229–S253. https://doi.org/10.1542/peds.2007-2329E
64. Spear BA, Barlow SE, Ervin C, et al. Recommendations for treatment of child and adolescent overweight and obesity. *Pediatrics*. 2007;120(suppl 4):S254–S288. https://doi.org/10.1542/peds.2007-2329F
65. Dietz WH, Gortmaker SL. Preventing obesity in children and adolescents. *Annu Rev Public Health*. 2001;22:337–353. https://doi.org/10.1146/annurev.publhealth.22.1.337
66. American Psychiatric Association. *Diagnostic and Statistical Manual of Mental Disorders*. 5th ed. American Psychiatric Publishing; 2013.
67. Yager J, Devlin M, Halmi KA, et al. *Practice Guideline for the Treatment of Patients With Eating Disorders*. 3rd ed. American Psychiatric Association; 2012.
68. Maternal and Child Health Bureau. Children and youth with special health care needs. Health Resources and Services Administration. Updated July 2023. https://mchb.hrsa.gov/programs-impact/focus-areas/children-youth-special-health-care-needs-cyshcn
69. Bayerl CT, Ries J, Bettencourt MF, Fisher P. Nutrition issues of children in early intervention programs: primary care team approach. *Semin Pediatr Gastroenterol Nutr*. 1993;4:11–15.
70. Dye BA, Thornton-Evans G, Li X, Iafolla TJ. *Dental Caries and Sealant Prevalence in Children and Adolescents in the United States 2011–2012*. NCHS Data Brief No. 191. National Center for Health Statistics; 2015. https://www.cdc.gov/nchs/data/databriefs/db191.htm
71. American Academy of Pediatric Dentistry. Policy on early childhood caries (ECC): classifications, consequences, and preventive strategies. In: *Reference Manual of Pediatric Dentistry*. American Academy of Pediatric Dentistry; 2020:79–81. https://www.aapd.org/media/policies_guidelines/p_eccclassifications.pdf
72. American Academy of Pediatric Dentistry. Fluoride therapy. Accessed October 18, 2023. https://www.aapd.org/globalassets/media/policies_guidelines/bp_fluoridetherapy.pdf.
73. Tang MLK, Mullins RJ. Food allergy: is prevalence increasing? *Intern Med J*. 2017;47(3):256–261. https://doi.org/10.1111/imj.13362
74. Smith P, Masilamani M, Sampson H. The false alarm hypothesis: food allergy is associated with high dietary advanced glycation end-products and proglycating dietary sugars that mimic alarmins. *J Allergy Clin Immunol*. 2017;139(2):429–437. https://doi.org/10.1016/j.jaci.2016.05.040
75. Kattan J. The prevalence and natural history of food allergy. *Curr Allergy Asthma Rep*. 2016 Jul;16(7):47. https://doi.org./10.1007/s11882-016-0627-4
76. Rusznak C, Davies RJ. Diagnosing allergy. *BMJ*. 1998;316(7132):686–689. https://doi.org/10.1136/bmj.316.7132.686

77. Michigan Medicine. Evaluation, testing and diagnosis for food allergies. University of Michigan Health. Accessed October 19, 2023. https://www.uofmhealth.org/conditions-treatments/food-allergy/diagnosis-testing
78. Partnership for Food Safety Education. Common foodborne pathogens. Accessed October 19, 2023. https://www.fightbac.org/food-poisoning/foodborne-pathogens/
79. American Psychological Association. Report of the APA Task Force on Advertising and Children. 2004. https://www.apa.org/pubs/reports/advertising-children
80. Batada A, Seitz MD, Wootan MG, Story M. Nine out of 10 food advertisements shown during Saturday morning children's television programming are for foods high in fat, sodium, or added sugars, or low in nutrients. *J Am Diet Assoc.* 2008;108(4):673–678. https://doi.org/10.1016/j.jada.2008.01.015
81. Ustjanaustkas AE, Harris JL, Schwartz MB. Food and beverage advertising on children's websites. *Pediatr Obes.* 2014;9:362–372. https://doi.org/10.1111/j.2047-6310.2013.00185.x
82. Centers for Disease Control and Prevention. Screen time vs. lean time infographic. Accessed October 19, 2023. https://www.cdc.gov/nccdphp/dnpao/multimedia/infographics/getmoving.html
83. National Institutes of Health. High amounts of screen time begin as early as infancy, NIH study suggests. November 25, 2019. https://www.nih.gov/news-events/news-releases/high-amounts-screen-time-begin-early-infancy-nih-study-suggests
84. De Jong E, Visscher TLS, HiraSing RA, Heymans MW, Seidell JC, Renders CM. Association between TV viewing, computer use, and overweight, determinants and competing activities of screen time in 4- to 13-year-old children. *Int J Obes.* 2013;37(1):47–53. https://doi.org/10.1038/ijo.2011.244
85. Wang D, van der Horst K, Jacquier EF, Afeiche MC, Eldridge AL. Snacking patterns in children: a comparison between Australia, China, Mexico, and the US. *Nutrients.* 2018;10(2):198. https://doi.org/10.3390/nu10020198
86. Duffey KJ, Popkin BM. Causes of increased energy intake among children in the US, 1977–2010. *Am J Prev Med.* 2013;44(2):e1–e8. https://doi.org/10.1016/j.amepre.2012.10.011
87. Peirnas C, Popkin BM. Food portion patterns and trends among U.S. children and their relationship to total eating occasion size, 1977–2006. *J Nutr.* 2011;141(6):1159–1164. https://doi.org/10.3945/jn.111.138727
88. Siega-Riz AM, Deming DM, Reidy KC, Fox MK, Condon E, Briefel RR. Food consumption patterns of infants and toddlers: where are we now? *J Am Diet Assoc.* 2010;110:S38–S51. https://doi.org/10.1016/j.jada.2010.09.001
89. Harnack L, Stang J, Story M. Soft drink consumption among U.S. Children and adolescents: nutritional consequences. *J Am Diet Assoc.* 1999;99:436–441. https://doi.org/10.1016/S0002-8223(99)00106-6
90. Hagan JF, Shaw JS, Duncan PM, eds. *Bright Futures: Guidelines for Health Supervision of Infants, Children, and Adolescents.* 3rd ed. American Academy of Pediatrics; 2008.
91. Bailey RL, Gahche JJ, Lentino CV, et al. Dietary supplement use in the United States, 2003–2006. *J Nutr.* 2011;141(2):261–266. https://doi.org/10.3945/jn.110.133025
92. Lohse B, Stotts JL, Priebe JR. Survey of herbal use by Kansas and Wisconsin WIC participants reveals moderate, appropriate use and identifies herbal education needs. *J Am Diet Assoc.* 2006;106:227–237. https://doi.org/10.1016/j.jada.2005.10.033
93. Black LI, Clarke TC, Barnes PM, Stussman BJ, Nahin RL. Use of complementary health approaches among children aged 4–17 years in the United States: National Health Interview Survey, 2007–2012. *Natl Health Stat Rep.* 2015;78:1–19. https://www.ncbi.nlm.nih.gov/pmc/articles/PMC4562218
94. Buck ML, Michael RS. Talking with families about herbal products. *J Pediatr.* 2000;136:673–678. https://doi.org/10.1067/mpd.2000.105234
95. De Cosmi V, Scaglioni S, Agostoni C. Early taste experiences and later food choices. *Nutrients.* 2017;9(2):107. https://doi.org/10.3390/nu9020107
96. Małachowska A, Jeżewska-Zychowicz M. Does examining the childhood food experiences help to better understand food choices in adulthood? *Nutrients.* 2021;13(3):983. https://doi.org/10.3390/nu13030983
97. World Health Organization. Social determinants of health. Accessed October 19, 2023. https://www.who.int/health-topics/social-determinants-of-health
98. Yue T, Zhang Q, Li G, Qin H. Global burden of nutritional deficiencies among children under 5 years of age from 2010–2019. *Nutrients.* 2022;14(13):2685. https://doi.org/10.3390/nu14132685
99. GBD 2019 Diseases and Injuries Collaborators. Global burden of 369 diseases and injuries in 204 countries and territories, 1990–2019: a systematic analysis for the Global Burden of Disease Study 2019. *Lancet.* 2020;396:1204–1222. https://doi.org/10.1016/S0140-6736(20)30925-9

100. World Health Organization, UNICEF. *Global Strategy for Infant and Young Child Feeding*. World Health Organization; 2003. https://www.who.int/publications/i/item/9241562218
101. World Health Organization. *Global Nutrition Targets 2025: Policy Brief Series*. World Health Organization; 2014. https://apps.who.int/iris/handle/10665/149018
102. Food Research & Action Center. *The Role of the Federal Child Nutrition Programs in Improving Health and Well-Being*. Food Research & Action Center; December, 2017. https://frac.org/wp-content/uploads/hunger-health-role-federal-child-nutrition-programs-improving-health-well-being.pdf
103. Logan C, Connor P, LeClair L, et al. *Study of Nutrition and Activity in Child Care Settings: Summary of Findings*. ABT Associates; 2021. https://researchconnections.org/childcare/resources/130746
104. Kenney EL, Poole MK, Cory H, Cradock AL. Impact of changes to the Child and Adult Care Food Program on children's dietary intake in family child care homes. *Public Health Nutr*. 2020;23(11): 2016–2023. https://doi.org/10.1017/S1368980019004646

6

ADOLESCENT NUTRITION: A PUBLIC HEALTH APPROACH

Kyle L. Thompson

LEARNING OBJECTIVES

At the end of this chapter, students will be able to:

1. Describe the growth and developmental patterns of adolescents and how they relate to life stage nutrition needs.
2. Identify key principles in promoting optimal nutrition intake for adolescents.
3. Name key nutrients and dietary issues of public health concern for adolescents.
4. Identify needs for nutrition intervention and referral for common dietary concerns among adolescents.
5. Describe influences on adolescents that influence dietary intake and disease risk.
6. Explain how social determinants of health affect the dietary intake of adolescents.
7. Recognize and describe governmental and nongovernmental resources available to assist adolescents in meeting nutrition needs.

INTRODUCTION

Adolescent development has been described as a roller coaster ride, with tumultuous ups and downs occurring at breathtaking speed! Human beings enter **adolescence** as children and leave as young adults, navigating immense physical, cognitive, emotional, and social changes during this life cycle phase.[1] The key developmental task of adolescence is to progress from dependence as a child to independence as an adult, with a myriad of factors influencing this journey. Successful adolescent development sets the stage for a happy, productive, and meaningful adult life. This chapter explores the crucial role of nutrition in supporting optimal adolescent growth and development, and presents a public health approach to adolescent nutrition.

OVERVIEW OF ADOLESCENT DEVELOPMENT

The adolescent life cycle phase has a potential duration of more than 10 years, and there is wide variation among individuals throughout the developmental timeline.[2]

Change and growth occur rapidly as adulthood approaches, and **growth velocity** is greater than that of any other life cycle stage with the exception of infancy.[3] About 16% of the world's population are adolescents, and a large majority live in low- to moderate-income countries.[4] The World Health Organization (WHO) has reported that the success of global child health initiatives, particularly initiatives to reduce mortality in children under the age of 5 years, has resulted in a substantial increase in the worldwide adolescent population.[4,5]

There is no standard definition of the ages that fall within adolescence, but there is overall agreement on the timing of the life phase. WHO defines *adolescence* as ages 10 to 19 years, and **youth** as 15 to 24 years, thus including the years of early adulthood in their definition.[6] The American Academy of Pediatrics (AAP) describes three phases of adolescence: **early adolescence** (in general, ages 10 or 11 to 13 or 14 years), **middle adolescence** (14–17 years), and **late adolescence** (18–21+ years).[2] Each phase has specific characteristics and developmental milestones. Typically, individuals' course through the phases of adolescence is not uniformly smooth. Challenges, setbacks, and conflicts are to be expected as young people encounter unfamiliar new roles, responsibilities, and relationships.[7]

Ten Tasks of Adolescent Development

In 2001, Dr. A. Rae Simpson published a now-classic report on successful parenting of teenagers, based on a synthesis of existing research.[8] The report found substantial congruence among researchers on the developmental tasks of adolescence and principles of effective parenting of adolescents. The results of this report are provided at a website called *Raising Teens* authored by Dr. Simpson and maintained by the Massachusetts Institute of Technology (MIT) Work-Life Center.[9] The Raising Teens website provides a distillation of the major findings of Dr. Simpson's report, presented to the general public in two documents entitled **Ten Tasks of Adolescent Development** and **Five Basics of Parenting Adolescents**. These documents have been found to be applicable to a broad range of academic disciplines and cultural perspectives.[10] The Ten Tasks of Adolescent Development are found in Table 6.1.[11]

In responding to the tasks of adolescent development, some writers have commented on the immense, overwhelming, and daunting nature of the transformations listed in Table 6.1.[12] It can be difficult to imagine completing the transition from child to adult in a few years' time. Indeed, the progression from childhood to adulthood is accompanied by life-altering changes. Those who work with adolescents in public health settings should demonstrate awareness, understanding, and empathy when confronting the significant challenges associated with the adolescent life cycle phase.

Five Basics of Parenting Adolescents

The Raising Teens Project provides research-based guidelines for the parents of adolescents.[13] These guidelines provide helpful suggestions for not only parents and guardians but also those who work with teens. Effective parenting of adolescents, according to the Raising Teens project, is supportive, attentive, and encouraging. Adolescents need clear but expanding boundaries to promote the development of adult independence, and mentors should guide the way toward healthy adulthood by example.[13] The Five Basics of Parenting Adolescents are found in Figure 6.1.[13]

It is difficult to overstate the importance of caring, consistent, supportive adult guidance and *mentorship* in every aspect of the progression from childhood to adulthood.[14]

Table 6.1. Ten Tasks of Adolescent Development

Task	Process Overview: From Early to Late Adolescence†
1. Adjust to sexually maturing bodies and feelings	Young people enter and complete puberty, attain most of their adult physical growth, and begin navigating life for the first time in an adult body.
2. Develop and apply abstract thinking skills	Thinking skills move from the very concrete toward the ability to conceptualize abstractions and understand their implications.
3. Develop and apply new perspectives on human relationships	Relationship-building skills progress from the more self-centered, dependent relationships of childhood to adult independence and the ability to consider the viewpoints, needs, and interests of others.[11]
4. Develop and apply new coping skills in areas such as decision-making, problem-solving, and conflict resolution	Basic and limited coping skills increase with physical, emotional, and neurologic growth.
5. Identify meaningful moral standards, values, and belief systems	Moral development begins with values upheld in the external environment, often that of the family, and progresses toward the ability to define and apply one's own personal moral and ethical framework to life decisions.
6. Understand and express more complex emotional experiences	Emotional development moves from a more self-focused approach to include a wider understanding of emotions in self and others, and an increased ability to address and manage one's own emotions.
7. Form friendships that are mutually close and supportive	As teens mature, peers become more important and the circle of acquaintances enlarges beyond the home; the basis of friendship tends to shift from common activities to shared values.
8. Establish key aspects of identity	From the beginning to the end of adolescence, individuality develops in relation to self and others. Identity includes but is not limited to ethnicity, sexuality, gender, physical characteristics, and approach to relationships.
9. Meet the demands of increasingly mature roles and responsibilities	Teens move from dependency to independence in the activities of living. Habits and skills that support the ability to meet adult roles and responsibilities develop throughout adolescence.
10. Renegotiate relationships with adults in parenting roles	Teens shift from dependence on parents/caregivers to freely chosen new relationships. Parent/caregiver relationships shift from a parenting focus to reciprocal adult interactions.

*With considerations for early (10–11 to 13–14 years), middle (14–17 years), and late adolescent (18–21+ years) developmental phases.

†For every task of adolescent development, appropriate instruction, guidance, support, and mentorship from caring adults is crucial.

Source: This table is based on and adapted from the work of Dr. A. Rae Simpson: Simpson AR. *Raising Teens: Ten Tasks of Adolescent Development*. MIT Work-Life Center; 2018. https://hr.mit.edu/static/worklife/raising-teens/ten-tasks.html

The Raising Teens Project identified five significant ways in which parents can influence healthy adolescent development—the Five Basics of Parenting Adolescents:

- **Love and Connect**
  Offer support and acceptance while affirming the teen's increasing maturity.
- **Monitor and Observe**
  Let teens know you are paying attention.
- **Guide and Limit**
  Uphold clear boundaries while encouraging increased competence.
- **Model and Consult**
  Provide continual support for decision-making, teaching by example and ongoing dialogue.
- **Provide and Advocate**
  Provide a supportive home environment and a network of caring adults.

Figure 6.1. The five basics of parenting adolescents from the **R**aising **T**eens **P**roject.
Source: This figure is taken from the work of Dr. A. Rae Simpson: Simpson AR. *Raising Teens: Five Basics of Parenting Adolescents*. MIT Work-Life Center; 2018. https://hr.mit.edu/static/worklife/raising-teens/five-basics.html

One of the U.S. Department of Health and Human Services (DHHS) *Healthy People 2030* goals is *Increase the proportion of adolescents who have an adult in their lives with whom they can talk about serious problems.*[15] In 2019, the DHHS estimated that about 78.3% of U.S teens had access to such an adult, nearly 5 percentage points below the desired goal of 82.9%.[15] Evidence indicates that effective adult mentorship of adolescents improves a variety of outcomes that persist into adulthood, including social, health, and academic outcomes.[15]

As adolescents grow closer to adulthood, they experience increasing opportunities to eat away from home and to make their own food choices. Effective mentors can help guide teens toward a healthy lifestyle by modeling positive behaviors such as making healthful food choices, engaging in regular physical activity, and avoiding smoking and excessive use of alcohol. While the provision of quality mentorship to emerging adults can be challenging, those who raise, guide, and mentor teens into productive adulthood can find great satisfaction in the knowledge that those teens will touch the future, hopefully creating a better world in the process.

OVERVIEW OF ADOLESCENT GROWTH

The rapid physical growth and development of adolescence require adequate and appropriate nutrients.[7] During adolescence, teens will add about 20% of their adult height, 40% of adult bone mass, and 50% of adult weight. The ability to think abstractly and to self-evaluate behaviors increases as neurologic capacity develops. The process of puberty, which takes place during adolescence, ends in the development of adult sexual characteristics and reproductive capacity, along with the growth and maturation of all body organs.[16]

Nutrition is a crucial component of achieving optimal growth and development prior to entering adulthood. Both under- and overnutrition in late childhood and adolescence set the stage for suboptimal growth and development, and can affect the timing of puberty with subsequent impacts on growth in height and body composition as well as lifetime risk for chronic disease.[16] Adolescent nutrient requirements are second only to those of infants in terms of calorie and protein needs per kilogram of body weight, but when described in actual amounts consumed, nutrient needs are at a peak.[2,3] In addition, adolescents are moving from dependence on adults for the provision of food and nutrients to self-efficacy in appropriately nourishing themselves. A multitude of sociocultural influences on adolescents, including but not limited to the increased importance of peer relationships, the surrounding nutrition environment, and media input can significantly impact nutrient intake.[17]

Growth in Height, Weight, and Bone Mass in Adolescence

Height

The adolescent growth spurt for males typically occurs between 12 and 16 years of age, with mean *peak height velocity* of 9.5 cm/year achieved at around 13 to 14 years.[16,18] For females, the growth spurt is typically seen between the ages of 9½ and 13½, with mean *peak height velocity* of 8.3 cm/year realized around age 11 to 12½.[16,18] On average, adolescents reach about 90% of their final adult height upon completing their period of rapid growth.[19] The growth spurt is considered an indicator of puberty, and poor nutrition during adolescence may result in failure to achieve genetic height potential.[16] Adolescent growth in stature is completed with the ossification of the *epiphyses,* or growth plates of the bones, in late puberty.

Weight

About 50% of adult weight is gained during adolescence.[20] In males, the growth spurt and peak weight gain velocity are roughly concurrent, averaging about 9 kg (~20 lb) per year. In females, peak weight gain tends to occur about 6 months after peak height velocity and averages around 8.3 kg (~18 lb) per year.[20] Normally, following the period of peak weight velocity, the rate of weight gain per year drops steadily through the remainder of adolescence. Accompanying adolescent weight gain are major changes in body composition, resulting in typical male and female adult characteristics including amounts and distribution of muscle, fat, and bone tissues.[20]

Bone Mass

By the age of 18, it is normal for adolescents to have acquired about 95% of their adult bone mass.[21] Acquisition of bone mass can be considered a critical period of pediatric development. As children and adolescents grow, they accumulate more bone tissue than they lose. Because adults lose more bone than they replace, maximizing the accumulation of bone mass in adolescence provides critical protection against osteomalacia and osteoporosis in later life.[22] Good nutrition and adequate physical activity are critical components of optimizing bone development in adolescence.[21]

During the adolescent growth spurt, teens may experience awkwardness and anxiety as they adjust to rapid physical changes and navigate the world for the first time in an adult body. Parents and caregivers may notice that their teen frequently expresses hunger and consumes increasingly large amounts of food. Teens experiencing their growth spurt may be moody, irritable, and want to sleep more than usual. As with other aspects of adolescence, understanding, empathy, and wise mentorship provided by trusted adults can help smooth the road to adulthood.

Pubertal Development

Puberty is a complex, intricate physiologic process. Its initiation and course are impacted mostly by genetics, with strong influences from hormones, environmental factors, and nutrient intake.[23] Puberty is characterized by rapid physical growth, maturation of organs, brain and neurologic development, and development of adult sexual characteristics and the capacity for reproduction.[24]

The relationships among the hypothalamus gland, the pituitary gland and its secreted hormones, and the gonads (ovaries in females, testes in males) are called the hypothalamic–pituitary–gonadal axis (HPG axis).[25] The HPG axis is active in the fetus during the gestational period, but activity subsides early in infancy and enters a period of dormancy that lasts throughout childhood.[25] The exact factor(s) that trigger the initiation of puberty are not well understood; however, it is known that renewed HPG axis activity, including the pituitary's resuming secretion of gonadotropin-releasing hormone (GnRH) in early adolescence, indicates that puberty has begun.[25]

The Stages of Puberty

The process of puberty occurs in sequential stages, although there is a range of ages at which initiation of puberty and completion of its subsequent developmental tasks is normal.[26] In females, puberty begins with the development of breast buds, and in males, with testicular enlargement.[16] Puberty ends with the near-completion of adult bone growth as the former adolescent becomes a young adult.

Healthcare professionals should be aware that in medical settings, the progress of puberty is often assessed by the use of *Tanner stages.* The Tanner stages were developed as the result of longitudinal observation studies conducted in England from the 1940s to the 1960s by Drs. J.M. Tanner and W.A. Marshall, with their classic studies for males and females published in 1969 and 1970, respectively.[27–29] Also known as Sexual Maturity Ratings (SMR), the Tanner stages provide medical practitioners with a five-stage reference standard for documenting the development of external genitalia throughout puberty.[28]

Variations in Pubertal Development

As previously mentioned, typical adolescent growth patterns are subject to wide variations among individuals.[7] The initiation of puberty is considered within normal limits when it occurs from ages 8 to 12 years in females, and from 9 to 14 years in males.[30] *Precocious puberty* is defined as the initiation of puberty prior to 8 years for females, and prior to 9 years for males.[30] *Delayed puberty* is defined as the initiation of puberty after the age of 12 for females, and after the age of 14 for males.[30] Children whose pubertal timing appears to fall outside these benchmarks should receive a medical consultation to rule out potential medical issues.

Those who work with adolescents should be aware that teens whose growth pattern differs from peers may suffer significant emotional distress. For all children, regular monitoring of height and weight should be conducted at well-child and adolescent visits to ensure that appropriate growth is occurring, and to provide opportunity for

Milestones in Sexual Development

During puberty, sexual development occurs in a set sequence. However, when the changes begin and how quickly they occur vary from person to person. For girls, puberty begins at age 8½ to 10 years and lasts about 4 years. The chart in Figure 6.2 shows a typical sequence and normal range of development for the milestones of sexual development for girls and boys.

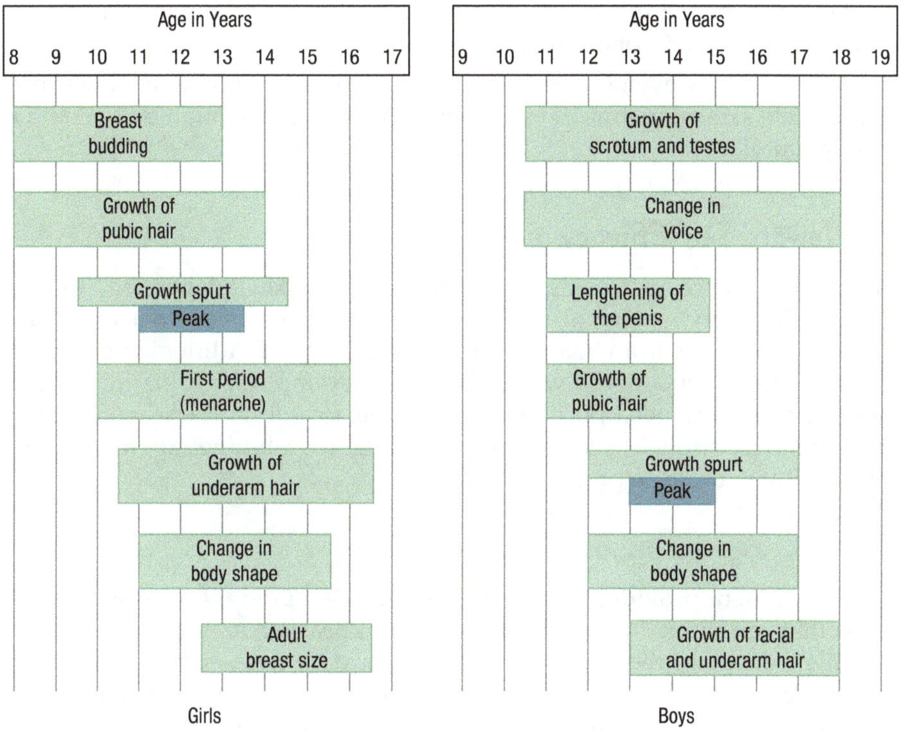

Figure 6.2. Milestones in sexual development, including normal timing of peak growth spurt for males and females.
Source: McLaughlin J. *Puberty in girls*. In: *Merck Manual: Consumer Version*. Merck; Updated September 2022. https://www.merckmanuals.com/home/women-s-health-issues/biology-of-the-female-reproductive-system/puberty-in-girls

intervention if appropriate. Pediatric growth charts for ages 2 to 20 years are found in **Appendix E**. Figure 6.2 illustrates the expected sequence of pubertal development in males and females, along with the timing of the peak growth spurt.[26]

NUTRITION TO SUPPORT HEALTHFUL GROWTH IN ADOLESCENCE

Goals for Adolescent Nutrition

Adolescence is the later phase of childhood, and overall goals for adolescent nutrition are similar to those for younger children. Adequate nutrient intake to support optimal growth and development is crucial. Throughout adolescence, however, a primary objective is to move from dependence on adults to meet nutrient needs to independence and self-efficacy in nourishing one's own adult body. Four major goals for adolescent nutrition are listed below:

- Achieve appropriate and adequate consumption of nutrients to support healthful puberty, optimal growth in height and weight, and maturation of all body systems.[16]
- Achieve appropriate and adequate consumption of nutrients to maintain and/or achieve healthful weight status, and to promote reduced risk of chronic disease in later life.[4]
- Move from dependency on adults to provide all food and nutrient needs, to independence in fulfilling one's own nutrient needs.
- Maintain and/or develop a healthful relationship with food that allows for both appropriate self-nourishment and enjoyment and appreciation of food and eating throughout life.

Growing Toward Self-Efficacy in Self-Nourishment

Adolescents experience increasing opportunities to make independent food choices as they grow. The food preferences of peers become more important in making food choices, and eating away from home becomes more frequent. Adult mentors should support this growing independence while setting the example for a lifetime of enjoyable self-nourishment. Teens need positive adult models for self-efficacy in effectively managing nutrition-related tasks such as meal planning, food budgeting, food buying, and food preparation in order to promote lifetime health.

Official Nutrition Guidance for Adolescents

The U.S. government provides several official nutrition guidance and *nutrition surveillance* tools that can inform public health nutrition practice among adolescents. These tools are aligned in that recommendations and/or data from each tool inform the development and application of the other tools. Examples of key official nutrition guidance and data gathering tools that are applied in adolescent nutrition settings are listed here:

- The Healthy Eating Index
- Youth Risk Behavior Surveillance System
- The Dietary Guidelines for Americans
- Dietary Reference Intakes
- MyPlate for Teens
- World Health Organization Guidelines for Adolescent Nutrition

Nutrition Surveillance Tools

The Healthy Eating Index: Evaluating the Quality of Adolescents' Nutrient Intake

The Healthy Eating Index (HEI) is a scoring tool that is used to assess populations' adherence to the U.S. Dietary Guidelines.[31] First developed in 1995, the current version of the HEI was developed in 2015 to align with the 2015–2020 U.S. Dietary Guidelines.[32] A new version of the HEI based on the 2020–2025 U.S. Dietary Guidelines is now in development. Data for the HEI are obtained from the *What We Eat in America* dietary interview survey administered as part of the National Health and Nutrition Examination Survey

(NHANES).[33] The HEI evaluates a set of foods using a defined system of scoring, and results in a score from 0 to 100, with a score of 100 indicating alignment with the Dietary Guidelines.[32]

The overall HEI for all Americans in 2022 is 58/100, indicating poor adherence to the Dietary Guidelines for Americans.[32] For children and adolescents, an interesting pattern is evident. The overall HEI score for young children (2–4 years) is 61, but by the time adolescence is reached (14–18 years), the average score drops to 51—a full 10 points.[34]

Adolescents consume proportionately lower amounts of fruits, vegetables, and dairy foods than younger children.[34]

Among life cycle groups, the differences between actual intake and recommended intake are higher for adolescents ages 14 to 18 than for any other life cycle group.[35] Based on data from the HEI and other federal health surveillance programs, the 2020–2025 Dietary Guidelines for Americans report that large majorities of older adolescents exceed recommendations for food constituents of concern. For example, adolescents ages 14 to 18 years as a population exceed guidelines for:

- Added sugar intake
  - Desired <10% total calories/day: guideline exceeded by 72% males, 76% females
- Sodium intake
  - Desired <2,300 mg/day: guideline exceeded by 97% males, 77% females
- Saturated fat intake
  - Desired <10% total calories/day: guideline exceeded by 85% males, 78% females[35]

Although percentages are lower than for older adolescents, findings are similar for young adolescents ages 9 to 13.[35] Because poor nutrition during one life cycle phase impacts health at subsequent life cycle phases, the importance of encouraging good nutrition in adolescents is evident.

The Youth Risk Behavior Surveillance System

The Youth Risk Behavior Surveillance System (YRBSS) is housed within the Centers for Disease Control and Prevention (CDC).[36] The YRBSS is conducted both nationally by the CDC as a school-based survey, and locally by state, territorial, local, and tribal governments.[35] The following six categories of risk behaviors, including poor diet, are included in the survey:

- Behaviors that contribute to unintentional injuries and violence
- Sexual behaviors related to unintended pregnancy and sexually transmitted diseases, including HIV infection
- Alcohol and other drug use
- Tobacco use
- Unhealthy dietary behaviors
- Inadequate physical activity[36]

The YRBSS may be useful for providing public health nutrition professionals with location-specific data regarding adolescent dietary behaviors. The *YRBS Explorer* provides a user-friendly tool for exploring national, state, and local data.[37]

Dietary Guidance Tools

Dietary Guidelines for Americans

Since 1980, the **Dietary Guidelines for Americans** (DGAs) have provided healthful diet recommendations for Americans ages 2 years and up.[38] The DGAs are developed jointly and updated every 5 years by the U.S. Department of Agriculture (USDA) and the DHHS, and are based on the best scientific evidence available at the time.[35] Written for a professional audience, the DGAs are used as the basis for U.S. food and nutrition policy; to support the development of nutrition guidance tools and nutrition education initiatives for a lay audience; to inform national, state, county, local, tribal, and territorial government programs at all levels; and to provide guidance for industry and organizations.[35] The four basic recommendations of the 2020–2025 DGAs are:

- Follow a healthy dietary pattern at every life stage.
- Customize and enjoy nutrient-dense food and beverage choices to reflect personal preferences, cultural traditions, and financial considerations.
- Focus on meeting food group needs with nutrient-dense foods and beverages, and stay within calorie limits.
- Limit foods and beverages higher in added sugars, saturated fat, and sodium, and limit alcoholic beverages.[39]

The 2020–2025 DGAs, for the first time, provide guidelines by stage of life from pregnancy through infancy through older adulthood, including adolescents.[40] Separate recommendations are provided for younger (ages 9–13) and older (ages 14–18) adolescents. Specific DGA recommendations for life cycle stages provide improved opportunities to tailor and apply the guidelines in nutrition interventions designed for adolescents. Table 6.2 provides a summary of food group intake recommendations based on the U.S. DGAs for early and late adolescents. Table 6.3 provides a sample meal plan for an adolescent. A summary of the DGAs can be found at www.dietaryguidelines.gov/sites/default/files/2021-03/DGA_2020-2025_Infographic_MakeEveryBiteCount.pdf.

Table 6.2. Food Group Intake Amounts Recommended for Early and Late Adolescents

Food Group	Early Adolescents (Ages 9–13 Years)*	Late Adolescents (Ages 14–18 Years)*
Vegetables (cups/day)	1.5–3.5	2.5–4
Fruits (cups/day)	1.5–2	1.5–2.5
Dairy (cups/day)	3–3	3–3
Grains (oz/day)	5–9	6–10
Protein foods (oz eq/day)†	4–6.5	5–7
Oils (g/day)	17–34	24–51

*Intake ranges vary by activity level, sex, and age.

†One oz eq (ounce equivalent) is defined by the U.S. Department of Agriculture as 1 oz lean meat, poultry, or seafood, 1 egg, ¼ cup cooked beans or tofu, 1 tbsp peanut butter, ½ oz nuts or seeds.

Source: Adapted from U.S. Department of Agriculture, U.S. Department of Health and Human Services. *Dietary Guidelines for Americans, 2020-2025*. 9th ed. U.S. Department of Health and Human Services; 2020. https://www.dietaryguidelines.gov

Dietary Reference Intakes

Table 6.3. Sample Menu for an Adolescent*

Meal	Sample Menu
Breakfast	Nut butter banana toast: 2 slices whole grain bread, 1 tsp butter, 2 tbsp nut butter, ½ sliced banana per bread slice, 1 cup low-fat yogurt or 1 cup milk
Lunch	Bean burrito: flour tortilla, ½ cup cooked seasoned beans, 2 tablespoons cheese, avocado slices; 1 oz taco chips, ¼ cup salsa, 1 cup milk
Afternoon snack	1 cup fruit/green vegetable smoothie, 2 tbsp walnuts
Dinner	4 oz rotisserie chicken, ½ cup mashed potatoes, 2 tbsp gravy, 1 cup dark green salad with 1 tbsp olive oil vinaigrette, ½ cup cooked peas and carrot mix, 1 dinner roll with 1 tsp butter, 1 cup milk
Evening snack	½ cup ice cream

*Based on requirement of about 2,500 kcal/day. Portions or serving sizes may be adjusted to meet lower or higher calorie needs. Water to drink if not otherwise indicated.

The Dietary Reference Intakes (DRIs) are a set of values that describe recommended ranges of intake for nutrients, energy, and fiber.[41] The DRIs are based on the latest scientific evidence available at a particular time a nutrient is reviewed, and are periodically updated. Until about 1990, the only recommended intake value provided in the United State was the RDA, or Recommended Dietary Allowance.[42] Around that time, it was recognized that a range of intake values for each nutrient would be useful for describing that nutrient's role in human health. Because the development of the DRIs is an ongoing process, not all values are available for every nutrient. The newest DRI value is the Chronic Disease Risk Reduction (CDRR) intake, which was determined for sodium in 2019.[43] **Appendix C** describes the current DRI values.

The DRIs include recommendations for males and females for a variety of age groups, including persons 4 to 18 years of age. For adolescents, DRI values are provided for males and females who are 9 to 13 years of age and 14 to 18 years of age. DRI values are also available for adolescents 14 to 18 years of age who are pregnant or lactating.[44] A link to access the DRIs is found in **Appendix C**.

MyPlate: Teens

MyPlate is the USDA consumer-oriented dietary guidance plan. MyPlate was launched in 2011, and was intended to replace the previous USDA Food Pyramid in providing consumers with information and resources to choose a healthful meal plan.[45] MyPlate is administered by the USDA Center for Nutrition Policy and Promotion (CNPP), which has been providing consumer nutrition guidance to the public since 1994.[46] MyPlate is revised every 5 years based on revisions of the DGAs. Current MyPlate resources are based on the 2020–2025 DGAs, and provide general nutrition guidance as well as targeted information for life stage groups, including teens.[47] The MyPlate resource is simple and flexible, and can accommodate a wide variety of personal likes and dislikes, cultural foodways, and budget needs.

MyPlate:Teens includes a wealth of developmentally appropriate dietary guidance, resources, and recommendations.[47] Instructions for obtaining a personalized MyPlate Plan as well as the *Start Simple with MyPlate* and *Shop Simple with MyPlate* computer applications are provided. The MyPlate plan provides protein options for those who choose to follow vegetarian or vegan meal plans. MyPlate: Teens also provides links to MyPlate Kitchen, which houses many nutritious and cost-effective recipes and cooking resources. MyPlate is available at myplate.gov.[48] **Appendix B** provides the MyPlate graphic used as the basis for dietary recommendations.

World Health Organization Guidelines for Adolescent Nutrition

In 2018, WHO published guidelines for improving adolescent nutrition across the globe: *Guideline: Implementing Effective Actions for Improving Adolescent Nutrition.*[49] As previously mentioned in this chapter, with progress in reducing early childhood mortality the population of adolescents has grown substantially worldwide.[5] Of the global adolescent population, about 90% live in moderate- to low-income countries.[5]

WHO guidelines are designed to address all types of malnutrition in adolescents, and were published to support an overall WHO strategic plan presented in *Every Woman, Every Child:* Every Woman, Every Child: The Global Strategy for Women's, Children's, and Adolescents' Health (2016–2030; Table 6.4).[49] Malnutrition in adolescents is described as occurring in three broad categories:

- Chronic undernutrition, which may present as stunting, underweight, or wasting
- Excessive or inadequate intake of micronutrients
- Overweight or obesity, which increases risk for a variety of chronic diseases[49]

Table 6.4. Major Recommendations for Improving Adolescent Nutrition Across the Globe

Major recommendations for improving adolescent nutrition across the globe are based on the following eight public health intervention actions:

- Promoting healthy diets
- Providing additional micronutrients through fortification of staple foods and targeted supplementation
- Managing acute malnutrition
- Preventing adolescent pregnancy and poor reproductive outcomes
- Promoting preconception and antenatal nutrition
- Providing access to safe environment and hygiene
- Promoting physical activity
- Disease prevention and management

Source: World Health Organization. *Guideline: Implementing Effective Actions for Improving Adolescent Nutrition.* World Health Organization; 2018. https://apps.who.int/iris/handle/10665/260297

Summary of Energy and Nutrient Needs for Adolescents

Macronutrients

Macronutrients include the **energy-yielding nutrients** protein, carbohydrate, and fat. Proportions of macronutrients in relation to total caloric intake are important to overall health. The DRIs provide acceptable macronutrient distribution ranges (AMDRs) for adolescents, found in Table 6.5.[50,51] Note that these recommendations are identical for all age/sex groups.

Table 6.5. Acceptable Macronutrient Distribution Ranges for Adolescents		
Age	Macronutrient, Percentage of otal Calories, Female*	Macronutrient, Percentage of Total Calories, Male*
9–13 years	Protein: 10%–30% Carbohydrate: 45%–65% Fat: 25%–35%	Protein: 10%–30% Carbohydrate: 45%–65% Fat: 25%–35%
14–18 years	Protein: 10%–30% Carbohydrate: 45%–65% Fat: 25%–35%	Protein: 10%–30% Carbohydrate: 45%–65% Fat: 25%–35%

*Needs also affected by activity levels or special conditions.
Source: U.S. Department of Agriculture, U.S. Department of Health and Human Services. Dietary Guidelines for Americans, 2020-2025. 9th ed. U.S. Department of Health and Human Services; 2020. https://www.dietaryguidelines.gov

Energy (Calorie) Needs

Energy (calorie) needs for adolescents vary based on age, sex, and level of activity.[35] Needs are also impacted by the presence of special medical conditions, for which adolescents should be referred to a physician or registered dietitian for comprehensive nutrition assessment. Adequacy of energy consumption—as well as energy balance—for adolescents is evaluated by steady progression along a standard growth chart trajectory, with no indications of excessive weight gain or undernutrition. Adequacy of energy intake via pediatric growth charts takes place at regular medical provider visits. Table 6.6 provides average calorie needs for adolescents.

Table 6.6. Average Calorie Needs for Adolescents		
Age	Calorie Needs, Female*	Calorie Needs, Male*
9–13 years	1,400–2,200	1,600–2,600
14–18 years	1,800–2,400	2,000–3,200

*Needs also affected by activity levels or special conditions.
Source: Adapted from U.S. Department of Agriculture, U.S. Department of Health and Human Services. *Dietary Guidelines for Americans, 2020-2025.* 9th ed. U.S. Department of Health and Human Services; 2020. https://www.dietaryguidelines.gov

Protein Needs

The HEI and the DGAs report that underconsumption of nutrient-dense foods by adolescents is a public health concern.[35] On average, protein consumption among female adolescents does not meet DRI recommendations, since females consume less meat, fish, eggs, beans, and lentils than male adolescents.[35] Protein foods include meats, poultry, fish, beans, and tofu, among others. Table 6.7 provides RDAs for protein for adolescents by age/sex groups.

Table 6.7. Recommended Dietary Allowances for Protein for Adolescents

Age	Protein Needs, Female (g/day)*	Protein Needs, Male (g/day)*
9–13 years	34	34
14–18 years	46	52

*Needs also affected by activity levels or special conditions.
Source: Adapted from U.S. Department of Agriculture, U.S. Department of Health and Human Services. *Dietary Guidelines for Americans, 2020-2025*. 9th ed. U.S. Department of Health and Human Services; 2020. https://www.dietaryguidelines.gov

Carbohydrate Needs

For both younger and older adolescents, consumption of whole grain carbohydrates does not meet population recommendations, while intake of refined grain carbohydrates exceeds recommendations. Large majorities of adolescents exceed recommendations for consumption of added sugars.[35] Note that carbohydrate recommendations are identical for all age/sex groups. Foods composed of primarily carbohydrates include grains, fruits, and some vegetables. Table 6.8 provides RDAs for carbohydrate for adolescents by age/sex groups.

Fat Needs

According to the HEI, saturated fat intake by younger and older adolescents exceeds the recommendation of 10% total calories per day. Overall fat needs are described as a percentage of total calories. It is recommended that saturated and trans-fat intake should be kept as low as possible while consuming a diet that meets nutritional needs. Alpha-linolenic acid (omega-3) and linoleic acid (omega-6) are fats required by humans and obtained from the diet. Adequate intakes (AIs) have been developed for these fats. Foods providing essential fats include nuts, seeds, oils such as olive and canola oil, fatty fish such as salmon, and avocados. Table 6.9 provides AMDRs and AIs for fat intake for adolescents by age/sex groups.

Table 6.8. Recommended Dietary Allowances for Carbohydrate for Adolescents*

Age	Carbohydrate Needs, Female (g/day)*	Carbohydrate Needs, Male (g/day)*
9–13 years	130	130
14–18 years	130	130

*Needs also affected by activity levels or special conditions.
Source: Adapted from U.S. Department of Agriculture, U.S. Department of Health and Human Services. *Dietary Guidelines for Americans, 2020-2025*. 9th ed. U.S. Department of Health and Human Services; 2020. https://www.dietaryguidelines.gov

Table 6.9. Acceptable Macronutrient Distribution Ranges and Adequate Intakes for Fat for Adolescents

Age	Fat Needs, Female*	Fat Needs, Male*
9–13 years	25%–35% of total kcal Linoleic acid: 10 g/day α-Linolenic acid: 1.0 g/day	25%–35% of total kcal Linoleic acid: 12 g/day α-Linolenic acid: 1.2 g/day
14–18 years	25%–35% of total kcal Linoleic acid: 11 g/day α-Linolenic acid: 1.1 g/day	25%–35% of total kcal Linoleic acid: 16 g/day α-Linolenic acid: 1.6 g/day

*Needs also affected by activity levels or special conditions.
Source: Adapted from U.S. Department of Agriculture, U.S. Department of Health and Human Services. *Dietary Guidelines for Americans, 2020-2025*. 9th ed. U.S. Department of Health and Human Services; 2020. https://www.dietaryguidelines.gov

Table 6.10. Recommended Dietary Allowances for Water for Adolescents

Age	Water Needs, Female*	Water Needs, Male*
9–13 years	2.1 L/day total water† includes 1.6 L (about 7 cups) water obtained from drinking water and beverages	2.4 L/day total water† includes 1.8 L (about 8 cups) water obtained from drinking water and beverages
14–18 years	2.3 L/day total water† includes 1.8 L (about 7 cups) water obtained from drinking water and beverages	3.3 L/day total water† includes 2.6 L (about 7 cups) water obtained from drinking water and beverages

*Needs also affected by activity levels or special conditions.
†*Total water* is water obtained from food, beverages, and drinking water.
Source: Otten JJ, Hellwig JP, Meyers LD, eds. *Dietary Reference Intakes: The Essential Guide to Nutrient Requirements*. The National Academies Press; 2006. https://doi.org/10.17226/11537.

Water Needs

Proper hydration is important in all life phases including adolescence. Humans obtain water from the consumption of liquids and foods. It is recommended that adolescents consume plain water as their primary beverage. Table 6.10 provides water and fluid intake RDAs for adolescents.

Micronutrients

A link to the DRIs for micronutrients for adolescents by age range is found in Appendix C. Because of the demonstrated gap between actual intake and recommended amounts of nutrient-dense foods such as fruits, vegetables, whole grains, and dairy, teens are at heightened risk for micronutrient deficiencies.[35] If micronutrient deficiencies are suspected in an adolescent, a complete nutrition assessment by a physician or registered dietitian is recommended. Any needed supplements should be prescribed with medical supervision. To impact adolescents' micronutrient status, public health nutrition interventions for adolescents should encourage consumption of healthful foods including fruits and vegetables, whole grains, lean proteins, and sources of calcium including dairy milk or fortified plant milk products. Three micronutrients of public health concern for adolescents are iron, calcium, and vitamin D, which are discussed next.

Iron

Adolescent iron needs are heightened by rapid growth, which includes increased blood volume as well as growth of other body tissues such as bone and muscle.[52] In adolescent females, iron needs are greater because of blood loss during menstruation. Suboptimal iron intake can result in subclinical iron deficiency, anemia, and suboptimal growth, including neurologic development. Good food sources of iron include meats and poultry, seafood, beans, dried fruits such as raisins, dark green leafy vegetables, and iron-fortified foods such as cereals. The RDA for iron for adolescent males ages 9 to 13 years and 14 to 18 years is 8 mg/day for both age groups. For adolescent females, the RDAs for ages 9 to 13 years and 14 to 18 years are 8 mg/day and 15 mg/day, respectively.[53]

Calcium

Because of rapid bone and muscle growth during adolescence, adequate calcium intake is key to optimal physical development and to prevention of osteoporosis in older adulthood.[54] Challenges to calcium intake in adolescents include the displacement of calcium-rich beverages such as diary milk by sugar-sweetened beverages as well as lower-than-recommended intakes of calcium-providing foods. Good food sources of calcium include dairy milk, calcium-fortified plant milks, calcium-fortified orange juice, canned salmon with bones, almonds, dark green leafy vegetables (such as kale, spinach, and other greens), and tofu made with calcium sulfate. The RDA for calcium for all adolescent age/sex groups is 1,300 mg/day.

Vitamin D

Vitamin D is an important nutrient for bone health and also appears to play a role in immune function. Because adolescence is the key life cycle phase for bone development for adulthood, the vitamin D status of adolescents is important. Humans obtain vitamin D from sun exposure—when exposure to sunlight triggers cells that produce vitamin D—and from food intake. The main source of vitamin D in American diets is fortified dairy milk and plant milk. There are only a small number of foods that are natural sources of vitamin D. Fatty fish such as salmon, tuna, and mackerel as well as fish oils are the richest food sources of vitamin D, and egg yolks and some mushrooms provide vitamin D in varying amounts.[55] The RDA for vitamin D for all adolescent age/sex groups is 15 mcg, or 600 IU, per day. Note that 1 IU = 0.025 mcg; therefore 15 mcg/0.025 = 600 IU.

Fiber and Exercise for Adolescents

Fiber

Adequate fiber consumption is important for optimal bowel function, the health of the digestive tract, regulation of blood glucose levels, and feelings of satiety, which may promote adequate but not excessive energy intake. Dietary fiber is provided by fruit, vegetable, and whole grain intake. Because overall teen consumption of these

Table 6.11. Adequate Intakefor Fiber for Adolescents

Age	Fiber Needs, Female (g/day)*	Fiber Needs, Male (g/day)*
9–13 years	31	38
14–18 years	26	26

*Needs also affected by special conditions.

Source: Adapted from U.S. Department of Agriculture, U.S. Department of Health and Human Services. *Dietary Guidelines for Americans, 2020-2025.* 9th ed. U.S. Department of Health and Human Services; 2020. https://www.dietaryguidelines.gov

fiber-containing foods does not meet recommendations, the adolescent population tends to consume inadequate fiber.[35] Table 6.11 provides AI recommendations for fiber intake for adolescents.

Physical Activity for Adolescents

The AAP recommends 60 minutes of daily physical activity for adolescents to promote overall health and physical, emotional, and social development.[56] At least 3 days per week, it is recommended that adolescents participate in physical activities that develop bone and muscle strength. Physical activity that includes opportunities to practice social skills is encouraged for adolescents.[56]

Effective Public Health Nutrition Interventions for Adolescents

The characteristics of adolescent development—rapid physical, emotional, and social growth coupled with growing independence—should be used to inform planning for public health nutrition interventions. In addition, interventions should consider the many environmental influences on adolescent nutrition. Hargreaves et al., in 2022, recommended that nutrition interventions focused on adolescents should encompass a number of societal sectors including healthcare, education, the digital world, and the food system and environment.[57]

Hargreaves et al. also suggested two major directions for public health nutrition interventions for adolescents: (1) impacting their surrounding nutrition environment; and (2) providing nutrition education to promote self-efficacy and independence in making nutrition decisions.[57] Examples of public health interventions to impact adolescents' nutrition environment include:

- Strengthening school meal programs to improve the school nutrition environment and the number of participating teens
- Implementing policy changes to promote reduced consumption of sugar-sweetened beverages, reduce adolescents' exposure to fast-food and junk food advertising, and the like
- Engaging in civic planning to provide safe and accessible walking/biking pathways to and from key locations in the community including schools
- Globally, providing fortified staple foods such as fortified maize to improve the nutritional profile of usual diets for families[57]

Examples of public health interventions focused on nutrition education to promote self-efficacy and independence include:

- Use schools to teach practical nutrition-related life skills such as cooking, gardening, meal planning, food budgeting, and the like
- Optimize the use of social media to promote healthful nutrition messages, to influence social norms, and to help make healthy choices the easiest choices[57]
- Use schools to impart basic nutrition knowledge and knowledge applications, such as label reading and principles of food safety[57]

Nutrition interventions among teens appear to be most effective when embedded within what might be called a "circle of support," including parents/caregivers and other caring adults. Interaction that involves direct participation of teens, as well as grounding in an understanding of adolescent development, also appear to improve the effectiveness of interventions.[58] Because of their growing competence and independence, it is recommended that adolescents be included as much as possible in the creation, planning, implementation, and evaluation of programs focused on them.[58]

SELECTED NUTRITION ISSUES AMONG ADOLESCENTS: A PUBLIC HEALTH PERSPECTIVE

This section highlights four public health nutrition issues among adolescents: disordered eating, displacement of healthful beverages with sugar-sweetened beverages, food insecurity, and support and resources—including nutrition resources—for adolescents with long-term chronic health conditions.

Disordered Eating

A complete discussion of the pathophysiology, diagnosis, and treatment of eating disorders is beyond the scope of this textbook. However, public health and nutrition professionals should be aware that adolescent populations are at increased risk for engaging in disordered eating behaviors. Eating disorders are severe illnesses with serious consequences for physical and mental health, including a high case fatality rate.[59] Duncan et al. reported in 2017 that the lifetime prevalence of eating disorders in the United States is 4.9% among women and 2.2% among men.[60] Over the past two decades, there has been progress in developing effective preventive interventions for eating disorders, but more research is needed.[61]

The AAP, in its 2021 Clinical Report, *Identification and Management of Eating Disorders in Children and Adolescents*, lists five diagnosable eating disorders that may affect children and adolescents:

- Anorexia nervosa (AN), characterized by severely restricted calorie intake and low body weight compared to recommendations for age and sex
- Bulimia nervosa (BN), characterized by recurring incidences of binge eating followed by purging behaviors such as self-induced vomiting or laxative use
- Binge eating disorder (BED), characterized by eating large amounts of food within a given period of time, without purging behaviors
- Avoidant/restrictive food intake disorder (ARFID), characterized by eating patterns showing avoidance or disinterest in food, resulting in sequelae such as weight loss, failure to grow, or nutrient deficiency
- Other eating disorders, often atypical variants on AN, BN, BED, or ARFID[62]

The overall goals of treatment for eating disorders are essentially the same as the nutritional goals for all adolescents: to attain and maintain good nutritional status, to achieve optimal growth, and to develop a healthy relationship with food that includes good mental health.[62] Eating disorder treatment combines a primary emphasis on psychological therapy with intensive nutritional therapy focused on repletion.[62]

Public Health Considerations Relevant to Eating Disorders

The YRBSS, administered throughout the United States by the CDC every 2 years, eliminated questions pertaining to eating disorders in 2015.[59] Thus, available uniformly collected data are over a decade old. While other datasets are available, they are not representative on a nationwide scale and may omit key population groups or questions. In addition, data from 2013 does not include findings from adolescents impacted by mental health stresses associated with the COVID-19 pandemic.[59]

In 2022, the U.S. Preventive Services Task Force announced the results of a review of the evidence surrounding routine screening for eating disorders in adolescents and adults, and found that there was insufficient evidence to evaluate either the benefits or harms of such screening.[63] This finding does not necessarily mean that screening for eating disorders is not beneficial; rather, it indicates that there is not enough evidence to make either a positive or negative recommendation.

Given the critical need for enhanced knowledge on eating disorder prevention, screening, and treatment among adolescents, public health and nutrition professionals' role includes:

- Advocating urgently for quality research on eating disorder prevention, screening, and treatment among adolescents
- Advocating urgently for improved access to high-quality care for adolescent patients with eating disorders
- Promoting healthful food and nutrition environments at all levels of the social ecological model, including the individual, family, community, and societal (policy) levels
- Focusing on encouraging healthful behaviors and habits such as family meals and promoting a healthful body image rather than norms centered around dieting, weight, and food restriction
- Educate parents and caregivers on ways to help children and adolescents develop a healthful relationship with food, including development of a healthful structure around eating in the home, avoidance of using food as a reward or punishment, and providing role modeling for appropriate self-nourishment and enjoyment of food

Displacement of Healthful Beverages With Sugar Sweetened Beverages

Sugar-sweetened beverages, as the name suggests, are drinks of various types that are sweetened with added sugars.[64,65] Sugar-sweetened beverages can include but are not limited to soft drinks such as soda, juice drinks, energy beverages, flavored milks, coffee beverages, and many others. According to the CDC, added sugars include a variety of nutritive sweeteners, including but not limited to table sugar, honey, molasses, high-fructose corn syrup, and others.[65] Sugar-sweetened beverages tend to have minimal nutritional value while providing excessive calories.[66] In addition, evidence indicates that sugar-sweetened beverages may not produce the same feeling of fulness, or **satiety**, that results from eating solid food.[66,67] WHO and the DGAs recommend that maximum intake of added sugars be no more than 10% of total calories; this benchmark can be quickly exceeded by overconsumption of sugary drinks.[35,68] Intake of added sugars appears at its highest in adolescence, when it reaches about 15% of total calories consumed on average, and about 32% of total calories from added sugars in adolescents come from sugar-sweetened beverages.[35]

A greater proportion of adolescents consume sugar-sweetened beverages than other age groups, although overall consumption has decreased somewhat among teens since 2000.[65] Risk of obesity, higher-than-recommended waist circumference, increased body fat percentage, abnormal blood lipid profiles, dental caries, and high blood pressure among children and adolescents have been associated with increased sugar-sweetened beverage consumption.[69–71] In adults, evidence indicates the possibility of association between suboptimal bone mineral density and excessive sugar-sweetened beverage intake; this association may be related to replacement of calcium-rich beverages with sugar-sweetened beverages in adolescence, since about 95% of adult bone mass is accrued by the end of the adolescent years.[21,72]

Interventions to Reduce Sugar-Sweetened Beverage Intake Among Adolescents

"Reduce consumption of added sugars by people aged 2 years and older" (NWS-10) is an objective from the *Healthy People 2030* project of the Office of Disease Prevention and Health Promotion.[73] Reduction of the consumption of sugar-sweetened beverages by teens will almost certainly be required to meet this goal. The DGAs recommend that children and adolescents shift from drinking sugar-sweetened beverages to healthful beverages such as:

- Water
- Unsweetened fat-free or low-fat milk including low-lactose options and fortified soy beverages
- 100% juice (limit to 4 oz/day for young children, 10 oz/day for older children and adolescents)[35]

A meta-analysis found that the types of interventions commonly used in public health settings, largely nutrition education and counseling, were of moderate success in reducing sugar-sweetened beverage intake in populations of children but resulted in only small reductions in adolescents.[74] Another meta-analysis found that school-based interventions among children and adolescents to reduce sugar-sweetened beverage consumption were effective.[58] Effective strategies incorporated interaction, integrated psychosocial factors, and involved parents and caregivers. Comprehensive approaches that consider environmental factors heightened the efficacy of interventions.[58]

Public Policy Approaches

The AAP has suggested six public policy strategies, based on current research evidence, to curtail sugar-sweetened beverage consumption among children and adolescents.[66] A summary of the recommendations follows:

- Tax sugar-sweetened beverages to make them more expensive.
- Government policy should seek to reduce the marketing of sugar-sweetened beverages to children and adolescents.
- Design government food assistance programs to reduce the purchase of sugar-sweetened beverages.
- Make nutrition information easily to access and understand on labels, menus, and marketing materials.
- Support policies that make healthful beverage choices the easiest choices by increasing access to healthful beverages.
- Encourage healthcare facilities such as hospitals to set the example of serving healthful beverages and discouraging sugary beverages.[66]

Both direct and environmental interventions that are effective in reducing the amount of sugar-sweetened beverages consumed by teens have the potential to confer substantial societal benefits by improving short- and long-term health outcomes.

Food Insecurity

In 2019–2020, the CDC National Center for Health Statistics reported that 11.2% of children age 12 to 17 years lived in food-insecure households.[75] Food insecurity, or the condition of lacking consistent access to adequate food, is associated with poor physical and mental health in adolescents.[76] Shankar et al., in a systematic review, found that food insecurity in children and adolescents was associated with poor behavioral, academic, and emotional outcomes even after controlling for confounding factors.[77] Another study found that the prevalence of obesity was higher among adolescents who lived in food-insecure households, but no causative relationship was found between the two factors, indicating a need for further research to understand potentially complex environmental influences.[78]

In 2016, the Urban Institute and Feeding America collaborated on two reports focused on teen food insecurity, completed as a result of the *Teens and Hunger Project* (THP).[79,80] The THP was a qualitative research effort that conducted focus-group interviews with 193 adolescents living in urban and rural lower-income communities across the United States. The researchers' goal was to learn more about the teens' experiences of food insecurity, their coping strategies, and perceived barriers to engaging in governmental and nongovernmental food insecurity programs. The collaboration found that food insecurity among adolescents is common and widespread.

Some of the major findings published in the Urban Institute and Feeding America reports were:

- Adolescents perceive stigma associated with food insecurity, and may seek to conceal their lack adequate food from others.
- While teens reported that their parents tried to protect them from lack of food, they also described coping with food insecurity by assuming adult responsibilities within their families, such as taking paid employment to contribute to the family food budget, or giving up their own food so that younger siblings could eat.
- Teens reported knowledge of incidents of criminal behavior in response to food insecurity such as shoplifting or selling substances/stolen goods to obtain money for food.[81]

- Adolescents had many comments on the U.S. federal school nutrition program, and offered many ideas for strengthening and improving these programs; many were unaware of available federal summer feeding programs, or thought that resources such as backpack programs were unavailable to them.
- Study participants often reported the perception that food assistance could be accessed only by adults.

Public health practitioners should be aware that adolescents impacted by food insecurity will likely benefit from supportive and sensitive adult guidance in facilitating connections with appropriate resources.

The AAP has provided guidelines for addressing food insecurity in pediatric populations, including adolescents[81]:

1. Pediatricians should screen for food insecurity risk at regular well-child and adolescent visits; the Hagar 2-question validated screening tool is recommended.[81,82]
2. Facilitate connections among food-insecure households and community food resources; resources most helpful to adolescents may include governmental programs such as SNAP and the National School Lunch and Breakfast Programs, as well as private resources such as local food pantries and backpack programs; of interest, some local elementary and secondary schools are now developing their own food pantries in response to student food insecurity.[83]
3. Advocate for policies and programs that promote access to adequate, healthful food for all people.[81]

In public health, the second and third guidelines, which promote community connections and advocacy for food-insecure adolescents, are of primary importance.

Public health professionals should be aware of the Hager 2-Question Food Insecurity Screen (H2QS), cited by the AAP in guideline 1. Also known as the Hunger Vital Sign, the H2QS is based on the first two questions of the USDA 18-item Household Food Insecurity Scale (HFSS).[84] The H2QS was developed from and validated against the gold-standard USDA 18-item HFSS, and has been validated in other settings as well.[82,85] In 2015, the H2QS was validated for use with youth and adolescents.[86] It is a useful tool in appropriate public health and nutrition programs, as it is very easy to administer in a variety of settings. The H2QS is provided in Figure 6.3.[82,84]

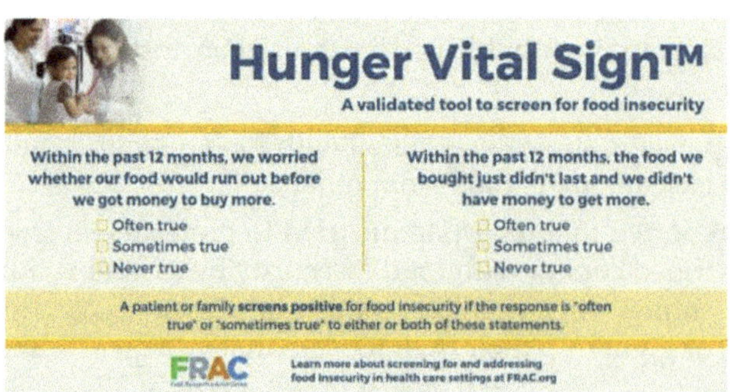

Figure 6.3. The Hager 2-Question Food Insecurity Screen, also known as the Hunger Vital Sign.
Source: Food Research & Action Center. Hunger Vital Sign. October 2019. https://frac.org/screen-intervene/hunger-vital-sign-graphic-oct-2019

Chronic Long-Term Health Conditions

The presence of chronic long-term health conditions in adolescence adds additional layers of challenge to a developmental phase that is already difficult, if not turbulent. A discussion of the medical and nutritional treatment of chronic diseases in adolescence is beyond the scope of this textbook. However, it is important for public health practitioners to be aware of the importance of appropriate support systems for all young people impacted by long-term health conditions, and to encourage the development of community health and organizational resources to address the needs of this population.

All adolescents with chronic conditions should be under the care of a physician. Because the course and management of many chronic diseases are affected by nutrition, individualized medical nutrition therapy and a nutritional plan should be provided by a registered dietitian nutritionist. Self-management is a key component of chronic disease care, and much research has been conducted among adults regarding best practices for self-management of chronic disease. While there is recognition of the importance of self-management among adolescents with chronic disease, to date not as much research informs these interventions.[87] Lozano and Houtrow stated the need for chronic disease self-management interventions specifically designed and developmentally appropriate for pediatric populations.[87] The authors also emphasized the importance of recognizing that in children, including adolescents, chronic disease self-management is a collaboration among the patient, parents/caregivers, and medical providers.[87] Interventions, therefore, should include all these stakeholders.

Effective interventions build self-efficacy and consider the unique physical, emotional, and social needs of adolescents. Community and organizational resources may include support groups, availability of mental health counseling, summer camps for children and teens such as the American Diabetic Association camping programs, publications and educational resources, and other resources available through schools, medical providers, governmental organizations such as county health departments and nongovernmental nonprofits such as the American Heart Association.[88,89]

SOCIAL DETERMINANTS OF HEALTH IN THE ADOLESCENT LIFE CYCLE STAGE

Social determinants of health (SDOH) impact every life cycle stage and every population around the globe, including adolescents. According to the CDC, five overall factors influence health: (1) genetics, (2) health behaviors, (3) environmental conditions, (4) access to medical care, and (5) SDOH.[90] In recent years research has underscored the importance of the fifth factor, social determinants, in impacting overall health.

The socioeconomic conditions in which people live can profoundly influence health and nutrition throughout the life cycle. During the adolescent life cycle stage, teens are forming lifelong habits that will either positively influence health and quality of life, or increase risk for debilitating health problems. It is difficult to overstate the importance of SDOH and their downstream effects on adolescents as they grow up because the overall well-being of nations and societies is determined by the health and productivity of its adults.[91]

SDOH and nutrition that impact teens include but are not limited to family income level, race and/or ethnicity, culture, access to healthful food and adequate housing, educational opportunities, access to caring adult mentors, safe air and water, access to medical care, access to health information leading to health literacy, access to technology, and safe neighborhoods. Teens' nutrition status is negatively impacted when social determinants include such factors as:

- Living in poverty or at a low income level, which impacts access to healthful food
- Habitual poor nutrition, perhaps resulting from food insecurity
- Lack of access to quality educational opportunities, including nutrition education
- Lack of access to ongoing, quality healthcare services to monitor growth and health
- Lack of health information leading to poor health literacy including poor nutrition literacy
- Living in unsafe or unstable housing, or being unhoused, which limits opportunities for the safe acquisition, storage, and preparation of food
- Exposure to violence or living in an unsafe neighborhood, which may prevent ready access to healthful food
- Lack of access to caring, positive adult mentors, which may lead to the lack of a positive structure around family meals and nutrition

Viner et al., in a well-known study of SDOH in adolescents, proposed that three major factors impacting global adolescent health include the overall financial status of one's nation, income disparities, and access to high-quality education.[91] According to Viner's study, effective interventions to improve SDOH globally include policies to broaden youth access to education and employment opportunities.[91] The CDC suggests that interventions addressing SDOH can be impactful in promoting **health equity**, which is defined as every person having the opportunity to achieve their highest possible health potential, with no social determinants preventing the achievement of that potential.[90]

Other Social Influences on Adolescent Nutrition Status

Many sociocultural influences, which may overlap with SDOH, impact the adolescent nutrition environment. Influences on teens' food choices, which impact consumption of healthful food include the increasing importance of the food preferences of peers, expanding opportunities to eat away from home, greater exposure to the community nutrition environment whether positive or negative, and media sources including food advertising and social media.[17]

The Social Ecological Model of Health

The social ecological model of health (SEM), first proposed by WHO in 1947, provides a framework for thinking of health within the complete social environment encompassing four stratifications for intervention: individuals, relationships, community, and society.[92] The model shows the relationships among the various stratifications and their location within the overall social environment. Because the SEM takes the social milieu into account, it provides helpful scaffolding for thinking through interventions that address SDOH. Figure 6.4 illustrates the SEM. Table 6.12 provides an example of interventions focused on adolescent food insecurity, placed within the four levels of the SEM.

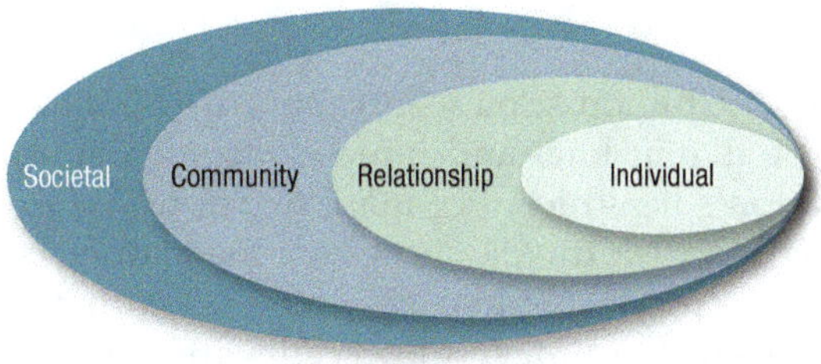

Figure 6.4. The social ecological model of health.
Source: Agency for Toxic Substances and Disease Registry. Models and frameworks for the practice of community engagement. U.S. Department of Health and Human Services. Updated June 15, 2015. https://www.atsdr.cdc.gov/communityengagement/pce_models.html

Table 6.12. Interventions Focused on Food Security for Adolescents*

Social Ecological Level	Proposed Intervention	Social Determinant of Health Targeted
Individual	*Individual Nutrition Education* (provided in school or by community organizations): Knowledge and skills including healthful diet, cooking skills, and food management skills such as food budgeting and acquisition	• Access to quality education • Access to healthful food • Health and nutrition literacy • Income level (optimizing resources)
Relationships	*Family Nutrition Education* (intentionally include adolescents' families in nutrition education efforts): Develop parent/caregiver–school nutrition communications and activities, look for opportunities to involve parents/caregivers in nutrition initiatives such as school food pantries, encourage adolescents to share nutrition knowledge and skills with their families.	• Access to healthful food • Health and nutrition literacy • Income level (optimizing resources) • Access to quality educations (by promoting parent/caregiver involvement)
Community	*Development of community food resources:* May include resources such as a school food pantry and backpack programs for students and their families, or a local food council to address local nutrition issues	• Access to healthful food • Access to quality education (good nutrition helps children get the most out of school)
Society	*Policy* focused on improved food security: Federal nutrition programs such as the Supplemental Nutrition Assistance Program (SNAP), the School Lunch and School Breakfast Programs, Expanded Food and Nutrition Education Program (EFNEP) for youth *Policy* to encourage the optimal functioning of nonprofit nongovernmental organizations such as food banks and their constituent food pantries	• Access to healthful food • Access to quality education (improved education outcomes associated with the School Lunch and Breakfast Programs) • Health and nutrition literacy

*These interventions address specific social determinants of health within each social ecological level.

POLICY: GLOBAL ISSUES AND CHALLENGES

Currently, an estimated 1.6 billion adolescents make up about 17% of the world's population, and about 90% live in low- and middle-income countries.[93] Overall, adolescents are usually a nation's healthiest population group.[4] WHO reports that interpersonal violence, suicide, and road travel injuries are the leading causes of the 1.1 million adolescent deaths that occur on average per year.[93] Health concerns for adolescents vary by age, sex, and location. Younger adolescents are more likely to be impacted by diseases associated with inadequate sanitation including contaminated water. Health behaviors in regards to alcohol and sexual activity contribute to a greater proportion of older adolescent morbidity and mortality. For all adolescents globally, poor nutrition and sedentary lifestyles adopted early in life often persist and negatively impact health throughout the lifespan.[93]

Recommendations for positively impacting global adolescent health include continued collection of data and information to support the development of evidence-based protocols, the provision of health education including nutrition education, and the development of policies to improve adolescents' access to health education, information, and services. A crucial component of improving global adolescent health is to recognize that adolescents are growing in competence and independence, and to include them as partners in the development of interventions that impact their health.[93]

PUBLIC HEALTH NUTRITION PROGRAMS FOR ADOLESCENTS

Table 6.13 provides information regarding several U.S. federal public health nutrition programs that are available to adolescents in the United States. In addition to U.S. federal nutrition programs, private organizations and initiatives such as food banks and their constituent food pantries and backpack programs are available to fill nutrition gaps for adolescents. Globally, the United Nations supports a number of programs that are available to adolescents, including micronutrient supplements and food fortification where needed, provision of safe and nutritious food and clean drinking water to increase accessibility, and nutrition education to promote self-efficacy in making nutritional improvements on individual and societal levels.[94]

WHAT WORKS: THE NATIONAL SCHOOL LUNCH AND BREAKFAST PROGRAMS

In the United States, adolescents attending public and many private schools have access to two nutrition intervention programs of proven effectiveness: the National School Lunch Program and the School Breakfast Program.[95] Public health nutrition professionals should encourage teens to utilize these programs, which provide healthful lunches and breakfasts that meet U.S. federal nutrition standards. Free and reduced-price options are available to children who meet income guidelines. Research indicates that the National School Lunch Program and the School Breakfast Program are associated with reductions in food insecurity, improved intake of key nutrients, reductions in obesity rates among low-income children, and better learning outcomes.[95]

Table 6.13. Summary of U.S. Federal Nutrition Programs Available to Adolescents

Program Name	Description	Reach of Services	Eligibility	Website
SNAP: Supplemental Nutrition Assistance Program	Provides supplemental income for the purchase of food for low-income families	The average SNAP benefit is $104 per month Over 248,000 participating food retailers	All ages Must be at or below 130% of the poverty line to qualify	www.fns.usda.gov/snap/supplemental-nutrition-assistance-program
TEFAP: The Emergency Food Assistance Program	Provides food items to food banks, food pantries, and soup kitchens to be given out to the community. Most participants who enroll are older adults and have an income high enough to not qualify for SNAP.	In 2020, TEFAP provided over 2.4 billion meals.	All ages	www.fns.usda.gov/tefap/emergency-food-assistance-program
School Meals: Breakfast, Lunch, Summer Feeding Program	Assists low-income families by providing reduced cost or free school lunches in public schools, nonprofit private schools, and child care facilities. During the summer adolescents also qualify for the Summer Food Service Program that provides nutritious meals and snacks.	About 7.1 million children participate in the school lunch program.	PreK–12 Students	www.fns.usda.gov/nslp

(*continued*)

Table 6.13. Summary of U.S. Federal Nutrition Programs Available to Adolescents (*continued*)

Program Name	Description	Reach of Services	Eligibility	Website
EFNEP: Expanded Food and Nutrition Education Program	Federal Extension (community outreach) program operating in every state, the District of Columbia, and the six U.S. territories by the 1862 and 1890 Land-Grant Universities. Nutrition education via hands-on learning and applied science, to support participants' efforts toward self-sufficiency, nutritional health, and well-being.	About 45,500 adults and 187,500 youth in 2022.	Children (5–12 years), youth (13–8 years), and adults of limited financial resources	www.nifa.usda.gov/grants/programs/capacity-grants/efnep/expanded-food-nutrition-education-program

SUMMARY

Adolescence is the key transitional period in the human life cycle: the time during which a child becomes an adult. Caring adult mentors play a key role throughout adolescence and are essential in helping teens navigate the tasks of adolescence successfully. Optimal physical, emotional, intellectual, and social development is supported by good nutrition, and without good nutrition adolescents' genetic potential for growth will not be reached. By focusing on nutrition issues of importance to teen populations and contextualizing adolescent development within an environmental milieu defined by SDOH, public health nutrition professionals can positively impact adolescents' journey to adulthood.

KEY CHAPTER CONCEPTS

1. Human beings enter *adolescence* as children and leave as young adults, navigating immense physical, cognitive, emotional, and social changes during this life cycle phase.[1]
2. The American Academy of Pediatrics describes three phases of adolescence: *early adolescence* (in general, ages 10 or 11 to 13 or 14 years), *middle adolescence* (14–17 years), and *late adolescence* (18–21+ years).[2] Each phase has specific characteristics and developmental milestones.
3. Evidence indicates that effective adult mentorship of adolescents improves a variety of outcomes that persist into adulthood, including social and academic outcomes.[15] Effective mentors can also help guide teens toward a healthy lifestyle by modeling positive health behaviors such as healthful eating, regular physical activity, and avoidance of smoking and excessive use of alcohol.
4. The rapid physical growth and development of adolescence require adequate and appropriate nutrients.[7] During adolescence, teens will add about 20% of their adult height, 40% of adult bone mass, and 50% of adult weight. The ability to think abstractly and to self-evaluate behaviors increases as neurologic capacity develops. The process of puberty ends in the development of adult sexual characteristics and reproductive capacity, along with the growth and maturation of all body organs.[16]
5. Examples of key official nutrition guidance and data gathering tools that are applied in adolescent nutrition settings include the Healthy Eating Index (HEI), the Dietary Guidelines for Americans (DGAs), the Dietary Reference Intakes (DRIs), MyPlate for Teens, the Youth Risk Behavior Surveillance Survey (YRBSS), and the World Health Organization (WHO) Guideline: Implementing Effective Actions for Improving Adolescent Nutrition.
6. Effective public health nutrition interventions for adolescents should be multifaceted, encompassing educational, health, environmental, and digital considerations. Two primary areas for intervention are the overall nutrition environment and nutrition education to promote self-efficacy and independence. Support from caring adults as well as consideration of developmental needs may increase the effectiveness of interventions. Involving teens as partners in the creation, management, and evaluation of interventions is likely to heighten their effectiveness.
7. Public health nutrition issues for adolescents include but are not limited to eating disorders, displacement of nutritious beverages with sugar-sweetened beverages, food insecurity, and the need for resources and supports, including nutrition resources, for adolescents with long-term medical conditions.
8. SDOH have a strong impact on teens' health and nutrition status. SDOH include including family income level, race and/or ethnicity, culture, access to healthful food and adequate housing,

educational opportunities, access to caring adult mentors, safe air and water, access to medical care, access to health information leading to health literacy, access to technology, and safe neighborhoods.

CASE STUDY

Your local high school has identified a need to provide resources and support to students who are living with food insecurity. As director of a large local food pantry, you have been asked to consider developing a satellite pantry housed at the high school. School administrators are highly supportive. The school board has approved the project and has asked you to write an implementation plan.

In preparation for designing your implementation plan, review this web page: www.feedingamerica.org/our-work/hunger-relief-programs/school-pantry. Then answer the following questions as though you are the project leader.

1. Write a brief mission statement for the school food pantry. Include: Who will the pantry serve? What is its purpose?
2. Which stakeholders will be important to include in your planning and why? List at least three. How will you invite each stakeholder into the process? What role will each stakeholder play in the implementation process?
3. What community collaborators will you include in your planning and why?
4. How will you determine funding needs for the pantry? What sources of funding are likely to be available? What sources of funding could be developed? How would you go about ensuring a sustainable funding base over time?
5. What kind of physical facility will be needed to host the pantry? What special equipment might be needed, and how could it be obtained?
6. How will you obtain food to stock the pantry? (Remember the possibility of collaborating with a food bank, as well as local businesses.)
7. What hours/days of the week would you suggest the pantry be open, and why?
8. List at least four food pantry policies that you will need to develop, along with a brief description of the purpose of each policy.

DISCUSSION QUESTIONS

1. Review the *10 Tasks of Adolescent Development.* If these tasks could be ranked in order of importance, what do you think would be the top three tasks? Discuss.
2. What are some best practices for mentoring adolescents? These can include practices that are recommended for parents/caregivers as well as those who work with adolescents in professional settings. How might these practices apply to nutrition intervention and guidance?
3. Official U.S. dietary data and guidance tools that can be used when working with teens include the Healthy Eating Index, the Dietary Guidelines for Americans, the Dietary Reference Intakes, and MyPlate for Teens. How can these tools inform the development of public health nutrition interventions for adolescents?

4. Nutrition plays a key role in supporting the rapid physical development that takes place during adolescence. What are possible short- and long-term consequences of poor nutrition during this life cycle phase?
5. Discuss typical environmental factors that influence adolescents' food choices. What are some strategies that could be implemented for improving the nutrition environment for teens in communities and schools?
6. What components do you think are important to include in an intervention to reduce sugar-sweetened beverage consumption among adolescents in your community?
7. How could access to food resources and support for adolescents with food insecurity be improved in your community? Discuss.
8. Discuss and list three or four characteristics of effective nutrition interventions for adolescents. For each listed item, describe an example of how that characteristic might be used in an intervention design.

SUGGESTED LEARNING ACTIVITIES

1. (Group or individual activity) Prepare a 25-minute inservice presentation on adolescent nutrition for school nutrition staff in a high school. Your planning for the presentation should include audience considerations, session objectives, a session outline, content to be included, methods for presenting your content, and supplementary materials to be prepared for distribution (such as a handout or post-quiz), if any. Present to fellow students and your instructor to receive feedback, and revise the presentation accordingly. If possible, present as an inservice in a high school food service setting.
2. Choose one of the body's systems, such as the neurologic, skeletal, reproductive, muscular, or digestive systems. Prepare a report on the development of your chosen system throughout adolescence, including the normal progression of development as well as desired outcomes of optimal development.
3. Review local middle and high school websites, or talk to school food service staff within those schools, to learn of any school-based food pantries in your community. Prepare a summary table for one pantry, including information such as:
    - Pantry location
    - Hours of operation
    - How can a student and/or student's family access the pantry?
    - Does the school offer additional services such as a backpack program?
    - What classes are available to promote the development of lifetime food-related competencies, such as food budgeting and shopping, cooking skills, and nutrition knowledge?
    - How does the school connect students who may be impacted by food insecurity with appropriate support and resources?

After completing your review of local resources, determine whether you can identify any opportunities for local middle and high schools to enhance food access services for adolescents with food insecurity. This learning activity may be used to provide background information for this chapter's case study.

4. Develop, prepare, and present a cooking skills class for either younger or older adolescents. Follow planning principles for effective cooking classes such as considering your audience, developing

objectives, thinking through details, and practicing class delivery prior to the actual class. Evaluate the delivery of your class, including audience input as appropriate. Make suggestions for future cooking skills classes for adolescents, based on your learning.

5. Use the social ecological model to plan a community-wide intervention to reduce sugar-sweetened beverage intake in adolescents. Include suggestions for appropriate interventions at each level of influence: individual, relationship, community, and societal.[96]
6. Prepare a list of the seven Dietary Reference Intake (DRI) values. For each DRI value, provide a corresponding instance of a situation in which that value would be useful for adolescents. Here is an example:
    - Tolerable upper intake level (UL): A teen athlete is drinking 5 to 6 glasses of milk per day in addition to taking a calcium supplement. A nutrition professional wishes to know if the teen is exceeding the safe UL for calcium for their age/sex group.

RESOURCES FOR FURTHER LEARNING

- USDA MyPlate for Teens: www.myplate.gov/life-stages/teens
    - Designed for use by teens, provides nutrition guidelines, access to MyPlate resources, and information on MyPlate-related apps
- *Healthy Eating for Teens* Tip Sheet: https://myplate-prod.azureedge.us/sites/default/files/2022-04/TipSheet_18_HealthyEatingForTeens.pdf
    - A one-page brochure based on *MyPlate for Teens* recommendations
- Raising Teens: Massachusetts Institute of Technology Work-Life Center: https://hr.mit.edu/static/worklife/raising-teens
    - Houses data and recommendations from the MIT Raising Teens research project; includes the Ten Tasks of Adolescent Development and the Five Basics of Parenting Adolescents
- Centers for Disease Control and Prevention, National Center for Health Services, CDC Growth Charts: www.cdc.gov/growthcharts
    - Standardized growth charts for children and adolescents ages 2 to 20 years
- Feeding America School Food Pantry Program: www.feedingamerica.org/our-work/hunger-relief-programs/school-pantry
    - Provides information on school-based food pantry programs and how to start such a program
- YRBS Explorer: https://yrbs-explorer.services.cdc.gov
    - A user-friendly tool that allows review of national, state, and local data from the YRBSS survey, including nutrition data
- American Academy of Pediatrics: www.aap.org
    - Information, resources, and guidelines on child and adolescent health
- Academy of Nutrition and Dietetics: www.eatright.org
    - Reliable nutrition information for all life cycle phases
- School Nutrition Association: https://schoolnutrition.org
    - Information, credentialing, resources, and networking for school nutrition professionals

- Child Nutrition Programs (National School Lunch, School Breakfast, Special Milk, Summer Food Service, and Child and Adult Care Food Programs): www.fns.usda.gov/child-nutrition-programs
  - Resources, information, and guidance on the U.S. government's child nutrition programs

SPRINGER PUBLISHING CONNECT™ | **A robust set of instructor resources designed to supplement this text is located at http://connect.springerpub.com/content/book/978-0-8261-8623-2. Qualifying instructors may request access by emailing textbook@springerpub.com.**

REFERENCES

1. Office of Population Affairs. *Adolescent Development Explained.* U.S. Department of Health and Human Services; 2018. https://opa.hhs.gov/sites/default/files/2021-03/adolescent-development-explained-download.pdf
2. Allen B, Waterman H. Stages of adolesence. American Academy of Pediatrics, healthy children.org. Updated March 28, 2023. https://www.healthychildren.org/English/ages-stages/teen/Pages/Stages-of-Adolescence.aspx
3. Balasundaram P, Avulakunta ID. Human growth and development. In: *StatPearls.* StatPearls Publishing; 2022. https://www.ncbi.nlm.nih.gov/books/NBK567767
4. Das JK, Salam RA, Thornburg KL, et al. Nutrition in adolescents: physiology, metabolism, and nutritional needs. *Ann N Y Acad Sci.* 2017;1393(1):21–33. https://doi.org/10.1111/nyas.13330
5. United Nations, Department of Economic and Social Affairs, Population Division. *World Population Prospects: The 2015 Revision—Key Findings and Advance Tables.* United Nations; 2015. https://esa.un.org/unpd/wpp/publications/files/key_findings_wpp_2015.pdf
6. Patton GC, Sawyer SM, Santelli JS, et al. Our future: a Lancet commission on adolescent health and wellbeing. *Lancet.* 2016;387(10036):2423–2478. https://doi.org/10.1016/S0140-6736(16)00579-1
7. Christie D, Viner R. Adolescent development. *BMJ.* 2005;330(7486):301–304. https://doi.org/10.1136/bmj.330.7486.301
8. Simpson AR. *Raising Teens: A Synthesis of Research and a Foundation for Action.* Center for Health Communication, Harvard School of Public Health; 2001.
9. Simpson AR. Raising teens. Massachusetts Institute of Technology Work-Life Center. Raising Teens Project. 2018. https://hr.mit.edu/static/worklife/raising-teens/index.html
10. Simpson AR. About the Raising Teens Project. Massechusetts Institute of Technology Work-Life Center. Raising Teens Project. 2018. https://hr.mit.edu/static/worklife/raising-teens/about.html
11. Simpson AR. Ten Tasks of Adolescent Development. Massachusetts Institute of Technology Work-Life Center. Raising Teens Project. 2018. https://hr.mit.edu/static/worklife/raising-teens/ten-tasks.html
12. Levenson L. Ten Tasks of Adolescent Development. Medium; January 4, 2022. https://medium.com/circle-dynamics/ten-tasks-of-adolescent-development-82d645facd36
13. Simpson AR. Raising teens: Five Basics of Parenting Adolescents. Massachusetts Institute of Technology Work-Life Center. Raising Teens Project. 2018. https://hr.mit.edu/static/worklife/raising-teens/five-basics.html
14. Paritosh K, Fisher M. Addressing key issues in adolescent health care. *Pediatrics.* 2020;145:S151–S152. https://doi.org/10.1542/peds.2019-2056B
15. Office of Disease Prevention and Health Promotion. Increase the proportion of adolescents who have an adult they can talk to about serious problems. *Healthy People 2030.* U.S. Department of Health and Human Services; 2020. https://health.gov/healthypeople/objectives-and-data/browse-objectives/adolescents/increase-proportion-adolescents-who-have-adult-they-can-talk-about-serious-problems-ah-03
16. Norris SA, Frongillo EA, Black MM, et al. Nutrition in adolescent growth and development. *Lancet.* 2022;399(10320):172–184. https://doi.org/10.1016/S0140-6736(21)01590-7

17. Ziegler AM, Kasprzak CM, Mansouri TH, et al. An ecological perspective of food choice and eating autonomy among adolescents. *Front Psychol*. 2021;12:654139. https://doi.org/10.3389/fpsyg.2021.654139
18. Graber EG. Physical growth and sexual maturation of adolescents. Merck Manual: Professional Version. Updated March 2023. https://www.merckmanuals.com/professional/pediatrics/growth-and-development/physical-growth-and-sexual-maturation-of-adolescents
19. Sanders JO, Qiu X, Lu X, et al. The uniform pattern of growth and skeletal maturation during the human adolescent growth spurt. *Sci Rep*. 2017;7(1):16705. https://doi.org/10.1038/s41598-017-16996-w
20. Rogol AD, Clark PA, Roemmich JN. Growth and pubertal development in children and adolescents: effects of diet and physical activity. *Am J Clin Nutr*. 2000;72(2):521S–528S. https://doi.org/10.1093/ajcn/72.2.521S
21. Min SK, Oh T, Kim SH, et al. Position statement: exercise guidelines to increase peak bone mass in adolescents. *J Bone Metab*. 2019;26(4):225–239. https://doi.org/10.11005/jbm.2019.26.4.225
22. Levine MA. Assessing bone health in children and adolescents. *Indian J Endocrinol Metab*. 2012;16(suppl 2):S205–S212. https://doi.org/10.4103/2230-8210.104040
23. Soliman A, De Sanctis V, Elalaily R, Bedair S. Advances in pubertal growth and factors influencing it: can we increase pubertal growth? *Indian J Endocrinol Metab*. 2014;18(suppl 1):S53–S62. https://doi.org/10.4103/2230-8210.145075
24. Viner RM, Allen NB, Patton GC. Puberty, developmental processes, and health interventions. In: Bundy DAP, de Silva N, Horton S, Jamison DT, Patton GC, eds. *Child and Adolescent Health and Development*. 3rd ed. International Bank for Reconstruction and Development/The World Bank; 2017:chap 9. https://doi.org/10.1596/978-1-4648-0423-6_ch9
25. Chulani VL, Gordon LP. Adolescent growth and development. *Prim Care*. 2014;41(3):465–487. https://doi.org/10.1016/j.pop.2014.05.002
26. McLaughlin J. Puberty in girls. Merck Manual: Consumer Version. Updated September 2022. https://www.merckmanuals.com/home/women-s-health-issues/biology-of-the-female-reproductive-system/puberty-in-girls
27. Emmanuel M, Bokor BR. Tanner stages. In: *StatPearls*. StatPearls Publishing; 2021. https://www.ncbi.nlm.nih.gov/books/NBK470280
28. Marshall WA, Tanner JM. Variations in the pattern of pubertal changes in boys. *Arch Dis Child*. 1970;45(239):13–23. https://doi.org/10.1136/adc.45.239.13
29. Marshall WA, Tanner JM. Variations in pattern of pubertal changes in girls. *Arch Dis Child*. 1969;44(235):291–303. https://doi.org/10.1136/adc.44.235.291
30. Abreu AP, Kaiser UB. Pubertal development and regulation. *Lancet Diabetes Endocrinol*. 2016;4(3):254–264. https://doi.org/10.1016/S2213-8587(15)00418-0
31. National Cancer Institute, Division of Cancer Control and Population Sciences. Overview & background of the healthy eating index. Updated July 28, 2023. https://epi.grants.cancer.gov/hei
32. U.S. Food and Nutrition Service. Healthy eating index (HEI). U.S. Department of Agriculture. Updated July 14, 2023. https://www.fns.usda.gov/healthy-eating-index-hei
33. Centers for Disease Control and Prevention. What we eat in America, DHHS-USDA dietary survey integration. National Health and Nutrition Examination Survey. Accessed March 6, 2023. https://www.cdc.gov/nchs/nhanes/wweia.htm
34. Anderson-Villaluz D. Giving children and adolescents a healthy start through nutrition. U.S. Departement of Health and Human Services, Office of Disease Prevention and Health Promotion. March 30, 2021. https://health.gov/news/202103/giving-children-and-adolescents-healthy-start-through-nutrition
35. U.S. Department of Agriculture, U.S. Department of Health and Human Services. *Dietary Guidelines for Americans, 2020-2025*. 9th ed. U.S. Department of Health and Human Services; 2020. https://www.dietaryguidelines.gov
36. Centers for Disease Control and Prevention. Adolescent and school health: Youth Risk Behavior Surveillance System (YRBSS). Accessed March 6, 2023. https://www.cdc.gov/healthyyouth/data/yrbs/index.htm
37. Centers for Disease Control and Prevention. YRBS Explorer. Accessed March 6, 2023. https://yrbs-explorer.services.cdc.gov
38. U.S. Department of Agriculture, U.S. Department of Health and Human Services. History of the *Dietary Guidelines*. Accessed February 25, 2023. https://www.dietaryguidelines.gov/about-dietary-guidelines/history-dietary-guidelines

39. U.S. Department of Agriculture. Make every bite count with the *Dietary Guidelines for Americans*. December 2020. https://www.dietaryguidelines.gov/sites/default/files/2020-12/DGA_2020-2025_Infographic_MakeEveryBiteCount.pdf
40. U.S. Department of Agriculture, U.S. Department of Health and Human Services. Top 10 things you need to know about the Dietary Guidelines for Americans, 2020–2025. Accessed February 25, 2023. https://www.dietaryguidelines.gov/resources/2020-2025-dietary-guidelines-online-materials/top-10-things-you-need-know-about-dietary
41. Office of Disease Prevention and Health Promotion. Dietary reference intakes. U.S. Department of Health and Human Services. Updated January 18, 2023. https://health.gov/our-work/nutrition-physical-activity/dietary-guidelines/dietary-reference-intakes
42. Office of Disease Prevention and Health Promotion. Dietary reference intakes development. U.S. Department of Health and Human Services. Updated January 18, 2023. https://health.gov/our-work/nutrition-physical-activity/dietary-guidelines/dietary-reference-intakes/dietary-reference-intakes-development
43. National Academies of Sciences, Engineering, and Medicine. Sodium and potassium dietary reference intake values updated in new report; introduces new category for sodium based on chronic disease risk reduction. March 5, 2019. https://www.nationalacademies.org/news/2019/03/sodium-and-potassium-dietary-reference-intake-values-updated-in-new-report
44. Otten JJ, Hellwig JP, Meyers LD, eds. 2006. *Dietary Reference Intakes: The Essential Guide to Nutrient Requirements*. The National Academies Press; 2006. https://doi.org/10.17226/11537
45. U.S. Department of Agriculture. USDA's MyPlate celebrates its first anniversary. Press release. May 30, 2012. https://www.usda.gov/media/press-releases/2012/05/30/usdas-myplate-celebrates-its-first-anniversary
46. U.S. Department of Agriculture Food and Nutrition Service. Center for Nutrition Policy and Promotion (CNPP). Accessed March 6, 2023. https://www.usda.gov/media/press-releases/2012/05/30/usdas-myplate-celebrates-its-first-anniversary
47. U.S. Department of Agriculture. MyPlate: teens. Accessed March 6, 2023. https://www.myplate.gov/life-stages/teens
48. U.S. Department of Agriculture. Learn how to eat healthy with MyPlate. Accessed March 6, 2023. https://www.myplate.gov
49. World Health Organization. *Guideline: Implementing Effective Actions for Improving Adolescent Nutrition*. World Health Organization; 2018. https://apps.who.int/iris/handle/10665/260297
50. Libretexts Medicine. Early adolescence and nutrition. University of California at Davis, Department of Education Open Textbook Pilot Project. June 7, 2023. https://med.libretexts.org/Courses/Metropolitan_State_University_of_Denver/Introduction_to_Nutrition_(Diker)/13%3A_Lifecycle_Nutrition%3A_Childhood_to_Late_Adulthood/13.03%3A_Puberty_and_Nutrition
51. Libretexts Medicine. Older adolescence and nutrition. University of California at Davis, Department of Education Open Textbook Pilot Project. June 7, 2023. https://med.libretexts.org/Courses/Metropolitan_State_University_of_Denver/Introduction_to_Nutrition_(Diker)/13%3A_Lifecycle_Nutrition%3A_Childhood_to_Late_Adulthood/13.04%3A_Older_Adolescence_and_Nutrition
52. Mesías M, Seiquer I, Navarro MP. Iron nutrition in adolescence. *Crit Rev Food Sci Nutr*. 2013;53(11):1226–1237. https://doi.org/10.1080/10408398.2011.564333
53. Institute of Medicine. *Dietary Reference Intakes for Vitamin A, Vitamin K, Arsenic, Boron, Chromium, Copper, Iodine, Iron, Manganese, Molybdenum, Nickel, Silicon, Vanadium, and Zinc*. National Academies Press; 2001. https://doi.org/10.17226/10026
54. Mesías M, Seiquer I, Navarro MP. Calcium nutrition in adolescence. *Crit Rev Food Sci Nutr*. 2011;51(3):195–209. https://doi.org/10.1080/10408390903502872
55. National Institutes of Health, Office of Dietary Supplements. Vitamin D: fact sheet for health professionals. Updated August 12, 2022. https://ods.od.nih.gov/factsheets/VitaminD-HealthProfessional
56. American Academy of Pediatrics. American Academy of Pediatrics urges physical activity prescriptions at doctor visits. healthychildren.org. February 24, 2020. https://www.healthychildren.org/English/news/Pages/Physical-Activity-Assessment-and-Counseling-.aspx#
57. Hargreaves D, Mates E, Menon P, et al. Strategies and interventions for healthy adolescent growth, nutrition, and development. *Lancet*. 2022;399(10320):198–210. https://doi.org/10.1016/S0140-6736(21)01593-2

58. Chiang WL, Azlan A, Mohd Yusof BN. Effectiveness of education intervention to reduce sugar-sweetened beverages and 100% fruit juice in children and adolescents: a scoping review. *Expert Rev Endocrinol Metab*. 2022;17(2):179–200. https://doi.org/10.1080/17446651.2022.2060818
59. Gaffney T. A decade without data: eating disorder researchers say a gap in CDC survey has left them flying blind. *STAT*. December 9, 2021. https://www.statnews.com/2021/12/09/eating-disorders-research-health-cdc
60. Duncan AE, Ziobrowski HN, Nicol G. The prevalence of past 12-month and lifetime DSM-IV eating disorders by BMI category in U.S. men and women. *Eur Eat Disord Rev*. 2017;25(3):165–171. https://doi.org/10.1002/erv.2503
61. Dakanalis A, Clerici M, Stice E. Prevention of eating disorders: current evidence-base for dissonance-based programmes and future directions. *Eat Weight Disord*. 2019;24(4):597–603. https://doi.org/10.1007/s40519-019-00719-3
62. Hornberger LL, Lane MA, Breuner CC, et al. Identification and management of eating disorders in children and adolescents. *Pediatrics*. 2021;147(1):e2020040279. https://doi.org/10.1542/peds.2020-040279
63. Attia E, Guarda AS. Prevention and early identification of eating disorders. *JAMA*. 2022;327(11):1029–1031. https://doi.org/10.1001/jama.2022.2458
64. Bennett AM, Murray K, Ambrosini GL, Oddy WH, Walsh JP, Zhu K. Prospective associations of sugar-sweetened beverage consumption during adolescence with body composition and bone mass at early adulthood. *J Nutr*. 2022;152(2):399–407. https://doi.org/10.1093/jn/nxab389
65. Centers for Disease Control and Prevention. Get the facts: sugar-sweetened beverages and consumption. February 13, 2023. https://www.cdc.gov/nutrition/data-statistics/sugar-sweetened-beverages-intake.html
66. Muth ND, Dietz WH, Magge SN, et al. Public policies to reduce sugary drink consumption in children and adolescents. *Pediatrics*. 2019;143(4):e20190282. https://doi.org/10.1542/peds.2019-0282
67. Shearrer GE, O'Reilly GA, Belcher BR, et al. The impact of sugar sweetened beverage intake on hunger and satiety in minority adolescents. *Appetite*. 2016;97:43–48. https://doi.org/10.1016/j.appet.2015.11.015
68. World Health Organization. *Guideline: Sugars Intake for Adults and Children*. World Health Organization; 2015. https://apps.who.int/iris/handle/10665/149782
69. Abbasalizad Farhangi M, Mohammadi Tofigh A, Jahangiri L, Nikniaz Z, Nikniaz L. Sugar-sweetened beverages intake and the risk of obesity in children: an updated systematic review and dose–response meta-analysis. *Pediatr Obes*. 2022;17(8):e12914. https://doi.org/10.1111/ijpo.12914
70. Farhangi MA, Nikniaz L, Khodarahmi M. Sugar-sweetened beverages increases the risk of hypertension among children and adolescence: a systematic review and dose–response meta-analysis. *J Transl Med*. 2020;18(1):344. https://doi.org/10.1186/s12967-020-02511-9
71. Nikniaz L, Abbasalizad-Farhangi M, Vajdi M, Nikniaz Z. The association between sugar sweetened beverages (SSBs) and lipid profile among children and youth: a systematic review and dose-response meta-analysis of cross-sectional studies. *Pediatr Obes*. 2021;16(7):e12782. https://doi.org/10.1111/ijpo.12782
72. Ahn H, Park YK. Sugar-sweetened beverage consumption and bone health: a systematic review and meta-analysis. *Nutr J*. 2021;20(1):41. https://doi.org/10.1186/s12937-021-00698-1
73. Office of Disease Prevention and Health Promotion. Reduce consumption of added sugars by people aged 2 years and over—NWS-10. *Healthy People 2030*. U.S. Department of Health and Human Services; 2020. https://health.gov/healthypeople/objectives-and-data/browse-objectives/nutrition-and-healthy-eating/reduce-consumption-added-sugars-people-aged-2-years-and-over-nws-10
74. Vargas-Garcia EJ, Evans CEL, Prestwich A, Sykes-Muskett BJ, Hooson J, Cade JE. Interventions to reduce consumption of sugar-sweetened beverages or increase water intake: evidence from a systematic review and meta-analysis. *Obes Rev*. 2017;18(11):1350–1363. https://doi.org/10.1111/obr.12580
75. Ullmann H, Weeks JD, Madans JH. Children Living in Households That Experienced Food Insecurity: United States, 2019–2020. NCHS Data Brief, no 432. National Center for Health Statistics; 2022. https://doi.org/10.15620/cdc:113966
76. Dush JL. Adolescent food insecurity: a review of contextual and behavioral factors. *Public Health Nurs*. 2020;37(3):327–338. https://doi.org/10.1111/phn.12708
77. Shankar P, Chung R, Frank DA. Association of food insecurity with children's behavioral, emotional, and academic outcomes: a systematic review. *J Dev Behav Pediatr*. 2017;38(2):135–150. https://doi.org/10.1097/DBP.0000000000000383

78. Fleming MA, Kane WJ, Meneveau MO, Ballantyne CC, Levin DE. Food insecurity and obesity in U.S. adolescents: a population-based analysis. *Child Obes.* 2021;17(2):110–115. https://doi.org/10.1089/chi.2020.0158
79. Popkin SJ, Scott MM, Galvez MM. *Impossible Choices: Teens and Food Insecurity in America.* Urban Institute; 2016. https://www.urban.org/research/publication/impossible-choices-teens-and-food-insecurity-america
80. Waxman E, Popkin SJ, Galvez M. *Bringing Teens to the Table: A Focus on Food Insecurity in America.* Urban Institute; 2016. https://www.feedingamerica.org/sites/default/files/research/teen-hunger-research/bringing-teens-to-the-table.pdf
81. Council on Community Pediatrics, Committee on Nutrition. Promoting food security for all children. *Pediatrics.* 2015;136(5):e1431–e1438. https://doi.org/10.1542/peds.2015-3301
82. Hager ER, Quigg AM, Black MM, et al. Development and validity of a 2-item screen to identify families at risk for food insecurity. *Pediatrics.* 2010;126(1):e26–e32. https://doi.org/10.1542/peds.2009-3146
83. Feeding America. School food pantry program. Accessed February 23, 2023. https://www.feedingamerica.org/our-work/hunger-relief-programs/school-pantry
84. Children's HealthWatch. Hunger Vital Sign. Boston Medical Center; 2022. https://childrenshealthwatch.org/public-policy/hunger-vital-sign
85. Radandt NE, Corbridge T, Johnson DB, Kim AS, Scott JM, Coldwell SE. Validation of a two-item food security screening tool in a dental setting. *J Dent Child.* 2018;85(3):114–119. https://www.ncbi.nlm.nih.gov/pmc/articles/PMC6419517
86. Baer TE, Scherer EA, Fleegler EW, Hassan A. Food insecurity and the burden of health-related social problems in an urban youth population. *J Adolesc Health.* 2015;57(6):601–607. https://doi.org/10.1016/j.jadohealth.2015.08.013
87. Lozano P, Houtrow A. Supporting self-management in children and adolescents with complex chronic conditions. *Pediatrics.* 2018;141(suppl 3):S233–S241. https://doi.org/10.1542/peds.2017-1284H
88. American Diabetes Association. Get involved: embrace the spirit of camp. Accessed March 15, 2023. https://diabetes.org/get-involved/camp
89. Stanford Medicine Children's Health. Psychological complications of chronic illness; 2023. https://www.stanfordchildrens.org/en/topic/default?id=psychological-complications-of-chronic-illness-in-teens-90-P01658
90. Centers for Disease Control and Prevention. NCHHSTP Social Determinants of Health: Frequently Asked Questions. U.S. Department of Health and Human Services. https://www.cdc.gov/nchhstp/socialdeterminants/faq.html#what-are-social-determinants
91. Viner RM, Ozer EM, Denny S, et al. Adolescence and the social determinants of health. *Lancet.* 2012;379(9826):1641–1652. https://doi.org/10.1016/S0140-6736(12)60149-4
92. Agency for Toxic Substances and Disease Registry. Models and frameworks for the practice of community engagement. U.S. Department of Health and Human Services. Published 2015. https://www.atsdr.cdc.gov/communityengagement/pce_models.html
93. World Health Organization. Adolescent health: impact. Accessed March 15, 2023. https://www.who.int/health-topics/adolescent-health#tab=tab_2
94. UNICEF. Nutrition in middle childhood and adolescence: preventing malnutrition in school-age children and adolescents. Accessed March 8, 2023. https://www.unicef.org/nutrition/middle-childhood-and-adolescence
95. Food Research & Action Center. Benefits of school lunch. Accessed March 15, 2023. https://frac.org/programs/national-school-lunch-program/benefits-school-lunch
96. Centers for Disease Control and Prevention. The social-ecological model: a framework for prevention. https://www.cdc.gov/violenceprevention/about/social-ecologicalmodel.html

7

YOUNG AND MIDDLE ADULT NUTRITION

Amy B. Dailey

LEARNING OBJECTIVES

At the end of this chapter, students will be able to:

1. Describe nutrition-related data trends and disparities in the U.S. adult population, using public health surveillance systems.
2. Explain the social determinants of health, such as economic instability and **food insecurity**, that affect adult nutrition-related behaviors and outcomes.
3. Apply the social ecological model to adult fruit and vegetable access and intake, including public policy, community, institutional, interpersonal, and individual/intrapersonal levels.
4. Explain how life stressors in adulthood, such as perceived racial/ethnic discrimination and weight stigma influence nutrition-related behaviors.
5. Describe public health nutrition policy initiatives and programs that have been designed to address multiple levels of the social ecological model to improve adult nutrition.
6. Discuss why a health equity approach matters for improving nutrition-related behaviors and health outcomes for adults.

INTRODUCTION

This chapter describes the dietary recommendations and intake patterns for adults with a focus on factors that may affect nutrition-related behaviors and health outcomes. Disparities in intake will be explored with a discussion of public health nutrition policies, programs, and resources available to improve adult nutrition. The public health nutrition goals during this stage of life include **health equity** and chronic disease prevention.

NORMAL NUTRITION SUMMARY

The **U.S. Department of Agriculture (USDA)** has a long history of communicating nutritional guidance for the adult population and works with the Department of Health and Human Services (DHHS) to provide **Dietary Guidelines for Americans (DGA)**.

The DGA provides nutritional advice for health promotion and disease prevention in the United States and is written for policy makers, healthcare providers, and nutrition educators to provide guidance on federal, state, and local nutrition policies and programs. Since the 1940s, educational materials have included basic food groups, wheels, and pyramids. The latest educational materials to emerge from the USDA food guidance system, called **MyPlate** (Figure 7.1),[1] includes colorful graphics of a plate divided into sections for fruits, vegetables, proteins, grains, and a circle for dairy to the side.[2] Their website materials provide information across all of the life stages. For young adults, the USDA acknowledges the responsibilities that come with making independent choices and building healthy habits.[3] They provide healthy eating tips and information on cooking basics. Adulthood includes a wide range of ages and circumstances, which comes with changes in nutritional and physical activity needs as bodies change over time. For adults, MyPlate.gov offers basic nutritional advice, provides the opportunity for people to download a tailored plan, and provides guidance for movement, too.[4] MyPlate.gov offers the following guidance for eating healthy: "Fruits, vegetables, whole grains, protein foods, and fat-free or low-fat dairy products are healthy choices. Include a variety of protein foods such as seafood, lean meats, poultry, beans, peas, lentils, nuts, seeds, and eggs. Limit foods and beverages higher in added sugars, saturated fat, and sodium."[4] Tailored MyPlate Plans provide information on food group targets and calorie allowances based on age, sex, height, weight, and physical activity levels.

From a population health perspective, it is important to know whether public health educational programs, such as MyPlate, are effective. According to some evidence, people using the MyPlate plan reported healthier diets than nonusers.[5] However, there is a lack of evidence for whether the MyPlate approach improves adult population nutritional outcomes. A review study, published in 2019,[6] discussed how systems and policy approaches, particularly federally instituted initiatives such as MyPlate, need to be rigorously evaluated to determine their impact, considering the vast resources allocated toward them and the potential for influencing outcomes. However, the authors concluded that such evidence is lacking for MyPlate, particularly for populations at high risk for nutrition disparities.

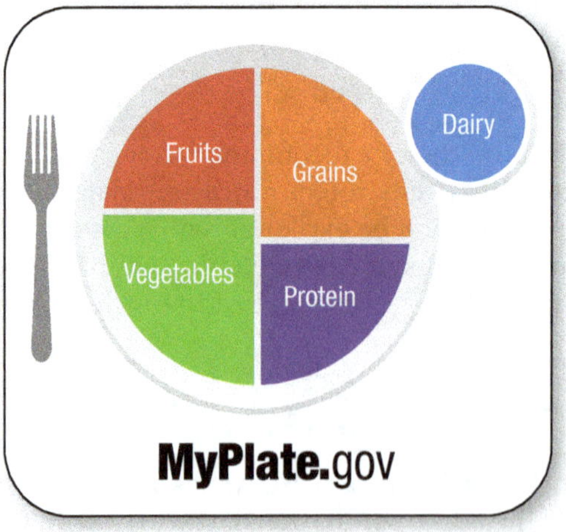

Figure 7.1. Basic MyPlate graphic.
Source: U.S. Department of Agriculture. MyPlate graphics. Accessed September 20, 2023. https://www.myplate.gov/resources/graphics/myplate-graphics

PUBLIC HEALTH NUTRITION SURVEILLANCE

In the United States, adult nutrition **surveillance** activities are carried out in numerous ways by different government agencies, including household sample surveys and administrative data. Surveillance activities allow for the monitoring of trends over time and help with public health nutrition policy making and community initiatives. The **Centers for Disease Control and Prevention (CDC)** houses the **National Center for Health Statistics (NCHS)**, which is responsible for producing health statistics for the country. The **National Health and Nutrition Examination Survey (NHANES)** is a program that provides statistics on many health conditions, including nutrition and nutrition-related health conditions.[7] The CDC also administers the **Behavioral Risk Factor Surveillance System (BRFSS)**, collaborating with U.S. state governments, to provide national and state-level data on many health and nutrition-related conditions including fruit and vegetable consumption and overweight and obesity prevalence measures. The **Economic Research Service (ERS)** provides information on food security in the United States, among other food and agricultural economic outcomes.[8]

Data from NHANES 2015–2018 show that overall, most American adults (95%) consumed some amount of vegetables on a given day and that fruit consumption was higher for women than men, and consumption increased with income.[9] During 2013–2016, over a third of U.S. adults consumed fast food on a given day and a higher percentage of non-Hispanic Black adults regularly consumed fast food, compared to other races/ethnicities.[10] An analysis of data from the 2019 BRFSS[11] also showed that most American adults consumed some fruits and vegetables on a daily basis (median frequency of fruit intake was once per day; median frequency of vegetable intake was 1.6 times per day). However, only 12.3% of adults met fruit intake recommendations and 10% met vegetable intake recommendations. Consumption varied by sociodemographic characteristics including gender, religion, age, race/ethnicity, and income status. Some of the barriers to fruit and vegetable consumption include costs, access to grocery stores, and general food insecurity. **Food insecurity** is defined as lack of consistent access to enough food to fuel a healthy lifestyle, typically due to lack of financial resources,[12] which is discussed in detail in Chapter 9. In 2021 the ERS reported[13] that most U.S. households had consistent, dependable access to enough food for healthy living. Yet, 13.5 million U.S. households were considered food insecure in 2021.

Public health surveillance systems also track nutrition-related health outcomes trends across the U.S. population over time. Some of the nutrition-related diseases that can begin in early or middle adulthood include obesity, type 2 diabetes, and cardiovascular conditions. Over 40% of U.S. adults are obese,[14] and obesity disproportionately impacts some racial and ethnic populations and income groups.[15] Furthermore, the COVID-19 pandemic worsened the preexisting epidemic of adult obesity in the United States.[16] Over 37 million Americans have been diagnosed with diabetes and 96 million U.S. adults have prediabetes.[17] Nearly 700,000 people died from heart disease in the United States in 2020 and over 20 million adults have coronary artery disease.[18] While genetic factors play roles in all of these conditions, nutritional risk factors are primary drivers of these outcomes. Thus, public health nutrition initiatives are crucial to reversing these trends on a population level.

SOCIAL DETERMINANTS OF HEALTH RELATED TO YOUNG AND MIDDLE ADULT NUTRITION

To understand life cycle nutrition for young and middle adults from the public health perspective, one must consider the **social determinants of health (SDOH)** that intersect with nutrition. SDOH are factors that affect health, function, and quality-of-life and they have been grouped by **Healthy People 2030** into five major domains: **economic stability**, education access and quality, healthcare access and quality, neighborhood and built environment, and social and community context.[19] For adults, major SDOH that relate to nutrition include access to nutritious foods, language and literacy skills, job opportunities, income, transportation, and ability to meet other basic needs, such as safe housing. Inequities across SDOH lead to increased risk of nutrition-related health conditions such as heart disease, diabetes, obesity, and reduced life expectancy.

One of the primary SDOH is economic stability, which is discussed in detail in Chapter 14. Approximately one in 10 people in the United States live in poverty,[20] which makes it difficult to afford housing, healthcare, healthy foods, and other basic needs. By the time adults have paid for rent, healthcare, child care, transportation costs, utilities, mobile phones, and so on, they may not have enough money to cover food costs. Food is often prioritized last, which can affect the quantity and the quality of food that people are able to purchase. Healthy People 2030 economic stability objectives for adults include reducing the proportion of people living in poverty,[21] increasing employment in working-age people,[22] and reducing household food insecurity and hunger.[23]

While some modest progress has been observed in reducing food insecurity, not all population subgroups have experienced reductions,[24] which points to the importance of equity and consistency in national programs, regulations, policies, and laws, some of which are discussed later in this chapter. Screening for food insecurity and connecting adults to food resources is an important public health approach that requires clinical and community partnerships.[25] Many hospital systems now screen for a variety of SDOH, including food insecurity, and connect patients with the appropriate community resources.

PUBLIC HEALTH NUTRITION ISSUES RELATED TO YOUNG AND MIDDLE ADULTHOOD

Chronic health conditions that can begin in young and middle adulthood include obesity, diabetes, and heart disease. Healthy People 2030 places a large emphasis on health behaviors that contribute to those conditions. The overarching goal of their nutrition and healthy eating objectives is to improve health by promoting healthy eating and making nutritious foods available.[26] From a public health perspective, this approach spans the different levels of the **social ecological model (SEM)** by linking policy and community-level access initiatives to individual-level consumption and health outcomes. The specific objectives include increasing fruit, vegetable, whole grain, and vitamin consumption, while other objectives focus on reducing consumption of added sugars, saturated fat, and sodium. The SEM provided in Figure 7.2 shows the factors that specifically shape fruit and vegetable access and intake, emphasizing the importance of public policy, community, and institutional drivers.[27]

While many approaches to nutrition focus primarily on individual and behavioral factors, a public health approach to nutrition across the life span emphasizes the importance of the public policy, community, and institutional factors that provide the environment and context in which the individual/intrapersonal and interpersonal factors operate. Consider the outermost circle of Figure 7.2: public policy. Public policy includes the social, political, and economic factors that, in this example, shape fruit and vegetable access and intake. One could substitute other nutrition-related outcomes into this model

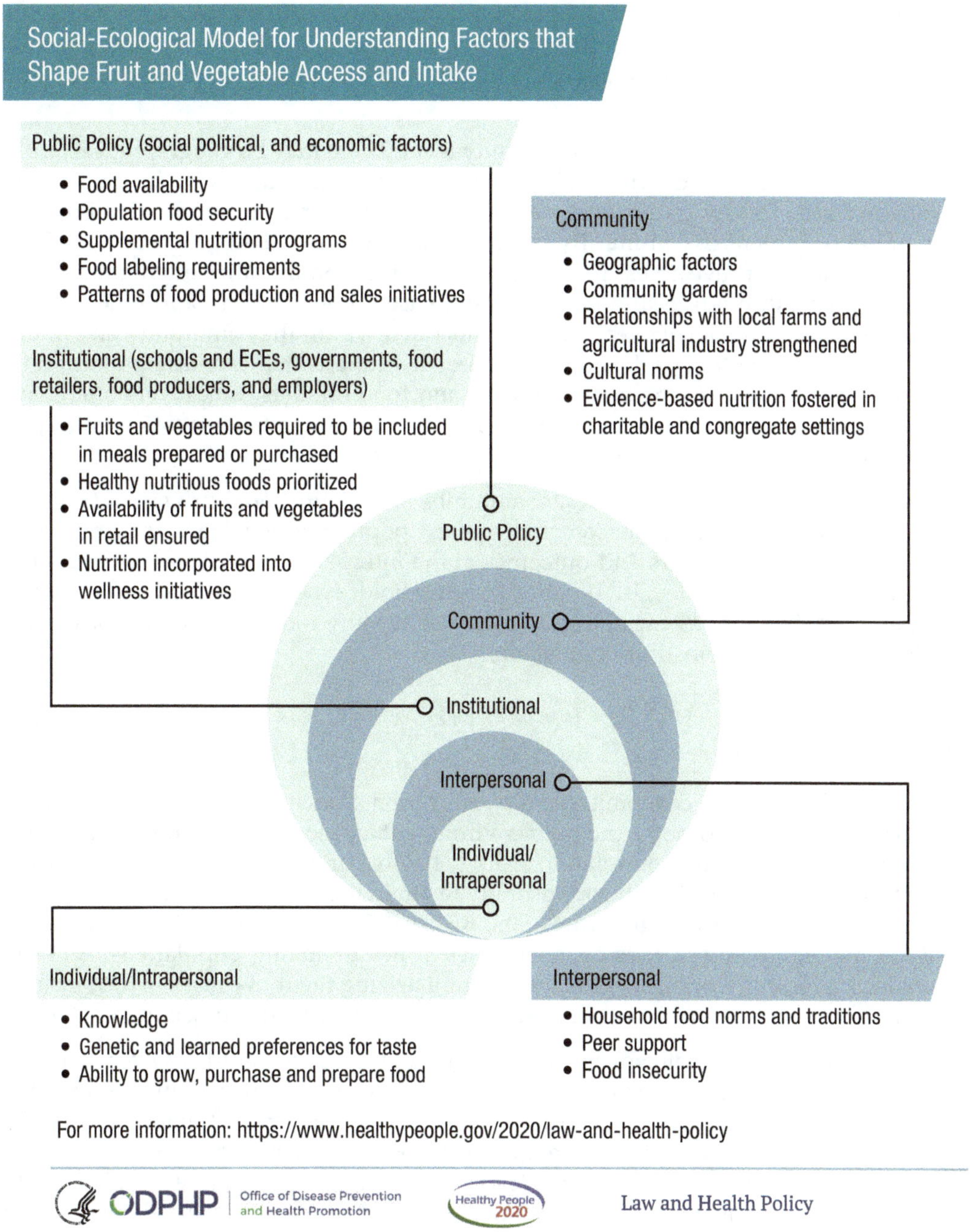

Figure 7.2. Social ecological model for understanding factors that shape fruit and vegetable access and intake.

Source: Office of Disease Prevention and Health Promotion. Law and health policy: social-ecological model. *Healthy People 2020*. U.S. Department of Health and Human Services. Accessed September 20, 2023. https://wayback.archive-it.org/5774/20220414114727/https://www.healthypeople.gov/2020/law-and-health-policy-social-ecological-model-graphic

(see Suggested Learning Activities). Later in the chapter we will discuss some of the major U.S. policies that influence food availability, population food security, supplemental nutrition programs, food labeling requirements, and patterns of food production and sales initiatives.

The next level of the SEM is the community level. There may be geographic factors of a community that influence fruit and vegetable access and intake, such as the number of supermarkets, transportation accessibility, and fast food restaurant density. Presence of community gardens or **community supported agriculture (CSA)** programs with local farmers can help improve access to local fresh produce. Communities often initiate food access programs through local nonprofits, faith-based organizations, and other institutions. The institutional level of the SEM is embedded within the community and public policy levels of the SEM. For the adult life state, institutions that can have an important influence on nutrition can include employers and food retailers. Employers often have wellness programs that include nutritional programming and retailers work within communities to ensure availability of fruits and vegetables.

When analyzing the public policy, community, and institutional drivers of fruit and vegetable access and intake, it becomes clear these population-level factors significantly influence nutrition behaviors and outcomes at the interpersonal (e.g., family or household) and/or individual levels. Whether a household experiences food insecurity or whether an individual has the ability to purchase healthy food is rooted in social, economic, community, and institutional factors.

SOCIAL DETERMINANTS OF HEALTH AND NUTRITION-RELATED HEALTH INEQUITIES

SDOH inequities such as economic stability, education access and quality, healthcare access and quality, neighborhood and built environment and social and community context produce inequities in nutrition-related health behaviors and outcomes. **Health equity** is the concept that everyone has the opportunity to attain their highest level of health[28] and is closely related to concepts of fairness and justice.[29] For many years, the public health field has highlighted disparities or inequalities in health among populations. A health equity lens takes this work a step further by emphasizing the root causes, which include structural and social determinants of health, many of which are discussed in this chapter.

Food insecurity is a major driver of nutrition outcomes for adults. Given that low income and race/ethnicity are factors associated with elevated rates of nutrition-related chronic diseases such as obesity, cardiovascular disease, and type 2 diabetes, addressing food insecurity is imperative for reducing socioeconomic and racial/ethnic disparities. Latinx, Black, and Indigenous people experience significantly more food insecurity than White households. It is important to note that socioeconomic status alone does not explain all of the existing racial disparities in nutrition. Root causes of lack of access to healthy foods stems from centuries of **racism**.[30] The lack of affordable, healthy food in communities of color is the result of long-standing discriminatory policies, some of which are discussed in the following section. In addition to racial/ethnic disparities, research has indicated there may be gender and age differences in responsiveness to media-based educational strategies and heart-healthy food labeling initiatives, with men and younger adults less likely to purchase healthful foods than women and older adults.[31] People living in rural communities also experience higher levels of food insecurity than those living in urban areas.

POPULATION CONSIDERATIONS: LIFE STRESSORS IN ADULTHOOD

The SDOH described here present numerous challenges and considerations for adult populations that can affect nutrition including life stressors, barriers to engaging in healthy behaviors, and balancing the numerous priorities that adults face in this stage of their life. Stress can manifest in different ways and create challenges for maintaining a healthy lifestyle.[32] As young adults take on more responsibilities in their jobs and families, stress can become particularly problematic in this life stage. Stressors can be acute in nature, but SDOH such as economic instability and food insecurity can lead to chronic stress that can influence physical health, mental health, and health behaviors.

The physical effects of stress can include changes in hormone releases and increases in heart rate and blood pressure, a process known as *fight-or-flight response*. Under acute stress circumstances, the body will return to normal relatively quickly. However, experiences of chronic stress can lead to persistent physical responses, which can lead to a range of adverse health problems, many related to nutrition. Chronic stress may lead to digestive issues, weight gain, and mental health problems, among other health conditions. Life stressors, most of which are related to the SDOH, such as unemployment, job strain, interpersonal conflict, and economic instability have been associated with weight gain and obesity. The relationships between stress, diet, and physical and mental health are complex and may be bidirectional.[33] Chronic stress can also affect eating patterns in response to the physical effects on the body. With increased demands on the body for oxygen, energy, and nutrients, it is common for people to reach for comforting foods to cope. Stressors can also place demands on time and motivation, which may make it more difficult for adults to prepare healthy meals. Stress can also influence sleep patterns, appetite levels, and adiposity. Stress, paired with ubiquitous highly palatable foods, may lead to overeating, which can influence fat metabolism, insulin sensitivity, and appetite hormones.[34]

A particular form of chronic stress that can be detrimental to nutrition-related health outcomes is experiences of racial/ethnic discrimination as a result of racism. A study in the U.S. South revealed **perceived discrimination** to be significantly associated with obesity.[35] While the mechanisms are not fully understood, the stress of discrimination may influence whether adults have the energy or resources to make healthy choices or participate in behaviors that promote good health. However, the relationship may be more complex. Results from the Black Women's Health Study have shown that perceived racism is associated with increased risk of type 2 diabetes and body mass index (BMI).[36] A study using data from the Family and Community Health Study found that optimism may moderate the relationship between perceived discrimination and BMI among African Americans.[37] There has been increased attention to the ways in which systemic racism is associated with nutrition and how traditional approaches to nutrition have perpetuated systemic racism. In many ways, food insecurity is a racial/ethnic equity issue.

It makes sense that one major way to cope with stress is to eat a healthy, balanced diet in a mindful manner to help support the immune system and counteract stress. However, as discussed earlier, many adults may find it difficult to engage in healthy eating behaviors because they have practiced coping with chronic stress by comforting through eating highly palatable and processed food and lowering intake of whole foods, fruits, and vegetables. Behavior change is notoriously difficult to achieve, and becomes even more difficult for individuals experiencing chronic stress.

Another potential life stressor for young and middle adults is discrimination due to **weight stigma**. Weight stigma refers to negative attitudes and beliefs that devalue people based on their weight status that may include bias, discrimination, stereotyping, and social exclusion.[38] The negative health consequences of weight stigma can include increased intake of high-calorie foods, healthcare avoidance, emotional overeating, and binge eating.[38] Weight stigma is perpetuated by **diet culture** or wellness culture, which is a set of social expectations related to expectations about how individuals should look and how they should eat, often linked to morality or worthiness, driven by systemic and structural factors.[39] Diet culture is a term that has become popular among advocacy groups and is being studying by researchers interested in weight stigma, body image, and how cultural norms around dieting are influencing physical and mental health among young and middle adults.

Public health approaches to reducing stigma and discrimination are needed to address these issues at the public policy level of the SEM. Public health policies to address weight stigma could include changing language in health policies to be less stigmatizing. Policies could also include creating legislation to include body size in antidiscrimination laws, and deescalating combative language about obesity in media (e.g., avoiding terms such as "the war on obesity").[38]

POLICY: GLOBAL ISSUES AND CHALLENGES

Food Justice

Addressing access to food, food behaviors, coping with life stressors, and improving population outcomes on nutrition-related health outcomes will require a focus on **food justice**. Food justice can be defined as the struggle against racism, exploitation, and oppression taking place within the food system that addresses the root causes of inequalities both within and beyond the food chain.[40] Efforts to address food justice with policy can happen at many levels. Referring back to the SEM (Figure 7.2), policies can include strengthening food programs, supporting food policy councils, supporting community retail programs to attract grocery stores and supermarkets to underserved communities, and implementing nutrition incentive programs. Farm-to-institution approaches that promote culturally preferred fruit and vegetable offerings in places of employment, hospitals, and food pantries; expanding land and resources for Black farmers; passing inclusive zoning policies; and investment in community food initiatives are all examples of policies that use a food justice approach.

Food justice approaches should address the root causes of food insecurity, which may include long-standing discriminatory policies such as zoning policies, supermarket redlining, and other factors that have impacted socioeconomic status at population levels.[30] Zoning policies in cities can often divide cities across racial lines, which then can influence food access. These policies are rooted in intentional efforts to prevent Black and other people of color from accessing loans and mortgages, leading to concentrated poverty across racial lines. A consequence of zoning policies and racial residential segregation can be supermarket redlining, where larger supermarket retailers avoid opening in low-income areas, limiting access to food along racial/ethnic lines. Absence of supermarkets and inadequate transportation force many communities of color to rely on convenience stores and fast food establishments that have limited healthy food options. These areas have been called **food deserts**, which are geographic regions with limited access to healthy and affordable food. This term has been criticized for implying that these situations arise naturally, when they are rooted in discriminatory policies.

A discussion of food justice policies would be incomplete without mentioning the enormous U.S. **farm bill**. The farm bill is a package of legislation that encompasses policies on farming, healthy food access, and food systems. It expires approximately every 5 years, at which point it goes through extensive review processes and must be passed by Congress and signed by the President. Many policies in the farm bill affect adult nutrition, including affordability of food and access to food programs. Nutrition programs can account for over 75% of farm bill budgets, some of which are described in the next section. Given the large federal budget for nutrition assistance programs, ongoing policy debates and research consider whether these policies and programs work. Large-scale nutritional program and policy reforms can be difficult to study.

Beyond the U.S. context, in examining food justice, one of the most persistent problems globally is the simultaneous prevalence of high rates of underweight and overweight within countries, communities, households, or even within an individual. In many countries, the prevalence of underweight adults has decreased over the past three decades, but the prevalence of overweight has increased. However, many low- and middle-income countries are projected to experience a double burden of malnutrition, which is defined as having both underweight and overweight prevalence greater than 20%.[41] In the United States, the double burden of having obesity coupled with malnutrition is prevalent in more than half of all malnourished households.[42] Policies to address these complex situations need to balance initiatives to reduce consumption of high energy-dense processed foods and initiatives that help support access to healthy foods such as fruits, vegetables, and whole grains. Some have suggested that nonprofit organizations, such as food banks, could eliminate sugary food products from their inventories; however, refusing donations to collect healthier products has been a controversial idea.[42] Other barriers that food assistance nonprofits face is refrigeration capacity, storage, and client preferences.

PUBLIC HEALTH NUTRITION PROGRAMS FOR ADULTS

Governmental: SNAP

The **Supplemental Nutrition Assistance Program (SNAP)** is the largest antihunger program in the United States and it provides food support to low-wage workers and people living with disabilities, among others. During 2021, over half of food-insecure households participated in one or more federal nutrition assistance programs, such a SNAP. SNAP provides monthly benefits to eligible low-income households based on financial and nonfinancial criteria. Eligibility for SNAP can be complicated and is administered at the state level. The U.S. government spent over $113 billion on SNAP in 2021, with an average benefit of about $218 per person per month.[8] SNAP also helps support the U.S. economy during high periods of unemployment and during periods of recession.[43] When participants spend money on food items, such as fruits and vegetables, using SNAP benefits, researchers have found that the program can free up budgets for people to spend money on nonfood items, which can help support local jobs and improve economic output.

Nongovernmental: Food Policy Councils, Food Scarcity Projects

Given the significant inequities described in this chapter and their relationship to the SDOH, systems and policy level approaches to food and nutrition are essential to achieve equity. Food policy councils, as defined by the Johns Hopkins **Center for a Livable Future's Food Policy Networks (FPN)**,[44] are networks that represent multiple stakeholders to address food-related issues and needs in a community. The establishment of food policy councils in the United States has grown rapidly in the past decade. Councils are complex, are heterogeneous, and address a wide range of issues under the umbrella of *food policy*, including food access, economic development, and antihunger, to name a few. Grounded in a commitment to racial and socioeconomic justice, the FPN is a resource for groups that are building food policy partnerships to help with capacity building, research, networking, and technical assistance. It has provided an important space for councils to connect with one another to help improve food systems through public policy. The FPN maintains a directory of active food policy councils across North America and conducts regular surveys to document progress and achievements.

One of the ways that food policy councils can influence food and nutrition policy is by keeping abreast of what federal policies are in the farm bill (the most recent being the Agricultural Improvement Act of 2018) and creating advocacy strategies.[45] Many policies in the enormous farm bill affect adult nutrition, including affordability of food and access to food programs. Nutrition programs can account for over 75% of farm bill budgets and include the following programs: SNAP, the Food Distribution Program on Indian Reservations (FDPIR), the Emergency Food Assistance Program (TEFAP), Community Food Projects (CFP), the **Gus Schumacher Nutrition Incentive Program (GusNIP**; discussed in more detail later), and others.

While SNAP is the largest nutrition assistance program at the federal level, communities often create programs to further supplement nutrition for adults and families. **Food voucher programs** are nutrition incentive programs that can come in a variety of forms, some of which leverage federal and state dollars with matched funds to use at local farmers markets or grocery stores. The USDA supports a program called the **Farmers Market Nutrition Program (FMNP)**,[46] which is affiliated with the WIC (Special Supplemental Nutrition Program for Women, Infants, and Children) program that is discussed in several earlier chapters. The program provides locally grown fruits and vegetables to participants while also helping to support local growers. Fruit and vegetable prescription programs and hospital-based voucher programs for high-risk populations, such as adults living with diabetes or cancer, have also become prevalent.

Food voucher and incentive programs can significantly reduce food insecurity, reduce chronic disease risk, and promote healthy diets. Some research has shown that vegetable prescription programs and hospital-based voucher programs can improve chronic disease management, reduce utilization of the healthcare system, and improve health outcomes.[47–49] Some food voucher programs attempt to restrict purchases to healthy foods, such as fresh fruits and vegetables. WIC, GusNIP, and many other state and local food voucher programs explicitly restrict purchases to foods considered healthy. While there are some indications that food and vegetable incentive programs can increase the purchase of fruits and vegetables, there is mixed evidence to suggest that placing restrictions on voucher programs improves nutrition outcomes.[50,51] Frequency of voucher distribution has also been an area of evaluation inquiry. There does not seem to be any benefit to a higher frequency (weekly) compared to monthly distributions in terms of nutrition outcomes.[50] Voucher programs and food policy networks have been important public health measures for addressing food insecurity during crises, such as the COVID-19 pandemic.[52,53]

Local farmers markets are important contributors to local food systems and play significant roles in connecting local populations to healthy food. They are often a place for participants to use food voucher programs (described earlier). Farmers market usage can have positive impacts on fruit and vegetable consumption and healthy behaviors, such as increasing the frequency of preparing meals at home.[54] Grocery stores are also often partners in a public health approach to improving nutrition in local populations. Some research indicates that there are gender and age differences in food purchasing behaviors and willingness to use grocery vouchers.[31] Household size can also be an important factor, and programs may need to adjust dollar amounts to account for sharing food among larger family sizes.[55]

Food banks are important community organizations that aim to provide hunger relief across the United States. A food bank is a nonprofit organization that collects and distributes food to local frontline hunger-relief organizations, such as food pantries. Many food banks are associated with a nationwide network called **Feeding America,**[56] whose mission is to ensure equitable access to nutritious food for all in partnership with food banks, policy makers, supporters, and the communities they serve. A *food pantry* is a distribution center where families can receive food supplied from food banks and other community food collection sources.[57] Different models of distribution from food banks and pantries exist. Some pantries employ preconstructed food parcels and some offer experiences for clients that are similar to shopping at a grocery store or offer delivery service. Food parcel models have been criticized for failing to meet individual needs, such as cultural and health preferences.[58]

WHAT WORKS: GusNIP

As discussed earlier, nutrition incentive programs can be powerful tools for improving fruit and vegetable intake and may improve chronic disease outcomes and improve health equity. GusNIP is a federal program that brings together stakeholders from various parts of the food and healthcare systems, providing incentives to income-eligible consumers to increase the purchase of fruits and vegetables.[59] It was designed to improve the health and nutrition behaviors and outcomes for participants, facilitate economic and food system growth in underrepresented communities, and identify broad-scale best practices. GusNIP administers three programs: a nutrition incentive program, a produce prescription program, and training and technical assistance grants. Recently, a group of researchers sought to gain a deeper understanding whether the federal GusNIP works using the **Theory of Change (TOC)** as a tool for understanding how and why a program works.[60] The TOC was used to identify what the GusNIP program hopes to achieve and how it achieves it. The researchers employed a health equity lens using a multistop process that included GusNIP document reviews, published evidence, and findings from interviews, workshops and focus groups with partners, practitioners, and GusNIP participants. Central themes to the design and success of the GusNIP program were equity and partnership, which were enhanced by community member involvement in project planning, implementation, and evaluation. GusNIP grantees implemented activities and demonstrated short-term outcomes knowing that: participants want fruits and vegetables and participate in nutrition incentive programs; food retailers are accessible, welcoming, and provide fruits and vegetables to participants; and local farmers supply fruits and vegetables to some retail food stores and at farm direct sites. These pathways can lead to long-term outcomes and the ultimate goals of the program, such as improvements in community health and economic well-being, decreases in health and wealth disparities, and sustained and expanded diverse and just food systems.

SUMMARY

Many adults are not meeting dietary recommendations and suffer the consequences of chronic health conditions. It is important that the public health nutrition professional understand the influence of various levels of the social ecological model on food choices of adults. Food justice and health equity approaches can guide the development of appropriate solutions for improving food access and nutritional intake among adults.

KEY CHAPTER CONCEPTS

1. Public health surveillance data show that most American adults do not meet dietary recommendations. The United States also has a high prevalence of nutrition-related chronic health conditions.
2. Social determinants of health, such as economic stability and food insecurity, drive nutrition-related behaviors and outcomes among adults.
3. Public policy, institutional, community, interpersonal, and individual levels of the social ecological model explain adult nutritional access and intake.
4. Life stressors, such as perceived discrimination and everyday challenges in adulthood, influence nutrition-related behaviors and outcomes.
5. Public health approaches to food justice include government nutrition programs (e.g., SNAP) and nongovernmental and/or community initiatives (e.g., food policy councils).

CASE STUDY: A RURAL COMMUNITY RESPONDS TO FOOD INSECURITY BY CREATING A FOOD POLICY COUNCIL

Adams County, located in south-central Pennsylvania, is a rural community that identified food insecurity as a significant unmet need, even after taking into account federal food programs. Low-wage jobs dominate the economic landscape, rates of obesity and chronic health conditions are high, and consumption of fruits and vegetables is low. After listening to participants of a community poverty-reduction program, it became clear many community members were living in a food gap, in which they did not qualify for federal food benefits, but they did not make enough money to provide healthy food for themselves or their families. Several community organizations came together to discuss strategies for addressing this problem; the idea of a local food policy council was generated, and the Adams County Food Policy Council (ACFPC) was created. The vision of the ACFPC is that all residents of Adams County will have access to a safe, nutritious, affordable, and adequate food supply. In the interest of health and sustainability, ACFPC promotes the integration of the individual, community, the economy, and the environment to develop food policy and take action.

Like the majority of food policy councils, healthy food access has been a policy priority of the ACFPC for over a decade. In addition to healthy food access, the ACFPC also prioritizes local food waste reduction and food systems. The all-volunteer council's core membership includes approximately 20 active members at any given time, representing local health organizations, social service agencies, farmers market associations, higher education, local government, and community members. The council also maintains communication with a wide extended network of governmental officials, growers, and retailers. The ACFPC convenes monthly meetings that are open to the public and anyone may become a member.

The primary elements that have contributed to sustaining the work of the ACFPC include having a common agenda; collaboration; maintaining independent but mutually supporting member organizational goals; valuing those who are most impacted; and continuous communication (Figure 7.3). In addition to drawing upon Kania and Kramer's collective impact work,[61] the ACFPC included an intentional focus on valuing those who are most affected and highlights the independent, but mutually reinforcing, goals of member organizations.

While valuing and listening to those most affected, the ACFPC brings people and organizations working independently on local foods and food access issues together to create a common food access agenda. An example of a change resulting from this collective work is the day-to-day operations of the local food pantry. Listening to participants' voices about how to foster dignity and autonomy in food choices, the organization remodeled the food pantry space to offer a shopping experience similar to going to a retail store, allowing families to choose the foods they prefer.

The ACFPC has also initiated collaborative healthy food access programs. Since 2011, the ACFPC has administered Healthy Options, a food voucher program that supports low-wage earners, immigrants, and senior citizens who experience food insecurity, yet are not eligible for SNAP. Another program they coordinate is Fruit and Vegetable Bucks,[19] which provides SNAP recipients additional food assistance in the form of produce discounts at a local commercial grocery. The local farmers market also began implementing strategies to provide a robust outlet for local farmers while establishing policies and programs that prioritized low-wage shoppers. These efforts included shifting location and hours, accepting SNAP benefits, and securing private funding to double SNAP and FMNP dollars.

More than 10 years from inception, the ACFPC remains active and engaged in local and regional food policy conversations and action, proving itself resilient despite many changes in membership and leadership over the years. In rural areas where there may be significant challenges with fewer people and limited resources, organizing around food policy issues can have important implications for addressing intersecting social justice issues. The council has been an important anchor for networking, connecting people and organizations extending far beyond their core membership, and facilitating communication to respond to community food needs quickly during typical times and during times of crisis such as the COVID-19 pandemic.

To read more about the ACFPC, please refer to the articles by Dailey et al.[52,62] and Calancie et al.[63]

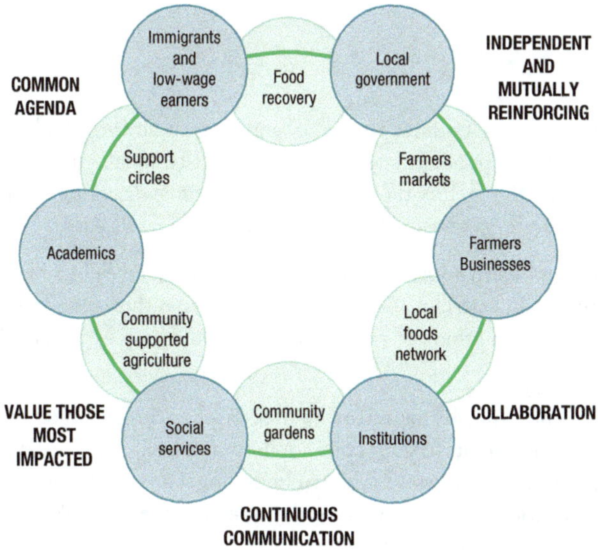

Figure 7.3. Adams County (PA) Food Policy Council collaboration model.

CASE STUDY QUESTIONS

1. Does your community have a food policy council? Search this directory: www.foodpolicynetworks.org/councils/directory/online/index.html. Choose a food policy council to learn more about. Who are the partners? What are their goals? How do they operate? How could you get involved?
2. In what ways is the work of the ACFPC a public health approach to nutrition in Adams County, PA?
3. Why is listening to and valuing those most affected important to ACFPC's collaboration model? How might their model align with health equity and food justice approaches?

DISCUSSION QUESTIONS

1. Do you think most adults have seen MyPlate? In what ways is this education tool accessible and useful to the adults who may be seeking nutritional advice? What are its limitations?
2. This chapter describes how one of the five major domains of social determinants of health from Healthy People 2030, economic stability, is related to food insecurity. Describe how one of the four remaining major domains (education access and quality, healthcare access and quality, neighborhood and built environment, or social and community context) may be related to food insecurity, access, or intake.
3. Referring to Figure 7.2, what additional community factors may influence fruit and vegetable access and intake?
4. What are the pathways by which perceived racial/ethnic discrimination and/or weight stigma may lead to adverse nutrition-related behaviors or outcomes?
5. How could changing language in health policies to be less stigmatizing toward obesity and body size be helpful in addressing nutrition-related behaviors and outcomes?
6. Consider the public health nutrition programs and policies described in this chapter. In what ways might these programs help communities achieve food justice and health equity? What are the gaps?
7. How does the GusNIP program address SDOH through different levels of the SEM?

SUGGESTED LEARNING ACTIVITIES

1. Figure 7.2 shows the SEM as it relates to understanding fruit and vegetable access and intake. Using the same framework (public policy, community, institutional, interpersonal, and individual), draw a figure that shows the factors that shape socioeconomic disparities in a nutrition-related chronic health condition (e.g., obesity, type 2 diabetes, or heart disease).
2. Watch this video about health equity produced by the American Public Health Association: www.youtube.com/watch?v=Arpzx6TJuQI. Apply the concepts in this video to food justice. Besides the baseball analogy, can you think of an analogy that could help explain health equity as it relates to food justice?
3. You or someone you know may be experiencing food insecurity. Search on the internet for food access programs for which adults in your community may be eligible. Did you find information on federal or state government programs? Did you find nongovernmental or nonprofit resources? Describe eligibility criteria, application requirements, and procedures. What are the challenges adults may face as they try to access these resources?

4. Suppose you work for a local hunger-relief nonprofit organization and they would like your help writing a grant to improve fruit and vegetable access for SNAP recipients in the community. Search GusNIP grantee projects for ideas: www.nutritionincentivehub.org/grantee-projects. Provide a brief list of ideas.

RESOURCES FOR FURTHER LEARNING

- *Dietary Guidelines for Americans*: www.dietaryguidelines.gov
  - The 2020–2025 DGAs provide evidence-based nutrition guidelines by life stage.
- *National Health and Nutrition Examination Survey* (NHANES): www.cdc.gov/nchs/nhanes/index.htm
  - Uses physical examinations and interviews to assess the physical and nutritional health of adults and children in the United States over time, and maintains a repository of data that can be used to track outcomes of interest over time
- *Behavioral Risk Factor Surveillance System*: www.cdc.gov/brfss/index.html
  - Uses telephone interviews to conduct continuous surveys on health risk behaviors in the United States; and maintains a data repository to track health risk behaviors over time
- *USDA Economic Research Service*: www.ers.usda.gov
  - Conducts economic research to obtain reliable information, identify trends, and support good decision-making in the areas of agriculture, food, the environment, and rural America.
- *Healthy People 2030*: health.gov/healthypeople
  - Sets objectives for improving health and well-being in the United States for the subsequent decade, based on available data; administered by the Office of Disease Prevention and Health Promotion, U.S. Department of Health and Human Services
- *Supplemental Nutrition Assistance Program*: www.fns.usda.gov/snap/supplemental-nutrition-assistance-program
  - Primary food assistance program in the United States; administered by the USDA
- *Johns Hopkins Center for a Livable Future*: https://clf.jhsph.edu
  - Works with a wide range of constituencies to work toward an equitable and sustainable food system
- *Nutrition Incentive Hub*: www.nutritionincentivehub.org/about/nutrition-incentive-hub
  - Funded by the USDA through the 2018 Farm Bill, provides support and assistance for nutrition incentive and produce prescription projects
- *USDA Farmers Market Nutrition Program*: www.fns.usda.gov/fmnp/wic-farmers-market-nutrition-program
  - Provides eligible WIC participants with coupons to purchase approved foods at participating farmers market vendors
- *Feeding America*: www.feedingamerica.org
  - The largest private hunger organization in the United States; provides support to a nationwide network of food banks; works to ensure equitable access to nutritious food for all

REFERENCES

1. U.S. Department of Agriculture. MyPlate graphics. Accessed September 20, 2023. https://www.myplate.gov/resources/graphics/myplate-graphics
2. U.S. Department of Agriculture. MyPlate. https://www.myplate.gov/resources/graphics/myplate-graphics
3. U.S. Department of Agriculture. MyPlate: young adults. Accessed October 13, 2023. https://www.myplate.gov/life-stages/young-adults.
4. U.S. Department of Agriculture. MyPlate: adults. Accessed October 13, 2023. https://www.myplate.gov/life-stages/adults
5. Schwartz JL, Vernarelli JA. Assessing the public's comprehension of dietary guidelines: use of MyPyramid or MyPlate is associated with healthier diets among U.S. adults. *J Acad Nutr Diet*. 2019;119(3):482–489. https://doi.org/10.1016/j.jand.2018.09.012
6. Chrisman M, Diaz Rios LK. Evaluating MyPlate after 8 years: a perspective. *J Nutr Educ Behav*. 2019;51(7):899–903. https://doi.org/10.1016/j.jneb.2019.02.006
7. Centers for Disease Control and Prevention. National Center for Health Statistics: about the National Health and Nutrition Examination Survey. Accessed October 23, 2023. https://www.cdc.gov/nchs/nhanes/about_nhanes.htm
8. Coleman-Jensen A, Rabbitt MP, Gregory CA, Singh A. *Household Food Security in the United States in 2021*. ERR-309. U.S. Department of Agriculture, Economic Research Service; 2022. http://www.ers.usda.gov/publications/pub-details/?pubid=104655
9. Ansai N, Wambogo EA. *Fruit and Vegetable Consumption Among Adults in the United States, 2015–2018*. NCHS Data Brief, No.397. National Center for Health Statistics; 2021. https://doi.org/10.15620/cdc:100470
10. Fryar CD, Hughes JP, Herrick KA, Ahluwalia N. *Fast Food Consumption Among Adults in the United States, 2013–2016*. NCHS Data Brief, no. 322. National Center for Health Statistics; 2018. https://stacks.cdc.gov/view/cdc/59582
11. Lee SH, Moore LV, Park S, Harris DM, Blanck HM. Adults meeting fruit and vegetable intake recommendations—United States, 2019. *MMWR Morb Mortal Wkly Rep*. 2022;71(1):1–9. https://doi.org/10.15585/mmwr.mm7101a1
12. Feeding America. Hunger in America: a definition of food security. Accessed October 13, 2023. https://www.feedingamerica.org/hunger-in-america/food-insecurity
13. Coleman-Jensen A, Rabbitt MP, Gregory CA, Singh A. Household food security in the United States in 2021. ERR-309, U.S. Department of Agriculture, Economic Research Service; 2022. http://www.ers.usda.gov/publications/pub-details/?pubid=104655
14. Centers for Disease Control and Prevention. Adult obesity facts: obesity is a common, serious, and costly disease. Accessed October 13, 2023. https://www.cdc.gov/obesity/data/adult.html
15. Centers for Disease Control and Prevention. Obesity, race/ethnicity, and COVID-19. Accessed October 13, 2023. https://www.cdc.gov/obesity/data/obesity-and-covid-19.html
16. Restrepo BJ. Obesity prevalence among U.S. adults during the COVID-19 pandemic. *Am J Prev Med*. 2022;63(1):102–106. https://doi.org/10.1016/j.amepre.2022.01.012
17. Centers for Disease Control and Prevention. National Diabetes Statistics Report: estimates of diabetes and its burden in the United States. Accessed October 13, 2023. https://www.cdc.gov/diabetes/data/statistics-report/index.html
18. Centers for Disease Control and Prevention. Heart disease facts. Accessed October 13, 2023. https://www.cdc.gov/heartdisease/facts.htm
19. Office of Disease Prevention and Health Promotion. Social determinants of health. *Healthy People 2030*. U.S. Department of Health and Human Services; 2020. October 13, 2023 https://health.gov/healthypeople/priority-areas/social-determinants-health
20. Semega J, Kollar M, Creamer J, Mohanty A. *Income and Poverty in the United States: 2018*. U.S. Census Bureau; 2020. https://www.census.gov/library/publications/2019/demo/p60-266.html

21. Office of Disease Prevention and Health Promotion. Reduce the proportion of people living in poverty—SDOH-01. *Healthy People 2030.* U.S. Department of Health and Human Services; 2020. Accessed October 13, 2023. https://health.gov/healthypeople/objectives-and-data/browse-objectives/economic-stability/reduce-proportion-people-living-poverty-sdoh-01
22. Office of Disease Prevention and Health Promotion. Increase employment in working-age people—SDOH-02. *Healthy People 2030.* U.S. Department of Health and Human Services; 2020. Accessed October 13, 2023. https://health.gov/healthypeople/objectives-and-data/browse-objectives/economic-stability/increase-employment-working-age-people-sdoh-02
23. Office of Disease Prevention and Health Promotion. Reduce household food insecurity and hunger—NWS-01. *Healthy People 2030.* U.S. Department of Health and Human Services; 2020. Accessed October 13, 2023. https://health.gov/healthypeople/objectives-and-data/browse-objectives/nutrition-and-healthy-eating/reduce-household-food-insecurity-and-hunger-nws-01
24. Coleman-Jensen A, Rabbitt MP, Gregory CA, Singh A. *Household Food Security in the United States in 2020. ERR-298. U.S. Department of Agriculture, Economic Research Service; 2021.* http://www.ers.usda.gov/publications/pub-details/?pubid=102075
25. Lundeen EA, Siegel KR, Calhoun H, et al. Clinical-community partnerships to identify patients with food insecurity and address food needs. *Prev Chronic Dis*. 2017;14:E113. https://doi.org/10.5888/pcd14.170343
26. Office of Disease Prevention and Health Promotion. Nutrition and healthy eating. *Healthy People 2030. U.S. Department of Health and Human Services*; 2020. https://health.gov/healthypeople/objectives-and-data/browse-objectives/nutrition-and-healthy-eating
27. Office of Disease Prevention and Health Promotion. Law and health policy: social-ecological model. *Healthy People 2020*. U.S. Department of Health and Human Services. Accessed October 13, 2023. https://wayback.archive-it.org/5774/20220414114727/https://www.healthypeople.gov/2020/law-and-health-policy-social-ecological-model-graphic
28. American Public Health Association. Health equity. Accessed October 13, 2023. https://www.apha.org/topics-and-issues/health-equity
29. Benfer EA. Health justice: a framework (and call to action) for the elimination of health inequity and social injustice. *Am Univ Law Rev*. 2015;65(2):275–351.
30. American Public Health Association. *Creating the Healthiest Nation: Food Justice*. American Public Health Association; 2022. https://apha.org/-/media/Files/PDF/advocacy/CHN_Food_Justice.ashx
31. Hardin-Fanning F, Gokun Y. Gender and age are associated with healthy food purchases via grocery voucher redemption. *Rural Remote Health*. 2014;14(3):2830. https://doi.org/10.22605/RRH2830
32. Harvard T.H. Chan School of Public Health. The nutrition source: stress and health. Updated October 2021. https://www.hsph.harvard.edu/nutritionsource/stress-and-health
33. Bremner JD, Moazzami K, Wittbrodt MT, et al. Diet, stress and mental health. *Nutrients*. 2020;12(8):E2428. https://doi.org/10.3390/nu12082428
34. Sinha R. Role of addiction and stress neurobiology on food intake and obesity. *Biol Psychol*. 2018;131:5–13. https://doi.org/10.1016/j.biopsycho.2017.05.001
35. Stepanikova I, Baker EH, Simoni ZR, et al. The role of perceived discrimination in obesity among African Americans. *Am J Prev Med*. 2017;52(1 suppl 1):S77–S85. https://doi.org/10.1016/j.amepre.2016.07.034
36. Bacon KL, Stuver SO, Cozier YC, Palmer JR, Rosenberg L, Ruiz-Narváez EA. Perceived racism and incident diabetes in the Black Women's Health Study. *Diabetologia*. 2017;60(11):2221–2225. https://doi.org/10.1007/s00125-017-4400-6
37. Gibbons FX, Gerrard M, Fleischli ME, Simons RL, Kingsbury JH. Perceived racial discrimination and healthy behavior among African Americans. *Health Psychol*. 2021;40(3):155–165. https://doi.org/10.1037/hea0001056
38. Brown A, Flint SW, Batterham RL. Pervasiveness, impact and implications of weight stigma. *EClinicalMedicine*. 2022;47:101408. https://doi.org/10.1016/j.eclinm.2022.101408
39. Jovanovski N, Jaeger T. Demystifying 'diet culture': exploring the meaning of diet culture in online 'anti-diet' feminist, fat activist, and health professional communities. *Womens Stud Int Forum*. 2022;90:1–10. https://doi.org/10.1016/j.wsif.2021.102558
40. Glennie C, Alkon AH. Food justice: cultivating the field. *Environ Res Lett*. 2018;13(7):073003. https://doi.org/10.1088/1748-9326/aac4b2
41. Hasan MM, Ahmed S, Soares Magalhaes RJ, Fatima Y, Biswas T, Mamun AA. Double burden of malnutrition among women of reproductive age in 55 low- and middle-income countries: progress

achieved and opportunities for meeting the global target. *Eur J Clin Nutr*. 2022;76(2):277–287. https://doi.org/10.1038/s41430-021-00945-y

42. Shifler Bowers K, Francis E, Kraschnewski JL. The dual burden of malnutrition in the United States and the role of non-profit organizations. *Prev Med Rep*. 2018;12:294–297. https://doi.org/10.1016/j.pmedr.2018.10.002
43. Miller C, Ralston K, Vogel S. USDA's Supplemental Nutrition Assistance Program (SNAP) contributed to rural economic output, jobs following the great recession. *Amber Waves.* December 07, 2021. https://www.ers.usda.gov/amber-waves/2021/december/usda-s-supplemental-nutrition-assistance-program-snap-contributed-to-rural-economic-output-jobs-following-the-great-recession
44. Johns Hopkins Center for a Livable Future. Food policy networks. Johns Hopkins Bloomberg School of Public Health. http://www.foodpolicynetworks.org
45. Pezzuti C. What food policy councils should know about the farm bill: a guide for advocacy. January 2022. https://assets.jhsph.edu/clf/mod_clfResource/doc/FarmbillGuide[7].pdf
46. U.S. Department of Agriculture Food and Nutrition Service. Farmers Market Nutrition Program. Accessed October 13, 2023. https://www.fns.usda.gov/fmnp/wic-farmers-market-nutrition-program
47. Veldheer S, Scartozzi C, Bordner CR, et al. Impact of a prescription produce program on diabetes and cardiovascular risk outcomes. *J Nutr Educ Behav*. 2021;53(12):1008–1017. https://doi.org/10.1016/j.jneb.2021.07.005
48. Sastre L, Wynn D, Roupe M, Jacobs M. Link between redemption of a medical food pantry voucher and reduced hospital readmissions. *Prev Med Rep*. 2021;23:101400. https://doi.org/10.1016/j.pmedr.2021.101400
49. Gany F, Melnic I, Wu M, et al. Food to overcome outcomes disparities: a randomized controlled trial of food insecurity interventions to improve cancer outcomes. *J Clin Oncol*. 2022;40(31):3603–3612. https://doi.org/10.1200/JCO.21.02400
50. Basu S, Gardner CD, White JS, et al. Effects of alternative food voucher delivery strategies on nutrition among low-income adults. *Health Aff (Millwood)*. 2019;38(4):577–584. https://doi.org/10.1377/hlthaff.2018.05405
51. Harnack L, Oakes JM, Elbel B, Beatty T, Rydell S, French S. Effects of subsidies and prohibitions on nutrition in a food benefit program: a randomized clinical trial. *JAMA Intern Med*. 2016;176(11):1610–1618. https://doi.org/10.1001/jamainternmed.2016.5633
52. Dailey A, Davidson K, Gaskin K, et al. Responding to food insecurity and community crises through food policy council partnerships in a rural setting. *Prog Community Health Partnersh*. 2022;16(2 suppl):39–44. https://doi.org/10.1353/cpr.2022.0037
53. Haidar A, Markham C, Marshall A, et al. Innovative partnerships to address food insecurity during the COVID-19 pandemic: the brighter bites produce voucher program. *Int J Environ Res Public Health*. 2021;18(17):9175. https://doi.org/10.3390/ijerph18179175
54. Hu X, Clarke LW, Zendehdel K. Farmers' market usage, fruit and vegetable consumption, meals at home and health–evidence from Washington, DC. *Sustainability*. 2021;13(13):7437. https://doi.org/10.3390/su13137437
55. White JS, Vasconcelos G, Harding M, et al. Heterogeneity in the effects of food vouchers on nutrition among low-income adults: a quantile regression analysis. *Am J Health Promot*. 2021;35(2):279–283. https://doi.org/10.1177/0890117120952991
56. Feeding America. Find your local food bank. Accessed October 13, 2023. https://www.feedingamerica.org/find-your-local-foodbank
57. Waite T. What is the difference between food banks and pantries? Feeding America. February 20, 2019. https://www.feedingamerica.org/hunger-blog/what-difference-between-food-bank-and-food-pantry
58. Oldroyd L, Eskandari F, Pratt C, Lake AA. The nutritional quality of food parcels provided by food banks and the effectiveness of food banks at reducing food insecurity in developed countries: a mixed-method systematic review. *J Hum Nutr Diet*. 2022;35(6):1202–1229. https://doi.org/10.1111/jhn.12994
59. U.S. Department of Agriculture. Gus Schumacher Nutrition Incentive Program (GusNIP). National Institute of Food and Agriculture. Accessed October 13, 2023. http://www.nifa.usda.gov/grants/programs/hunger-food-security-programs/gus-schumacher-nutrition-incentive-program

60. Leng KH, Yaroch AL, Nugent NB, Stotz SA, Krieger J. How does the Gus Schumacher nutrition incentive program work? A theory of change. *Nutrients*. 2022;14(10):2018. https://doi.org/10.3390/nu14102018
61. Kania J, Kramer M. Collective impact. *Stanf Soc Innov Rev*. 2011;9(1):36–41. https://doi.org/10.48558/5900-KN19 https://ssir.org/articles/entry/collective_impact
62. Dailey AB, Hess A, Horton C, et al. Healthy options: a community-based program to address food insecurity. *J Prev Interv Community*. 2015;43(2):83–94. https://doi.org/10.1080/10852352.2015.973248
63. Calancie L, Stritzinger N, Konich J, et al. Food policy council case study describing cross-sector collaboration for food system change in a rural setting. *Prog Community Health Partnersh*. 2017;11(4):441–447. https://doi.org/10.1353/cpr.2017.0051

8

OLDER ADULT NUTRITION: A POPULATION APPROACH TO HEALTHY AGING

Kyle L. Thompson

Note on terminology: Both aging *and* ageing *are correct spellings, with* ageing *being used primarily in the United Kingdom. In this chapter,* aging *is used except when referring to the World Health Organization's* Decade on Healthy Ageing: Baseline Report.[1]

LEARNING OBJECTIVES

At the end of this chapter, students will be able to:

1. Define **global population aging**.
2. Explain the concept of **healthy aging**.
3. Describe three determinants of healthy aging: **functional ability**, **intrinsic capacity**, and **environments**.
4. Develop an understanding of the physiologic changes associated with aging of each body system.
5. Explain seven specific goals for older adult nutrition.
6. Identify available nutrition guidance tools for older adults.
7. Recall macronutrient and micronutrient intake concerns among older adults.
8. Identify public health nutrition issues of concern for older adults.
9. Describe public health nutrition programs available to promote health and longevity for older adults.

INTRODUCTION

The final life cycle stage, **older adulthood**, is a time when the health and nutrition behaviors and practices of earlier life cycle stages are likely to have their greatest impact. The older adult population is growing rapidly both in the United States and globally.

In 2004, the global population of adults older than 65 years was about 461 million; by 2050 it is projected that those over 65 years will number 2 billion.[2] In the United States in 2019 there were about 54.1 million older adults representing 16% of the total population, indicating a 36% increase since 2009.[3] Notably, the under-65 population increased by only 3% during the same time period.[3] The number of older adults in the United States is expected to grow to over 80 million by 2040. The implications of *global population aging* for healthcare systems and society as a whole are enormous; some have called this demographic shift the single most important medical challenge the world faces.[4]

Older adulthood is ideally a time of fulfillment and the culmination of a life well lived. Like all the other life cycle stages, it is a developmental stage during which persons continue to live, learn, and grow as human beings. Older adults bring tremendous gifts and value to society, including but not limited to their lifetime of experience, knowledge of history, lessons learned, and wisdom gained. Those who work with older adults know that each one is a unique individual. The focus of public health nutrition interventions among older adults is to utilize the power of nutrition to maximize each person's functional ability, overall well-being, and quality of life.

Nutrition is a crucial factor in promoting optimal outcomes as one ages. This chapter covers the concept of *healthy aging* (also called **successful aging**) as a model for nutrition practice in public health, normal nutrition for older adults, the importance of nutrition in promoting active participation in life and quality of life, and the impact of social determinants of health on older adults, along with associated public health issues and strategies for addressing those issues.

HEALTHY AGING AS AN APPROACH TO OLDER ADULTHOOD

The concept of healthy aging begins with the assumption that chronic disease and debilitation are not normal accompaniments to getting older. Often, persons enter a period of marked decline and poor health early in older adulthood and experience a years-long battle with poor health and increasing disability before death. The healthy aging approach recognizes that death is an inevitable part of life and seeks to promote an active, healthy life up until the final months, weeks, or days before death.

The World Health Organization (WHO) has defined healthy aging as "the process of developing and maintaining the functional ability that enables well-being in older age."[1] The concept of healthy aging has been evolving since at least the early 1900s.[5] According to Michel and Sadana, there is a prolific literature on the topic—much of it recent—that explores aging in two primary ways: first, from the viewpoints of older adults themselves on what constitutes successful aging, and second, from the perspective of measurements, standards, and data collected by investigators. The first perspective tends to envision healthy aging as the process of successfully adapting to the life changes characteristic of aging, while the second focuses on the maintenance of healthful metabolic and functional parameters.[5,6] Michel and Sadana posit that the WHO definition of healthy aging incorporates both perspectives in framing a healthy aging approach based on (1) a comprehensive view of health and well-being as more than the absence of disease, (2) a focus on functional ability as the primary indicator of successful aging, and (3) alignment with the life course theory, which views every stage of life as a preparation for healthy older adulthood.[5,6]

Decade of Healthy Ageing Report

In 2016, WHO published the *Decade of Healthy Ageing Report* (DHAR).[1] As of the writing of this chapter, the *Decade of Healthy Ageing* (2021–2030) is underway. The DHAR describes three determinants of healthy aging: functional ability, intrinsic capacity, and environments. Each is described here:

- **Functional ability:** Functional ability is the ability for a person to do what they want to do. According to the DHAR, functional ability encompasses abilities such as being able to meet one's own basic needs, to continue learning and growing as a person, to make one's own decisions, to be mobile, to participate in relationships, and to contribute to society.[1] Nutrition-related functional abilities include such capacities as being able to obtain food, observe food safety guidelines, plan and prepare meals, and meet one's own nutrition needs.
- **Intrinsic capacity**: Intrinsic capacity describes the personal capacities and resources a person can draw on during the aging process, such as physical abilities, the senses including vision and hearing, one's energy level, and psychological functioning including mental health.[1] The life course theory implies that lifelong habits have a strong impact on older adults' intrinsic capacities, as attention to health and good nutrition across the **life span** can help maintain and even improve capacities, ideally building reserve capacity when possible.
- **Environments:** Environments are the places where people live, including their homes, communities, and societies. Environment interacts with the intrinsic capacities of older adults to impact the ability to age successfully. Aspects of the environment that help or hinder healthy aging include but are not limited to:
  - The natural or built environment, including access to the outdoors, facility accessibility, distance to necessary services such as grocery stores, and neighborhood safety
  - Access to services and technology to enhance functional ability; for example, the ability to access medical care and treatment for vision and hearing, or medical nutrition therapy for chronic disease management
  - The availability of social support and relationships as well as needed assistance; for example, the availability of congregate meal programs to improve nutritional intake and socialization
  - Availability and access to community services to promote healthy aging; for example, access to a community senior center that serves as a hub for information sharing, socialization, and services, which may include nutrition services such as food assistance and congregate meals[1]

Figure 8.1 provides a diagram showing WHO's three components of healthy aging.[1] Note that the figure illustrates the impact that intrinsic capacity and environment have on the key determinant of healthy aging: functional ability.

THE OLDER ADULT LIFE CYCLE PHASE: PHYSIOLOGY

The older adult life cycle phase is generally considered to extend from the age of 65 years until death. The vast majority of older adults in the United States are community-living; that is, they reside, work, or are retired and care for themselves within their communities rather than living in care facilities. In 2019, about 19% of older adults

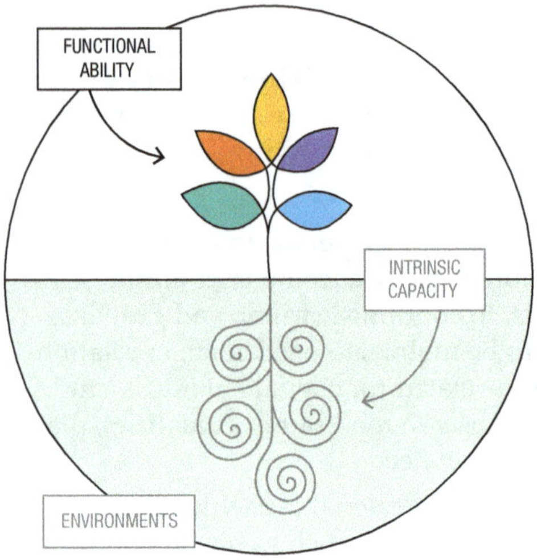

Figure 8.1. The World Health Organization three components of healthy aging.
Source: Adapted from World Health Organization. *Decade of Healthy Ageing: Baseline Report.* World Health Organization; 2020.

overall reported any disability, with varying numbers reporting challenges in one of six major functional areas: vision, hearing, mobility, cognition, communication, and/or self-care.[3] A small number of older adults reside within care facilities such as nursing homes largely due to disability and difficulties managing self-care. About half of those residing in care homes suffer from Alzheimer disease or related dementias.[7] According to the Agency on Aging *2020 Profile of Older Americans*, about 1% of those age 65 to 74, 2% of those age 75 to 84, and 8% of those age 85 years and up reside in care facilities.[3]

As noted in the preceding sentence, the 2020 *Profile of Older Americans* describes older adults' living arrangements by utilizing three stratifications of age:

- 65 to 74 years, sometimes called the **young-old**
- 75 to 84 years, sometimes called the **old**
- 85 years and older, sometimes called the **old-old**

Older adulthood from the age of 65 can extend for more than 30 years, and there is a nearly twofold worldwide increase in the number of **centenarians**, or persons 100 years of age, over the past two decades.[8] It is important to remember that between the ages of 65 years and 85 years, there is a period of 20 years. The differences between a 65-year-old and an 85-year-old in terms of functional ability, life focus, and healthcare needs can be as pronounced as the differences between an older adolescent and a middle-aged person.

At the same time, health practitioners must also keep in mind that each older adult is a unique individual with unique capabilities. There is great variation in the capabilities of individual older adults. For example, a particular 80-year-old person may be completely independent in activities of daily living and able to participate fully in the community, while a particular 65-year-old person in the same community may suffer poor health and be completely dependent on others for care. A popular saying among those who work with older adults is "If you've seen one 80-year-old, you've seen one 80-year-old."[9] Successfully working with older adults in public health settings requires professionals to avoid generalizations and instead get to know people as individuals.

It is important, too, to consider the role of **resilience** in aging. Often described as the ability to "bounce back," resilience is the process and outcome of successfully adapting to difficult or challenging life experiences. Resilience is often demonstrated by utilizing one's capacities to be flexible, to accept and adjust to change, and to reframe negative situations in positive ways. As humans age, their ability to bounce back from physical insults such as illness and injury decreases, and the body gradually loses reserve capacity to deal with physical stress. However, older adults who age successfully often have great reserves of mental and emotional strength that they use, even at very advanced ages, to demonstrate resilience in dealing with the challenges and progressive losses of growing old.

Physiologic Changes of Older Adulthood

Senescence, or aging, is a normal biological process that takes place over a lifetime, and results in the gradual loss of physiologic capabilities, including healing and recovery processes, that ultimately leads to death.[10] The process of aging is poorly understood, but several theories have been posited, including the idea that aging is a genetically programmed process; WHO describes aging as the generalized accumulation of cellular damage over time.[10,11]

Regardless of the reasons for which aging occurs, it is a universally recognized fact of life. Modern medicine has greatly extended average human life spans; at the turn of the 20th century, the average U.S. life span was about 47 years, compared with 76.4 years in 2023.[12,13] Parenthetically, it should be noted that the 2023 average life span represents a substantial decrease from the 2018 average life span of 78.7 years, and may reflect the COVID-19 pandemic, including its impacts on the entire U.S. healthcare system.[12] Medical technology has not always, however, extended the **health span**, or the period of life during which one is able to enjoy good health, make one's own decisions, and participate fully in one's desired life's activities.

The physiologic changes of aging impact every body system, and eventually result in death. Genetics is a crucial factor in the rate and characteristics of an individual's aging process, but general healthful lifestyle habits play an important role. Lifestyle practices may prevent, delay, or ameliorate the decline of aging for a long period of time by extending and enhancing the ability to be resilient. Regular interactions with healthcare providers are essential during aging, as many age-related challenges can be addressed with lifestyle or medical interventions.

Public health practitioners should not assume that decline and disability are a normal part of aging, but should actively intervene to improve nutrition-related functional ability and quality of life in older adult populations. Many older adults experience a years-long or even decades-long gradual deterioration of health, spending a large portion of their older adult life cycle stage battling illness and disability. The ideal for healthy aging is to enjoy good health until shortly before death, with a period of decline lasting a few months, weeks, or days rather than years. While genetics may prevent some from achieving this goal, healthful habits can be a powerful support to extend the health span. Table 8.1 provides a list of body systems and age-associated changes to those systems.

Interventions, including lifestyle interventions, focused on increasing the health span show promise for increasing the health span and improving quality of life for millions of older adults.

Table 8.1. Examples of Body Systems, Age-Associated Changes, and Possible Modifications

Body System	Age-Associated Changes	Modifiable Factors	Possible Modifications
Cellular aging	One theory of aging posits that the effects of aging become evident when the proportion of senescent, or aging, cells in the body becomes sufficiently large to impair the processes of normally functioning cells.[10]	It is possible (and hopeful) that all or parts of the cellular aging process can be modified. Research is ongoing; as knowledge accumulates and genetic technology improves, it is hoped that specific aspects of aging will become modifiable. It is already known that certain health habits are associated with an improved course of aging.	Cellular aging is a topic of great interest to researchers, and a number of possible accumulated effects of aging on cells have been identified.
Cardio-vascular	The most common cardiovascular change that occurs with aging is stiffening of the blood vessels, called **arteriosclerosis**, which leads to *hypertension*, or high blood pressure. High blood pressure and increasing age heighten the risk of *atherosclerosis*, in which the blood vessels become blocked by the buildup of plaque. Buildup of plaque in the blood vessels leads to decreased blood flow, and thus a decreased oxygen supply to the heart.[14]	Some risk factors are modifiable; in particular, hypertension can be treated medically and/or with lifestyle interventions. Lifestyle interventions include diet and physical activity. Increasing age is a nonmodifiable risk factor.	Heart disease is not always inevitable with aging; maintaining healthful behaviors such as regular physical activity, a healthful diet, and not smoking can be helpful in reducing the risk of heart disease as one grows older.
Pulmo-nary	In healthy persons, most changes in the lungs are due to muscular and physical aging rather than disease. For example, the general muscle loss associated with aging impacts the major breathing muscle, the diaphragm. The aging immune system is less able to protect against infectious diseases that impact the lungs, such as COVID-19.[15]	In healthy persons, there are several modifiable risk factors that can positively impact and maintain lung health. The main modifiable risk factor for prevention of lung disease is avoidance of smoking. Increasing age is a nonmodifiable risk factor.	The first recommendation for preventing and ameliorating pulmonary decline is to not smoke. Support and resources for quitting smoking are available from the Centers for Disease Control and Prevention at this link: www.cdc.gov/tobacco/quit_smoking/index.htm. Following general guidelines for good health is helpful for lung health.

Neurologic	In normal aging, nerve tissue including the spinal cord and brain atrophies. Thought processes may slow, and reaction time decreases. Sensory deficits may occur. Neurologic changes are not always evident. The process is highly individualized, with some individuals experiencing few evident changes and others experiencing many. Some brain functions may improve with age. Capacity to detect and understand issues at a macro level may increase with age.[16] Dementias such as Alzheimer disease are not a normal part of aging.[17]	In healthy persons, there are several modifiable risk factors that can positively impact and maintain neurologic health. Moving from a sedentary to an active lifestyle is a controllable risk factor, as is consuming a healthful diet, and regularly participating in mental activities and paying attention to mental health. Increasing age is a nonmodifiable risk factor.	Following general guidelines for good health is helpful for neurologic health. Staying physically active and engaging in regular physical activity is important for brain health and helps in transporting oxygen and nutrients to brain tissue. Staying mentally active is also recommended to maintain neurologic health; activities such as reading, learning new skills, taking classes, learning a language, and doing word and math puzzles may be helpful. Regular socialization is an important part of maintaining brain health. Acting to treat mental health conditions such as depression is of vital importance, as depressive conditions are associated with worse cognitive status in older adults.[18]
Digestive	Aging can lead to alterations in sensory perceptions of taste and smell, making eating less enjoyable. Nerve and smooth muscle changes that reduce the speed at which food passes through the digestive tract (reduced gut motility) can promote constipation. Changes in the gut microbiome can alter nutrient metabolism; together, these changes can result in unintended weight loss and/or malnutrition.[10]	In healthy persons, there are several modifiable risk factors that can positively impact and maintain digestive health. Increasing age is a nonmodifiable risk factor.	Good nutritional status is a foundational component of maintaining functional ability and quality of life for older adults. For specific challenges, nutrition assessment provided by a physician or registered dietitian nutritionist can be very helpful in providing an individualized nutrition plan that addresses digestive difficulties. Medical treatment for digestive problems is essential. For population health, interventions to positively impact older adults' access to nutritious food, relieve food insecurity, promote adequate fruit and vegetable intake, develop congregate meal and home-delivered meal programs, and promote socialization during meals can be very helpful.

(*continued*)

Table 8.1. Examples of Body Systems, Age-Associated Changes, and Possible Modifications (*continued*)

Body System	Age-associated Changes	Modifiable?	Possible Modifications
Musculoskeletal	A normal part of the aging process is an inevitable loss of bone and muscle mass, accompanied by loss of cartilage tissue and loss/compression of intervertebral tissue leading to loss of height.[19] These losses take places in all people, both males and females, of all races and ethnicities. Results of musculoskeletal aging can include **osteoarthritis**, **osteoporosis**, and sarcopenia.	In healthy persons, there are several modifiable risk factors that can positively impact and maintain musculoskeletal health. Levels of physical activity, along with healthful dietary practices, are controllable risk factors. Increasing age is a nonmodifiable risk factor.	Loss of bone and muscle tissue can be slowed and ameliorated, and in some cases even reversed for a time by engaging in regular physical activity and consuming a healthful diet with particular attention to adequate intake of protein and micronutrients. Assessment of musculoskeletal issues by a qualified physician followed by evidence-based treatment can have a profound positive impact on quality of life. Effective lifestyle changes and medical and surgical treatments are available for many musculoskeletal issues. Relief from pain and improvements in functional ability can drastically improve an older adult's overall outlook on life.
Sensory	Some degree of hearing loss is very common among older adults, with about half of those over age 75 years experiencing hearing impairments.[20] Cataracts, or clouding of the lens of the eye, is very common in older adults and is related to aging. About 36% of older adults age 70 to 74 years will experience cataracts, and this number rises to about half in those 75 to 79 years old.[21]	Increasing age is a nonmodifiable risk factor for sensory impairment in older adults, and some loss is likely inevitable although widely variable among individuals, probably due to genetics. Modifiable risk factors for sensory impairment include engaging in regular physical activity, consuming a healthful diet, and not smoking. Additional modifiable risk factors include lifetime exposure to loud noise, use of ear protection, and wearing sunglasses to protect the eyes.	Regular vision and hearing examinations are vital to the process of healthy aging. Effective treatments for many vision and hearing problems are available, and can have major positive impacts on functional ability and quality of life.

Immune	As part of normal aging, the immune system declines in function, resulting in greater susceptibility to infections, complications from infectious disease, and cancer, and reduced resilience to recover from infections and other physiologic insults.[22]	In healthy persons, there are several modifiable risk factors that can positively impact and maintain immune health in the face of aging's inevitable decline. Engaging in regular physical activity and consuming a healthful diet are controllable risk factors, as is not smoking. Maintaining a regular vaccination schedule is helpful in enhancing immune system function.	Regular physical activity and consumption of a healthful diet are helpful in promoting immune system function in older adults. Research indicates that older adults' immune response is heightened by vaccines specially developed for older adults; for example, flu vaccines designed for older adults provide greater protection than those designed for younger adults. Specialization of vaccines for older adults demonstrates that immune function in older adults can be enhanced.[22]
Endocrine	In normal aging, the function of endocrine organs such as the thyroid and pancreas gradually declines. Metabolism slows, so older adults require fewer calories than younger adults to meet energy needs. Glucose metabolism becomes less responsive, increasing the risk of diabetes.[10]	In healthy persons, there are several modifiable risk factors that can positively impact and help to maintain endocrine health. Engaging in regular physical activity and consuming a healthful diet are controllable risk factors, as is not smoking.	While the risk of endocrine dysfunction increases with age, general healthful lifestyle practices such as engaging in regular physical activity, consuming a healthful diet, and not smoking can help maximize endocrine function. Diabetes and endocrine disease are not inevitable in aging adults. Regular medical encounters to check endocrine function are important to identify and treat problems early before complications occur.

(continued)

Table 8.1. Examples of Body Systems, Age-Associated Changes, and Possible Modifications (*continued*)

Body System	Age-associated Changes	Modifiable?	Possible Modifications
Genitourinary	The reserve capacity of the kidneys declines, the bladder becomes less flexible, and risk of genitourinary problems such as incontinence, sexual dysfunction, urinary tract infections, and prostate problems increases.[23]	In healthy persons, there are several modifiable risk factors that can positively impact and help to maintain endocrine health. Engaging in regular physical activity and consuming a healthful diet including adequate water consumption are controllable risk factors, as is not smoking. Controlling high blood pressure is an important modifiable risk factor for kidney function.	While the risk of endocrine dysfunction increases with age, general healthful lifestyle practices such as engaging in regular physical activity, consuming a healthful diet, and not smoking can help maximize genitourinary function. Regular medical encounters to check genitourinary function are important to identify and treat problems early. Typically, urinary control problems have a substantial negative impact on quality of life, and appropriate treatment can substantially increase an older adult's enjoyment of daily activities.

THE OLDER ADULT LIFE CYCLE PHASE: NUTRITION TO SUPPORT HEALTHY AGING

Goals for Older Adult Nutrition

Older adulthood is the final life cycle stage and ideally is the culmination of a life well lived. Nutrition plays a crucial role in older adult health and quality of life. Seven major goals for older adult nutrition are listed here:

1. Achieve appropriate and adequate consumption of nutrients to support the healthy aging process and promote optimal quality of life.
2. Consume a diet aligned with the prevention, delay, or management of chronic disease to promote healthy aging and an active lifestyle, and to extend the health span.
3. Prevent involuntary and inappropriate weight loss, in order to support adequate immune function, maintain or improve functional ability, prevent weakness and falls, and maintain a healthy weight.
4. Consume adequate protein and engage in regular physical activity to maintain muscle mass and prevent and/or attenuate **sarcopenia**.
5. Maintain nutrition-related functionality for as long as and to the fullest extent possible: this includes the tasks involved in self-nourishing such as planning, preparing, and consuming meals.
6. Enjoy the many benefits of socializing around food, which include better nutrient intake, opportunities to make new friends, and improved physical and mental health.
7. Maintain a healthful relationship with food that allows for both appropriate self-nourishment and enjoyment and appreciation of food and eating throughout the life span.

Official Nutrition Guidance for Older Adults

The U.S. government provides several official nutrition surveillance and guidance tools that can inform public health nutrition practice among older adults. Examples of key official nutrition gathering and guidance tools that are applied in older adult nutrition settings include the Healthy Eating Index (HEI), the Dietary Guidelines for Americans (DGAs), the Dietary Reference Intakes (DRIs), and MyPlate for Older Adults. WHO also provides Guidelines for Older Adult Nutrition. Each tool is described in this chapter:

The Healthy Eating Index: Evaluating the Quality of Older Adults' Nutrient Intake

The HEI was first developed in 1995 and is a dietary scoring tool that is used to compare U.S. populations' usual food consumption to the DGAs.[24] The current version of the HEI was revised in 2015 to align with the 2015–2020 DGAs.[25] The *What We Eat in America* dietary interview survey is administered as part of the National Health and Nutrition Examination Survey (NHANES) and provides data for the HEI.[26] The HEI algorithm results in a score from 0 to 100, with a score of 100 indicating complete alignment with the Dietary Guidelines.[24]

The overall HEI for all Americans in 2022 is 58/100, indicating poor adherence to the DGAs.[24] Older adults' overall score of 61 points is second only to 2- to 4-year-olds' score of 62 points, but still indicates room for substantial improvement.

Older adults' usual intakes differ from recommended intakes in several important ways.[27] In general, older adults do not meet recommendations for intake of fruits, vegetables, and dairy, and older adult females consume slightly less protein than recommended. Other dietary areas of concern include:

- Added sugar intake
  - Desired ≤10% total calories/day: guideline exceeded by 54% older adult males and 58% older adult females
- Sodium intake
  - Desired <2,300 mg/day: guideline exceeded by 94% older adult males, 72% older adult females
- Saturated fat intake
  - Desired ≤10% total calories/day: guideline exceeded by 85% older adult males, 78% older adult females[27]

Because good nutrition is a key contributor to health and quality of life in older adulthood, population-wide nutrition interventions, which encourage adherence to the DGAs' recommendations, are an important focus for public health nutrition and should help to increase the population's HEI scores.

The Dietary Guidelines for Americans

Since 1980, the DGAs have provided healthful dietary guidance for Americans ages 2 years and up.[28] The DGAs are updated every 5 years by the USDA and the DHHS, and are based on the best scientific evidence available at the time of the update.[27] The DGAs are used as the basis for U.S. food and nutrition policy, and support the development of tools to assist lay audiences in applying the guidelines. The four basic recommendations of the 2020–2025 DGAs are:

- Follow a healthy dietary pattern at every life stage.
- Customize and enjoy nutrient-dense food and beverage choices to reflect personal preferences, cultural traditions, and financial considerations.
- Focus on meeting food group needs with nutrient-dense foods and beverages, and stay within calorie limits.
- Limit foods and beverages higher in added sugars, saturated fat, and sodium, and limit alcoholic beverages.[29]

Guidelines specific to the stage of life from pregnancy through older adulthood are provided for the first time by the 2020–2025 DGAs.[30] Specific DGA recommendations for life cycle stages provides improved opportunities to tailor and apply the guidelines in nutrition interventions designed for older adults. Table 8.2 provides a summary of food group intake recommendations based on the U.S. DGAs for older adults. Table 8.3 provides a sample meal plan for an older adult. An infographic providing a summary of the 2020–2025 DGAs can be found at www.dietaryguidelines.gov/sites/default/files/2021-03/DGA_2020-2025_ExecutiveSummary_English.pdf.

Table 8.2. Food Group Amounts Recommended for Older Adults for Two Calorie Intake Levels

Food Group	Older Adults (60 + Years),* 1,800 Kcal/Day	Older Adults (60 + Years),* 2,200 Kcal/Day
Vegetables (cups/day)	2.5	3
Fruits (cups/day)	1.5	2.0
Dairy (cups/day)	3	3
Grains (oz/day)	6	7
Protein foods (oz eq/day)†	5	6
Oils (g/day)	24	29

*Intake ranges vary and should be adapted for activity level, sex, and age.
†One oz eq (ounce equivalent) is defined by the U.S. Department of Agriculture as 1 oz lean meat, poultry, or seafood, 1 egg, ¼ cup cooked beans or tofu, 1 tbsp peanut butter, ½ oz nuts or seeds.
Source: Adapted from U.S. Department of Agriculture, U.S. Department of Health and Human Services. *Dietary Guidelines for Americans, 2020-2025*. 9th ed. U.S. Department of Health and Human Services; 2020. https://www.dietaryguidelines.gov

Table 8.3. Sample Menu for Healthy Older Adult*

Meal	Sample Menu†
Breakfast	1 cup cooked oatmeal with ½ sliced banana, 2 tbsp chopped walnuts and 1 tsp brown sugar; 1 scrambled egg
Lunch	Turkey and cheese sandwich: 2 slices whole grain bread, 2 oz sliced turkey, 1 oz sliced cheese, 2 tsp mayonnaise; Salad: 1 cup dark leafy greens with ½ cup sliced cherry tomatoes, 1 tbsp vinaigrette-type dressing; ½ cup mandarin oranges canned in their own juice, 1 cup milk
Afternoon snack	1 medium apple, sliced, with 1 tbsp peanut butter used as dip
Dinner	Chili, 1 cup: made with pinto or kidney beans, ground beef or turkey, canned tomatoes (lower sodium preferred), diced onion, diced green peppers, chili seasonings; ½ cup green beans, cornbread, 2" by 2" piece, 1 tsp butter, 1 cup milk
Evening snack	¼ cup nuts of choice

*Requiring about 1,800 kcal/day. Adjust number of servings/portion sizes to meet lower or higher calorie needs.
†Water to drink if not otherwise indicated.

Dietary Reference Intakes

Recommended ranges of intake for nutrients, energy, and fiber are provided by the DRIs.[31] The DRIs are established by the Food and Nutrition Board of the National Academies of Science, Engineering, and Medicine, and are updated periodically based on the best available scientific evidence. Around 1990, it was recognized that the Recommended Dietary Allowance (RDA), the only nutrient value available at that time, was inadequate to completely describe nutrient recommendations.[32] Thus, a set of values for each nutrient was proposed. Because the development of the DRIs is an ongoing process dependent on available research, not all values are available for every nutrient. The Chronic Disease Risk Reduction (CDRR) intake, which was determined for sodium in 2019, is the newest DRI value.[33]

DRI values are provided for adults ages 51 to 70 years as well as for adults older than 70 years. Definitions of the current DRI values, and a link to access the various DRI tables, are found in Appendix C.

MyPlate: Older Adults

The USDA's consumer-focused dietary guidance plan is called MyPlate. Implemented in 2011 to replace the previous U.S. Department of Agriculture (USDA) Food Pyramid, MyPlate is a computer-based platform that provides practical assistance in choosing a healthful meal plan.[34] MyPlate is in alignment with the 2020–2025 DGAs, and provides targeted information by life stage group. MyPlate is administered by the USDA Center for Nutrition Policy and Promotion (CNPP).[35] MyPlate is revised every 5 years in alignment with DGA revisions. The MyPlate resource is designed to be user-friendly, flexible, and inclusive of a wide range of cultural foods and budget levels.

MyPlate: Older Adults includes nutrition guidance and recommendations, including descriptions of the nutrition needs of older adults, nutrition tips, suggestions for remaining physically active, and resources.[36] Instructions for obtaining a personalized MyPlate Plan as well as the *Start Simple with MyPlate* computer application are provided. Tips for healthy eating on a budget, reading the Nutrition Facts label, and food safety are provided. The older adult MyPlate web page provides a link to MyPlate Kitchen for access to many healthful and cost-effective recipes and cooking tips. The web page also provides information on accessing MyPlate information through technology such as smart speakers.[36]

The World Health Organization and Older Adult Nutrition

WHO is currently coordinating the *Decade of Healthy Ageing*, a worldwide initiative designed to improve the lives of older adults, their families, and their communities.[1] The *Decade of Healthy Ageing: Baseline Report* integrates and emphasizes the importance of nutrition as a key determinant of vitality and functional ability in older adulthood. WHO supports initiatives to improve the availability, access, and quality of food and nutrition resources available to older adults.

Summary of Energy and Nutrient Needs for Older Adults

Macronutrients

Macronutrients include the *energy-yielding nutrients* protein, carbohydrate, and fat. Proportions of macronutrients in relation to total caloric intake are important to overall health. The DRIs provide acceptable macronutrient distribution ranges (AMDRs) for older adults, found in Table 8.4. Note that these recommendations are identical for all age/sex groups.

Energy (Calorie) Needs

Older adults' energy (calorie) needs vary based on age, sex, and level of activity.[27] The presence of medical conditions may affect energy needs, and older adults with medical conditions should be referred to a physician or registered dietitian nutritionist (RDN) for an comprehensive, individualized nutrition assessment. In general, adequacy of energy intake for healthy older adults can be evaluated by ongoing monitoring of weight; the usual goal is steady weight maintenance without sudden substantial loss or gain of weight. Table 8.5 provides average calorie needs for older adults.

Protein Needs

On average, protein consumption among older adult females does not meet DRI recommendations.[27] Adequate protein intake is especially important for older adults to promote healing and repair of body tissues (both from daily use ("wear and tear") and from injuries or illness), proper physiologic function, and—along with appropriate physical activity—amelioration of age-related muscle loss, or **sarcopenia**. Older adults may consume inadequate protein for a variety of reasons, including the cost of protein foods, poor chewing ability/dental problems, and functional impairments impacting the ability to cook.

Table 8.4. Acceptable Macronutrient Distribution Ranges for Older Adults*

Age	Macronutrient Range (Percent of Total Calories), Females	Macronutrient Range (Percent of Total Calories), Males
≥51 years	Protein: 10%–35% Carbohydrate: 45%–65% Fat: 20%–35%	Protein: 10%–35% Carbohydrate: 45%–65% Fat: 20%–35%

*Needs also affected by activity levels or special conditions.

Source: U.S. Department of Agriculture, U.S. Department of Health and Human Services. *Dietary Guidelines for Americans, 2020-2025*. 9th ed. U.S. Department of Health and Human Services; 2020. https://www.dietaryguidelines.gov

Table 8.5. Estimated Energy Requirement for Older Adults*

Age	Energy Needs (kcal/day), Females	Energy Needs (kcal/day), Males
≥60 years	1,600–2,200	2,000–2,600

*Needs also affected by activity levels or special conditions.
Source: Adapted from U.S. Department of Agriculture, U.S. Department of Health and Human Services. *Dietary Guidelines for Americans, 2020-2025*. 9th ed. U.S. Department of Health and Human Services; 2020. https://www.dietaryguidelines.gov

Another reason older adults' protein intake may be inadequate is that evidence indicates older adults may have a physiologic need for a higher protein level than the RDA to maintain muscle mass and function. The RDA of 0.8 g protein per kilogram per day for all adults was developed based on the amount of protein required to prevent a loss of lean body tissue. In addition to maintaining lean body tissue, older adults need adequate protein to promote muscle health and prevent sarcopenia—a debilitating loss of muscle mass—and preserve strength and functional ability. Investigators have posited that older adults may require as much as 1.2 to 2.0 g protein per kilogram per day to meet these goals.[37] Research is ongoing.

Protein foods to encourage among healthy older adults include lean meats, fish and seafood, poultry, eggs, beans and legumes, tofu, dairy products such as Greek yogurt and cottage cheese, nuts and seeds, and nut butters. Note that while nuts, seeds, and nut butters provide protein and healthful fats, portion control is important because the fat content in these foods also increases their calorie content. One portion of nuts is about 1 oz, usually about a handful or 2 tbsp. Table 8.6 provides RDAs for protein for older adults by age/sex groups.

Carbohydrate Needs

Carbohydrate foods are the body's main source of energy as they supply the body's primary fuel, glucose. Notably, adequate carbohydrate consumption is essential for optimal brain function, as carbohydrates are the brain's preferred source of energy. Indigestible carbohydrates called fiber are components of fruits, vegetables, and grains, and these make important contributions to human health.

According to the HEI, older adults meet guidelines for total grain consumption, but do not meet guidelines for consumption of whole grains and exceed recommendations for consumption of refined grains.[27] Well over half of older adults exceed guidelines for consumption of added sugars.[27] Note that carbohydrate recommendations are identical for all age/sex groups. Carbohydrate foods include grains, fruits, and vegetables, as well as table sugar, fructose, and honey. Dairy milk provides carbohydrate as well as protein. Table 8.7 provides RDAs for carbohydrate for older adults.

Table 8.6. Recommended Dietary Allowances for Protein for Older Adults*

Age	Protein Needs (g/day), Females	Protein Needs (g/day), Males
≥51 years	46	56

*Needs also affected by activity levels or special conditions.
Source: Adapted from U.S. Department of Agriculture, U.S. Department of Health and Human Services. *Dietary Guidelines for Americans, 2020-2025.* 9th ed. U.S. Department of Health and Human Services; 2020. https://www.dietaryguidelines.gov

Table 8.7. Recommended Dietary Allowances for Carbohydrate for Older Adults*

Age	Carbohydrate Needs (g/day), Females	Carbohydrate Needs (g/day), Males
≥51 years	130	130

*Needs also affected by activity levels or special conditions.
Source: Adapted from U.S. Department of Agriculture, U.S. Department of Health and Human Services. *Dietary Guidelines for Americans, 2020-2025.* 9th ed. U.S. Department of Health and Human Services; 2020. https://www.dietaryguidelines.gov

Fiber

Dietary fiber, or the indigestible components of plants, is provided by fruit, vegetable, and whole grain intake. Adequate fiber consumption is important for optimal bowel function throughout life. Fiber intake promotes digestive health, helps regulate blood glucose levels, and provides feelings of satiety (fullness), which may promote healthful weight management. Overall consumption of these fiber-containing foods by older adults does not meet DGA recommendations.[27] Intake of fiber-providing plant foods by older adults should be encouraged. Table 8.8 provides adequate intake (AI) recommendations for fiber intake for older adults.

Fat Needs

The HEI reports that 80% of older adult males and 77% of older adult females exceed the recommended saturated fat intake of 10% of total calories.[27] The AMDR for fat is 20% to 35% of total calories. Alpha-linolenic acid (omega-3) and linoleic acid (omega-6) are essential fats required by humans and obtained only from the diet, and AI values have been developed for these fats. Foods providing the essential fats include nuts, seeds, oils such as olive and canola oil, fatty fish such as salmon, mackerel, and sardines, and avocados. Healthy older adults should be encouraged to consume healthful fats on a daily basis. Table 8.9 provides AIs for fat intake for older adults by age/sex groups.

Water Needs

Adequate hydration is essential to optimal body function. Humans obtain water from the consumption of liquids and foods. It is recommended that older adults consume plain water as their primary beverage. Table 8.10 provides water and fluid intake AIs for older adults.

Table 8.8. Adequate Intake for Fiber for Older Adults*

Age	Fiber Needs (g/day), Females	Fiber Needs (g/day), Males
51 to 70 years	21	30
>70 years	21	30

*Needs also affected by special conditions.
Source: Adapted from U.S. Department of Agriculture, U.S. Department of Health and Human Services. *Dietary Guidelines for Americans, 2020-2025*. 9th ed. U.S. Department of Health and Human Services; 2020. https://www.dietaryguidelines.gov

Table 8.9. Adequate Intake for Fat for Older Adults*

Age	Fat Needs, Females	Fat Needs, Males
≥51 years	Total fat: no adequate intake determined Linoleic acid: 11 g/day α-Linolenic acid: 1.1 g/day	Total fat: no adequate intake determined Linoleic acid: 14 g/day α-Linolenic acid: 1.6 g/day

*Needs also affected by activity levels or special conditions.
Source: Adapted from U.S. Department of Agriculture, U.S. Department of Health and Human Services. *Dietary Guidelines for Americans, 2020-2025*. 9th ed. U.S. Department of Health and Human Services; 2020. https://www.dietaryguidelines.gov

Table 8.10. Recommended Dietary Allowances for Water for Older Adults*

Age	Water Needs, Females	Water Needs, Males
19–70 years	2.7 L/day total water† includes 2.2 L (about 9 cups) water obtained from drinking water and beverages	3.7 L/day total water† includes 3 L (about 13 cups) water obtained from drinking water and beverages

*Needs also affected by activity levels or special conditions.
†*Total water* is water obtained from food, beverages, and drinking water.
Source: Adapted from U.S. Department of Agriculture, U.S. Department of Health and Human Services. *Dietary Guidelines for Americans, 2020-2025*. 9th ed. U.S. Department of Health and Human Services; 2020. https://www.dietaryguidelines.gov

Micronutrients

To access the DRIs for micronutrients including vitamins and minerals for older adults, see Appendix C. Older adults overall consume less than recommended amounts of fruits, vegetables, and whole grains, and so are at risk for micronutrient deficiencies. The best source of micronutrients is an overall healthful diet providing recommended amounts of nutritious foods. If a comprehensive nutrition assessment reveals a need for nutrient supplementation, this should be supervised by a physician or RDN due to risks including but not limited to medication–nutrient interactions and/or the possibility of exceeding the tolerable upper intake limit (UL) of supplemented nutrients. Public health nutrition interventions for older adults should encourage the consumption of healthful foods providing key nutrients to promote health and functional ability. Four micronutrients of public health concern for older adults are iron, calcium, vitamin D, and vitamin B_{12}, which are discussed in the following sections.

Iron

Suboptimal iron intake in older adults can be a contributing factor to **subclinical iron deficiency** and **anemia**.[38] Anemia occurs when there are too few red blood cells to adequately carry oxygen throughout the body, or there are enough red blood cells but they do not work properly.[38] The prevalence of older adults with anemia increased in the United States during the years 2013 to 2016, and the prevalence rose sharply with increasing age: for example, the rate was 7.4% among men age 65 to 74 years, but rose to 39.5% for men >85 years of age.[39] While the increase was not as dramatic for women, the trajectory was similar. Anemia is associated with a number of poor outcomes in older adults including cognitive problems, increased falls and broken bones, higher rates of cardiovascular disease, lower quality of life, and higher risk of mortality.[38] Regular evaluation of the iron status of older adults by a medical professional is essential to determine the cause of anemia, along with a treatment strategy, which may include supplementation and medical nutrition therapy. Iron supplementation should be supervised by a physician or RDN.

Older adults may consume inadequate dietary iron for a variety of reasons that parallel those underlying low protein intake, as many high-iron foods are also high protein foods. Cost of high-iron foods, poor chewing ability/dental problems, and functional impairments impacting the ability to cook may impair iron intake. Sources of iron from foods include poultry, meats, seafood, iron-fortified cereals, beans, dried fruits, and dark green leafy vegetables. The RDA for iron for males 51 to 70 years and >70 years is 8 mg/day for both age groups. For females in the same age groups, the RDA is also 8 mg/day.[27]

Calcium

Calcium is the most abundant stored nutrient in the human body, with 99% deposited in the bones and teeth, and the remaining 1% serum calcium playing an essential role in crucial body processes such as nerve signal transmission, heart contraction, and muscle function.[40] Notably, serum calcium levels remain constant whatever the dietary intake of calcium, and so cannot be used to evaluate calcium nutriture. If calcium is needed in the serum to support crucial body processes, the body takes calcium from the bones to maintain the appropriate level.

Calcium is essential for bone health throughout the life span. Bone formation and maintenance begin during the embryonic and fetal stages and continue throughout the remainder of the life cycle. In older adults, the life course theory applies to calcium nutriture: adequate calcium intake during the years of childhood, adolescence, and adulthood make it more likely that the resulting older adult will maintain healthy bones.

About 30% of the total calcium consumed in food or supplements is absorbed by the human body.[40] Older adult females who are postmenopausal and persons who avoid dairy products, such as those with lactose intolerance, are most at risk for calcium deficiency. In postmenopausal females, the lack of estrogen results in decreased calcium absorption and increased calcium excretion.[41] Persons with lactose intolerance may consume none or very small amounts of dairy products, the richest source of dietary calcium, because of unpleasant digestive symptoms caused by a lack of the milk sugar–digesting enzyme lactase. Both groups may benefit from calcium supplementation supervised by a healthcare professional.

The U.S. Preventive Services Task Force has determined that evidence is inadequate to determine if calcium or calcium/vitamin D supplements prevent fractures in older adults, and further research is needed.[41] However, consumption of adequate calcium at the RDA level throughout older adulthood is known to be important for bone health and for health in general.

Older adults should be encouraged to promote the health of their bones by consuming adequate amounts of calcium and vitamin D (see the following section), engaging in weight-bearing exercise, avoiding smoking, and consuming alcohol not at all or in moderation.[42] Food sources of calcium include dairy milk, the richest source of calcium. Other sources include calcium-fortified plant milks and juices, canned salmon with bones, almonds, dark green leafy vegetables, and tofu made with calcium sulfate.

Nutrition professionals should be aware that the UL for calcium for both males and females ages 51+ years is 2,000 mg/day. Older adults who take dietary supplements and regularly consume fortified foods in addition to consuming calcium-rich foods may easily exceed this level. Excessive calcium intake may be associated with increased risk of heart disease, prostate cancer, and kidney stones, though evidence is mixed and further research is needed.[41] The RDA for calcium for males ages 51+ is 1,000 mg/day. The RDA for females 51 to 70 years and >70 years is 1,200 mg/day.[41]

Vitamin D

Vitamin D is an important nutrient for bone health in older adults, and also appears to play a role in the function of the immune system. Adequate vitamin D is needed to promote the mineralization of bone, to prevent **osteomalacia**, or bone softening, in adults, and to enhance calcium absorption in the gut.[43]

Humans obtain the fat-soluble vitamin D from two sources: sun exposure, when sunlight triggers photosensitive cells in the skin to produce a vitamin D, and from diet including supplements and fortified foods.[43] Vitamin D obtained from the sun, food, or supplements is a precursor that must undergo conversion in the body to transform it into a biologically usable form. Older adults may be at risk for vitamin D deficiency as a result of lack of sun exposure if they do not often go outdoors. One study conducted in Switzerland found that 1,000 IU vitamin D was synthesized in 10 to 15 minutes of sun exposure in summer and spring with 22% of the skin uncovered.[44] Amounts of sun exposure needed vary by latitude and season throughout the globe, as well as by skin type. Persons with dark skin tones do not absorb as much vitamin D from the sun due to the skin pigment melatonin.[45]

No definitive cutoff levels for serum vitamin D deficiency have been established, but an expert committee of the National Institute of Medicine has suggested that risk of deficiency exists at levels <30 nmol/L, and that vitamin D status is adequate for most people at levels >50 nmol/L.[43] Guidelines differ at this time among professional organizations and countries.

Only a small number of foods are natural sources of vitamin D. In the United States, fortified dairy and plant milks are the richest source. Salmon, tuna, and mackerel, egg yolks, and some mushrooms also provide varying amounts.[43] The RDA for vitamin D for older adult males and females ages 51 to 70 years is 15 mcg, or 600 IU, per day. The RDA for vitamin D for older adult males and females ages 70+ is 20 mcg, or 800 IU, per day. As a note, 1 IU = 0.025 mcg; therefore, 15 mcg/0.025 = 600 IU.

Vitamin B_{12}

Vitamin B_{12} is crucial for the generation of red blood cells and for normal neurologic function.[46] It is a water-soluble vitamin that is found in nature only in animal foods. Some plant-based foods such as cereals are fortified with vitamin B_{12}, and fortified nutritional yeast is a source of vitamin B_{12} for those who follow vegetarian or vegan meal plans.[47] Food sources of vitamin B_{12} include meats, liver, poultry, fish, dairy, eggs, and fortified cereals/other fortified foods.[48]

Crucial steps to absorb vitamin B_{12} occur in the stomach, where acid breaks down the nutrient so it can be digested. The ability of older adults to absorb vitamin B_{12} declines naturally with age as production of stomach acid declines, and some medications can also negatively impact the nutrient's absorption. Conditions affecting the stomach's ability to absorb nutrients may precipitate a vitamin B_{12} deficiency. *Pernicious anemia* is an autoimmune condition that reduces vitamin B_{12} absorption by attacking the stomach cells needed to absorb the vitamin.[48] Older adults may consume inadequate amounts of vitamin B_{12} foods due to cost, poor chewing and/or dental status, or decreased functional ability impacting the ability to prepare one's own meals.

Ongoing, severe vitamin B_{12} deficiency—from whatever cause—is associated with irreversible neurologic dysfunction in older adults, including symptoms that impair the ability to ambulate.[46] The treatment for most deficiencies is medically supervised supplementation with the vitamin, often by intramuscular injection to bypass the stomach. After adequate vitamin B_{12} status is restored, high-dose oral supplementation usually maintains a satisfactory level of nutriture.[48] Adequate consumption of protein foods can enhance dietary intake of vitamin B_{12}.[27] Assessment of vitamin B_{12} status should be included in regular medical encounters with older adults, and supplementation should be prescribed as needed. The RDA for vitamin B_{12} for males 51 to 70 years and >70 years is 2.4 mcg/day for both age groups. For females in the same age groups, the RDA is also 2.4 mcg/day.[27]

Physical Activity for Older Adults

Physical activity is an essential lifestyle intervention to help older adults delay and ameliorate age-related physical decline to the greatest extent possible. Virtually every body system is positively impacted by regular physical activity. By engaging in exercise to preserve bone health, muscle mass, and strength, older adults have a better opportunity to maintain functional ability and independence. The benefits of appropriate physical activity are substantial, and can greatly improve quality of life as one ages. As one famous older adult, the actor Dick Van Dyke, has said, "Keep moving!"[49]

Older adults should consult with their medical provider regarding participation in physical activity. The CDC recommends that older adults ages 65+ years engage in moderate-intensity exercise (an example is brisk walking) at least 150 minutes per week, or 75 minutes per week of vigorous exercise such as hiking or jogging.[50] Engaging in strength training to promote muscle strength is recommended at least 2 days each week, and activities to improve balance are recommended as well.[50] For those who have health conditions impeding the ability to engage in exercise, consultation with a medical provider is imperative in regard to specific recommendations, adaptations, and further interventions such as physical therapy.

SOCIAL DETERMINANTS OF HEALTH FOR OLDER ADULTS

Social determinants of health, according to the CDC, are "the nonmedical factors that influence health outcomes."[51] Evidence indicates that of the major determinants of health—social, environmental, behavioral, and clinical—social determinants account for anywhere from 30% to 60% of health outcomes.[52–54] Public health professionals work at the community and policy levels to improve social determinants of health that impact the nutrition status of older adults. Table 8.11 provides a list of factors considered by WHO to be social determinants of health, along with examples of the determinants' nutritional implications for the older adult life stage.[55,56]

PUBLIC HEALTH AND NUTRITION ISSUES AMONG OLDER ADULTS

This portion of the chapter returns full circle to the WHO DHAR, presented at the beginning of the chapter. Three determinants of healthy aging were described, and their brief definitions are reviewed here:

1. Functional ability: The ability for a person to do what they want to do
2. Intrinsic capacity: The personal capacities and resources a person can draw on during the aging process, including physical abilities, the senses including vision and hearing, energy level, and psychological functioning including mental health
3. Environments: The places where people live, including their homes, communities, and societies

Table 8.11. Social Determinants of Health and Related Nutrition Implications for the Older Adult

Social Determinant of Health	Nutrition Implications: Older Adult Life Cycle Stage
Income and social protection	Adequate income, whether through employment or social protections, is essential to acquire sufficient nutritious food to promote health and quality of life.
Education	Evidence indicates that higher education levels, in general, are associated with higher incomes and better health outcomes over the life span; there are likely associations with improved nutrient intake.[53,55]
Unemployment and job insecurity	Steady/secure employment and associated benefits over the life span imply better nutrient intake and better health outcomes in older adulthood, and the opposite is implied as well.
Working life conditions	Over the life span, safe working conditions with appropriate worker protections imply reduced risk of chronic disease and subsequent poor nutrient intake in older adulthood.
Food insecurity	Inability to access adequate nutritious food is associated with poor health outcomes in older adults. In the United States, 7.1%, or 5.5 million, older adults were estimated to be food insecure in 2021.[56]
Housing, basic amenities, and the environment	A lack of housing or substandard housing, lack of access to appropriate food preparation and storage equipment, and unsafe neighborhoods may impede older adults' ability to safely acquire, store, prepare, and consume food needed to maintain health.
Early childhood development	According to the life course theory, the health of older adults is affected by nutritional intake and behaviors during each of the previous life cycle phases.
Social inclusion and nondiscrimination	Racism and discrimination underlie many nutritional inequities and disparities among older adults.
Structural conflict	Wars and political conflicts in the areas/regions where older adults live can have a profound negative impact on the ability to obtain and consume adequate food.
Access to affordable health services of decent quality	Access to healthcare and medical nutrition therapy services aids older adults in prevention and management of chronic disease and of conditions that impair food intake.

Source: Adapted from World Health Organization. Social determinants of health. Health Topics. Accessed June 18, 2023. https://www.who.int/health-topics/social-determinants-of-health#tab=tab_1

Public health issues among older adults are described here within the WHO DHAR threefold framework, and they are aligned with a public health and nutrition initiative and programming examples. The examples are organized according to the levels of the social-ecological model: individual, relationship, community, and society.

Initiative 1: Functional Ability and Public Health Nutrition

Older adults value being able to live independently, care for themselves adequately, and participate in life fully. Good nutrition is a key component to maintaining the functional ability needed to live with autonomy and independence. Public health nutrition professionals can help support the maintenance of functional ability in older adults by focusing on an initiative such as the following:

Initiative: Work at all levels of the social-ecological model (individual, relationship, community, society) *to promote access to adequate, nutritious food for all, including older adults*, to enhance the ability to live and participate successfully in the community throughout the entire life span.

- Individual level:
  - Develop mobile food pantries that serve areas where older adults live, and are designed to increase individuals' access to healthful foods although they may have difficulty traveling to a grocery store.
- Relationship level:
  - Provide opportunities for older adults to eat with others to develop friendships and relationships that engender social support that increases access to food, such as congregate meal settings, community and faith-based settings, and special events. Notably, a body of research indicates that older adults' dietary intake improves when eating with others rather than eating alone.
- Community:
  - Collaborate with healthcare providers throughout the community to deliver a "produce prescription" program for older adults with chronic disease.
- Society:
  - Work at the governmental and policy levels to develop food access–friendly initiatives to improve social and economic conditions that promote health and good nutrition in communities for all life stage populations, such as walkable neighborhoods with foot access to grocery stores and farmers markets, effective public safety measures, community gardens, Americans with Disabilities Act–compliant facilities for exercise, safe and attractive public parks, and the like.

Initiative 2: Intrinsic Capacity and Public Health Nutrition

Good nutrition supports, enhances, and fuels older adults' intrinsic capacities—that is, the personal physical, mental, and emotional resources they bring to the aging process. Public health nutrition professionals can help encourage the intrinsic capacities of older adults by focusing on an initiative such as the following:

Initiative: Work at all levels of the social-ecological model (individual, relationship, community, society) *to utilize the power of nutrition to preserve, fully utilize, and enhance the intrinsic capacities of older adults* to improve their ability to fully participate in the community and enjoy the highest possible quality of life.

- Individual level:
  - Collaborate with appropriate professionals as needed to work with older adults to assess needs and implement adjustments and home modifications to promote *aging-in-place* and allow them to maximize independence in meal preparation.

- Relationship level:
  - Implement group cooking skills classes to enhance older adults' capacity to prepare their own meals while allowing valuable opportunities for socialization and friendship building.
- Community:
  - Work within the community to ensure the access and availability of mental health services to older adults. Poor mental health is often associated with reduced capacity to take part in normal life activities and with nutrition problems such as losing interest in eating or excessive emotional eating that can lead to **malnutrition** or exacerbate health problems.
- Society:
  - Work at the governmental and policy levels to ensure the availability and access of appropriate maintaining/rehabilitating resources to all older adults to promote overall quality of life including the ability to nourish oneself. Access to rehabilitative medical care is paramount, including ophthalmology and audiology services, medical care to preserve and/or restore mobility, physical and occupational therapy, and mental healthcare.

Initiative 3: Environments and Public Health Nutrition

The environments in which we live have a tremendous influence on whether or not older adults are able to engage in the process of healthy aging. Public health nutrition professionals should be active in participating in broad initiatives designed to impact the overall systems that affect older adults' health and quality of life in their communities.

Initiative: Work at all levels of the social-ecological model (individual, relationship, community, society) to bring systemwide change to community environments *to allow all older adults the opportunity to engage in a healthy aging process* to the extent possible.

- Individual level:
  - Work at the policy level to ensure that every individual older adult in a community has the opportunity for access to comprehensive information on the nutrition environment and nutrition resources within the community; this could include an app prepared by the local health department, a social media campaign, public service announcements, and/or information provided at community or faith-based organizations, food resource centers such as food pantries, and others.
- Relationship level:
  - Provide opportunities for older adults to gather with friends to discuss nutrition issues in the community; gather their input and suggestions for action items to improve the nutrition environment. These discussions may take place at senior centers or other community venues in congregate meal settings. It is not unknown for such a group to decide to implement an initiative(s) themselves.
- Community:
  - Initiate or participate in a community health assessment through your local health department, and ensure that nutrition issues and older adults are included as a focus along with other health topics and populations. Invite older adults to participate in the assessment as volunteer staff if appropriate. Use assessment results to prioritize and plan for public health nutrition interventions and nutrition environment shifts likely to be helpful to the community.

- Society:
    - Work at the governmental and policy levels to implement change that reduces barriers to nutrition security for all people, including older adults.

MALNUTRITION IN OLDER ADULTS: A PUBLIC HEALTH AND NUTRITION ISSUE

Malnutrition is common in older adults around the world, and is a topic of great importance to public health nutrition professionals. WHO defines **malnutrition** as either inadequate or excessive intake of nutrients, imbalance of nutrients consumed (e.g., very high consumption of carbohydrates but little intake of protein), or physiologic inability to utilize nutrients consumed.[57] Inadequate nutrient intake results in undernutrition, while excessive nutrient intake results in overnutrition. The Administration for Community Living (ACL) of the DHHS has estimated the prevalence of malnutrition in U.S. older adults—both under- and overnutrition—to be around 50%.[58] Malnutrition and its precursors are key targets for screening, programming, and advocacy and policy development by public health nutrition professionals in order to promote the highest quality of life for older adult populations in the United States and globally.

In older adults, undernutrition is associated with overall decline as evidenced by inappropriate weight loss, sarcopenia, and resultant **frailty**. Undernutrition is also related to immune dysfunction, greater numbers of infections, longer hospital stays, increased risk of falls, and higher morbidity and mortality rates.[59] One of the early signs of undernutrition is significant weight loss, defined by the Centers for Medicare and Medicaid Services for long-term care residents as a weight loss of 5% or more of usual weight within 1 month, or 10% or more within 6 months in a person not following a weight loss plan prescribed by a physician.[60] Older adults exhibiting signs of malnutrition should be seen promptly by a physician for a thorough evaluation, and referred to an RDN for medical nutrition therapy if indicated.

Public health professionals play a role in advocacy for population health measures designed to impact societal conditions and risk factors that may lead to malnutrition and premature and/or accelerated physical decline in older adults. Areas for advocacy and policy intervention include but are not limited to:

- *Eating alone/loneliness*: While further research is needed to determine causality, evidence indicates that older adults' food intake is negatively impacted by eating alone, and appears to improve when eating with others.[61–63] For many, food has positive associations with emotions and life events. These associations can include comfort, memories of family and friends, reminders of happy social events, and even aspects of one's spirituality. There is some evidence that congregate meal programs for older adults are associated with improved functional ability, socialization, and nutrient intake—all of which may promote improved mental and physical health and higher quality of life.[64]

  The social and emotional aspects of eating are important considerations when planning nutrition interventions for older adults. Measures designed to strengthen and encourage access to congregate and home-delivered meal programs, to promote participation in social functions that include eating, and to enhance older adults' ability to participate in community life and socialization are preventive measures that reduce risk for malnutrition. Public health and public health nutrition professionals will do well to align the positive socialization aspects of food and meals with population nutrition interventions for older adults whenever appropriate.

- *Food insecurity:* According to Feeding America, in the United States in 2021 about 7.1%, or 5.5 million persons, ages 60 and over were food insecure.[56] This is about one in 14 older adults. Food insecurity is linked to many poor outcomes for older adults, including health problems, increased disability, chronic disease, and malnutrition.[56]

  Public health nutrition professionals can make a difference by working to increase awareness of and access to federal nutrition programs such as the Supplemental Nutrition Assistance Program (SNAP),[65] the Senior Farmers Market Nutrition Program,[66] Older Americans Act Nutrition Programs such as congregate and home-delivered meals,[67] and the Commodity Supplemental Foods Program.[68] Private organizations such as local food pantries and food banks can help to fill nutrition gaps. Advocacy for healthful food for all, including older adults, is an important function of public health nutrition professionals.

- *Oral health:* While further research is needed to determine causality, it appears evident that there is a relationship between malnutrition and oral health.[69] Conditions that result in difficult or painful eating, such as chewing problems; missing, decaying, and/or broken teeth; mouth and/or tongue sores; gum disease; oral cancers; poorly fitting and/or painful dentures; and **xerostomia**, or dry mouth, can make adequate nutritional intake difficult to achieve and overt malnutrition more likely. Higher risk of oral health problems is associated with lower income, lack of dental insurance, being homebound or living in a care facility, being a member of a racial or ethnic minority, and/or having chronic disease(s).[70] Older adults are less likely than younger adults to have dental insurance, as dental benefits are often lost at retirement and government insurance programs such as Medicare and Medicaid do not provide dental benefits.[70] The cost of dental care puts it out of reach for many seniors. Because of the strong connections between oral health, overall health, and quality of life, public health professionals should provide educational interventions for older adults on maintaining oral health, as well as advocating for policies which improve access to dental services for older adults.

- *Polypharmacy:* Literally meaning "many medications," **polypharmacy** is common among older adults who consume a variety of prescribed and unprescribed pharmaceuticals on a daily basis. A recent systematic review found a statistically significant association between polypharmacy and malnutrition in older adults.[71] While there is no standard definition of polypharmacy, many experts consider it to be the taking of at least five prescribed drugs per day.[72]

  Many commonly used drugs have possible nutrition-related side effects that can discourage eating, including but not limited to nausea, diarrhea, stomach discomfort, xerostomia, taste changes such as metallic tastes or "off" tastes, and decreased appetite. Helpful strategies include advocacy for policies to strengthen senior adults' access to regular medical care that includes evaluation of all medications taken in order to determine the regimen least likely to interfere with nutritional intake, as well as associated medical nutrition therapy. General wellness initiatives to prevent and manage chronic disease among older adults, and thus decrease the overall need for prescription medications, will be helpful as well.

OLDER AMERICANS ACT NUTRITION PROGRAMS FOR OLDER ADULTS

The **Older Americans Act** (OAA) became law in the United States in 1965 as the result of a perceived need to improve resources and social services available to older adults.[73] The OAA established grants to states to provide services, conduct research, and train personnel with a focus on aging. The Administration on Aging was established by the OAA, housed within what was then the Department of Health, Education, and Welfare (now the DHHS), and was charged with administering the state grant programs.[73] In 1972, Title VII was established within the OAA for the purpose of funding nutrition programs for older adults.[73] Over the years, the older adult nutrition programs have been consolidated with several other programs within Title III. The OAA, through the ACL's Administration on Aging, provides grants to state and community programs on aging to fund the nutrition programs. Title VI funds older adult nutrition programs for Alaskan Natives, Native Hawaiians, and American Indians.[67] In addition to federal grant funding, OAA programs may receive support from a variety of other entities including state and local governments, direct payment from participants, charitable foundations, volunteer assistance, and the like.[74]

The overarching purpose of the OAA older adult nutrition programs is to provide crucial nutrition services that support older adults' ability to live independently in their communities.

Meals provided by the OAA are in alignment with the DGAs, and provide one third of the daily nutrients recommended by the DRIs. These programs are widely available in a variety of settings frequented by seniors, such as senior centers, faith-based organizations, and healthcare facilities such as hospital dining rooms. The home-delivered nutrition program is available to homebound older adults. Public health professionals should be familiar with OAA nutrition program resources in their areas, as they are an important resource for supporting older adults' well-being. There are two major OAA nutrition programs, described here:

The Congregate Nutrition Program

The **Congregate Nutrition Program** provides opportunities for older adults to enjoy socializing over a nutritious meal. Congregate meal participation can also be a jumping-off place for involvement in many other activities that promote healthy aging, since so many programs take place in community-based settings such as senior centers that offer comprehensive older adult services. Participants can be made aware of available resources and assistance in accessing them. Congregate meal participants may have opportunities to engage in volunteer activities that draw on their lifetime of experience and skills. They may be able to access a wide variety of educational programs, exercise classes, health screenings, and group travel opportunities. Thus, the benefits of congregate meal programs include not only the health benefits of good nutrition but also the health benefits of new friendship connections and the resulting social support.

Eligibility for OAA nutrition programs is determined by the states and localities administering the programs. Age is the only requirement specified by federal law. Older Americans aged 60 and older, and their spouses of any age are eligible to participate in congregate meals. In addition, persons who have disabilities and live with eligible older adults in home settings, and in group settings in many cases, are eligible by law.[74] No income test is applied to program eligibility; however, program sites are prioritized in areas of greatest need in order to promote optimal use of resources and provision of assistance to the most vulnerable older adult populations.[75] Older adult populations of particular concern include those who are low income, of minority status, living in rural areas, of lower English proficiency, and at high risk for needing institutional care.[74]

The Home-Delivered Nutrition Program

Congregate meals are recommended for older adults who are able to participate in order to reap the benefits of social interaction. Older adults who are unable to travel to congregate meal programs for health and/or mobility reasons are eligible to participate in the OAA **home-delivered meals program**. Eligibility requirements are the same as for participation in congregate meals, and home-delivered meals adhere to the same nutritional standards as congregate meals. Meal delivery staff routinely engage in socialization with participants, and are encouraged to report any issues or concerns they may note during encounters.[67] Participants often look forward to their daily encounters with meal delivery staff.

WHAT WORKS: OAA NUTRITION PROGRAMS

The OAA nutrition programs for older adults are described in preceding sections of this chapter. The specific goals of the programs include (1) reducing hunger and food insecurity among older adults; (2) encouraging social interactions; (3) promoting good health outcomes and overall wellness; and (4) delaying negative health conditions.[67] Currently, about 5,000 U.S. providers serve around 900,000 nutritious meals per day to older adults.[67]

Data from the *2021 National Survey of OAA Participants*, conducted by the Administration on Community Living, indicates a number of positive outcomes from the OAA nutrition programs, including achievement of program objectives. Of those participating in the survey, 80% of congregate meal participants and 89% of home-delivered meal participants reported that the OAA meal programs helped them to continue living independently, 74% of congregate meals participants stated that program participation resulted in health improvements, and 70% of congregate and 76% of home-delivered participants said that they ate more healthfully because of the program. In addition, 91% of congregate and 85% of home-delivered meal participants rated their meals as good to excellent, indicating a high degree of satisfaction with the meals provided.[74] Effective use of resources and targeting of services toward more vulnerable older adults is indicated by survey results demonstrating that 57% of participants in both congregate and home-delivered programs are 75 years of age or older, and more than 50% of both groups live alone.[74]

SUMMARY

The older adult population is growing rapidly both in the United States and globally. The implications of *global population aging* for healthcare systems and society as a whole are enormous; some have called this demographic shift the single most important medical challenge the world faces.[4] The older adult life cycle phase is generally considered to extend from the age of 65 years until death. The vast majority of older adults in the United States are community-living, that is, they reside, work or are retired, and care for themselves within their communities rather than living in care facilities. *Senescence,* or aging, is a normal biological process that takes place over a lifetime and results in the gradual loss of physiologic capabilities, including healing and recovery processes, that ultimately leads to death.[10]

Public health and public health nutrition practitioners should not assume that decline and disability are a normal part of aging, but should actively intervene to improve nutrition-related functional ability and quality of life in older adult populations. The ideal for healthy aging is to enjoy good health until shortly before death, with a period of decline lasting a few months, weeks, or days rather than years. While genetics may prevent some from achieving this goal, healthful habits can be a powerful support to extend the health span. Healthy aging can be the culmination of a long and healthy life.

KEY CHAPTER CONCEPTS

1. The older adult population is growing rapidly in the United States and globally.
2. WHO defines healthy aging as "the process of developing and maintaining the functional ability that enables well-being in older age." Thus, the concept of healthy aging is focused on being able to do what one wants to do. The **WHO** *Decade of Healthy Ageing Report* (DHAR) provides the framework to support WHO's definition.
3. *The* DHAR describes three determinants of healthy aging: functional ability, intrinsic capacity, and environment.
4. The physiologic changes of aging affect every body system, several with direct impacts on nutritional intake and status.
5. Seven nutrition areas of concern are presented in the chapter and are related to intake quality, functional ability, weight status, protein consumption, food access and preparation, socialization and mental health, and relationship with food.
6. The HEI, DGAs, DRIs, and MyPlate are official nutrition guidance tools for older adults.
7. Dietary patterns of older adults indicate low intakes of fruits, vegetables, whole grains, and protein, and excess intakes of added sugars, sodium, and saturated fat.
8. Four micronutrients of public health concern for older adults are iron, calcium, vitamin D, and vitamin B_{12}.
9. Physical activity is an essential lifestyle intervention to help older adults delay and ameliorate age-related physical decline.
10. Many public health nutrition issues among older adults fall within the WHO DHAR threefold framework of functional ability, intrinsic capacity, and environments.
11. Malnutrition is a major public health nutrition issue highlighted in the chapter and interrelated to eating alone/loneliness, food insecurity, oral health, and polypharmacy.
12. Many public health nutrition programs for older adults, including the congregate meals program and home-delivered meals program, fall under the OAA, which became law in 1965. The overarching purpose of the OAA older adult nutrition programs is to provide crucial nutrition services that support older adults' ability to live independently in their communities.

CASE STUDY AND QUESTIONS

JP is a 78-year-old man who is retired and has lived in a small town in the United States all his life. He lost his beloved wife 2 years ago to a stroke. He lives in the small home they built in the 1960s. JP has three children and five grandchildren, all of whom live within 2 hours of his home. JP's family has been concerned about him living alone for the past 2 years, but they are especially concerned now about his recent weight loss. He is 6' tall and weighs 150 lbs. He has lost about 25 lbs since his wife died. He is still independent for all activities of daily living. He is determined to remain in his own home. When his wife was alive, they gardened every year and put up many fresh vegetables; however, JP has not gardened since her death. He used to enjoy several hobbies, but now spends much of his time watching television. Once in a while he takes his boat out on a nearby river to fish alone. He does not socialize much.

JP has enjoyed a fairly healthy life until recently. He has arthritis and frequently complains of constipation. He quit smoking in 1975 and does not consume alcohol. He has maintained his mental status fairly well, but is slowly becoming more forgetful. The only medication he has taken for an extended period of time is an antacid.

JP's typical food intake is the following: black coffee in the morning with a sausage and egg biscuit, or sometimes biscuits and gravy that he gets at a local fast-food restaurant. His noon meal is usually a can of soup and perhaps a cheese sandwich. He keeps bananas on hand and usually has one at lunch. He consumes mostly soft drinks at home, rather than water. For his evening meal he may fry himself some bologna and potatoes, but that is the extent of his cooking. His wife always did the meal preparation and he is just not bothered with it much himself. He does keep some frozen dinners on hand that he eats occasionally. On the weekends, his children invite him over for dinner, but he doesn't always feel like going.

1. Do you feel JP is living out the definition of healthy aging? Why or why not?
2. Which determinant of healthy aging do you feel is having the greatest impact on JP: functional ability, intrinsic capacity, or environment? Provide a rationale for your answer.
3. What evidence in this case supports physiologic changes of aging based on the information provided in this chapter (i.e., which body systems are affected and how)?
4. Review JP's dietary intake information. Are there areas of inadequacy that match the information provided in this chapter? Consider food groups, macronutrients, and micronutrients in your answer.
5. Does JP have any risk factors for malnutrition? Please explain.
6. What social determinants of health are affecting JP?
7. Identify at least one public health nutrition program that may be helpful to JP and consider how you might go about referring him to this resource.

DISCUSSION QUESTIONS

1. Consider the growth in the aging population. How will this impact your career as a public health professional?
2. What components do you think should be addressed in a definition of healthy aging?
3. Explore how the three determinants of healthy aging—functional ability, intrinsic capacity, and environment—relate to nutrition for older adults.
4. Select physiologic changes of aging for three body systems from Table 8.1 that you think will most impact the nutritional status of older adults.

5. Select one of the official nutrition guidance tools provided in this chapter and explore how you could use it to work with an older adult to improve dietary intake.
6. Describe the common nutritional concerns among older adults, including macronutrients and micronutrients.
7. Summarize the physical activity recommendations for older adults.
8. Consider malnutrition as a public health nutrition issue that affects older adults. Describe the social determinants of health that impact this issue, which level of the WHO DHAR this issue applies to, and one initiative or current public health nutrition program that is aimed at improving this issue.
9. Describe the two older adult nutrition programs that are part of the OAA. What is the key difference between these programs? In what ways have these programs been effective for older adults?

SUGGESTED LEARNING ACTIVITIES

1. Interview an older adult in your life about their typical dietary intake. Comment on your overall impression of their diet. What factors are contributing to nutritional status (good or bad)? This can include specific foods, but also psychological, physiologic, and social determinants. Are any food groups lacking? If so, what nutrients are present in these groups that are common problems for the aging population? What suggestions would you make for improving the diet? Could this individual benefit from any of the public health nutrition programs presented in the chapter?
2. Create a nutrition education tool or lesson plan outline for older adults that could be presented at your local senior center. What topics would you be sure to include based on the information in this chapter?
3. Spend some time volunteering with a community agency that serves older adults. This could be a senior center, assisted living or nursing home, adult day care, congregate meals center, or even a church event. What can you observe that brings the chapter concepts to life? These may be related to the physiologic changes of aging, food intake, health/nutrition concerns or questions, or public health nutrition issues.
4. Research one of the public health nutrition programs for older adults in greater depth (e.g., Meals on Wheels, the Senior Farmers Market Program, or the Child and Adult Care Food Program). How do the services offered by the program align with the specific targets for improving older adult nutrition discussed in this chapter?

RESOURCES FOR FURTHER LEARNING

- U.S. Department of Agriculture, Nutrition Programs for Seniors: www.nutrition.gov/topics/food-security-and-access/food-assistance-programs/nutrition-programs-seniors
    - Provides a comprehensive list of food and nutrition programs that focus on the needs of older adults, ages 60 and over
- U.S. Department of Agriculture, Aging resources: www.fns.usda.gov/assistance-seniors
    - Links to resources for older adults such as caregiver information, Medicare enrollment, and Social Security resources
- National Institute on Aging: www.nia.nih.gov
    - Leads a broad scientific effort to understand the nature of aging and to extend the healthy, active years of life

- MyPlate for Older Adults: www.myplate.gov/life-stages/older-adults
  - Nutrition tips and resources for those ages 60 and over
- Academy of Nutrition and Dietetics, for Seniors: www.eatright.org/for-seniors
  - Information and resources to support healthy aging.
- Administration for Community Living, Nutrition and Aging Resource Center: https://acl.gov/senior-nutrition
  - The purpose of the Nutrition and Aging Resource Center is to build the capacity of senior nutrition programs funded by the OAA to provide high-quality, person-centered services, and to assist the ACL and stakeholders to identify current and emerging issues and opportunities to enhance program sustainability and resiliency.
- Dietary Guidelines for Americans: www.dietaryguidelines.gov
  - Chapter 6, Older Adults, provides information about healthy eating patterns, current intakes, and special considerations for older adults.
- World Health Organization, Aging: www.who.int/news-room/fact-sheets/detail/ageing-and-health
  - Fact sheets, databases, initiatives, and resources regarding older adults, including the *Decade of Healthy Ageing Report*
- Administration on Community Living, Find a Local Nutrition Site button: https://acl.gov/programs/health-wellness/nutrition-services
  - Provided by the Administration on Community Living, this button on the web page provides a gateway to locate older adult resources including local OAA nutrition programs.
- My Dietary Supplement and Medicine Record: https://ods.od.nih.gov/pubs/DietarySupplementandMedicineRecord.pdf
  - A printable form that can be used by an older adult to record all medications and dietary supplements regularly used; may be helpful for medical appointments

SPRINGER PUBLISHING CONNECT™ | **A robust set of instructor resources designed to supplement this text is located at http://connect.springerpub.com/content/book/978-0-8261-8623-2. Qualifying instructors may request access by emailing textbook@springerpub.com.**

REFERENCES

1. World Health Organization. *Decade of Healthy Ageing: Baseline Report*. World Health Organization; 2020.
2. Brivio P, Paladini MS, Racagni G, Riva MA, Calabrese F, Molteni R. From healthy aging to frailty: in search of the underlying mechanisms. *Curr Med Chem*. 2019;26(20):3685–3701. https://doi.org/10.2174/0929867326666190717152739
3. The Administration on Aging. *2020 Profile of Older Americans*. Administration for Community Living; 2021.
4. Rudnicka E, Napierała P, Podfigurna A, Męczekalski B, Smolarczyk R, Grymowicz M. The World Health Organization (WHO) approach to healthy ageing. *Maturitas*. 2020;139:6–11. https://doi.org/10.1016/j.maturitas.2020.05.018
5. Michel J-P, Sadana R. "Healthy aging" concepts and measures. *J Am Med Dir Assoc*. 2017;18(6):460–464. https://doi.org/10.1016/j.jamda.2017.03.008
6. Kusumastuti S, Derks MG, Tellier S, et al. Successful ageing: a study of the literature using citation network analysis. *Maturitas*. 2016;93:4–12. https://doi.org/10.1016/j.maturitas.2016.04.010
7. Centers for Disease Control and Prevention. Dementia and mental health: Alzheimer disease. FastStats. Accessed June 20, 2023. https://www.cdc.gov/nchs/fastats/alzheimers.htm
8. Perls T. Centenarian statistics. New England Centenarian Study. Boston University. Updated January 1, 2023. https://www.bumc.bu.edu/centenarian/statistics

9. Aronson L. An anti-ageism fail. *Louise Aronson Blog*. February 17, 2020. https://louisearonson.com/2253-2/
10. Flint B, Tadi P. Physiology, aging. In: *StatPearls*. StatPearls Publishing; 2023. https://www.ncbi.nlm.nih.gov/books/NBK556106
11. World Health Organization. Fact sheet: ageing and health. October 1, 2022. https://www.who.int/news-room/fact-sheets/detail/ageing-and-health
12. Arias E, Xu J. United States life tables, 2018. *Natl Vital Stat Rep*. 2020;69(12):1–45.
13. Harvard T.H. Chan School of Public Health. What's Behind 'Shocking' U.S. Life Expectancy Decline—and What To Do About It. Harvard University; 2023. https://www.hsph.harvard.edu/news/hsph-in-the-news/whats-behind-shocking-u-s-life-expectancy-decline-and-what-to-do-about-it
14. National Institute on Aging. Heart health and aging. National Institutes of Health. https://www.nia.nih.gov/health/heart-health-and-aging
15. American Lung Association. Your aging lungs. *Each Breath Blog*. April 24, 2018. https://www.lung.org/blog/your-aging-lungs
16. Harvard Medical School. How Memory and Thinking Ability Change with Age. Harvard Health Publishing. August 30, 2017. https://www.health.harvard.edu/mind-and-mood/how-memory-and-thinking-ability-change-with-age
17. Medline Plus. Aging changes in the nervous system. National Library of Medicine. July 21, 2022. https://medlineplus.gov/ency/article/004023.htm
18. Dominguez LJ, Veronese N, Baiamonte E, et al. Healthy aging and dietary patterns. *Nutrients*. 2022;14(4):889. https://doi.org/10.3390/nu14040889
19. Roberts S, Colombier P, Sowman A, et al. Ageing in the musculoskeletal system. *Acta Orthop*. 2016;87(supp 363):15–25. https://doi.org/10.1080/17453674.2016.1244750
20. Fuller-Thomson E, Nowaczynski A, MacNeil A. The association between hearing impairment, vision impairment, dual sensory impairment, and serious cognitive impairment: findings from a population-based study of 5.4 million older adults. *J Alzheimers Dis Rep*. 2022;6(1):211–222. https://doi.org/10.3233/ADR-220005
21. National Eye Institute. Cataract tables. Updated February 7, 2020. https://www.nei.nih.gov/learn-about-eye-health/eye-health-data-and-statistics/cataract-data-and-statistics/cataract-tables
22. Haynes L. Aging of the immune system: research challenges to enhance the health span of older adults. *Front Aging*. 2020;1:602108. https://doi.org/10.3389/fragi.2020.602108
23. Hardy CC. The aged lower urinary tract: deficits in neural control mechanisms. *Front Aging*. 2021;2:791833. https://doi.org/10.3389/fragi.2021.791833
24. U.S. Department of Agriculture Food and Nutrition Service. Healthy eating index (HEI). Updated July 14, 2023. https://www.fns.usda.gov/healthy-eating-index-hei
25. National Cancer Institute, Division of Cancer Control and Population Sciences. Overview & background of the healthy eating index. Updated July 28, 2023. https://epi.grants.cancer.gov/hei
26. Centers for Disease Control and Prevention. What we eat in America, DHHS-USDA dietary survey integration. National Health and Nutrition Examination Survey. Accessed June 13, 2023. https://www.cdc.gov/nchs/nhanes/wweia.htm
27. U.S. Department of Agriculture, U.S. Department of Health and Human Services. *Dietary Guidelines for Americans 2020–2025*, 9th ed. U.S. Department of Health and Human Services; 2020. https://www.dietaryguidelines.gov
28. U.S. Department of Agriculture, U.S. Department of Health and Human Services. Dietary Guidelines for Americans: history of the Dietary Guidelines. https://www.dietaryguidelines.gov/about-dietary-guidelines/history-dietary-guidelines
29. U.S. Department of Agriculture. Make every bite count with the Dietary Guidelines for Americans. December 2020. https://www.dietaryguidelines.gov/sites/default/files/2020-12/DGA_2020-2025_Infographic_MakeEveryBiteCount.pdf
30. U.S. Department of Agriculture, U.S. Department of Health and Human Services. Top 10 things you need to know about the *Dietary Guidelines for Americans, 2020–2025*. https://www.dietaryguidelines.gov/resources/2020-2025-dietary-guidelines-online-materials/top-10-things-you-need-know
31. Office of Disease Prevention and Health Promotion. Dietary reference intakes. U.S. Department of Health and Human Services. Updated January 18, 2023. https://health.gov/our-work/nutrition-physical-activity/dietary-guidelines/dietary-reference-intakes
32. Office of Disease Prevention and Health Promotion. Dietary Reference intakes development. U.S. Department of Health and Human Services. Updated January 18, 2023. https://health.gov/our

-work/nutrition-physical-activity/dietary-guidelines/dietary-reference-intakes/dietary-reference-intakes-development
33. National Academies of Sciences, Engineering, and Medicine. Sodium and potassium dietary reference intake values updated in new report; introduces new category for sodium based on chronic disease risk reduction. March 5, 2019. https://www.nationalacademies.org/news/2019/03/sodium-and-potassium-dietary-reference-intake-values-updated-in-new-report
34. U.S. Department of Agriculture. USDA's MyPlate celebrates its first anniversary. Press release. May 30, 2012. https://www.usda.gov/media/press-releases/2012/05/30/usdas-myplate-celebrates-its-first-anniversary
35. U.S. Department of Agriculture Food and Nutrition Service. Center for Nutrition Policy and Promotion (CNPP). Accessed June 13, 2023. https://www.fns.usda.gov/cnpp
36. U.S. Department of Agriculture. MyPlate: older adults. Accessed June 13, 2023. https://www.myplate.gov/life-stages/older-adults
37. Baum JI, Kim IY, Wolfe RR. Protein consumption and the elderly: what is the optimal level of intake? *Nutrients*. 2016;8(6):359. https://doi.org/10.3390/nu8060359
38. Stauder R, Thein SL. Anemia in the elderly: clinical implications and new therapeutic concepts. *Haematologica*. 2014;99(7):1127–1130. https://doi.org/10.3324/haematol.2014.109967
39. Seitz AE, Chen TC, Lukacs SL. QuickStats: prevalence of anemia among adults aged ≥65 years, by sex and age group—National Health and Nutrition Examination Survey, 2013–2016. *MMWR Morb Mortal Wkly Rep*. 2018;67(42):1198. https://doi.org/10.15585/mmwr.mm6742a8
40. Beto JA. The role of calcium in human aging. *Clin Nutr Res*. 2015;4(1):1–8. https://doi.org/10.7762/cnr.2015.4.1.1
41. National Institutes of Health, Office of Dietary Supplements. Calcium: fact sheet for health professionals. Updated October 6, 2022. https://ods.od.nih.gov/factsheets/Calcium-HealthProfessional
42. Centers for Disease Control and Prevention. Genomics & precision health: does osteoporosis run in your family? U.S. Department of Health and Human Services. Accessed June 14, 2023. https://www.cdc.gov/genomics/disease/osteoporosis.htm
43. National Institutes of Health, Office of Dietary Supplements. Vitamin D: fact sheet for health professionals. Updated August 12, 2022. https://ods.od.nih.gov/factsheets/VitaminD-HealthProfessional
44. Religi A, Backes C, Chatelan A, et al. Estimation of exposure durations for vitamin D production and sunburn risk in Switzerland. *J Expo Sci Environ Epidemiol*. 2019;29(6):742–752. https://doi.org/10.1038/s41370-019-0137-2
45. Guo J, Lovegrove JA, Givens DI. A narrative review of the role of foods as dietary sources of vitamin D of ethnic minority populations with darker skin: the underestimated challenge. *Nutrients*. 2019;11(1):81. https://doi.org/10.3390/nu11010081
46. Stover PJ. Vitamin B12 and older adults. *Curr Opin Clin Nutr Metab Care*. 2010;13(1):24–27. https://doi.org/10.1097/MCO.0b013e328333d157
47. Obeid R, Heil SG, Verhoeven MMA, van den Heuvel E, de Groot L, Eussen S. Vitamin B12 intake from animal foods, biomarkers, and health aspects. *Front Nutr*. 2019;6:93. https://doi.org/10.3389/fnut.2019.00093
48. Cleveland Clinic. Pernicious anemia. Accessed June 14, 2023. https://my.clevelandclinic.org/health/diseases/22377-pernicious-anemia
49. Van Dyke D. *Keep Moving: And Other Tips and Truths About Aging*. Weinstein Books; 2015.
50. Centers for Disease Control and Prevention. How much physical activity do older adults need? U.S. Department of Health and Human Services. Accessed June 14, 2023. https://www.cdc.gov/physicalactivity/basics/older_adults/index.htm
51. Centers for Disease Control and Prevention. Social determinants of health at CDC. Accessed June15, 2023. https://www.cdc.gov/about/sdoh/index.html
52. Hood CM, Gennuso KP, Swain GR, Catlin BB. County health rankings: relationships between determinant factors and health outcomes. *Am J Prev Med*. 2016;50(2):129–135. https://doi.org/10.1016/j.amepre.2015.08.024
53. Perez FP, Perez CA, Chumbiauca MN. Insights into the social determinants of health in older adults. *J Biomed Sci Eng*. 2022;15(11):261–268. https://doi.org/10.4236/jbise.2022.1511023
54. World Health Organization. Social determinants of health. Health Topics. Accessed June 18, 2023. https://www.who.int/health-topics/social-determinants-of-health#tab=tab_1
55. Wolla SA, Sullivan J. *Education, Income, and Wealth*. Page One Economics; 2017.

56. Ziliak JP, Gundersen C. *The State of Senior Hunger in 2021*. Feeding America; 2023. https://www.feedingamerica.org/research/state-senior-hunger
57. World Health Organization. Malnutrition. Accessed June 19, 2023. https://www.who.int/health-topics/malnutrition#tab=tab_1
58. Greuling HK. Combatting senior malnutrition. Administration for Community Living. Updated May 7, 2020. https://acl.gov/news-and-events/acl-blog/combatting-senior-malnutrition
59. Norman K, Hass U, Pirlich M. Malnutrition in older adults-recent advances and remaining challenges. *Nutrients*. 2021;13(8):2764. https://doi.org/10.3390/nu13082764
60. Centers for Medicare & Medicaid Services. *MDS 3.0 Quality Measures User's Manual (v15.0)*. Centers for Medicare & Medicaid Services; 2022.
61. Björnwall A, Mattsson Sydner Y, Koochek A, Neuman N. Eating alone or together among community-living older people—a scoping review. *Int J Environ Res Public Health*. 2021;18(7):3495. https://doi.org/ 10.3390/ijerph18073495
62. Tkatch MT, Towers AJ, Keller HH, Wham CA. Nutrition risk prevalence and associated health and social risk factors in Māori and non-Māori: results from the New Zealand health, work and retirement study. *Australas J Ageing*. 2022;41(1):59–69. https://doi.org/10.1111/ajag.12952
63. Hata T, Seino S, Yokoyama Y, et al. Interaction of eating status and dietary variety on incident functional disability among older Japanese adults. *J Nutr Health Aging*. 2022;26(7):698–705. https://doi.org/10.1007/s12603-022-1817-5
64. Banerjee S, Loshak H. *Congregate Meal Programs for Older Adults Living in the Community: A Review of Clinical Effectiveness*. Canadian Agency for Drugs and Technologies in Health; 2019. https://www.ncbi.nlm.nih.gov/books/NBK541210
65. U.S. Department of Agriculture Food and Nutrition Service. Supplemental Nutrition Assistance Program (SNAP). Accessed June 20, 2023. https://www.fns.usda.gov/snap/supplemental-nutrition-assistance-program
66. U.S. Department of Agriculture Food and Nutrition Service. Senior Farmers' Market Nutrition Program. Accessed June 20, 2023. https://www.fns.usda.gov/sfmnp/senior-farmers-market-nutrition-program
67. Administration on Aging. Older Americans Act nutrition programs Administration for Community Living. Updated July 15, 2016. https://acl.gov/sites/default/files/news%202017-03/OAA-Nutrition_Programs_Fact_Sheet.pdf
68. U.S. Department of Agriculture Food and Nutrition Service. Commodity Supplemental Food Program. Accessed June 20, 2023. https://www.fns.usda.gov/csfp/commodity-supplemental-food-program
69. Algra Y, Haverkort E, Kok W, et al. The association between malnutrition and oral health in older people: a systematic review. *Nutrients*. 2021;13(10):3584. https://doi.org/10.3390/nu13103584
70. Centers for Disease Control and Prevention. Facts about older adult oral health. Accessed June 19, 2023. https://www.cdc.gov/oralhealth/basics/adult-oral-health/adult_older.htm
71. Kok WE, Haverkort EB, Algra YA, et al. The association between polypharmacy and malnutrition (risk) in older people: a systematic review. *Clin Nutr ESPEN*. 2022;49:163–171. https://doi.org/10.1016/j.clnesp.2022.03.007
72. Wastesson JW, Morin L, Tan ECK, Johnell K. An update on the clinical consequences of polypharmacy in older adults: a narrative review, *Expert Opinion on Drug Safety*. 2018;17(12):1185–1196. https://doi.org/10.1080/14740338.2018.1546841.
73. Administration for Community Living. Older Americans Act. U.S. Department of Health and Human Services. Updated July 10, 2023. https://acl.gov/about-acl/authorizing-statutes/older-americans-act
74. Administration for Community Living. Nutrition services. health, wellness, and nutrition. Updated August 29, 2023. https://acl.gov/programs/health-wellness/nutrition-services
75. Beasley JM, Sevick MA, Kirshner L, Mangold M, Chodosh J. Congregate meals: opportunities to help vulnerable older adults achieve diet and physical activity recommendations. *J Frailty Aging*. 2018;7(3):182–186. https://doi.org/10.14283/jfa.2018.21

III

PUBLIC HEALTH AND NUTRITION: KEY TOPICS AND TRENDS

9

FOOD INSECURITY THROUGHOUT THE LIFE CYCLE

Jessica Soldavini and Joshua D. Miller

LEARNING OBJECTIVES

At the end of this chapter, students will be able to:

1. Define food insecurity.
2. Describe methods for measuring and monitoring food insecurity.
3. Describe the differential impacts of food insecurity throughout the life cycle.
4. Describe factors and policies that influence food insecurity.
5. Identify public health policies, resources, and interventions for addressing food insecurity throughout the life cycle.
6. Explain global issues and challenges related to reducing the burden of food insecurity.

INTRODUCTION

Food security creates an enabling environment for good nutrition and health, but millions of individuals are unable to reliably access sufficient food for well-being. The prevalence and severity of **food insecurity** are increasing globally due to climate change and the demands of a growing population, with marked disparities by gender and socioeconomic status. As such, there is an urgent need to understand the causes and consequences of food insecurity to develop policies and programs that sustainably reduce its burden. We therefore review the importance of experience-based measures, identify tools for measuring food insecurity, examine trends across settings and time, discuss the differential impacts of food insecurity across the life course, and conclude by describing current strategies for addressing food insecurity.

OVERVIEW OF FOOD INSECURITY IN THE UNITED STATES AND GLOBALLY

History and Definitions

Food insecurity—the inability to reliably access and benefit from safe, nutritious, and preferred foods through culturally and socially acceptable means[1]—affects nutrition, physical health, and mental well-being. Numerous tools have been developed to measure analogous concepts such as **dietary diversity** (the variety or the number of different food groups people eat over a given time), **hunger** (a consequence of severe food insecurity that results in a physiologic sensation of discomfort), and **malnutrition** (a surfeit or deficit of nutrients), but tools for comparably measuring food insecurity across time and populations have only been developed and widely implemented in the prior two decades (Table 9.1).[2–5] This is important given that accurate measurement of food insecurity is needed to assess progress toward achieving universal access to adequate food for good health, a human right recognized by the United Nations.[6]

Until the late 1970s, food insecurity was primarily conceptualized in terms of food production and availability at the national scale.[7] During this period, policy makers and nongovernmental actors focused on reducing hunger, a consequence of severe food insecurity. Less attention was given to food quality or diversity. The number of calories available per capita, calculated using food balance sheets that estimate the total amount of food produced and imported into a country, was used as the primary nutrition indicator. But such measures mask inequities at subnational levels. For instance, while the United States produces sufficient food to meet the energy requirements of all individuals in the country,[8] more than 10% of households are unable to access adequate food for part of the year due to financial or other constraints.[9] Limitations in supply-focused tools, including growing evidence of persistent malnutrition in regions with sufficient food availability, led to a call for the development of scales that capture lived experiences with food availability and use at the household and individual levels.[10]

The first experience-based food insecurity scale was developed in the early 1990s using data from women with children in New York State.[11] Findings from this research inspired the U.S. Department of Agriculture (USDA) to develop a nationally comparable measure of household food insecurity—the United States Household Food Security Survey Module—that has been included in the National Health and Nutrition Examination Surveys (NHANES) since 1999.[12] Numerous tools to measure food insecurity among specific populations or regions have been developed in the following decades. Application of these tools has demonstrated that food insecurity is a prevalent condition and revealed new policy and programmatic strategies for improving malnutrition.[13]

Nutrition security, which builds off the concept of food insecurity, refers to "consistent access, availability, and affordability of foods and beverages that promote well-being, prevent diseases, and, if needed, treat disease, particularly among racial/ethnic minority populations, lower income populations, and rural and remote populations including Tribal communities and Insular areas."[14] The concept recognizes that most individuals are not meeting nutrition and physical activity guidelines, which help prevent diet-related disease. Nutrition security emphasizes using an equity lens to understand how structural issues, such as systemic racism, creates barriers to accessing affordable and diverse high-quality foods, thus contributing to higher prevalence of food insecurity and diet-related chronic diseases in populations that are historically underserved or

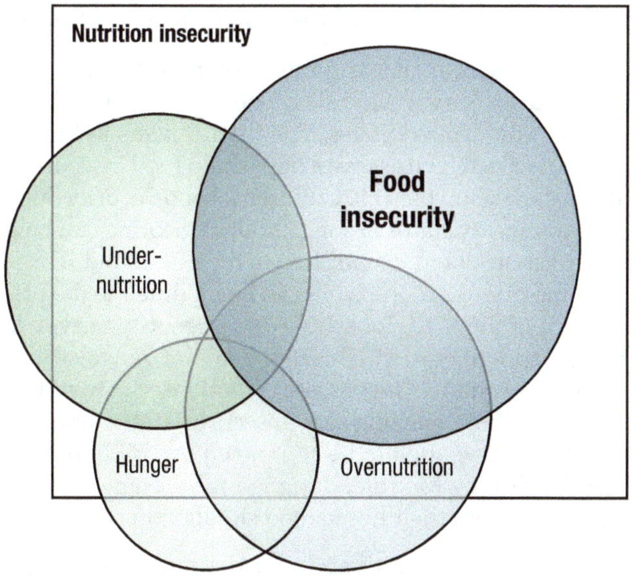

Figure 9.1. Relationship between food insecurity and allied concepts.

persecuted. In March 2022, the USDA announced actions to address nutrition security, which are organized under four pillars:

- Meaningful support: Providing nutrition support throughout all life stages.
- Healthy food: Connecting all Americans with healthy, safe, affordable food.
- Collaborative action: Developing, translating, and enacting nutrition science through partnership.
- Equitable systems: Prioritizing equity every step of the way.

Figure 9.1 highlights the relationship between food insecurity and allied concepts.

Measurement of Food Insecurity

Level of Analysis

Experiential food insecurity scales have primarily been developed for use at the household level. What defines a "household," however, has not been standardized, although most consider food sharing and common residency to be key characteristics.[15] Application of these tools has demonstrated that issues with food access and use are more prevalent than suggested by less granular indicators (e.g., national food sufficiency). Importantly, though, intra-household variations in food division and consumption are not captured by household-level measures. For instance, work in Jaipur, India found that mothers were more likely to affirm experiences of food insecurity than fathers from the same household, and that mothers more frequently affirmed food insecurity experiences than their children (supporting the theory that mothers buffer children against the most severe experiences of food insecurity).[16] Other work has also reported heterogeneous food insecurity experiences by gender[17] and age.[18] Therefore, depending on the aims of the project, individual measures of food insecurity may be preferred (Table 9.1). Recognizing that adults may not be able to report on all experiences of their children (e.g., hunger), a tool has been developed to comparably measure food insecurity among school-age children and adolescents across diverse contexts.[19]

Data Sources and Measures of Food Insecurity in the United States

The USDA has a variety of tools available for assessing food security status.[20] The 18-item U.S. Household Food Security Survey Module is one of the most common tools for measuring food security status in the United States. The first 10 items in the module make up the U.S. Adult Food Security Scale, which assesses household food insecurity among adults, and the remaining eight items make up the U.S. Children's Food Security Survey Scale, which assesses household food insecurity status among children. Scoring can be done for the household overall, adults in the household, or children in the household. The reference period for the survey is generally the prior 12 months but can be modified to the prior 30 days. There is also a six-item short form of the U.S. Household Food Security Survey Module, which was developed to reduce respondent burden. This tool does not, however, ask specifically about children in the household. Most tools for assessing food insecurity status are designed to be completed by adults (even those assessing food insecurity status among children), although there have been some tools developed to be completed by children. For instance, the nine-item Child Food Security Survey Module, designed for use among children ages 12 years and older, asks adolescents about their home food situation in the prior month.

The severity of food insecurity can vary, and the tools described in the prior paragraph allow for the assessment of ranges of food security status. The USDA has used the following categories of food security status since 2006[21]:

- High food security: No limitations to accessing food are reported.
- Marginal food security: Some indications of food access challenges are reported, and these are often related to anxiety around having enough food.
- Low food security: Variety, quality, or desirability of foods eaten are reduced.
- Very low food security: Multiple indications of reduced food intake and disrupted eating patterns are reported.

Often, individuals experiencing high and marginal food security are considered food secure while those experiencing low and very low food security are considered food insecure. Collapsing these categories, however, may lead to an underestimation of those experiencing food access challenges and associated negative impacts of food insecurity. Some researchers have expressed concern around collapsing categories and recommend looking at them separately, especially the marginally food secure group, as differences have been found in the characteristics and health outcomes of these groups.[22,23]

The Hunger Vital Sign is a two-question screener that is based on the U.S. Household Food Security Survey Module. Given its brevity and utility, the Hunger Vital Sign is increasingly used in both research and practice. For instance, healthcare providers and affiliated organizations like the American Academy of Pediatrics and AARP now recommend use of the screener to identify at-risk populations and provide more tailored health messaging.[24]

National and state estimates of food insecurity in the United States are released in the annual *Household Food Security in the United States* report by the USDA Economic Research Service.[9] Statistics in this report are based on data gathered from the Current Population Survey Food Security Supplement, which assesses food insecurity status using the U.S. Household Food Security Survey Module. Other national surveys, such as the NHANES, also collect data on food insecurity. Public health nutrition practitioners may also be interested in the *Map the Meal Gap* tool from Feeding America, which provides estimates of food insecurity by geographic levels, such as states, counties, and congressional districts.[25]

Food insufficiency is a concept related to food insecurity that is sometimes assessed. It is used to assess whether households have enough to eat and is considered similar to very low food security. Food insufficiency is assessed through a single question that asks respondents to indicate if their household has "enough of the kinds of foods we wanted to eat," "enough, but not always the kinds of foods we wanted to eat," "sometimes not enough to eat," or "often not enough to eat."[26] Households are considered food insufficient if they sometimes or often do not have enough to eat. This measure has been used in a variety of national surveys, including the U.S. Census Bureau's Household Pulse Survey that has tracked food insufficiency rates throughout the COVID-19 pandemic.

Data Sources and Measures of Food Insecurity Globally

Numerous site-specific scales have been developed and validated for use in particular regions or populations. Given the high cost, time burdens, and complex analytic procedures associated with scale development[27] only a few tools have been created to comparably measure food insecurity across diverse populations (Table 9.1). The Household Food Insecurity Access Scale was the first indicator developed to measure food insecurity globally and is still in wide use by academics and governmental organizations, such as USAID. But the scale is not cross-culturally comparable and performs poorly in some settings[28] (e.g., Bangladesh).[29] A subset of three items in this tool have been shown to perform comparably across diverse contexts and were packaged together as the Household Hunger Scale. Given the brevity of the tool, it can only discern between little, moderate, or severe household hunger and is therefore recommended for use in areas with substantial food insecurity. In contrast, the Latin American and Caribbean Food Security Scale has been shown to comparably measure food insecurity across South America, Central America, and the Caribbean.[30]

Table 9.1. Validated Tools for Measuring Food Insecurity

Scale	Level of Analysis	Number of Items	Recall Period	Regional Focus	Key Publications
Household Food Security Survey Module	House-hold	18	1 month or 1 year	United States	Bickel et al. (2000)[2]
Household Food Insecurity Access Scale (HFIAS)	House-hold	9	1 month	Global	Coates et al. (2007)[3]
Food Insecurity Experiences Scale (FIES)	Individ-ual or house-hold	8	1 month or 1 year	Global	Food and Agriculture Organization (2016)[4]
Latin American and Caribbean Food Security Scale (ELCSA)	House-hold	8 (house-holds without children), 15 (households with children)	3 months	Latin Ameri-can and Carib-bean	Food and Agriculture Organization (2012)[5]

The Voices of the Hungry project was initiated in 2012 by the Food and Agriculture Organization to develop a tool that could effectively measure all components of food insecurity across all contexts. The resultant eight-item Food Insecurity Experiences Scale is currently one of the indicators used to measure progress toward Sustainable Development Goal (SDG) 2.1: "end hunger and ensure access by all people to safe, nutritious and sufficient food all year round." Results from application of the tool in national surveys are annually reported in *The State of Food Security and Nutrition in the World* report.

Measures of Nutrition Security

The U.S. Household Food Security Survey Module focuses primarily on the ability of households to afford food in general. The Gretchen Swanson Center for Nutrition recently developed new measures to assess nutrition security and other related concepts. They developed four items to assess household nutrition security, three items to assess household healthfulness choice (perceived level of control over obtaining healthful foods), and three items to assess household dietary choice (perceived control over obtaining foods they prefer).[31] Measures to assess household resilience, perceived limited availability, utilization barriers, and food insecurity stability have also been developed.[32]

Temporal Trends in Food Insecurity

United States

In 2021, 10.2% of U.S. households experienced food insecurity.[9] There were 33.8 million individuals (9.3 million children and 24.6 million adults) living in 13.5 million food-insecure households. The prevalence of food insecurity was higher among households with children, although this differed based on household composition. Overall, 12.5% of households with children experienced food insecurity in 2021; however, the prevalence was 12.9% for those with children 6 years and younger, 16.2% for households headed by a single male, 24.3% for households headed by a single female, and 7.4% for married couples with children. In 6.3% of households with children, only adults experienced food insecurity and in 6.2% households, both adults and children were food insecure. Households with older adults had a lower prevalence, with 7.1% of households with older adults experiencing food insecurity. Among older adults living alone, 9.5% experienced food insecurity.

The prevalence of household food insecurity in the United States did not significantly change between 2019 and 2021 despite the COVID-19 pandemic. Policies and programs introduced during the COVID-19 pandemic (described later) may have helped keep food insecurity rates from rising, although there have been changes in the prevalence of food insecurity over the past 20 years. In 2001, the prevalence of household food insecurity was 10.7%. This increased to 11.9% in 2004 and decreased to 11% from 2005 to 2007. During the recession, the prevalence of food insecurity increased to 14.6% in 2008 and remained above 14% until 2014. In 2015, the prevalence of food insecurity decreased to 12.7% and continued to decrease from 2016 to 2019 (Figure 9.2).[33]

Globally

The burden of food insecurity is growing globally and is not borne equally across geographic location and social status. The prevalence of moderate or severe food insecurity has increased annually since the Food and Agriculture Organization first started monitoring experiential food insecurity in 2014. It was estimated that 29.3% of the population experienced moderate or severe food insecurity in 2021, compared to 21.2% 5 years prior.[34]

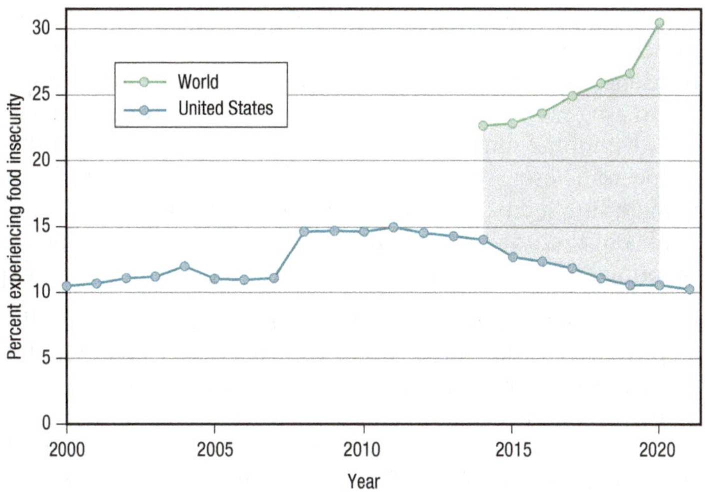

Figure 9.2. Temporal trends in food insecurity, measured using the Household Food Security Survey Module (United States) and Food Insecurity Experiences Scale (World).

Sources: Data from Food and Agriculture Organization, International Fund for Agricultural Development, UNICEF, World Food Programme, World Health Organization. *The State of Food Security and Nutrition in the World 2022: Repurposing Food and Agricultural Policies to Make Healthy Diets More Affordable.* Food and Agriculture Organization; 2022. doi:10.4060/cc0639en; U.S. Department of Agriculture Economic Research Center. Food security in the U.S.: key statistics & graphics. Updated June 20, 2023. https://www.ers.usda.gov/topics/food-nutrition-assistance/food-security-in-the-u-s/key-statistics-graphics

Worsening food availability and accessibility is due, in part, to the negative impacts of climate change on agricultural schedules, growing economic inequality, and supply chain disruptions from the COVID-19 pandemic[35] and war between Russian and Ukraine (both of which are major producers of fertilizer and grains).[36] There are, however, notable inequities. For instance, 57.9% of individuals throughout Africa experienced moderate or severe food insecurity in 2021 compared to only 8.0% of individuals in Northern America and Europe.[34] Gender differences in food insecurity also exist and are growing globally, with 31.9% of women experiencing moderate or severe food insecurity in 2021 compared to 27.6% of men.[34]

IMPACTS OF FOOD INSECURITY THROUGHOUT THE LIFE CYCLE

Across life stages, food insecurity has been demonstrated to be associated with elevated risk of noncommunicable disease,[37] changes in body composition,[38,39] lower cognitive function,[40] and psychological distress.[41] Social and biological changes throughout the life course modify these relationships. That is, there are periods when experiences of food insecurity more acutely impact health and morbidities that can only develop during sensitive phases.

First 1,000 Days

The first 1,000 days is a critical developmental window from 1 year prior to delivery through 2 years postpartum. Poor health during this period can have lifelong consequences both for caregivers and infants. For instance, pregnant caregivers have elevated nutrient demands to support a developing fetus and may be limited in their ability to access needed social support or resources, making them particularly susceptible to the detrimental consequences of food insecurity.[42] Studies have found that pregnant persons from food-insecure households are more likely to be malnourished, have suboptimal gestational weight gain[43] and adverse body composition changes,[39] experience pregnancy-induced hypertension and gestational diabetes, and suffer from poor mental health[44] compared to their food-secure peers. These issues can persist after delivery and also contribute to poor neonatal health, including increased risk of neonatal mortality,[45] birth defects,[46] and small birth size.[47] Future cohort studies should investigate whether consequences and their severity vary depending on the trimester during which food insecurity is experienced.

Lactating individuals also have high nutrient demands to promote lactogenesis and maintain normal physiologic function. Food insecurity is associated with lower breastfeeding self-efficacy and perceived breast milk sufficiency.[48] Consequently, infants in food-insecure households are less likely to be exclusively breastfed to 6 months[49,50] and consume less breast milk (due to fewer feeding episodes or decreased milk production) than their counterparts from food-secure households.[51] This is important given that exclusive breastfeeding to 6 months is protective against diarrheal disease—a leading cause of death among children under 5—and provides needed nutrients and microbes for optimal growth.[52,53] Food insecurity can also limit the quality and diversity of complementary foods available[54] as well as the psychological capacity of caregivers to implement optimal feeding practices,[55] such that food-insecure infants are less likely to have adequate diets.[56] This may be one mechanism through which food insecurity contributes to increased risk of stunting (low weight for age) and underweight,[57] as well as overweight and obesity.[58,59] This is important given that exposures during infancy can have lifelong impacts on metabolic functioning, including fat oxidation, which can influence risk of obesity in adulthood.[60]

Children and Adolescents

Food insecurity in children and adolescents has been associated with a variety of mental health outcomes, including greater risk of depression, hyperactivity, externalizing behaviors (directing problematic or harmful behaviors outward), and internalizing behaviors (directing problematic or harmful behaviors inward).[61,62] Food insecurity has also been shown to negatively impact academic performance.[62] Some studies have found food insecurity to be associated with poorer dietary outcomes; however, the evidence is less consistent for children than adults.[63,64] Studies suggest that food insecurity may be associated with negative outcomes related to eating behaviors, academic performance, and self-rated health in college students.[65]

Adults and Older Individuals

Food insecurity in adults is associated with poor diet quality, including lower consumption of fruits, vegetables, dairy, and certain micronutrients.[64] Adults who are food insecure are more likely to experience mental health challenges such as stress,[61,63] depression,[61,66,67] anxiety,[61,67] and sleep disorders[61,67] than food-secure adults. Food insecurity has also been found to be associated with a variety of chronic health conditions, although associations vary between self-report and clinical diagnosis for conditions such as type 2 diabetes[68] and hypertension.[69,70]

In older adults, food insecurity is associated with malnutrition, including protein-energy malnutrition, low weight, and overweight.[71] Older adults who are food insecure have been shown to consume less fruits, vegetables, dairy, energy, and many macro- and micronutrients compared to food-secure peers.[71] Food insecurity in older adults is also associated with higher risk of depression.[66,67] Individuals who are food insecure often need to choose between purchasing medicine or food. Studies suggest that food insecurity is related to cost-related medication nonadherence in older adults.[72]

POLICY PERSPECTIVES

United States

The USDA Food and Nutrition Service administers 15 nutrition assistance programs that reach different populations throughout the life cycle. The programs aim to "increase food security and reduce hunger by providing children and low-income people access to food, a healthful diet and nutrition education in a way that supports American agriculture and inspires public confidence."[73] These programs are generally administered at state, local, territory, or tribal levels.

The Supplemental Nutrition Assistance Program (SNAP) serves all ages and is the largest nutrition assistance program in the United States. SNAP provides monthly benefits to low-income individuals through the electronic benefit transfer (EBT) system to purchase food. Households must meet certain requirements (e.g., income limits) to qualify for SNAP. The number of benefits received is based on household income and size. Households can use SNAP benefits to purchase food as well as seeds and plants to grow food. Most food items are eligible, although SNAP benefits cannot be used for alcoholic beverages, vitamins and supplements, and nonfood items. Generally, SNAP benefits cannot be used to purchase hot prepared foods, unless recipients are participating in the Restaurant Meals Program, which states can provide to recipients who are homeless, 60 years or older, or disabled. The Food Distribution Program on Indian Reservations (FDPIR) is another program that serves individuals across the life cycle. The program provides USDA foods to low-income households who live on Indian Reservations and American Indian households who live in approved areas. Households that are unable to easily access SNAP offices or authorized retail locations may participate in FDPIR as an alternative to SNAP. The Emergency Food Assistance Program (TEFAP) additionally serves individuals across the life cycle. This program provides USDA foods, which are U.S.-grown and produced foods that USDA purchases, to states that provide them to local agencies (e.g., food banks) that distribute the foods to local organizations (e.g., food pantries, soup kitchens) to be given to individuals in the community.

The Special Supplemental Nutrition Assistance Program for Women, Infants, and Children (WIC) serves infants and children ages 5 years and younger, and pregnant, breastfeeding, and nonbreastfeeding postpartum individuals who are low income and at nutritional risk. Nutritional risk includes medically based risks such as history of pregnancy complications, poor pregnancy outcomes, underweight, anemia, or other dietary risks such as not meeting the current Dietary Guidelines for Americans recommendations or inappropriate feeding practices. Recipients of WIC receive nutritious supplemental foods; nutrition education and counseling; breastfeeding support and promotion; and screening and referrals to other social, welfare, and health services. The WIC Farmers Market Nutrition Program provides coupons to WIC recipients to purchase locally grown fruits, vegetables, and herbs from authorized farmers markets, individual farmers, or roadside stands.

The Child and Adult Care Food Program (CACFP) serves children ages 12 and younger in day-care homes and child care centers; children 18 years and younger in afterschool programs and emergency shelters; and adults who are physically or mentally impaired or 60 years or older who are enrolled in an adult day-care program. The program reimburses day-care homes, child care centers, afterschool programs, emergency shelters, and adult day-care centers for serving meals and snacks to eligible participants who meet meal pattern guidelines. The National School Lunch Program (NSLP) and School Breakfast Program (SBP) serve school-age children. These programs reimburse schools and residential child care programs for providing meals and snacks to students that meet meal pattern guidelines. For NSLP, SBP, and centers participating in CACFP, meals are served to participants at a free, reduced-price, or paid rate. Eligibility is generally based on household income: those whose incomes are 130% or more below the federal poverty level qualify for free meals while those with incomes between 130% and 185% of the federal poverty level qualify for reduced-price meals. Individuals may also be eligible for free meals if they are a migrant, homeless, or foster child or participate in certain federal assistance programs such as SNAP. Meals are served free to all children at day-care homes, afterschool programs, and emergency shelters participating in CACFP. Many schools provide meals for free to all students regardless of individual family income. The Community Eligibility Provision is an example of an option for schools and school districts with many students eligible for free meals to serve meals at no cost to all students without collecting household applications. Some states have also passed legislation to address costs not covered by federal reimbursements to serve meals at no cost to all students.

The Summer Food Service Program and NSLP Seamless Summer option provide free meals and snacks to children ages 18 and younger in low-income areas during the summer. The Special Milk Program reimburses schools, child care programs, and eligible camps that do not participate in other USDA child nutrition programs for serving milk to children. The Fresh Fruit and Vegetable Program provides funding to elementary schools to offer additional fresh fruits and vegetable snacks to children. The program prioritizes schools with a high percentage of children eligible for free and reduced-price meals.

The Senior Farmers Market Nutrition Program provides coupons to low-income individuals 60 years and older to purchase fruits, vegetables, herbs, and honey from authorized farmers markets, roadside stands, farmers, and community-supported agriculture programs. The Commodity Supplemental Food Program provides adults 60 years and older with healthy USDA foods.

The Farm Bill is a comprehensive piece of legislation that governs a variety of food and agriculture programs. It is typically reauthorized every 5 years. The Farm Bill includes 12 titles, with nutrition being the largest. Programs covered under the nutrition title include SNAP, the Commodity Supplemental Food Program, TEFAP, and FDPIR. The Farm Bill also allowed for the Gus Schumacher Nutrition Incentive Program, which provides funding to conduct and evaluate programs that provide incentives at the point of purchase for SNAP recipients to purchase fruits and vegetables and produce prescription programs. Reauthorization of the Farm Bill is an opportunity to make modifications to these programs as well as introduce new opportunities for addressing food and nutrition security.

The Richard B. Russell National School Lunch Act and Child Nutrition Act of 1966 are the primary pieces of legislation that govern the USDA child nutrition programs and WIC. Child nutrition reauthorization is the process Congress uses to change these pieces of legislation. This is supposed to occur every 5 years; however, sometimes it occurs less frequently.

The Older Americans Act Nutrition Program aims to reduce food insecurity, hunger, and malnutrition; promote health and well-being; and promote socialization among adults ages 60 years and older. The Administration for Community Living's Administration on Aging provides grants to states to administer programs. Services provided include both meals served in congregate settings and home-delivered meals as well as nutrition services such as screening, assessment, counseling, and education. Meals served must follow the current Dietary Guidelines for Americans, provide at least one-third of the Dietary Reference Intakes, appeal to older adults, and follow local and state food safety guidelines.

Federal Policies and Programs During the COVID-19 Pandemic

Multiple policies were passed throughout the COVID-19 pandemic, such as the Families First Coronavirus Response Act (P.L. 116-127); Coronavirus Aid, Relief, and Economic Security (CARES) Act (P.L. 116-136); and American Rescue Plan Act of 2021 (P.L. 117-2), which included provisions to address food insecurity. Congress made modifications to some USDA nutrition assistance programs and granted USDA the authority to issue nationwide waivers to a variety of regulations to better support participants and make it more feasible for programs to operate during the pandemic. Examples related to SNAP included temporary increases in SNAP benefits, expansion of SNAP online purchasing, and modifying eligibility rules so that more college students could qualify. The USDA issued a variety of waivers related to the WIC program that allowed for modifications such as the ability to offer services and issue benefits remotely, allow for food package substitutions if WIC-approved items are not available, and waive minimum stocking requirements if stores face supply chain issues. Due to USDA waivers, parents were able to pick up meals for their children, children were not required to eat meals onsite, multiple meals could be served at once, and meals could be made available at no cost to all students regardless of their family income among a variety of other modifications to child nutrition programs.

In addition to modifications to existing programs, the USDA also administered programs specific to the pandemic. Pandemic Electronic Benefit Transfer (P-EBT) was similar to Summer Electronic Benefit Transfer for Children (see What Works 9.2 later in the chapter) in that it provided EBT ssistance to families of children eligible for free and reduced-price school meals when they were not physically in school to help cover the costs of meals they would have had access to if they were at school. An average of 6.9 million children received benefits each month in March through September of 2020 and around 8.8 million children received benefits each month between October 2020 and September 2021.[74] Emergency Meals to You mailed shelf-stable meals to children in rural communities who would have otherwise been able to receive free or reduced-price meals in school. More than 40 million meals were delivered between March 2020 to August 2020 to around 400,000 children.[74] The Farmers to Families Food Box program provided organizations with fresh fruits and vegetables, meat, and dairy products to distribute to families. Between May 15, 2020 and April 30, 2021, more than 173 million boxes were distributed.[75]

The Child Tax Credit can be claimed by taxpayers with dependents under 17 when filing federal taxes. The American Rescue Plan Act of 2021 temporarily increased the amount of tax credit most families can receive, allowed families with very low incomes to receive the full amount, and allowed families to receive up to half of the tax credit as monthly payments from July to December 2021, prior to filing their tax return. These changes were associated with declines in food insecurity, food insufficiency, and child poverty.[76] Increases in the prevalence of food insufficiency among households with children were seen after the expiration of these temporary changes.[77]

Global

The Food and Agriculture Organization (FAO), World Food Programme (WFP), and the International Fund for Agricultural Development (IFAD) are specialized United Nations agencies that have a shared vision of improving nutritional well-being globally through distinct, but coordinated, mechanisms.[78] FAO was created in 1945 to improve diets and livelihoods by investing in and supporting farmers' capacities to implement sustainable agricultural and aquacultural practices. Such initiatives are intended to increase crop diversity and yields, strengthen agrifood supply chains, expand incomes, and improve well-being while preserving land and water ecosystems. FAO is also responsible for tracking progress toward Sustainable Development Goal 2 (creating a world free of hunger by 2030) and oversees numerous databases that aggregate diverse food, agricultural, and climatologic data intended to help inform the development of more effective policies and programs.

WFP, the world's largest humanitarian organization, was established in 1963 to address acute nutritional issues during regional and national emergencies. Since its creation, WFP has expanded its aim to end global hunger by providing direct food aid to communities experiencing or recently recovering from political, social, environmental, or economic turmoil (e.g., natural disasters, widespread disease outbreak). As a nonpartisan organization, WFP works with diverse actors and governmental groups to safely deliver and distribute food in war zones and areas of active conflict. Increasingly, WFP is offering cash-based transfers, which provide individuals with greater autonomy than in-kind food distributions. WFP also seeks to move beyond experiences of abject hunger by providing diverse, nutrient-dense foods that can reduce the risk of malnutrition. This is accomplished, in part, by the implementation of projects that consider underlying determinants of famine and poor nutrition, including the resilience of local supply chains.[79]

IFAD similarly aims to improve food systems and nutrition but exclusively focuses on rural communities given stark health and developmental disparities compared to urban regions. Recognizing that millions of families in rural areas throughout low- and middle-income countries primarily rely on smallholder farming for their livelihoods, IFAD has been investing in agricultural research and development since 1977. The organization funds diverse projects that target different sectors and agricultural pathways, from expanding youth engagement in agriculture (the youth population is growing fastest in low- and middle-income countries) to improving market access.

The U.S. Agency for International Development (USAID) was established in 1961 to reduce hunger internationally.[80] In the half century since its inception, USAID has expanded its scope to include increasing access to quality education, empowering women, and promoting economic growth. It manages its own portfolio of programs and provides funds for projects led by other institutions. In 2010, following the global recession and rapidly increasing food prices, the U.S. government launched Feed the Future. The initiative, coordinated by USAID, aims to reduce food insecurity and malnutrition in target countries. Countries are selected based on the prevalence of chronic hunger, political will and resource commitment from the host government, and possibility to scale up sustainable agricultural practices.[81] Currently, Feed the Future operates in Central America, Africa, and South Asia.

FOOD INSECURITY: EFFECTIVE PUBLIC HEALTH NUTRITION INTERVENTIONS

United States

Most food assistance in the United States is provided through government-supported programs, such as those previously described, although the charitable food systems also play a role in addressing food insecurity. Feeding America estimates that in 2021, 53 million individuals received charitable food assistance.[82] This is less than the more than 60 million who received charitable food assistance in 2020, but more than the over 40 million who received it in 2019 prior to the COVID-19 pandemic.[82] Food banks and food pantries often come to mind when thinking about food assistance programs. Food banks are nonprofit organizations that receive, store, and distribute food to local food programs, such as food pantries. Food pantries are sites where food is distributed to individuals and families. While food banks and food pantries can be a helpful source of food for those facing food insecurity, there are a variety of limitations to their ability to reduce food insecurity.[83] For instance, they do not address the root causes of food insecurity and many individuals fear potential stigma if their friends or family know they access food pantries.

School food pantries are becoming more common across the United States. These pantries are located at schools and provide food to students and their families. Weekend backpack programs are another growing intervention to address food insecurity among school-age children, primarily those in elementary and middle school. These programs provide foods that do not require parental assistance to prepare for students over weekends. Limited research exists on backpack programs; however, early studies suggest positive benefits, including improved academic outcomes. There is concern related to backpack programs having potentially negative consequences including creating stigma, shame, and stress for participating students.[84]

A variety of interventions exist for addressing food insecurity among college students. Examples include campus food pantries, campus gardens, and meal swipe programs. There is currently limited research evaluating the efficacy of campus-based food insecurity interventions.

Meals on Wheels programs provide home-delivered meals to older adults in communities across the United States. These types of programs have been shown to reduce food insecurity and improve diet quality.[85] Programs may also offer other services such as congregate meals, safety and wellness checks, socialization, nutrition assessments, nutrition education and counseling, and assistance with SNAP applications. More than 144 million meals are served annually to over 3.9 million individuals through Meals on Wheels programs across the United States.[86]

Global

Global nutrition programs and policies have been shown to be effective, cost-effective strategies for reducing stunting and improving well-being.[87] Yet development aid for nutrition initiatives is typically quite low; approximately 1% of the U.S. global health budget is directed toward nutrition-focused projects.[88] To achieve SDGs related to nutrition, increased funding is needed from public and private donors.[89] Improved governance is also needed to ensure equitable progress toward universal food security, including "1) multisectoral participatory decision making, 2) transparency and accountability, 3) equity in resource allocation and service delivery, and 4) multisectoral and multilevel policies and corresponding programs."[90] Programs are typically most effective at reducing food insecurity if they address its root causes (e.g., investing in agriculture to improve production and livelihoods), have an equity focus, and use sustainable practices that do not exacerbate climate change and ensure success continues after external partners leave.

The role of water in nutrition has historically been overlooked and minimally targeted but may be central to improving food security globally. Research has found that improving access to irrigation technologies can expand yields and crop diversity while also improving the incomes of smallholder farmers, who typically rely on rainfed operations.[91] Increasingly, such initiatives must compete with growing water demands from other sectors. Addressing other aspects of **water security**—the ability to reliably access sufficient water for all household uses[92]—also has the potential to improve food security. There is growing evidence that household water issues impact what foods are purchased and prepared, restrict the ability of caregivers to implement optimal infant and young child feeding practices, and exacerbate the deleterious effects of food insecurity.[93] As such, policies and programs are likely to be most effective if they address food and water issues concurrently.[94] Regular monitoring of water insecurity is also needed to identify vulnerable populations and better target resources.[95]

WHAT WORKS

What Works 9.1: Singida Nutrition Agroecology Project

To address persistent malnutrition and widespread food insecurity in rural Tanzania, researchers and government officials partnered together to develop a participatory curriculum that was implemented among smallholder farmers in 2015. Mentor farmers were selected from each community and trained in sustainable agroecological practices, nutrition, and social equity. These individuals then held monthly meetings where they communicated their findings to other local farmers. In addition to these trainings, participating households received a few legume seeds for crop experimentation. At the end of two growing seasons, the proportion of households experiencing moderate or severe food insecurity decreased, child dietary diversity increased, and the proportion of women with probable depression decreased.[96,97] This project demonstrates that a low-input intervention can meaningfully improve agricultural outcomes and nutritional well-being among smallholder farmers.

What Works 9.2: Summer Electronic Benefit Transfer for Children

The Summer Electronic Benefit Transfer for Children (SEBTC) was a USDA demonstration project that aimed to address food insecurity and nutrition among low-income children in the United States during the summer when they are not receiving free and reduced-price meals through schools. The program was implemented as a USDA demonstration project in selected states beginning in 2011. Households from participating school districts were eligible to participate if they had at least one child in prekindergarten through 12th grade who was certified for free or reduced-price school meals during the prior school year. The USDA assessed both a $60- and $30-per-month-per-child benefit that was provided on an EBT card. States had the option of administering the program using a SNAP model, where participants could purchase SNAP-eligible foods at SNAP-authorized retailers, or a WIC model, where participants could purchase foods from a specific food package at WIC-authorized retailers. Participation in SEBTC has been associated with a significant decrease in the prevalence of very low food security and significant improvements in dietary quality, including increased consumption of fruits and vegetables, whole grains, and dairy, and decreased consumption of sugar-sweetened beverages. Summer EBT was made a permanent program beginning summer 2024.[98]

SUMMARY

Food insecurity is a national and global public health concern, with the examination of both causes and consequences driving policies and programmatic solutions to its burden.

Exploration of food insecurity in this chapter identifies tools for measuring food insecurity, examines trends across settings and time, and discusses the differential impacts of food insecurity across the life course. Federal nutrition assistance programs, as well as international agencies working to alleviate the burden of food insecurity, are presented as resources for the public health nutrition professional.

KEY CHAPTER CONCEPTS

- Food insecurity is a serious public health concern in the United States and globally.
- A variety of tools have been developed to assess food insecurity, with most measuring at the household level.
- Food insecurity has been shown to have various negative impacts across the life course, including poor dietary intake, physical health, mental well-being, and academic performance.
- The USDA administers numerous federal nutrition assistance programs, including SNAP, WIC, and the National School Lunch and Breakfast Programs, that help to support individuals across the life cycle.
- A variety of agencies, including the FAO, WFP, IFAD, and USAID, are working to address food insecurity across the life cycle on a global level.

CASE STUDY: STARTING A COUNTYWIDE TASK FORCE TO ADDRESS FOOD INSECURITY

The county health department where you work is concerned about the high prevalence of food insecurity in the county. Recent data demonstrate that 20% of households in the area experience food insecurity, 19% of households participate in SNAP, and over 80% of students are eligible for free and reduced-price meals. The county has a population of approximately 200,000, of which 25% are under the age of 18 and 20% are over the age of 85. The population is approximately 50% non-Hispanic White, 15% African American, 10% Asian, 20% Hispanic, and 5% American Indian or Alaska Native. The county has a mix of urban and rural areas. You recently started your position and are new to the county. As part of your role, you have been asked to start a countywide task force to address the issue of food insecurity. Being new to the county and your role, you do not know much about the issue of food insecurity or current strategies for addressing it within the county.

1. What steps would you take to learn more about food insecurity and available resources within the county?
2. What types of programs would you investigate to learn more about the ways this issue is being addressed for individuals across the life cycle?
3. What types of individuals or groups would you want to involve in the task force? Why?
4. What items would you include on the agenda for the first task force meeting?
5. How would you develop goals for the task force? How would you ensure that the goals and strategies of the task force support all community members, considering differences in age, race, ethnicity, culture, and urbanicity?

DISCUSSION QUESTIONS

1. How are the concepts of food insecurity, nutrition insecurity, and hunger related? How do they differ?
2. What are advantages and disadvantages of measuring household, compared to individual, food insecurity? Which study questions are best suited for each?
3. What factors, from the individual to national level, influence food insecurity risk? What are the social and biological mechanisms through which food insecurity contributes to poor health and nutrition?

SUGGESTED LEARNING ACTIVITIES

1. Explore Feeding America's Map the Meal Gap tool: map.feedingamerica.org. What is the prevalence of food insecurity overall and for children in the state, county, and district where you are? How many individuals are estimated to be food insecure? What is the average cost of a meal? Are there differences in the prevalence of food insecurity for different demographic groups?
2. Create a handout that includes available food assistance programs in your local community. For each program, identify the services provided and eligibility criteria, including which age groups can participate.
3. Conduct an informational interview with someone who does work related to food insecurity to learn more about the issue, their role, and strategies they use for addressing the issue.
4. Volunteer at a local food bank, food pantry, summer meals site, or other food assistance program.
5. Select one country to examine using the World Food Programme's HungerMap: https://hungermap.wfp.org. Describe variations in food consumption across time and regions within the country. Add additional layers to the map and comment on any trends you notice between food consumption, rainfall, vegetation, hazards, and documented conflicts.

RESOURCES FOR FURTHER LEARNING

- USDA Food and Nutrition Service: www.fns.usda.gov
  - In collaboration with U.S. states, territories, and tribal organizations, oversees 15 nutrition assistance programs designed to promote equitable access to safe and adequate food for all
- USDA Food and Nutrition Security: www.usda.gov/nutrition-security
  - Highlights nutrition security as well as food security; describes USDA initiatives to promote nutrition security
- USDA Food Security in the United States: www.ers.usda.gov/topics/food-nutrition-assistance/food-security-in-the-u-s
  - Provides U.S. food security data from the USDA Economic Research Service (ERS)
- Food Research & Action Center: https://frac.org
  - A nonprofit organization focused on food security; addresses poverty-related hunger issues through advocacy, policy recommendations, and collaborations
- International Dietary Data Expansion Project: https://inddex.nutrition.tufts.edu
  - Develops, implements, and maintains tools for global dietary data assessment to support the development of effective agricultural and food policies to improve the lives of people worldwide

REFERENCES

1. Jones AD, Ngure FM, Pelto G, Young SL. What are we assessing when we measure food security? A compendium and review of current metrics. *Adv Nutr*. 2013;4(5):481–505. https://doi.org/10.3945/an.113.004119
2. Bickel G, Nord M, Price C, Hamilton W, Cook J. *Guide to Measuring Household Food Security, Revised 2000*. U.S. Department of Agriculture Food and Nutrition Service; 2000. https://ageconsearch.umn.edu/record/337157
3. Coates J, Swindale A, Bilinsky P. *Household Food Insecurity Access Scale (HFIAS) for Measurement of Household Food Access: Indicator Guide (v. 3)*. FHI 360/FANTA; 2007. https://www.fantaproject.org/monitoring-and-evaluation/household-food-insecurity-access-scale-hfias
4. Food and Agriculture Organization. *Methods for Estimating Comparable Rates of Food Insecurity Experienced by Adults Throughout the World*. Food and Agriculture Organization; 2016. https://www.fao.org/publications/card/fr/c/2c22259f-ad59-4399-b740
5. Food and Agriculture Organization. *Escala Latinoamericanay Caribeña de Seguridad Alimentaria (ELCSA): Manual de Uso y Aplicación*. Food and Agriculture Organization; 2012. https://www.fao.org/3/i3065s/i3065s.pdf
6. United Nations Human Rights. *The Right to Adequate Food*. Fact Sheet No. 34. Office of the United Nations High Commissioner for Human Rights, Food and Agriculture Organization; 2010. https://www.ohchr.org/sites/default/files/Documents/Publications/FactSheet34en.pdf
7. Webb P, Coates J, Frongillo EA, Rogers BL, Swindale A, Bilinsky P. Measuring household food insecurity: why it's so important and yet so difficult to do. *J Nutr*. 2006;136(5):1404S–1408S. https://doi.org/10.1093/jn/136.5.1404S
8. Putnam J, Allshouse J, Kantor LS, Putnam J, Allshouse J, Kantor LS. *U.S. Per Capita Food Supply Trends: More Calories, Refined Carbohydrates, and Fats*. Vol 25. U.S. Department of Agriculture, Economic Research Service; 2002:1–14. https://doi.org/10.22004/ag.econ.234624
9. Coleman-Jensen A, Rabbit MP, Gregory CA, Singh A. *Household Food Security in the United States in 2021* (ERR-309). U.S. Department of Agriculture, Economic Research Service. September 2022. https://www.ers.usda.gov/webdocs/publications/104656/err-309.pdf
10. Cafiero C, Melgar-Quiñonez HR, Ballard TJ, Kepple AW. Validity and reliability of food security measures. *Ann N Y Acad Sci*. 2014;1331:230–248. https://doi.org/10.1111/nyas.12594
11. Radimer KL, Olson CM, Greene JC, Campbell CC, Habicht J-P. Understanding hunger and developing indicators to assess it in women and children. *J Nutr Educ*. 1992;24(1):36S–44S. https://doi.org/10.1016/S0022-3182(12)80137-3
12. Radimer KL, Radimer KL. Measurement of household food security in the USA and other industrialised countries. *Public Health Nutr*. 2002;5(6A):859–864. https://doi.org/10.1079/PHN2002385
13. Pérez-Escamilla R, Gubert MB, Rogers B, Hromi-Fiedler A. Food security measurement and governance: assessment of the usefulness of diverse food insecurity indicators for policy makers. *Glob Food Sec*. 2017;14:96–104. https://doi.org/10.1016/j.gfs.2017.06.003
14. U.S. Department of Agriculture Food and Nutrition Service. *USDA Actions on Nutrition Security*. U.S. Department of Agriculture; 2022. https://www-usda-gov.libproxy.lib.unc.edu/sites/default/files/documents/usda-actions-nutrition-security.pdf
15. Beaman L, Dillon A. Do household definitions matter in survey design? Results from a randomized survey experiment in Mali. *J Dev Econ*. 2012;98(1):124–135. https://doi.org/10.1016/j.jdeveco.2011.06.005
16. Maxfield A. Testing the theoretical similarities between food and water insecurity: buffering hypothesis and effects on mental wellbeing. *Soc Sci Med*. 2020;244:112412. https://doi.org/10.1016/j.socscimed.2019.112412
17. Jung NM, de Bairros FS, Pattussi MP, Pauli S, Neutzling MB. Gender differences in the prevalence of household food insecurity: a systematic review and meta-analysis. *Public Health Nutr*. 2017;20(5):902–916. https://doi.org/10.1017/S1368980016002925

18. Kuku O, Gundersen C, Garasky S. Differences in food insecurity between adults and children in Zimbabwe. *Food Policy*. 2011;36(2):311–317. https://doi.org/10.1016/j.foodpol.2010.11.029
19. Frongillo EA, Fram MS, Ghattas H, et al. Development, validity, and cross-context equivalence of the child food insecurity experiences scale for assessing food insecurity of school-age children and adolescents. *J Nutr*. 2022;152(9):2135–2144. https://doi.org/10.1093/jn/nxac127
20. U.S. Department of Agriculture Economic Research Service. Survey tools. Updated October 17, 2022. https://www.ers.usda.gov/topics/food-nutrition-assistance/food-security-in-the-u-s/survey-tools
21. U.S. Department of Agriculture Economic Research Service. Definitions of food security. Updated October 17, 2022. https://www.ers.usda.gov/topics/food-nutrition-assistance/food-security-in-the-u-s/definitions-of-food-security
22. Cook JT, Black M, Chilton M, et al. Are food insecurity's health impacts underestimated in the U.S. population? Marginal food security also predicts adverse health outcomes in young U.S. children and mothers. *Adv Nutr*. 2013;4(1):51–61. https://doi.org/10.3945/an.112.003228
23. Soldavini J, Berner M. The importance of precision: differences in characteristics associated with levels of food security among college students. *Public Health Nutr*. 2020;23(9):1473–1483. https://doi.org/10.1017/S1368980019004026
24. Food Research & Action Center. Screen & intervene. Accessed September 12, 2022. https://frac.org/screen-intervene
25. Hake M, Engelhard E, Dewey A. *Map the Meal Gap 2023*. Feeding America; 2023. https://map.feedingamerica.org
26. U.S. Department of Agriculture Economic Research Center. Food insecurity in the U.S.: measurement. Updated October 17, 2022. https://www.ers.usda.gov/topics/food-nutrition-assistance/food-security-in-the-u-s/measurement
27. Boateng GO, Neilands TB, Frongillo EA, Melgar-Quiñonez HR, Young SL. Best practices for developing and validating scales for health, social, and behavioral research: a primer. *Front Public Health*. 2018;6:149. https://doi.org/10.3389/fpubh.2018.00149
28. Leroy JL, Ruel M, Frongillo EA, Harris J, Ballard TJ. Measuring the food access dimension of food security: a critical review and mapping of indicators. *Food Nutr Bull*. 2015;36(2):167–195. https://doi.org/10.1177/0379572115587274
29. Coates JC, Webb P, Houser RF, Rogers BL, Wilde P. "He said, she said": who should speak for households about experiences of food insecurity in Bangladesh? *Food Sec*. 2010;2(1):81–95. https://doi.org/10.1007/s12571-010-0052-9
30. Perez-Escamilla R, Paras P, Acosta MJ, Peyrou S, Nord M, Hromi-Fiedler A. Are the Latin American and Caribbean Food Security Scale (ELCSA) items comparable across countries? *FASEB J*. 2011;25(suppl 1):226.8. https://doi.org/10.1096/fasebj.25.1_supplement.226.8
31. Calloway EE, Carpenter LR, Gargano T, Sharp JL, Yaroch AL. Development of new measures to assess household nutrition security, and choice in dietary characteristics. *Appetite*. 2022;179:106288. https://doi.org/10.1016/j.appet.2022.106288
32. Gretchen Swanson Center for Nutrition. Other 3 pillars: availability, utilization, and stability pillars of food security. https://www.centerfornutrition.org/food-insecurity-measures/other-3-pillars
33. U.S. Department of Agriculture Economic Research Center. Food security in the U.S.: key statistics & graphics. Updated June 20, 2023. https://www.ers.usda.gov/topics/food-nutrition-assistance/food-security-in-the-u-s/key-statistics-graphics
34. Food and Agriculture Organization, International Fund for Agricultural Development, UNICEF, World Food Programme, World Health Organization. *The State of Food Security and Nutrition in the World 2022: Repurposing Food and Agricultural Policies to Make Healthy Diets More Affordable*. Food and Agriculture Organization; 2022. https://doi.org/10.4060/cc0639en
35. Béné C, Bakker D, Chavarro MJ, Even B, Melo J, Sonneveld A. Global assessment of the impacts of COVID-19 on food security. *Glob Food Sec*. 2021;31:100575. https://doi.org/10.1016/j.gfs.2021.100575
36. Behnassi M, El Haiba M. Implications of the Russia-Ukraine war for global food security. *Nat Hum Behav*. 2022;6(6):754–755. https://doi.org/10.1038/s41562-022-01391-x
37. Vercammen KA, Moran AJ, McClain AC, Thorndike AN, Fulay AP, Rimm EB. Food security and 10-year cardiovascular disease risk among U.S. adults. *Am J Prev Med*. 2019;56(5):689–697. https://doi.org/10.1016/j.amepre.2018.11.016
38. Benjamin-Neelon SE, Allen C, Neelon B. Household food security and infant adiposity. *Pediatrics*. 2020;146(3):e20193725. https://doi.org/10.1542/peds.2019-3725

39. Widen EM, Tsai I, Collins SM, et al. HIV infection and increased food insecurity are associated with adverse body composition changes among pregnant and lactating Kenyan women. *Eur J Clin Nutr*. 2019;73(3):474–482. https://doi.org/10.1038/s41430-018-0285-9
40. Royer MF, Guerithault N, Braden BB, Laska MN, Bruening M. Food insecurity is associated with cognitive function: a systematic review of findings across the life course. *Int J Technol Manag*. 2021;1(3):205–222. https://doi.org/10.3390/ijtm1030015
41. Myers CA. Food insecurity and psychological distress: a review of the recent literature. *Curr Nutr Rep*. 2020;9(2):107–118. https://doi.org/10.1007/s13668-020-00309-1
42. Ivers LC, Cullen KA. Food insecurity: special considerations for women. *Am J Clin Nutr*. 2011;94(6):1740S–1744S. https://doi.org/10.3945/ajcn.111.012617
43. Arzhang P, Ramezan M, Borazjani M, et al. The association between food insecurity and gestational weight gain: a systematic review and meta-analysis. *Appetite*. 2022;176:106124. https://doi.org/10.1016/j.appet.2022.106124
44. Laraia BA, Siega-Riz AM, Gundersen C. Household food insecurity is associated with self-reported pregravid weight status, gestational weight gain, and pregnancy complications. *J Am Diet Assoc*. 2010;110(5):692–701. https://doi.org/10.1016/j.jada.2010.02.014
45. Augusto ALP, de Abreu Rodrigues AV, Domingos TB, Salles-Costa R. Household food insecurity associated with gestacional and neonatal outcomes: a systematic review. *BMC Pregnancy Childbirth*. 2020;20(1):229. https://doi.org/10.1186/s12884-020-02917-9
46. Carmichael SL, Yang W, Herring A, Abrams B, Shaw GM. Maternal food insecurity is associated with increased risk of certain birth defects. *J Nutr*. 2007;137(9):2087–2092. https://doi.org/10.1093/jn/137.9.2087
47. Chowdhury M, Dibley MJ, Alam A, Huda TM, Raynes-Greenow C. Household food security and birth size of infants: analysis of the Bangladesh demographic and health survey 2011. *Curr Dev Nutr*. 2018;2(3):nzy003. https://doi.org/10.1093/cdn/nzy003
48. Webb-Girard A, Cherobon A, Mbugua S, Kamau-Mbuthia E, Amin A, Sellen DW. Food insecurity is associated with attitudes towards exclusive breastfeeding among women in urban Kenya. *Matern Child Nutr*. 2012;8(2):199–214. https://doi.org/10.1111/j.1740-8709.2010.00272.x
49. Macharia TN, Ochola S, Mutua MK, Kimani-Murage EW. Association between household food security and infant feeding practices in urban informal settlements in Nairobi, Kenya. *J Dev Orig Health Dis*. 2018;9(1):20–29. https://doi.org/10.1017/S2040174417001064
50. Orr SK, Dachner N, Frank L, Tarasuk V. Relation between household food insecurity and breastfeeding in Canada. *Can Med Assoc J*. 2018;190(11):E312–E319. https://doi.org/10.1503/cmaj.170880
51. Miller JD, Young SL, Boateng GO, Oiye S, Owino V. Greater household food insecurity is associated with lower breast milk intake among infants in western Kenya. *Matern Child Nutr.* 2019;15(4):e12862. https://doi.org/10.1111/mcn.12862
52. Berti C, Agostoni C, Davanzo R, et al. Early-life nutritional exposures and lifelong health: immediate and long-lasting impacts of probiotics, vitamin D, and breastfeeding. *Nutr Rev.* 2017;75(2):83–97. https://doi.org/10.1093/nutrit/nuw056
53. Dieterich CM, Felice JP, O'Sullivan E, Rasmussen KM. Breastfeeding and health outcomes for the mother-infant dyad. *Pediatr Clin North Am*. 2013;60(1):31–48. https://doi.org/10.1016/j.pcl.2012.09.010
54. Ali NB, Tahsina T, Hoque DME, et al. Association of food security and other socio-economic factors with dietary diversity and nutritional statuses of children aged 6-59 months in rural Bangladesh. *PLoS One*. 2019;14(8):e0221929. https://doi.org/10.1371/journal.pone.0221929
55. Saha KK, Frongillo EA, Alam DS, Arifeen SE, Persson LA, Rasmussen KM. Household food security is associated with infant feeding practices in rural Bangladesh. *J Nutr.* 2008;138(7):1383–1390. https://doi.org/10.1093/jn/138.7.1383
56. Agbadi P, Urke HB, Mittelmark MB. Household food security and adequacy of child diet in the food insecure region north in Ghana. *PLoS One*. 2017;12(5):e0177377. https://doi.org/10.1371/journal.pone.0177377
57. Moradi S, Mirzababaei A, Mohammadi H, et al. Food insecurity and the risk of undernutrition complications among children and adolescents: a systematic review and meta-analysis. *Nutrition*. 2019;62:52–60. https://doi.org/10.1016/j.nut.2018.11.029
58. Bronte-Tinkew J, Zaslow M, Capps R, Horowitz A, McNamara M. Food insecurity works through depression, parenting, and infant feeding to influence overweight and health in toddlers. *J Nutr.* 2007;137(9):2160–2165. https://doi.org/10.1093/jn/137.9.2160

59. Gross RS, Mendelsohn AL, Fierman AH, Racine AD, Messito MJ. Food insecurity and obesogenic maternal infant feeding styles and practices in low-income families. *Pediatrics*. 2012;130(2):254–261. https://doi.org/10.1542/peds.2011-3588
60. Nettle, D., Andrews, C., Bateson, M. (2017). Food insecurity as a driver of obesity in humans: The insurance hypothesis. *Behavioral and Brain Sciences*. 40:e105. https://doi.org/10.1017/S0140525X16000947
61. Cain KS, Meyer SC, Cummer E, et al. Association of food insecurity with mental health outcomes in parents and children. *Acad Pediatr*. 2022;22(7):1105–1114. https://doi.org/10.1016/j.acap.2022.04.010
62. Shankar P, Chung R, Frank DA. Association of food insecurity with children's behavioral, emotional, and academic outcomes: a systematic review. *J Dev Behav Pediatr*. 2017;38(2):135–150. https://doi.org/10.1097/DBP.0000000000000383
63. Eicher-Miller HA, Zhao Y. Evidence for the age-specific relationship of food insecurity and key dietary outcomes among U.S. children and adolescents. *Nutr Res Rev*. 2018;31(1):98–113. https://doi.org/10.1017/S0954422417000245
64. Hanson KL, Connor LM. Food insecurity and dietary quality in U.S. adults and children: a systematic review. *Am J Clin Nutr*. 2014;100(2):684–692. https://doi.org/10.3945/ajcn.114.084525
65. Bruening M, Argo K, Payne-Sturges D, Laska MN. The struggle is real: a systematic review of food insecurity on postsecondary education campuses. *J Acad Nutr Diet*. 2017;117(11):1767–1791. https://doi.org/10.1016/j.jand.2017.05.022
66. Pourmotabbed A, Moradi S, Babaei A, et al. Food insecurity and mental health: a systematic review and meta-analysis. *Public Health Nutr*. 2020;23(10):1778–1790. https://doi.org/10.1017/S136898001900435X
67. Arenas DJ, Thomas A, Wang J, DeLisser HM. A systematic review and meta-analysis of depression, anxiety, and sleep disorders in U.S. adults with food insecurity. *J Gen Intern Med*. 2019;34(12):2874–2882. https://doi.org/10.1007/s11606-019-05202-4
68. Beltrán S, Arenas DJ, Pharel M, Montgomery C, Lopez-Hinojosa I, DeLisser HM. Food insecurity, type 2 diabetes, and hyperglycaemia: a systematic review and meta-analysis. *Endocrinol Diabetes Metab*. 2022;5(1):e00315. https://doi.org/10.1002/edm2.315
69. Beltrán S, Pharel M, Montgomery CT, López-Hinojosa IJ, Arenas DJ, DeLisser HM. Food insecurity and hypertension: a systematic review and meta-analysis. *PLoS One*. 2020;15(11):e0241628. https://doi.org/10.1371/journal.pone.0241628
70. Liu Y, Eicher-Miller HA. Food insecurity and cardiovascular disease risk. *Curr Atheroscler Rep*. 2021;23(6):24. https://doi.org/10.1007/s11883-021-00923-6
71. Pereira MHQ, Pereira MLAS, Campos GC, Molina MCB. Food insecurity and nutritional status among older adults: a systematic review. *Nutr Rev*. 2022;80(4):631–644. https://doi.org/10.1093/nutrit/nuab044
72. Caouette S, Boss L, Lynn M. Original research: the relationship between food insecurity and cost-related medication nonadherence in older adults: a systematic review. *Am J Nurs*. 2020;120(6):24–36. https://doi.org/10.1097/01.NAJ.0000668732.28490.c1
73. U.S. Department of Agriculture Food and Nutrition Service. *USDA Food and Nutrition Service*. 2022. https://www.fns.usda.gov/
74. Aussenberg RA, Billings KC, Falk G. *USDA Nutrition Assistance Programs: Response to the COVID-19 Pandemic.* CRS Report No. R46681. Congressional Research Service; 2023.
75. U.S. Department of Agriculture. USDA Farmers to Families Food Box. Accessed November 19, 2022. https://www.ams.usda.gov/selling-food-to-usda/farmers-to-families-food-box
76. Karpman M, Maag E, Zuckerman S, Wissoker D. *Child Tax Credit Recipients Experienced a Larger Decline in Food Insecurity and a Similar Change in Employment as Nonrecipients Between 2020 and 2021*. Urban-Brookings Tax Policy Center; 2022. https://www.urban.org/research/publication/child-tax-credit-recipients-experienced-larger-decline-food-insecurity
77. Bovell-Ammon A, McCann NC, Mulugeta M, Ettinger de Cuba S, Raifman J, Shafer P. Association of the expiration of child tax credit advance payments with food insufficiency in U.S. households. *JAMA Netw Open*. 2022;5(10):e2234438. https://doi.org/10.1001/jamanetworkopen.2022.34438
78. Food and Agriculture Organization, International Fund for Agricultural Development, World Food Programme. *Working Together to Fight Hunger and Poverty*. Food and Agriculture Organization, International Fund for Agricultural Development, World Food Programme; 2001.
79. World Food Programme. *WFP Strategic Plan (2022–2025)*. World Food Programme; 2021. https://executiveboard.wfp.org/document_download/WFP-0000132205

80. U.S. Agency for International Development. *USAID'S Legacy in Agriculture Development: 50 Years of Progress*. U.S. Agency for International Development; 2016. https://www.usaid.gov/agriculture-and-food-security/document/usaids-legacy-agricultural-development-50-years-progress
81. Ho MD, Hanrahan CE. *The Obama Administration's Feed the Future Initiative* (CRS Report No. R41612). Congressional Research Service; 2011.
82. Feeding America. *Charitable Food Assistance Participation in 2021*. Feeding America; 2022. https://www.feedingamerica.org/sites/default/files/2022-06/Charitable%20Food%20Assistance%20Participation%20in%202021.pdf
83. Bazerghi C, McKay FH, Dunn M. The role of food banks in addressing food insecurity: a systematic review. *J Community Health*. 2016;41(4):732–740. https://doi.org/10.1007/s10900-015-0147-5
84. Fram MS, Frongillo EA. Backpack programs and the crisis narrative of child hunger—a critical review of the rationale, targeting, and potential benefits and harms of an expanding but untested model of practice. *Adv Nutr*. 2018;9(1):1–8. https://doi.org/10.1093/advances/nmx008
85. Zhu H, An R. Impact of home-delivered meal programs on diet and nutrition among older adults: a review. *Nutr Health*. 2013;22(2):89–103. https://doi.org/10.1177/0260106014537146
86. Meals on Wheels America. *More Than a Meal: A Story of Meals on Wheels in Communities Across the Country*. Meals on Wheels America; 2019. https://www.mealsonwheelsamerica.org/docs/default-source/research/comprehensive-network-study-public-summary_may-2020.pdf
87. Khalid H, Gill S, Fox AM. Global aid for nutrition-specific and nutrition-sensitive interventions and proportion of stunted children across low- and middle-income countries: does aid matter? *Health Policy Plan*. 2019;34(suppl 2):ii18–ii27. https://doi.org/10.1093/heapol/czz106
88. Kaiser Family Foundation. Fact sheet: breaking down the U.S. global health budget by program area. April 18, 2023. https://files.kff.org/attachment/Fact-Sheet-Breaking-Down-US-Global-Health-Budget-by-Program-Area.pdf
89. Díaz-Bonilla E. *Financing SGD2 and Ending Hunger.* Center for Development Research ; 2021. https://doi.org/10.48565/scfss2021-ba75
90. Pérez-Escamilla R. Food security and the 2015–2030 sustainable development goals: from human to planetary health: perspectives and opinions. *Curr Dev Nutr*. 2017;1(7):e000513. https://doi.org/10.3945/cdn.117.000513
91. Ringler C, Dias P. *Water and Nutrition: Harmonizing Actions for the United Nations Decade of Action on Nutrition and the United Nations Water Action Decade*. United Nations System Standing Committee on Nutrition; 2020. https://www.unscn.org/uploads/web/news/document/Water-Paper-EN-WEB-25mar.pdf
92. Jepson WE, Wutich A, Collins SM, Boateng GO, Young SL. Progress in household water insecurity metrics: a cross-disciplinary approach. *WIREs Water*. 2017;4(3):e1214. https://doi.org/10.1002/wat2.1214
93. Miller JD, Workman CL, Panchang SV, et al. Water security and nutrition: current knowledge and research opportunities. *Adv Nutr*. 2021;12(6):2525–2539. https://doi.org/10.1093/advances/nmab075
94. Young SL, Frongillo EA, Jamaluddine Z, et al. Perspective: the importance of water security for ensuring food security, good nutrition, and well-being. *Adv Nutr.* 2021;12(4):1058–1073. https://doi.org/10.1093/advances/nmab003
95. Young SL. Viewpoint: the measurement of water access and use is key for more effective food and nutrition policy. *Food Policy*. 2021;104:102138. https://doi.org/10.1016/j.foodpol.2021.102138
96. Cetrone H, Santoso M, Petito L, et al. A participatory agroecological intervention reduces women's risk of probable depression through improvements in food security in Singida, Tanzania. *Curr Dev Nutr*. 2020;4(suppl 2):819. https://doi.org/10.1093/cdn/nzaa053_024
97. Santoso MV, Bezner Kerr RN, Kassim N, et al. A nutrition-sensitive agroecology intervention in rural Tanzania increases children's dietary diversity and household food security but does not change child anthropometry: results from a cluster-randomized trial. *J Nutr.* 2021;151(7):2010–2021. https://doi.org/10.1093/jn/nxab052
98. U.S. Department of Agriculture. Summer EBT. Accessed October 20, 2023. https://www.fns.usda.gov/sebt

10

PEDIATRIC OVERWEIGHT AND OBESITY: A GLOBAL PUBLIC HEALTH PRIORITY

Linda L. Knol and Caroline Brantley

LEARNING OBJECTIVES

At the end of this chapter, students will be able to:

1. Evaluate weight status of children and adolescents at the individual and population levels.
2. Locate population-based obesity statistics.
3. Describe the biological, social, familial, neighborhood, and media factors associated with childhood obesity.
4. Select strategies that may be appropriate to use in your community to address childhood obesity.
5. Describe treatment strategies for childhood obesity.

INTRODUCTION

Over the past three decades, the United States and many developing and developed countries have reported an increase in childhood **obesity** rates. Many social and health consequences are associated with obesity during childhood, including the risk of adult **overweight** or obesity. The current childhood obesity epidemic has resulted from a complex set of societal changes including family life, food availability, eating and **physical activity** patterns, and use of media. Given the complexity of this priority public health problem, prevention and treatment measures need to address energy imbalance (food and beverage intake versus physical activity) through multifaceted interventions within settings frequented by children and their families. This chapter discusses the causes and consequences of childhood obesity and effective interventions and treatment protocols.

OVERVIEW OF U.S. AND GLOBAL CHILDHOOD OBESITY ISSUES

National and Worldwide Health Objectives

Both the United States and the World Health Organization (WHO) have created plans to address childhood obesity. **Healthy People 2030**, a set of data-driven, national objectives for improvements in health and well-being, identifies the reduction of childhood and adolescent obesity as a national public health priority for the United States.[1] The United Nations Sustainable Development Goals (SDGs) includes 17 goals with 169 target indicators.[2] All 191 member states have agreed that reduction of obesity in children under 5 years age is a priority health issue.[3]

Measurement of Obesity

Although **body mass index (BMI)** does not directly measure excess body fat, it is highly correlated with direct measures of adiposity such as dual energy x-ray absorptiometry, skinfold thickness, and underwater weighing and is associated with poor health outcomes.[4] Because of the ease in obtaining height and weight measures, BMI is commonly used to assess weight status. BMI is calculated as follows:

$$\text{BMI} = \text{weight (kg)}/\text{height (m)}^2$$

See Appendix F for the BMI table. The established cut-offs used to determine adult overweight and obesity status cannot be used with children and adolescents because BMI changes substantially as children age, and these changes differ by biological sex. For example, a male with a BMI of 17.8 kg/m^2 would be considered obese at age 4 and underweight at age 19. Therefore, in children and adolescents, BMI must be plotted to a BMI-for-age growth chart. These charts, developed by the Centers for Disease Control and Prevention (CDC) and WHO, provide references depicting national and worldwide growth patterns of normally developing children. The American Academy of Pediatrics (AAP) recommends using BMI to screen for overweight and obesity in children starting at 2 years of age using the BMI-for-age 2000 CDC growth charts. For children under 2 years of age, the WHO charts can be used to assess weight-for-length. Growth charts are available on the CDC website.[5,6]

The CDC also recommends the following steps be used when assessing growth in children and adolescents.

Step 1: Obtain accurate measurements of height, weight, and age. The accuracy of these measures is extremely important.

- Age: For age in months, subtract date of measures from date of birth.
- Height: Standing height should be measured to ⅛ inch or 0.1 cm using a **stadiometer**. To assess height, a child should be able to stand on their own with line of sight parallel to the floor, and feet (heels), buttocks, shoulders, and back of the head resting against the stadiometer. Shoes and any hair decorations or hats should be removed.
- Weight: To assess weight, heavy clothing and shoes should be removed. Weight should be taken on a calibrated scale with the child standing in the middle of the scale. Weight should be recorded to the nearest decimal such as 55.5 lb or 25.1 kg.

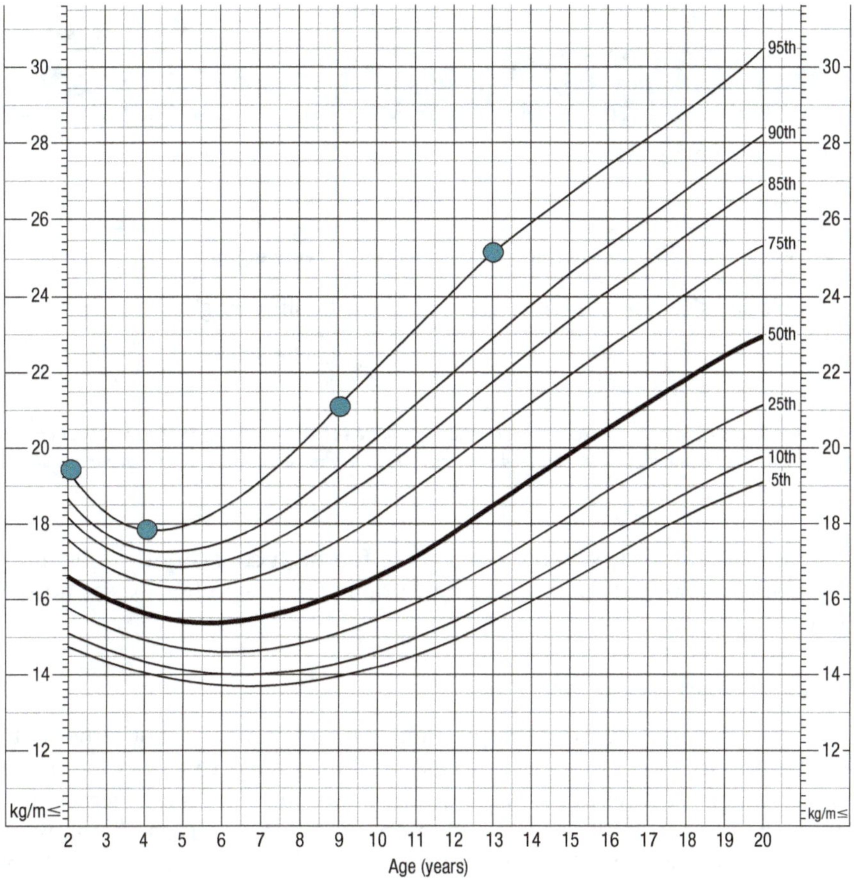

Figure 10.1. Center for Disease Control and Prevention growth chart: BMI-for-age for boys ages 2 to 20 years. Plot points show the curve of a boy measured at ages 2, 4, 9, and 13; he has consistently plotted at the 95th percentile.

BMI, body mass index.

Source: Adapted from Centers for Disease Control and Prevention. *Clinical* growth charts. Accessed October 16, 2023. https://www.cdc.gov/growthcharts/clinical_charts.htm

Step 2: Record the data. Calculate BMI.

Step 3: Select the appropriate growth chart. Plot measurements by finding the BMI on the *y*-axis and the age in months or years on the *x*-axis of the chart. Mark where the two lines intersect (Figure 10.1).

Step 4: Carefully interpret the plot. Each growth chart contains a series of growth curves with labels such as 5th or 95th percentile. Plots may fall directly on a line or between lines. When the plot falls between two lines, the plot indicates that the child is between two percentiles. For the child plotted in Figure 10.1, the plot shows that this child has consistently plotted at the 95th percentile, which means that the child's BMI is higher than 95% of boys his age.[7]

BMI-for-age percentile is used to help identify children and adolescents at risk for obesity-related chronic disease (Table 10.1).[7] For children and adolescents, BMI-for-age percentile is not a diagnostic tool but rather a screening tool. A series of plots are needed

Table 10.1. Interpretation of BMI-for-Age Percentiles From Growth Charts

BMI for Age	Nutritional Status
BMI ≥120% of the 95th percentile	Severely obese
≥95th percentile	Obese
≥85th percentile and <95th percentile	Overweight
≥5th percentile and <85th percentile	Healthy weight
<5th percentile	Underweight

BMI, body mass index.

Source: Centers for Disease Control and Prevention. Measuring children's height and weight accurately at home. Accessed October 16, 2023. https://www.cdc.gov/healthyweight/assessing/bmi/childrens_bmi/measuring_children.html/#Height

to establish a growth trend. When a child plots too high consistently, a healthcare provider may want to conduct further testing to determine whether excess adiposity is a health concern.

Prevalence of Childhood Obesity

In an effort to define the extent of the problem for policy makers and other community members, the public health nutrition professional may need to assess the overall **prevalence** of obesity or rates within specific groups, and monitor trends across time. These data may also be used to evaluate planned or ongoing interventions.[8] In many instances, these statistics may have already been captured through global, national, state, and local **surveillance** programs.

Global rates of child obesity are monitored by WHO and reported by region, country, age, and biological sex. WHO has also worked with other organizations to develop a tracking tool to monitor the six nutrition indicators associated with the Sustainable Development Goals.[9] Among children at or below 5 years or age, the prevalence of childhood obesity was 5.7% in 2020 representing 38.9 million children. Rates of obesity among children under 5 years worldwide are lowest in the least developed countries.[10]

In the United States, the prevalence of obesity is estimated using data collected in the National Health and Nutrition Examination Survey (NHANES). NHANES is a unique study that includes physical examination and interview data and samples noninstitutionalized infants, children, adolescents, and adults residing in the United States.[11] NHANES data are captured periodically. Therefore, these data can be used to assess changes in the prevalence of disease states such as obesity. Height and weight data are measured in person by highly trained staff. Using data from the 2017–2018 NHANES, the prevalence of overweight and obesity among children and adolescents, ages 2 to 19 years, was estimated at 16.1% and 19.3%, respectively. Figure 10.2 depicts the rise in U.S. obesity rates since 1963–1965. Between the 1966–1970 and the 2017–2020 NHANES, rates of obesity among U.S. adolescents have increased from 4.6% to 22.2%.[12]

Disparities in obesity rates exist by age, race and ethnicity, and family income in the United States. In 2017–2020, rates of obesity among children and adolescents ages 2 to 5, 6 to 11, and 12 to 19 years were 12.7, 20.7%, and 22.2%, respectively.[13] Youth identified as Hispanic (26.2%) and non-Hispanic Black (24.5%) had higher rates of obesity than their non-Hispanic

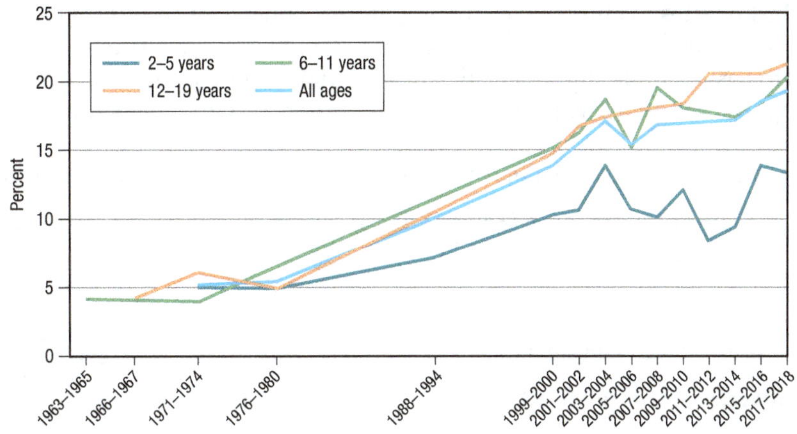

Figure 10.2. Trends in obesity among U.S. children and adolescents by age group: National Health and Nutrition Examination Survey (NHANES) 1963–1965 to 2017–2018.
Source: Fryar CD, Carroll MD, Afful J. Prevalence of overweight, obesity, and severe obesity among children and adolescents aged 2–19 years: United States, 1963–1965 through 2017–2018. Updated January 29, 2021. https://www.cdc.gov/nchs/data/hestat/obesity-child-17-18/obesity-child.htm

White (16.6%) and non-Hispanic Asian (9.0%) counterparts.[13] As family income increases in the United States, the rate of childhood obesity decreases. The prevalence of childhood obesity in youth living in low-income households, defined as a household with an overall income of less than 130% of the federal poverty threshold, was significantly higher than the rates of youth living in higher income households (25.8% versus 11.5%, respectively).[13]

At the state and local level, population-based obesity data for children and adolescents is limited and may rely on self- or parent-report, which introduces measurement bias and the potential for misclassification of weight status.[14] In-person measurement is the gold standard. However, it may be difficult to develop and coordinate in-person BMI measurement programs for many reasons. Self-report of height and weight has been used in public health surveillance projects such as the Youth Risk Behavior Surveillance System (YRBSS).[15] This survey is completed every 2 years by students attending public high schools across the United States. Obesity rates are reported by state. Although the rates are based on self-report, data are captured the same way across years and states. Thus, these data can be used to identify trends and compare rates between states.

Data for younger children are difficult to obtain because the child or parent may not be able to accurately self-report height and/or weight. If local data are needed, the public health interventionist may need to conduct in-person measurement of children in locations where children and adolescents congregate, such as schools. BMI measurement programs in schools may be completed for many reasons including surveillance of trends in weight status among a population over time or the identification of those at risk (screening). When surveillance is the goal of the program, data are usually anonymous, aggregated, and used to track trends. When screening is the goal, parents typically receive information about their child's weight status with the goals of helping correct parental misperceptions of the child's weight, motivating parents to make lifestyle changes, or referring parents to a healthcare provider for further evaluation.[8,16]

Critics of screening programs have argued that they may cause harm by increasing stigma, body dissatisfaction among youth, and the uptake of unsafe weight control behaviors.[8] To date, there is not enough evidence to suggest that BMI screening programs are reducing obesity rates in children or causing harm.[8] Thus, data collection for the purpose of surveillance is less controversial. Both the AAP and CDC have provided guidance for safeguards to ensure student privacy and confidentiality, protect against harm, and ensure that the program will generate positive outcomes. These safeguards include the following:

1. Inform parents about the program and obtain active parental and student consent for participation.
2. Ensure that personnel have the training needed to accurately obtain height and weight data while minimizing stigmatization.
3. Collect data in private.
4. Use accurate and reliable equipment.
5. Ensure BMI calculations are correct.
6. Coordinate data collection times with school personnel to ensure the process goes smoothly.
7. Do not use BMI for age percentiles to evaluate student performance in class.
8. Evaluate the BMI measurement program by assessing the process, outcomes, and potential harm.
9. Ensure resources are available for referral and follow-up.
10. Provide a respectful explanation of the results to parents with an appropriate list of follow-up activities.[8,16]

DETERMINANTS OF CHILDHOOD OBESITY

WHO defines social determinants of health as "the conditions in which people are born, work, live, and age, and the set of forces and systems shaping the conditions of daily life."[17] Thus, factors such as household income, family structure, parental education, housing, child care, and neighborhood characteristics have powerful effects on the health of the child.[17] Obesity is due to complex interactions between genetic, biological, developmental, behavioral, and environmental factors.[18] Many theories have emerged to explain the complex interactions among these factors. The social ecological model addresses the interaction of the individual with the larger social, cultural, economic, and environmental contexts that may shape the individual's health. In this model, the child's weight status may be influenced by individual factors (interpersonal), which are shaped by peer or family interactions (intrapersonal), household and neighborhood characteristics (community), social norms and media, and policy supporting physical activity and eating behavior in local settings the child frequents (e.g., schools, early child care facilities, afterschool programs).[19]

Biological Factors

Child level factors (individual factors) may include age, sex, race, genetics, developmental factors, and individual behaviors.[19] As discussed previously, disparities in childhood obesity rates exist by age, biological sex, and race.[10,13]

Genetic Factors

Genetic causes of obesity are classified as either monogenic or polygenic types.[18] Mongenic obesity, caused by a single gene mutation, is rare and typically presents before 2 years of age as **severe obesity** with abnormal eating behaviors. Genetic causes of obesity may include defects affecting regulation of hunger and satiety cueing, body weight, or energy metabolism. Other genetic causes of severe obesity include Prader–Willi syndrome, Bardet–Biedl syndrome, and Alström syndrome. Polygenic obesity, caused by a combination of genetic variants, is the common form of obesity. It is the result of the interaction between genetic susceptibility to obesity and environmental conditions that promote obesity. These genetic variants may increase food intake, decrease physical activity, decrease resting metabolic rate, or increase the ability to store body fat easily.[18,20] Individuals with a high genetic predisposition for obesity may be more likely to gain weight in excess when placed in an **obesigenic environment,** while individuals resistant to obesity may not gain weight or may gain less weight in the same environment.[18–20]

Epigenetics is the study of heritable changes in gene expression that are not caused by changes in the DNA sequence.[21] While DNA contains the instructions for building proteins that carry out many functions in the cell, the epigenome consists of proteins and chemical compounds that attach to the DNA and modify its instruction. Different cells have different **epigenetic** marks, which may or may not be replicated when the cell divides. When the genome is passed from parents to child, most but not all of the epigenome is reset. Environmental stressors, adverse childhood experiences (ACEs), and lifestyle factors (e.g., smoking or poor nutrition) may lead to changes that alter or damage the epigenome. Some adjustments to the epigenome may be helpful and allow humans to thrive in a changing environment (famine or feast) while others may increase the risk of disease. Additionally, there may be critical periods in development where over- and undernutrition may promote or impede disease development.[18,21,22]

Developmental Factors

Life course theory (LCT) suggests that health outcomes occur due to a *complex interplay* of social and environmental factors mixed with biological, behavioral, and psychological factors across the course of a person's life. *Each life stage exerts influence on the next stage and exposures accumulate over time to affect health.* Health trajectories are affected by social determinants of health during critical and sensitive periods of growth. These periods may include times of rapid growth, such as fetal development, early infancy, childhood, and adolescence. LCT can help explain disparities in obesity rates unrelated to genetics and individual choice.[21,23–26]

Fetal Growth and Birth Weight

According to the Pregnancy Risk Assessment Monitoring System (PRAMS), approximately 26% and 27% of U.S. women who gave birth in 2020 were overweight or obese, respectively.[27] Women who are overweight or obese prior to pregnancy are more likely to gain weight in excess of recommendations for optimal fetal and maternal health.[25,26] Maternal obesity, excessive gestational weight gain, and diet during pregnancy are independent risk factors for childhood adiposity and later cardiovascular and metabolic risk.[25,26] Obesity during pregnancy leads to altered hormonal and inflammatory activity. Thus, maternal obesity may lead to insulin resistance and gestational diabetes, which may lead to excess or rapid fetal growth and an infant that is large for gestational age (LGA) at birth.[28] LGA infants are at risk for birth trauma, cesarean delivery, and metabolic syndrome (obesity, insulin resistance, and hyperlipidemia) in childhood.[29] The proinflammatory state triggered by obesity may also lead to vascular injury, preeclampsia, preterm birth, and low birth weight. Low birth weight is associated with decreased risk of obesity later in life.[28] However, rapid catch-up growth in infants born with low birth weights may lead to increased risk of childhood obesity.[28]

First 1,000 Days

The first 1,000 days is an important time for brain development, as well as a period in which a normal growth trajectory can be established.[30] The AAP recommends that infants be exclusively breastfed for approximately 6 months after birth. The AAP also supports the continuation of breastfeeding up to 2 years of age or as long as mutually desired with the addition of appropriate complementary foods. In two recent meta-analyses, breastfeeding was associated with reduced risk of obesity.[31,32] When compared to children never breastfed, Qiao et al. found any breastfeeding reduced the risk of obesity in children ages 2 to 6 years by 17%.[32] Additionally, exclusive breastfeeding for at least 4 months reduced the risk for early childhood obesity by 47%. Horta et al. found similar results in children, ages 1 to 9 years, regardless of whether the studies were completed in high-income or middle/low-income countries.[31] Several mechanisms may explain this relationship. First, the components of breast milk may influence the development of a gut microbiome profile that is associated with a lower risk of obesity.[30] Second, breast milk is lower in protein than most of the human milk substitute (HMS) on the market. A few recent studies have shown that reducing the protein in HMS to mimic that found in breast milk prevented excessive early weight gain and obesity risk among preschool children.[33–36] More studies are needed to understand the long-term health effects of lowering the protein content of HMS. Third, infants who are breastfed may learn to honor their hunger and satiety cues, which may lead to better regulation of appetite and satiety cues later in life.[25,31,32] Breastfeeding mothers are also more likely to delay the introduction of complementary foods (CF).[37] However, studies assessing the early introduction of CF (less than 4 months) and types of CF introduced and later obesity show mixed results.[38]

Early Adiposity Rebound and Puberty

Rapid accumulation of body fat early in life may contribute to obesity later in life. Typically, BMI begins to decrease after 1 year of age, falls to its lowest value around 3 to 8 years of age, and then continues to increase. This is a normal pattern of growth, and is illustrated by the shape of the CDC growth chart curve (Figure 10.1). The age in which BMI is at its lowest value is the age of adiposity rebound (AR). Early AR, age of adiposity rebound below 5 years, is on the rise worldwide. Early AR may contribute to the development of obesity later in life. Causes of early AR need further investigation.[39] In addition, obesity may lead to early onset of puberty (early menarche and breast bud development) among girls. More research is needed to understand the relationship between puberty and obesity in boys.[40] Overweight and obesity prior to puberty increases the risk for adult overweight/obesity.[39,40]

Behavioral Factors

Dietary Behaviors

Researchers have assessed the relationship between childhood obesity and intake of specific foods, nutrients, and dietary patterns. Many of these studies were cross-sectional or prospective cohort studies. Thus, it may be difficult to determine whether consumption of a specific food, food group, or nutrient leads to obesity.[41] For example, in a recent systematic review, authors found that whole milk consumption compared to low-fat milk consumption lowered the risk of childhood obesity by 39% in children ages 1 to 18 years. Another interpretation of this study's results is that parents of children with overweight and obesity attempted to control the weight of their child by replacing high-fat milk for lower fat milk.[42] Different definitions of family meal, sugar-sweetened beverage, breakfast, and fast food make it difficult to draw conclusions about the contribution of these behaviors or foods on the risk of childhood obesity. Given these limitations, several dietary factors have emerged as targets for interventions. First, consumption of sugar-sweetened beverages (SSBs), or beverages that contain added caloric sweeteners, has a positive association with obesity in a large number of studies.[42] Skipping breakfast, defined as not eating between 6 a.m. and 9 a.m., and less frequent family meals are eating behaviors in children that increase in frequency as the child ages. Both behaviors are associated with lower dietary quality and obesity. Additionally, higher consumption of meals is associated with lower risk for obesity while snacking, especially on energy-dense food items, may contribute to obesity. Additional high-quality intervention studies are needed to evaluate the effect of alterations in diet or dietary patterns and childhood obesity.[42]

Physical Activity and Sedentary Behavior

Physical activity is defined as body movement produced by skeletal muscles that contribute to an increase in energy expenditure.[42,43] **Sedentary behaviors** are defined by researchers as any waking behavior that is completed in a sitting or reclining posture. Physical activity and sedentary behaviors are independent risk factors of obesity. However, these two behaviors are not highly correlated.[42,43] In other words, one can be very active and also engage in high amounts of sedentary activity. Among sedentary behaviors, recreational **screen time** and long periods of uninterrupted sedentary behaviors are associated with obesity and cardiometabolic risk. Additionally, high screen time is associated with eating habits that may favor weight gain.[43]

Sleep Behaviors

In children and adolescents, sleep requirements are related to developmental age. The National Sleep Foundation suggests that preschoolers, children 6 to 13 years old, and adolescents 14 to 17 years old get 10 to 13, 9 to 11, and 8 to 10 hours of sleep per day, respectively.[44] However, the CDC reports approximately one third of children, ages 4 months to 17 years, slept less than the recommended amounts.[45] Short sleep duration, below recommendations, is associated with obesity in children and adolescents.[46,47] Sleep duration appears to play a role in the blood glucose levels and the orexin system, which controls appetite, wakefulness, and energy expenditure. Low sleep duration may be related to obesity by increasing energy intake and decreasing energy expenditure. Low sleep duration leads to an increase in ghrelin and decrease in leptin, which increase appetite. Additionally, longer periods of wakefulness may also lead to more opportunities to eat. Short sleep duration may also lead to voluntary reduction in physical activity throughout the day due to sleepiness. Sleep duration and quality may also be influenced by screen time, low levels of physical activity, poor spacing of meals, late night eating habits, and caffeine use.[44–46]

Home Environment

Children spend a large portion of their day in the home environment. The *Home Food Environment Model of Childhood Obesity* suggests that the home microenvironment is enmeshed within the larger community or macro environment and family determinants of childhood obesity can be placed into three domains: political and economic environment, social and cultural environment, and built environment.[48] The three domains influence one another and collectively or independently influence children's dietary and physical activity behaviors, which influences the child's weight status.

Political and Economic Home Environment

Family socioeconomic status, household food security status, and participation in food assistance programs are components of the political and economic environments. These factors may shape the types of foods that are brought into the home and consumed, and physical and sedentary activity.[48] Children growing up in households with low socioeconomic status are also at greater risk for developing obesity and mental health problems.[49–51] Families living in low-income neighborhoods may not have access to healthy foods or opportunities for physical activity. Financial hardship is usually coupled with the reasons that caretakers cannot gain employment. These factors may be related to where the family lives or individual parental characteristics such as job training or education. When the parent is not gainfully employed or enjoying their job or jobs, it can lead to low self-esteem or self-worth, feeling as if nothing will ever change, food and financial insecurity, and negative emotions. When financial hardship is combined with low self-esteem, disempowerment, stress, and negative emotions, individuals find themselves making hasty decisions about food, coping with negative emotions with food, and may become more susceptible to food marketing or environmental cues to eat. If a child spends the first few years of their life in this type of environment, then these behaviors are learned and difficult to unlearn.[49–51] In addition, food insecurity and poor access to food are predictors of poor intake, especially parental intake—a role model for healthy or unhealthy food choices for children.[49–51]

Social and Cultural Environment

The social and cultural environment of the home is influenced by family structure, stress, and schedules; parenting styles and rules; parental role modeling of eating and physical activity habits; and parental food preparation skills and nutrition knowledge.[48] Research suggests that early childhood adversity (e.g., socioeconomic adversity, family dysfunction, neglect, and abuse or child maltreatment), is an independent risk factor for obesity and can lead to poor self-esteem, chronic stress, poor mental health, chronic inflammation, and increased appetite.[49] Financial hardship can lead to relationship problems among the adults, and lack of family cohesion. Mental health problems, addiction, and financial hardship can occur simultaneously. These disruptions in family life lead to disturbances in social, psychological, and emotional nurturing of the child. Young children internalize their external environment. They do not know how to cope with the emotions they are feeling and can become highly sensitive. These reactions may lead to more stress, which raises cortisol levels and increases chronic inflammation.[49–51] Family dysfunction may encourage the young child to adopt maladaptive coping mechanisms such as stress-related and emotional eating.[49–51] Lastly, interpersonal violence in childhood is also a risk factor for obesity. Interpersonal violence can be defined as physical abuse, sexual abuse, domestic violence within the home, bullying by peers, and neighborhood crime. Children who experienced interpersonal violence may report emotional difficulties, negative affect, disordered eating, and physical inactivity. These factors may play a role in the relationship between interpersonal violence and obesity. Additionally, overweight and obese children and adolescents are often victims of bullying by peers.[51]

Parenting styles, feeding practices, and parental role modeling of dietary and physical activity behaviors are also aspects of the social and cultural home environment.[52,53] Parenting style refers to the general interaction between the parent and child. There are four styles based on two dimensions: warmth/responsiveness and control/demandingness. Authoritative parents (high warmth/high control) have high expectations, show

Table 10.2. Types of Parenting Styles and Feeding Styles

Authoritative (High Control/High Warmth)	Authoritarian (High Control, Low Warmth)	Permissive (Indulgent or Neglectful)
• Balance healthful intake with child's food preferences • Take responsibility • Encourage healthful intake, monitor child's intake • Role model appropriate behaviors	• Restricting specific foods • Controlling child's intake without thinking about preferences • Pressure to eat • Monitoring in a negative manner	• Indulgent, nonrestricting • Possibly neglectful • Allows child to make decisions • Role modeling inappropriate behaviors

Source: Hubbs-Tait L, Kennedy TS, Page MC, Topham GL, Harrist AW. Parental feeding practices predict authoritative, authoritarian, and permissive parenting styles. *J Am Diet Assoc* 2008;108:1154–1161. https://doi.org/10.1016/j.jada.2008.04.008

high parental affection, and set respectful limits. Authoritarian parents (high control/low warmth) may be strict, and insensitive to their child's needs. This type of parenting may result in a child who is motivated by external controls. Permissive parents are categorized as indulgent or neglectful (low control with either high or low warmth). These parents have low expectations for the child's self-control and/or set few limits. This parenting style may lead to poor self-regulation of behavior in the child. Each parenting style is associated with characteristic feeding practices (Table 10.2).[54] In a systematic review of prospective studies, Sokol and colleagues found five out of eight prospective studies that assessed parenting style and later risk of obesity found that when compared to other styles, maternal and/or paternal authoritative parenting was associated with less risk of obesity among both boys and girls. However, results were inconsistent between styles and minority groups were not well represented in the selected studies.[52]

Built Environment

For the child, the home food and physical activity environments are created by the caregivers, which are influenced by access to safe, nutritious, and affordable foods; safe housing; adequate recreational opportunities; and a safe water supply. Thus, the built environment includes availability and accessibility of "healthy" (e.g., fruits, vegetables, low-fat milk and proteins, and whole grains) and "unhealthy" (e.g., SSBs, chips, snack cakes, sweets, and candy) foods, kitchen appliances, home gardens, and media equipment and electronic devices.[48] Researchers have attempted to assess the characteristics of the home environment associated with child overweight and identified three domains: home food environment (foods availability and accessibility), home physical activity environment (physical activity and facilities availability and accessibility), and home media environment (media equipment availability and accessibility). Parental practices and role modeling of specific behaviors influence availability and accessibility.[55]

In their systematic review of home environment and child obesity, Kininmonth and colleagues found the home media environment had the most consistent association with child obesity across all studies.[55] Among the 29 studies assessed, 21 suggested a positive relationship between availability and access to electronic media equipment and child obesity. Two strong predictors of child obesity included a higher number of electronic or screen devices in the home and having a television in the child's bedroom. In their review of 15 studies on the relationship between the home food environment and child obesity, six studies showed an association between food or drink availability and child obesity while eight did not. When assessing the seven available studies on the home physical activity environment and child obesity, they found that only three out of seven studies suggest that the availability and access to equipment was associated with lower rates of child overweight.[55]

CONSEQUENCES OF CHILDHOOD OBESITY

Childhood obesity is linked with multiple comorbidities previously thought of as "adult" diseases and affects almost every system in the body.[18,56] Children with obesity are at increased risk for cardiometabolic and cardiovascular disorders such as insulin resistance, prediabetes, type 2 diabetes mellitus, elevated blood pressure, low levels of high-density lipoprotein (HDL) cholesterol, and high levels of triglycerides.[56] Additionally, children with severe obesity are at greater risk of obstructive sleep apnea, which may affect the quality and duration of sleep, attention span, daytime wakefulness, and risky decision-making. Obesity is the leading cause of nonalcoholic fatty liver disease (NAFLD) in children. Childhood obesity also increases the risk of musculoskeletal problems that may lead to poor mobility, joint pain, lower extremity malalignment, and increased risk for fracture. Lastly, child obesity is associated with higher risk of pseudotumor cerebri, menstrual irregularities, early puberty in girls, and polycystic ovaries.[18,56] Persistence of obesity into adulthood depends on the age of onset of obesity during childhood, severity of obesity, and genetic predisposition or parental obesity.[56]

Children with obesity are at increased risk for several psychosocial health issues including depression, dissatisfaction with body image, low self-esteem, and social isolation.[18,56] Body dissatisfaction can lead to disordered eating habits (e.g., meal skipping, dieting, and binge eating), depression, and low self-esteem. When compared with children at a **healthy weight**, children with obesity are also likely to be teased or bullied as a result of their weight status, which can have severe and lasting emotional consequences.[18,56] Weight stigmatization is defined as the devaluation of others based on weight.[57] Weight stigmatization is often tolerated in society because of the belief that stigma and shame may motivate people to lose weight. Children who are overweight/obese often experience weight stigma such as peer bullying and teasing. However, other sources may include parents/caregivers, educators, healthcare providers, and the media. For example, characters in the media who are slim are often portrayed as kind, loving, and attractive while those with larger body sizes are mean, unintelligent, and unpopular with unhealthy behaviors.[57] Media consumed by children often portrays the larger characters as the target of jokes or ridicule. Weight stigmatization can lead to binge eating, substance use, social isolation, decreased physical activity, avoidance of healthcare services, school absenteeism, increased weight gain, and poor quality of life.[57]

POLICY PERSPECTIVES: GLOBAL ISSUES AND CHALLENGES

As stated previously, both the United States and WHO have created plans to address childhood obesity. In the United States, the National Collaborative on Childhood Obesity Research (NCCOR) coordinates efforts to reduce obesity in the United States by bringing together the four leading funders of research: Division of Nutrition, Physical Activity, and Obesity within the CDC, U.S. Department of Agriculture, National Institutes of Health, and Robert Wood Johnson Foundation.[58] Additionally, the Institutes of Medicine Committee on Progress in Prevention of Childhood Obesity suggests the use of the social ecological model with interventions aimed to address more than one level within the model to promote a healthy marketplace and media environment, healthy communities, healthy schools, and healthy homes.[59] WHO suggests a similar strategy.[60]

EFFECTIVE PUBLIC HEALTH NUTRITION INTERVENTIONS TO PREVENT AND TREAT PEDIATRIC OBESITY

Prevention of Pediatric Overweight and Obesity

The interventionist should look to the literature to guide the selection of obesity-preventive interventions that may work best for a given population. Given the complexity of the problem, a multilevel approach is needed. To this end, the CDC has suggested 24 recommendations within six categories to promote obesity prevention.[61]

Category 1: Promote the Availability and Affordability of Healthy Food and Beverages. Strategies in this domain focus on improving access to healthy foods in public venues (e.g., schools, early child care settings, afterschool programs, city and county buildings, recreation centers, parks, playgrounds, and juvenile detention centers) and making these items affordable. Also included under this domain was increasing the availability of supermarkets in lower income neighborhoods, improving the number of healthy options offered at food retailers such as corner stores, and improving farm-to-table programs such as farmers market programs or community supported agriculture (CSA) programs.

Category 2: Support Healthy Food and Beverage Choices. This set of strategies focus on restricting availability of less healthy items, instituting smaller portion sizes at public venues, limiting media messages about less healthy foods and beverages, and discouraging SSB intake.

Category 3: Encourage Breastfeeding. Strategies in this category focus on improving breastfeeding policy in the workplace and maternity care centers, availability of breastfeeding education programs and lactation consultants, and revising laws that prohibit breastfeeding in public.

Category 4: Encourage Physical Activity and Limit Sedentary Activity. Suggested strategies include requiring physical education in schools, improving the quality of these programs, and reducing screen time in public venues.

Category 5: Create Safe Communities That Support Physical Activity. These strategies include increasing access to outdoor recreational facilities and the number of activities offered, improving infrastructure to support bicycling and walking, locating schools in walking distances of residential areas, improving access to public transportation, and enhancing safety in high traffic areas and unsafe neighborhoods.

Category 6: Community Organization to Promote Change. This strategy focusesd on the development of local planning and implementation teams. These teams should take the time to build a sustainable infrastructure and advocate for changes.[61]

To address their recommendations, the CDC has published guidance on the implementation of effective strategies to:

- Increase physical activity in the community
- Increase fruit and vegetable consumption
- Increase breastfeeding rates
- Develop and implement school health guidelines
- prepare a community guide (a booklet that helps the public health nutrition professional select appropriate programs and polices appropriate for their specific community)
- Establish healthful food and nutrition practices in early child care settings[62]

Treatment of Pediatric Overweight and Obesity

Overview

In public health nutrition, our role is to ensure an adequately trained workforce, provide resources to that workforce, ensure referrals, and ensure adequate numbers of treatment facilities. Public health nutrition professionals may work in schools and other local community organizations where they may encounter children and adolescents with obesity who need referrals. Additionally, when community resources are limited public health nutrition professionals may assist in providing secondary and tertiary care treatment options. Therefore, while public health nutrition professionals may not provide care or services directly, it is important that they are aware of the treatment options and recommendations by the AAP.[63,64]

Evaluation of Pediatric Patients for Overweight or Obesity

The AAP suggests that all children and adolescents be universally assessed for obesity risk to improve early detection of elevated BMI, medical risks, and unhealthy eating and physical activity habits.[63] Under this recommendation, annual, routine care from a primary healthcare provider for all children ages 2 and older would include the following: assessment of healthy eating and active living behaviors, prevention messages with ongoing positive reinforcement for healthy behaviors, and weight classifications using CDC BMI growth charts, which would be used in decision-making for additional screenings and treatment.[63]

Several validated tools have been used by providers to screen and assess healthy eating and lifestyle behaviors. Such tools are used to evaluate intake of various food groups, SSBs, screen time, physical activity, and other family environmental factors. The Family Nutrition and Physical Activity (FNPA) screening tool is designed to assess family environmental and behavioral factors that may predispose a child to obesity.[65] This tool can be used by pediatricians, pediatric obesity clinics, school-based projects, and researchers (Table 10.3).

The APP additionally recommends providers deliver prevention messages at every well-child checkup to all children and adolescents and their parents.[63] Prevention messages focus on the promotion of a healthy diet and lifestyle. Let's Go! 5–2–1–0 has been promoted locally and nationally for broad utilization. The program focuses on simple messages that can be delivered by primary healthcare providers at a child's annual wellness visit: eat 5 or more servings of fruits and vegetables per day, limit screen time to 2 hours or less per day, get 1 hour or more of physical activity per day, and drink almost no sugary beverages.[66]

Table 10.3. Family Nutrition and Physical Activity Screening Tool

For each question, answer NEVER, SOMETIMES, OFTEN, or ALWAYS. Select the answer that best fits your child or your family. It is important to indicate the most common or typical pattern for your family, and not what you would like to happen. Scoring: Each item should be scored on a scale of 1 to 4 where 4 represents the more favorable practice. Questions 3,4,5,7,10, and 13 are reversed coded so values should be flipped before developing a summary score.

Family Meals

1. How often does your child eat breakfast, either at home or at school?
2. How often does your child eat at least one meal a day with at least one other family member?

Family Eating Practices

3. How often does your child eat while watching TV?
4. How often does your family eat "fast food"?

Food Choices

5. How often does your family use packaged "ready to eat" foods?
6. How often does your child eat fruits and vegetables at meals or snacks?

Beverage Choices

7. How often does your child drink soda pop or sweetened beverages?
8. How often does your child drink low-fat milk for meals or snacks?

Restriction/Reward

9. How often does your family monitor the amount of candy, chips, and cookies your child eats?
10. How often does your family use candy, ice cream, or other foods as a reward for good behavior?

Screen Time

11. How often does your child have less than 2 hours of "screen time" in a day?
12. How often does your family monitor the amount of "screen time" your child has?

Healthy Environment

13. How often does your child engage in screen time in his/her bedroom?
14. How often does your family provide opportunities for physical activity?

Family Activity

15. How often does your family encourage your child to be physically active?
16. How often does your child do physical activities with at least one other family member?

Child Activity

17. How often does your child do something physically active when he/she has free time?
18. How often does your child participate in organized sports or physical activities with a coach or leader?

Family Schedule/Sleep Routine

19. How often does your child follow a regular routine for your child's bedtime?
20. How often does your child get enough sleep at night?

Source: Ihmels MA, Welk GJ, Eisenmann JC, Nusser SM. Development and preliminary validation of a Family Nutrition and Physical Activity (FNPA) screening tool. *Int J Behav Nutr Phys Act*. 2009;6:14. https://doi.org/10.1186/1479-5868-6-1466

Child Obesity Management and Treatment Stages

Often there is a strong emphasis on weight loss with the narrowed focus advice to just eat less. Temporary and restrictive diets, often referred to as fad diets, are strategies adopted for adult weight loss, promising quick results but poor long-term improved health outcomes. Fad diets lack scientific rigor and tend to emphasize a singular food component to increase, reduce, or eliminate. Due to the popularity of fad diets, healthcare providers should be concerned that children or adolescents may engage in these restrictive eating behaviors without proper medical management. Therefore, it is important for primary care providers to understand the potential harm of fad dieting for children and how to motivate children and families to follow suggested advice under medical management, which would include assessment and screening of adequacy of the diet, growth, and BMI measurement.[63]

BMI measurement is the main tool used to screen for obesity and therefore the AAP uses BMI percentiles within its treatment algorithm to help make decisions regarding the need for additional screenings and initial steps for treatment.[63,64] Laboratory screenings and assessment for current medical conditions or future risk are suggested as a part of routine care requiring all children to receive a nonfasting lipid profile between the ages of 9 and 11 and again between the ages of 18 and 21.[67] However, for children who are diagnosed with overweight, obesity, or severe obesity, additional laboratory tests (fasting lipid profile, fasting glucose, and liver enzymes) may be needed depending on the child's age, family and medical history, and the presence of risk factors for type 2 diabetes mellitus and NAFLD (Table 10.4).

For treatment of overweight or obesity, the AAP suggests concurrent treatment of obesity and comorbid conditions for which the goals may include weight loss or avoidance of

Table 10.4. Components of Comprehensive Evaluation Based on Age and Weight Status of the Child/Adolescent

Component	Overweight		Obese	
	<10 years	≥10 years	<10 years	≥10 years
Comprehensive history including medical, social, nutrition, and physical activity; assessment of motivation to change; mental and behavioral health screening; physical exam; and diagnostic studies	x	x	x	x
Blood pressure	x	x	x	x
Fasting lipid panel		x		x
Fasting plasma glucose, oral glucose tolerance test, hemoglobin A1c		Depends on family history and medical presentation		x

Source: Hampl SE, Hassink SG, Skinner AC, et al. Clinical practice guideline for the evaluation and treatment of children and adolescents with obesity. *Pediatrics*. 2023;151:e2022060640. https://doi.org/10.1542/peds.2022-060640

Table 10.5. Components of Comprehensive Treatment by Age and Weight Status of the Child

Components	Overweight			Obesity		
	<6 years	6–<12 years	≥12 years	<6 years	6–<12 years	≥12 years
Motivational interviewing	x	x	x	x	x	x
Intensive health behavior and lifestyle treatment		x	x		x	x
Weight loss pharmacotherapy						x
Offer referral to comprehensive pediatric metabolic & bariatric surgery programs						x

Source: Hampl SE, Hassink SG, Skinner AC, et al. Clinical practice guideline for the evaluation and treatment of children and adolescents with obesity. *Pediatrics*. 2023;151:e2022060640. https://doi.org/10.1542/peds.2022-060640

further weight gain and improvements in obesity-related comorbidities.[64] Additionally, the primary healthcare practitioner should attempt to address underlying causes of obesity using social determinants of health and a family-centered approach. Components of a comprehensive treatment plan will depend on the child's age and weight status (Table 10.5). Motivational interviewing (MI), a patient-centered approach to counseling, should be used. This approach identifies and reinforces a patient's motivation to change goal behaviors. The target of MI should be the person who is responsible for behavior change. For the young child, this may be the parent.

Intensive Health Behavior and Lifestyle Treatment

For children 6 years of age or older, the primary healthcare practitioner should refer patients and their families as soon as possible to an evidence-based Intensive Health Behavior and Lifestyle Treatment (IHBLT) program led by a multidisciplinary team.[64] These intensive programs, 3 to 12 months in duration with more than 26 contact hours, focus on behavioral therapy and health education. These programs may be offered in group, individual family, or both situations and may be conducted either face to face or virtually. When intensive programs are not available, the public health nutrition professional may want to develop a list of resources available for primary healthcare provider referrals.

Pharmacotherapy

The AAP recommends pediatricians and other primary healthcare providers may use pharmacotherapy or medication in addition to health and lifestyle treatment in children with overweight, 12 years of age or older, or in children, 8 to 11 years with more life-threatening obesity-related comorbidities.[64] Medications are considered adjunctive therapy because if discontinued without significant behavioral changes, weight loss may be regained. There is no evidence to support weight loss medication as a monotherapy. There are not many medications approved by the Food and Drug Administration (FDA) for children and adolescents yet.[64]

Orlistat and phentermine are two of the medications approved for children and adolescents. Orlistat is FDA approved for long-term management of obesity in individuals ages 12 to 16 and is considered the first-line pharmacotherapy for adolescents with BMIs two or more units above the 95th percentile who continue to gain weight despite lifestyle modifications.[68] When studied in children, orlistat decreased BMI by 0.5 to 4.2 kg/m^2 compared to baseline or placebo.[69] Orlistat is an intestinal lipase inhibitor, which means it acts by decreasing hydrolysis of ingested triglycerides, reducing gastrointestinal (GI) absorption of fat by 30%.[68] Due to the unabsorbed fat excreted in the feces, side effects may include transient diarrhea, abdominal discomfort, and flatulence. A diet containing no more than 30% calories from fat and rich in dietary fibers is recommended to reduce GI side effects.[68–70] Alli is an over-the-counter form of orlistat at half the prescription strength.

Phentermine is FDA approved for short-term management of obesity (12 weeks or less) in individuals ages 16 and up.[71,72] Phentermine is an amphetamine analog that acts to suppress appetite by increasing catecholamines and serotonin activity in the central nervous system. Side effects of concern include increased blood pressure, rapid heart rate, anxiety, and headache.[72] When treating adolescents, phentermine with lifestyle therapy resulted in statistically significant reductions in weight and BMI percentile compared to lifestyle therapy alone.[72] While proved to be a powerful weight loss aid, without significant lifestyle changes weight is likely to be regained when phentermine is discontinued.

Pediatric Metabolic and Bariatric Surgery

Pediatricians and primary healthcare providers should offer referrals for adolescents, 13 years or older, with severe obesity for evaluation for metabolic and bariatric surgery to comprehensive multidisciplinary pediatric metabolic and bariatric surgery centers.[64] Three different surgeries are commonly performed, all of which have pros and cons.[73–75]

Laparoscopic adjustable gastric band is a restrictive surgery whereby an inflatable band is placed around the top part of the stomach, creating a small pouch with an adjustable opening. This procedure can be adjusted and reversed and poses the least risk of all the surgeries. However, one may have less weight loss compared to other surgeries and require more follow-up for band adjustments.

Vertical sleeve gastrectomy, also known as gastric sleeve, is a restrictive surgery as it requires removal of 80% of the stomach, creating a long vertical pouch. There is no change to the intestines within this surgery; however, due to the removal of a large portion of the stomach, one is at a greater risk for vitamin and iron deficiency. The gastric sleeve has potential for a greater amount of weight loss than the gastric band, but it is an irreversible surgery.

The *Roux-en-Y gastric bypass* is a bariatric surgical procedure whereby a small pouch is created in the top part of the stomach and is reattached to the small intestine. This surgery proposes the greatest amount of weight loss; however, it also has the greatest risk of surgery-related problems, and it is difficult to reverse. Due to the reconfiguration of the stomach, there is a high chance of vitamin and iron deficiency.

As surgery is a serious and often irreversible procedure, there are specific criteria for eligibility. The AAP discourages age limits for bariatric survey and more recent guidance advises that neither sexual maturation nor linear growth should be used as criteria for patient selection.[73] Therefore, selection largely mirrors that of adults, which includes having class 2 obesity (BMI >35, or 120% of the 95th percentile for age and sex) with an obesity-related health condition or class 3 obesity (BMI >40, or 140% of the 95th percentile for age and sex) without an obesity-related health condition.[64] Obesity-related conditions include obstructive sleep apnea, type 2 diabetes, Blount disease, slipped capital femoral epiphysis (SCFE), gastroesophageal reflux disease (GERD), and hypertension. In addition to BMI and comorbid conditions, physiologic, psychological, and developmental maturity are confirmed from a psychologist and physician. Children and adolescents must understand the risks and benefits of surgery and commit to adhere to lifelong dietary modifications. Additionally, children and adolescents must have family and social support leading up to and after surgery.[73–75]

WHAT WORKS

What Works 10.1: Let's Go! 5–2–1–0

Let's Go! 5–2–1–0 began as an initiative to support healthy eating and physical activity, major factors known to influence obesity in children.[66] Let's Go! 5–2–1–0 is a communication campaign to distribute the message regarding recommendations for healthy behaviors. Eat five or more servings of fruits and vegetables per day, limit screen time to 2 hours or less per day, get 1 hour or more of physical activity per day, and drink almost no sugary beverages. This communication campaign originally initiated in Nemours Children's Health in Delaware and later adopted by the Maine Youth Overweight Collaborative is supported by the AAP as the mantra recommended for counseling by primary care providers.

The specific components of the Maine Youth Overweight Collaborative Let's Go! 5–2–1–0 involved deploying this simple, yet consistent message across multiple community settings to remind families and children how to make healthy choices and to implement changes to the environment that support healthy behaviors within six major settings where families gather most.

Goals and Objectives

The goals of Let's Go! 5–2–1–0 were to:

1. Increase the awareness, knowledge, and practice of healthy behaviors by changing environments to support healthy choices and exposing families and children to a consistent health message.
2. Assess the strength of the environmental and policy changes implemented in three of the six settings.

Target Audience

The Let's Go 5–2–1–0 project was designed for all staff, patrons, and families involved at the participating sites. Settings of interest included child care programs, schools, afterschool programs, community sites, healthcare practices, and worksites within 12 communities near Portland, Maine.

Rationale for the Intervention

Let's Go 5–2–1–0 was initiated as a result of concern about the health and economic impacts of child obesity in Maine. While evidence is lacking on approaches that can be implemented and sustained at the community level, the research is clear that prevention strategies need to involve population-based interventions that are practical and target the places where people spend time. The Maine Youth Overweight Collaborative launched Let's Go! 5–2–1–0 program to improve healthy eating and physical activity, which are the main underlying health behaviors known to impact overweight and obesity.

Methodology

The Let's Go! 5–2–1–0 program was a 5-year demonstration project that consisted of a communication campaign and community-based intervention in six settings: schools, child care programs, afterschool programs, healthcare practices, community sites, and worksites. Eight public health professionals managed the design, implementation, and evaluation of the multifaceted project. From 2007 to 2011 a media campaign was executed to increase awareness of the 5–2–1–0 message among children and their families with advertisements broadcast on TV and spread through other targeted marketing approaches. Additionally, Let's Go! aligned with various partners around the community to promote 10 strategies within their own sites. Examples of these strategies included encouraging healthy choices for snacks, incorporating physical activity into the school day, collaborating with the School Nutrition Program, and developing a 5–2–1–0 friendly staff and wellness program.

Telephone interviews were conducted with parents at the midpoint and the end of the 5-year demonstration. A total of 800 parents of children, ages newborn to 18, living in the communities where Let's Go! was implemented were selected for each set of interviews. The survey covered domains on parent knowledge of the 5–2–1–0 recommendations, parent behaviors, child behaviors, awareness of and receptivity to program communications, intentions to change behaviors, and demographics.

Results

Over the 5-year program parent-survey data revealed statistically significant increases in parent awareness of the program message, knowledge in the four recommendations, and child adherence with two of the recommendations, consuming five or more fruits and vegetables and limiting sugary beverages each day. Following completion of the program in 2011, a majority of parents reported the reaction to the program as very positive. Surveys collected regarding site-based implementation revealed that there was a widespread implementation of Let's Go! strategies in child care programs, elementary schools, and afterschool programs. The three strategies that were implemented more frequently were encouraging healthy choices for snacks, encouraging drinking water, and increasing physical activity during the day.

Lessons Learned

A community-based environmental change program with a simple message is a feasible approach to reach families in multiple settings and can positively improve healthy eating and physical activity behaviors. Specific implementation strategies included providing toolkits for schools, child care, and afterschool programs on how to promote the 5–2–1–0 message and strategies, encouraging healthcare practices to hang posters in waiting rooms and hold conversations with their patients and families about healthy habits and the 5–2–1–0 message, and increased access to drinking water and improved local trails within community sites.

5–2–1–0 has continued to be adopted by states across the country. Several health departments utilize this message within their programs and provide toolkits and resources for use in a variety of sectors, such as child care, schools, afterschool programs, healthcare, workplaces, and parents and caregivers. Examples of some of these programs are the Kentucky

Department for Public Health Nutrition, Physical Activity, and Obesity Program (chfs.ky.gov/agencies/dph/dpqi/cdpb/hpdocs/5210Toolkitoptimized.pdf), the Healthiest State Initiative in Iowa (www.iowahealthieststate.com/resources/individuals/5210/resources), and the Nemours Children's Health program (www.nemours.org/services/health/growuphealthy/521almostnone.html). 5-2-1-0 is also an easy mantra for healthcare providers to use when counseling parents, children, and teens.

What Works 10.2: Coordinated Approach to Child Health

Coordinated Approach to Child Health (CATCH) is a coordinated school health program that integrates classroom learning with changes in the school environment.76,77 Across the United States, more than 10,000 school have used CATCH from preschool to eighth grade. The goals of CATCH are to:

promote physical activity and healthy food choices for children.

promote an environment that allows children the opportunity to engage in physical activity and select healthy food choices.

The program includes:

Classroom instruction promoting healthy behaviors

Lessons for physical education teachers

Cafeteria intervention to modify school meals

Family events.

Approximately 130 peer-reviewed research articles describe the effectiveness of CATCH at reducing childhood obesity. Coordinators and guides are available for implementation guidance. Workshops are available to train faculty and staff on the program.

SUMMARY

Childhood overweight and obesity have been identified as a priority public health issue globally and in the United States. A complex and multifactorial condition, childhood overweight and obesity are impacted by multiple biological, genetic, developmental, behavioral, and environmental factors including social determinants of health. Public health nutrition professionals impact child overweight and obesity through advocating for and resourcing effective public policy and programs, educating stakeholders in the issues surrounding pediatric obesity, and participating in pediatric obesity interventions as appropriate per one's scope of practice.

KEY CHAPTER CONCEPTS

1. Childhood obesity rates are on the rise in both developed and developing nations.
2. The current childhood obesity epidemic has resulted from a complex set of societal changes including family life, food availability, eating and physical activity patterns, and use of media.
3. Prevention and treatment measures need to address energy imbalance (food and beverage intake versus physical activity) through multifaceted interventions within settings frequented by children and their families.

4. Childhood obesity is linked with multiple comorbidities previously thought of as adult diseases and affects almost every system in the body.
5. Treatment of childhood obesity should be completed by a well-trained multidisciplinary team.
6. The role of the public health nutrition professional in addressing child overweight and obesity is to advocate for and resource effective public policy and programs, educate stakeholders in the issues surrounding pediatric obesity, and participate in pediatric obesity interventions as appropriate per one's scope of practice.

CASE STUDY AND QUESTIONS

MK is a 12-year-old boy seen by his pediatrician for an annual checkup. At his visit, MK measured 158 cm in height and 61 kg in weight, which is a significant increase in weight since his visit last year. During the visit, MK's provider asked about his diet and physical activity. MK's mother shared that they are a busy family; she works two jobs and typically picks something up for dinner on the way home from work. MK likes to have snacks after school and they are usually a soda and chips. MK's mother reports he is not active after school, but he does have physical education in school.

MK's parents are both obese with comorbidities including hyperlipidemia and hypertension. Today MK's blood pressure readings were also high, diagnosing him with pediatric hypertension. As a part of the AAP guidelines, MK received a fasting lipid panel when he was 10 years old, which was normal. However, due to significant weight gain, high blood pressure, and parental obesity factors, his provider followed the AAP algorithm and ordered another fasted lipid panel.

Answer the following questions regarding MK and the suggested treatment regimen.

1. Plot MK's BMI on the correct growth chart. What is his BMI percentile?
2. Following the AAP guidance, what should the provider suggest as the first line of treatment for MK?
3. MK and his mother return to follow-up 9 months after his initial visit. MK has been making many changes at home but continues to gain weight. He weighs 68 kg and is 160 cm tall. His mother asks about potential medications to help with weight loss. Are there medications with FDA approval for children? Does MK meet the guidelines to receive treatment?
4. MK's provider has started him on orlistat. Following medication therapy for 1 week, MK began experiencing abdominal discomfort, gas, and diarrhea. What dietary suggestions are recommended to help relieve GI side effects?
5. Is MK eligible for bariatric surgery? What selection criteria does he meet?

DISCUSSION QUESTIONS

1. What is the prevalence of childhood obesity in the United States?
2. Name several factors that may influence childhood obesity.
3. Describe how childhood obesity can affect health and mental health.
4. If your community does not have an IHBLT program, what should you do as the public health nutrition professional? How would you go about setting up such as program?

SUGGESTED LEARNING ACTIVITIES

1. Use the CDC Data and Statistics Tools at www.cdc.gov/datastatistics/index.html to find the prevalence of child and adolescent obesity in your state.
2. Plot a 4-year-old boy with BMI of 16.8 kg/m^2 on the WHO and CDC growth charts. Note the differences in the plot. Explain this difference.
3. Suggest three additional strategies to address obesity based on developmental risk factors.
4. Plan a multilevel intervention for a community using the strategies suggested by the CDC.
5. View a television show made specifically for children. Describe the nutrition, physical activity, and body image themes. Did you note any weight bias?
6. Describe the factors you may need to take into consideration when completing a nutrition assessment on a child who is overweight or obese.
7. Write a letter to a parent/caregiver about the results of a recent school BMI screening. (See safeguards listed by the CDC: www.cdc.gov/healthyweight/assessing/bmi/childrens_bmi/tool_for_schools.html.)

RESOURCES FOR FURTHER LEARNING

- CDC Data and Statistics Tools: www.cdc.gov/datastatistics/index.html
  - Provides population-level data and statistics for a variety of public health concerns in the United States, including overweight and obesity
- CDC 2000 Clinical Growth Charts: www.cdc.gov/growthcharts/clinical_charts.htm
  - Developed by the CDC, these are growth charts for children from birth to 20 years of age; CDC recommends use in children ages 2 years and up in the United States.
- WHO Growth Charts: www.cdc.gov/growthcharts/who_charts.htm
  - Developed by WHO, these are growth charts for children from birth to 59 months of age; CDC recommends use in children up to 2 years of age in the United States.
- CDC, Overweight and obesity: prevention strategies and guidelines: www.cdc.gov/obesity/resources/strategies-guidelines.html
  - Provides links to recommended obesity prevention resources, strategies, and guidelines
- U.S. Department of Health and Human Services, Office of Disease Prevention and Health Promotion, *Healthy People 2030*: Building a Healthier Future for All: https://health.gov/healthypeople
  - 10-year goals and objectives for public health in the United States
- CDC, Measuring children's height and weight accurately at home: www.cdc.gov/healthyweight/assessing/bmi/childrens_bmi/measuring_children.html
  - Instructions for parents/caregivers on how to accurately measure children's height and weight at home; can be used as an educational tool for parents and caregivers by public health professionals

SPRINGER PUBLISHING CONNECT™ **A robust set of instructor resources designed to supplement this text is located at http://connect.springerpub.com/content/book/978-0-8261-8623-2. Qualifying instructors may request access by emailing textbook@springerpub.com.**

REFERENCES

1. Office of Disease Prevention and Health Promotion. Healthy People 2030: building a healthier future for all. U.S. Department of Health and Human Services; 2020. https://health.gov/healthypeople
2. World Health Organization. Working for better health for everyone, everywhere. Accessed October 16, 2023. https://www.who.int/about/what-we-do/who-brochure
3. World Health Organization. The triple billion targets: a visual summary of the methods to deliver impact. Accessed October 16, 2023. https://www.who.int/data/stories/the-triple-billion-targets-a-visual-summary-of-methods-to-deliver-impact
4. Centers for Disease Control and Prevention. Defining adult overweight & obesity. Accessed October 16, 2023. https://www.cdc.gov/obesity/basics/adult-defining.html
5. Centers for Disease Control and Prevention. Clinical growth charts. Accessed October 16, 2023. https://www.cdc.gov/growthcharts/clinical_charts.htm
6. Centers for Disease Control and Prevention. WHO growth standards are recommended for use in the U.S. for infants and children 0 to 2 years of age. Accessed October 16, 2023. https://www.cdc.gov/growthcharts/who_charts.htm
7. Centers for Disease Control and Prevention. Measuring children's height and weight accurately at home. Accessed October 16, 2023. https://www.cdc.gov/healthyweight/assessing/bmi/childrens_bmi/measuring_children.html/#Height
8. Nihiser AJ, Lee SM, Wechsler H, et al. Body mass index measurement in schools. *J Sch Health*. 2007;77(10):651–724. https://doi.org/10.1111/j.1746-1561.2007.00249.x
9. World Health Organization. Global health estimates. Accessed October 16, 2023. https://www.who.int/data/global-health-estimates
10. World Health Organization. Overweight prevalence among children under 5 years of age (%) (% weight-for-height >+2 SD) (survey-based estimates). Global Health Observatory. Updated April 17, 2023. https://www.who.int/data/gho/data/indicators/indicator-details/GHO/gho-jme-overweight-prevalence
11. Centers for Disease Control and Prevention. About the National Health and Nutrition Examination Survey. National Center for Health Statistics. Accessed October 16, 2023. https://www.cdc.gov/nchs/nhanes/about_nhanes.htm
12. Fryar CD, Carroll MD, Afful J. Prevalence of overweight, obesity, and severe obesity among children and adolescents aged 2–19 years: United States, 1963–1965 through 2017–2018. Updated January 29, 2021. https://www.cdc.gov/nchs/data/hestat/obesity-child-17-18/obesity-child.htm
13. Stierman B, Afful J, Carroll MD, et al. National Health and Nutrition Examination Survey 2017–March 2020 prepandemic data files—development of files and prevalence estimates for selected health outcomes. National Health Statistics Reports, no 158. National Center for Health Statistics; 2021. https://doi.org/10.15620/cdc:106273
14. Brault M, Turcotte O, Aimé A, Côté M, Bégin C. Body mass index accuracy in preadolescents: can we trust self-report or should we seek parent report? *J Pediatr* 2015;167(2):366–371. https://doi.org/10.1016/j.jpeds.2015.04.043
15. Centers for Disease Control and Prevention. Youth Risk Behavior Surveillance System (YRBSS). Accessed October 16, 2023. https://www.cdc.gov/healthyyouth/data/yrbs/index.htm
16. Centers for Disease Control and Prevention. Body mass index (BMI) measurement in schools. Accessed October 16, 2023. https://www.cdc.gov/healthyschools/obesity/bmi/bmi_measurement_schools.htm
17. Solar O, Irwin A. *A conceptual framework for action on the social determinants of health*. World Health Organization; 2010.
18. Kansra AR, Lakkunarajah SM, Jay MS. Childhood and adolescent obesity: a review. *Front Pediatr*. 2021;8:581461. https://doi.org/10.3389/fped.2020.581461

19. Ohri-Vachaspati P, DeLia D, DeWeese RS, Crespo NC, Todd M, Yedidia MJ. The relative contribution of layers of the Social Ecological Model to childhood obesity. *Public Health Nutr*. 2015;18(11):2055–2066. https://doi.org/10.1017/S1368980014002365
20. Loos RJF, Rankinen T. Gene-diet interactions on bodyweight changes. *J Am Diet Assoc*. 2005;105: S29–S34. https://doi.org/10.1016/j.jada.2005.02.015
21. Jang H, Serra C. Nutrition, epigenetics, and diseases. *Clin Nutr Res*. 2014;3:1–8. https://doi.org/10.7762/cnr.2014.3.1.1
22. National Human Genome Research Institute. Epigenomics fact sheet. National Institutes of Health. Updated August 16, 2020. https://www.genome.gov/about-genomics/fact-sheets/Epigenomics-Fact-Sheet
23. Richards J, Pickett OK, Wilhite BC. Life course and social determinants. Maternal and Child Health Library; 2017. https://www.mchlibrary.org/professionals/lifecourse.php
24. Cockerham WC. Theoretical approaches to research on the social determinants of obesity. *Am J Prev Med*. 2022;63:S8–S17. https://doi.org/10.1016/j.amepre.2022.01.030
25. Koletzko B, Godfrey KM, Poston L, et al. Nutrition during pregnancy, lactation, and early childhood and its implications for maternal and long-term child health: the EarlyNutrition Project recommendations. *Ann Nutr Metab*. 2019;74:93–106. https://doi.org/10.1159/000496471
26. Stang J, Huffman LG. Position of the Academy of Nutrition and Dietetics: obesity, reproduction, and pregnancy outcomes. *J Acad Nutr Diet*. 2016;116:677–691. https://doi.org/10.1016/j.jand.2016.01.008
27. Centers for Disease Control and Prevention. Prevalence of selected maternal and child health indicators for all Pregnancy Risk Assessment Monitoring System (PRAMS) sites 2016–2020. Accessed October 16, 2023. https://www.cdc.gov/prams/prams-data/mch-indicators/states/pdf/2020/All-Sites-PRAMS-MCH-Indicators-508.pdf
28. Yu ZB, Han SP, Zhu GZ, et al. Birth weight and subsequent risk of obesity: a systematic review and meta-analysis. *Obes Rev*. 2011;12:525–542. https://doi.org/10.1111/j.1467-789X.2011.00867.x
29. Lakshman R, Elks CE, Ong KK. Childhood obesity. *Circulation*. 2012;126(14):1770–1779. https://doi.org/10.1161/CIRCULATIONAHA.111.047738
30. Pietrobelli A, Agosti M, MeNu Group. Nutrition in the first 1000 days: ten practices to minimize obesity emerging from the published science. *Intern J Environ Res Public Health*. 2017;14:1491. https://doi.org/10.3390/ijerph14121491
31. Horta BL, Rollins N, Dias MS, Garcez V, Escamilla R. Systematic review and meta-analysis of breastfeeding and later overweight or obesity expands on previous study for World Health Organization. *Acta Paediatr*. 2023;112:34–41. https://doi.org/10.1111/apa.16460
32. Qiao J, Dai LJ, Zhang Q, Ouyang YQ. A meta-analysis of the association between breastfeeding and early child obesity. *J Pediatr Nurs*. 2020;53:57–66. https://doi.org/10.1016/j.pedn.2020.04.024
33. Koletzko B, von Kries R, Closa R, et al. Lower protein in infant formula is associated with lower weight up to age 2 y: a randomized clinical trial. *Amer J Clin Nutr*. 2009;89:1836–1845. https://doi.org/10.3945/ajcn.2008.27091
34. Weber M, Grote V, Closa-Monasterolo R, et al. Lower protein content in infant formula reduced BMI and obesity risk at school-age: follow-up of a randomized trial. *Am J Clin Nutr*. 2014;99:1041–1051. https://doi.org/10.3945/ajcn.113.064071
35. Putet G, Labaune JM, Mace K, et al. Effect of dietary protein on plasma insulin-like growth factor-1, growth, and body composition in healthy term infants: a randomized, double-blind, controlled trial (Early Protein and Obesity in Childhood (EPOCH study). *Br J Nutr*. 2016;115:271–284. https://doi.org/10.1017/S0007114515004456
36. Inostroza J, Haschke F, Steenhout P, Grathwohl D, Nelson SE, Ziegler EE. Low-protein formula slows weight gain in infants of overweight mothers. *J Pediatr Gastroenterol Nutr*. 2014;59:70–77. https://doi.org/10.1097/MPG.0000000000000349
37. Huh SY, Rifas-Shiman SL, Taveras EM, Oken E, Gillman MW. Timing of the solid food introduction and risk of obesity in preschool children. *Pediatrics*. 2011;127(3):e544–e551. https://doi.org/10.1542/peds.2010-0740
38. Patro-Gołąb B, Zalewski BM, Kołodziej M, et al. Nutritional interventions or exposures in infants and children up to three years and their effects on subsequent risk of overweight, obesity, and body fat: a systematic review of systematic reviews. *Obes Rev*. 2016;17(12):1245–1257. https://doi.org/10.1111/obr.12476
39. Zhou J, Zhang F, Qin X, et al. Age at adiposity rebound and the relevance for obesity: a systematic review and meta-analysis. *Int J Obes*. 2022;44:1413–1424. https://doi.org/10.1038/s41366-022-01120-4

40. Li W, Liu Q, Deng X, Chen Y, Liu S, Story M. Association between obesity and puberty timing: a systematic review and meta-analysis. *Int J Environ Res Public Health*. 2017;14(10):1266. https://doi.org/10.3390/ijerph141012266
41. Verduci E, Bronsky J, Embelton N, et al. Role of dietary factors, food habits, and lifestyle in childhood obesity development: a position paper from the European Society for Paediatric Gastroenterology, Hepatology and Nutrition Committee on Nutrition. *J Pediatr Gastroenterol Nutr*. 2021;72:769–783. https://doi.org/10.1097/MPG.0000000000003075
42. Vanderhout SM, Aglipay M, Toarabi N, et al. Whole milk compared with reduced-fat milk and childhood overweight: a systematic review and meta-analysis. *Am J Clin Nutr*. 2020;111:266–279. https://doi.org/10.1093/ajcn/nqz276
43. Julian V, Ring-Dimitriou S, Wyszynska J, et al. There is a clinical need to consider the physical activity: sedentary pattern in children with obesity—position paper of the European Childhood Obesity Group. *Ann Nutr Metab*. 2022;78:236–241. https://doi.org/10.1159/000524570
44. National Sleep Foundation. How much sleep do you really need? October 1, 2020. https://www.thensf.org/how-many-hours-of-sleep-do-you-really-need
45. Wheaton AG, Claussen AH. Short sleep duration among infants, children, and adolescents aged 4 months to 17 years—United States, 2016–2018. *MMWR Morb Mortal Wkly Rep*. 2021;70(38):1315–1321. https://doi.org/10.15585/mmwr.mm7038a1
46. Sluggett L, Wagner SL, Harris RL. Sleep duration and obesity in children and adolescents. *Can J Diabetes*. 2019;43:146–152. https://doi.org/10.1016/j.jcjd.2018.06.006
47. Li L, Zhang S, Huang Y, Chen K. Sleep duration and obesity in children: a systematic review and meta-analysis of prospective cohort studies. *J Paediatr Child Health*. 2017;53:378–385. https://doi.org/10.1111/jpc.13434
48. Rosenkranz RR, Dzewaltowski DA. Model of the home food environment pertaining to childhood obesity. *Nutr Rev*. 2008;66:123–140. https://doi.org/10.1111/j.1753-4887.2008.00017.x
49. Hemmingsson E. Early childhood obesity risk factors: socioeconomic adversity, family dysfunction, offspring distress, and junk food self-medication. *Curr Obes Rep* 2018;7:204–209. https://doi.org/10.1007/s13679-018-0310-2
50. Sahoo K, Sahoo B, Choudhury AK, Sofi NY, Kumar R, Bhadoria AS. Childhood obesity: causes and consequences. *J Fam Med Prim Care*. 2015;4:187–195. https://doi.org/10.4103/2249-4863.154628
51. Porter RM, Tindall A, Gaffka BJ, et al. A review of modifiable risk factors for severe obesity in children ages 5 and under. *Child Obes*. 2018;14:468–476. https://doi.org/10.1089/chi.2017.0344
52. Sokol RL, Qin B, Poti JM. Parenting styles and body mass index: a systematic review of prospective studies among children. *Obes Rev*. 2017;18:281–292. https://doi.org/10.1111/obr.12497
53. Savage JS, Orlet Fischer JO, Birch LL. Parental influence on eating behavior: conception to adolescence. *J Law Med Ethics*. 2007;35:22–34. https://doi.org/10.1111/j.1748-720X.2007.00111.x
54. Hubbs-Tait L, Kennedy TS, Page MC, Topham GL, Harrist AW. Parental feeding practices predict authoritative, authoritarian, and permissive parenting styles. *J Am Diet Assoc*. 2008;108:1154–1161. https://doi.org/10.1016/j.jada.2008.04.008
55. Kininmonth AR, Smith AD, Llewellyn CH, Dye L, Lawton CL, Fildes A. The relationship between home environment and child adiposity: a systematic review. *Int J Behav Nutr Phys Act*. 2021;18(4):1–20. https://doi.org/10.1186/s12966-020-01073-9
56. Kumar S, Kelly AS. Review of childhood obesity: from epidemiology, etiology, and comorbidities to clinical assessment and treatment. *Mayo Clin Proc*. 2017;92:251–265. https://doi.org/10.1016/j.mayocp.2016.09.017
57. Pont SJ, Puhl R, Cook SR, Slusher W. Stigma experienced by children and adolescents with obesity. *Pediatrics*. 2017;140:e20173034. https://doi.org/10.1542/peds.2017-3034
58. National Collaborative on Childhood Obesity Research. Accelerating progress to reduce childhood obesity. Accessed October 16, 2023. https://www.nccor.org
59. Institute of Medicine. *Progress in Preventing Childhood Obesity: How Do We Measure Up?* National Academies Press; 2007. doi.org/10.17226/11722
60. World Health Organization. Controlling the global obesity epidemic. Accessed October 16, 2023. https://www.who.int/activities/controlling-the-global-obesity-epidemic
61. Khan LK, Sobush K, Keener D, et al. Recommended community strategies and measurements to prevent obesity in the United States. *MMWR Morb Mortal Wkly Rep*. 2009;58(RR-7):1–26. https://www.cdc.gov/mmwr/pdf/rr/rr5807.pdf

62. Centers for Disease Control and Prevention. Overweight and obesity: prevention strategies and guidelines. Accessed October 16, 2023. https://www.cdc.gov/obesity/resources/strategies-guidelines.html
63. Barlow SE, Expert Committee. Expert Committee recommendations regarding the prevention, assessment, and treatment of child and adolescent overweight and obesity: summary report. *Pediatrics*. 2007;120(suppl 4):S164–S192. https://doi.org/10.1542/peds.2007-2329C
64. Hampl SE, Hassink SG, Skinner AC, et al. Clinical practice guideline for the evaluation and treatment of children and adolescents with obesity. *Pediatrics*. 2023;151(2):e2022060640. https://doi.org/10.1542/peds.2022-060640
65. Ihmels MA, Welk GJ, Eisenmann JC, Nusser SM. Development and preliminary validation of a Family Nutrition and Physical Activity (FNPA) screening tool. *Int J Behav Nutr Phys Act*. 2009;6:14. https://doi.org/10.1186/1479-5868-6-14
66. Rogers VW, Hart PH, Motyka E, Rines EN, Vine J, Deatrick DA. Impact of Let's Go! 5–2–1–0: a community-based, multisetting childhood obesity prevention program. *J Pediatr Psychol*. 2013;38(9):1010–1020. https://doi.org/10.1093/jpepsy/jst057
67. National Heart, Lung, and Blood Institute. *Expert Panel on Integrated Guidelines for Cardiovascular Health and Risk Reduction in Children and Adolescents*. Summary Report. U.S. Department of Health and Human Services; 2012.
68. Dunican KC, Desilets AR, Montalbano JK. Pharmacotherapeutic options for overweight adolescents. *Ann Pharmacother*. 2007;41(9):1445–1455. https://doi.org/10.1345/aph.1K022
69. Rogovik AL, Goldman RD. Pharmacologic treatment of pediatric obesity. *Can Fam Physician*. 2011;57(2):195–197.
70. Cavaliere H, Floriano I, Medeiros-Neto G. Gastrointestinal side effects of orlistat may be prevented by concomitant prescription of natural fibers (psyllium mucilloid). *Int J Obes Relat Metab Disord*. 2001;25(7):1095–1099. https://doi.org/10.1038/sj.ijo.0801645
71. Woodard K, Louque L, Hsia DS. Medications for the treatment of obesity in adolescents. *Ther Adv Endocrinol Metab*. 2020;11:2042018820918789. https://doi.org/10.1177/2042018820918789
72. Ryder JR, Kaizer A, Rudser KD, Gross A, Kelly AS, Fox CK. Effect of phentermine on weight reduction in a pediatric weight management clinic. *Int J Obes*. 2017;41:90–93. https://doi.org/10.1038/ijo.2016.185
73. Pratt JSA, Browne A, Browne NT, et al. ASMBS pediatric metabolic and bariatric surgery guidelines, 2018. *Surg Obes Relat Dis*. 2018;14(7):882–901. https://doi.org/10.1016/j.soard.2018.03.019
74. Armstrong SC, Bolling CF, Michalsky MP, Reichard KW, Section on Obesity, Section on Surgery. Pediatric metabolic and bariatric surgery: evidence, barriers, and best practices. *Pediatrics*. 2019;144(6):e20193223. https://doi.org/10.1542/peds.2019-3223
75. Styne DM, Arslanian SA, Connor EL, et al. Pediatric obesity-assessment, treatment, and prevention: an Endocrine Society Clinical Practice Guideline. *J Clin Endocrinol Metab*. 2017;102(3):709–757. https://doi.org/10.1210/jc.2016-2573
76. CATCH.org. Welcome to CATCH.org! Accessed October 16, 2023. https://letsgo.catch.org
77. Centers for Disease Control and Prevention. CATCH–Coordinated Approach to Child Health: curriculum & training. Accessed October 16, 2023. https://www.cdc.gov/prc/resources/tools/catch.html

11

CHRONIC DISEASE PREVENTION IN POPULATIONS ACROSS THE LIFE CYCLE

Soghra Jarvandi and David R. Buys

LEARNING OBJECTIVES

At the end of this chapter, students will be able to:

1. Describe the impact of chronic diseases on an individual, national, and global level.
2. Identify common risk factors, including nutritional factors, associated with chronic disease.
3. Differentiate among primary, secondary, and tertiary prevention efforts.
4. Describe common chronic conditions affecting each life stage.
5. Discuss the effects of the COVID-19 pandemic on chronic diseases.
6. Apply the social-ecological model as an approach to chronic disease policy and interventions.
7. Discuss current challenges to chronic disease prevention and management; consider global challenges and opportunities to inform directions of public health nutrition professionals in the United States.
8. Describe the components of a community-engaged chronic disease prevention and management intervention model.

INTRODUCTION

Chronic diseases are a national and global burden on the public health sector, yet an area for targeted prevention and management efforts implemented by public health nutrition professionals. This chapter provides an overview of the most salient **chronic conditions** affecting individuals in various life stages. Risk factors, preventive measures, and implications for public health nutrition policies and programs that can alleviate this burden are explored further.

OVERVIEW OF CHRONIC DISEASE IMPACTS: U.S. AND GLOBAL

Chronic diseases include a variety of health conditions of long duration. The Centers for Disease Control and Prevention (CDC) defines a **chronic condition** as a condition that lasts for at least 1 year and is associated with the need for ongoing medical care and/or limitations in activities of daily living.[1] Chronic diseases are also referred to as noncommunicable diseases, to differentiate these conditions from infectious diseases. With advances in overall health and living conditions in recent decades, the burden of infectious diseases has been decreasing, while the burden of chronic conditions has been increasing.

Chronic conditions are a global crisis. Based on World Health Organization (WHO) data, chronic conditions account for 74% of deaths worldwide, of which more than three quarters occur in low- and middle-income countries.[2] Four major categories of chronic conditions are: cardiovascular disease (diseases of the heart and/or blood vessels, such as stroke), cancers, chronic respiratory diseases, and diabetes. These four conditions collectively account for more than 80% of chronic disease–related deaths.[2] In the United States, about 60% of adults have at least one chronic disease, and 40% have two or more chronic diseases simultaneously.[1]

Measuring the Burden of Chronic Disease

Chronic conditions have negative impacts on people's health and quality of life and are the leading causes of death and disability. The burden of chronic diseases is higher in low-resource communities.[3] Figure 11.1 illustrates the changes in the burden of chronic disease over the past three decades, prior to the COVID-19 pandemic.[4]

Chronic diseases are costly. The economic burden of chronic conditions to the healthcare system is mostly related to disabilities resulting from chronic conditions. Researchers quantify the burden of disease as **disability-adjusted life years (DALYs)** by measuring the health loss resulting from disability; a higher value of DALYs represent greater disease burden.[5] One DALY is equivalent to 1 year of health lost, and is calculated as: Years lost due to disability + Years of life lost.[5] For example, the burden of ischemic heart disease and diabetes increased globally between 1990 and 2019, measured as a 50% and 148% increase in the number of DALYs due to ischemic heart disease and diabetes, respectively.[6] In the United States, the corresponding values are a 100% increase in DALYs due to ischemic heart disease and a 1,000% increase due to diabetes over the same time period.[7] DALY data can be gathered for populations, analyzed, and used to develop policy.[5] Figure 11.2 illustrates how DALYs are measured.[5]

From the 20th century to the 21st century, the burden of disease has shifted from infectious disease to chronic conditions. In 2019, chronic conditions accounted for about 64% of total disease burden globally with variations among countries. Figure 11.3a illustrates the global disease burden by cause and Figure 11.3b shows the U.S. burden of disease by cause.[8]

In the United States chronic conditions accounted for more than 80% of the chronic disease burden in 2019.[7] The shift from infectious disease to chronic conditions has created a need for new approaches/strategies in the healthcare system. People with chronic conditions need care over the long term to manage their disease, and ideally slow disease progression and complications. In addition, risk factors for chronic conditions differ

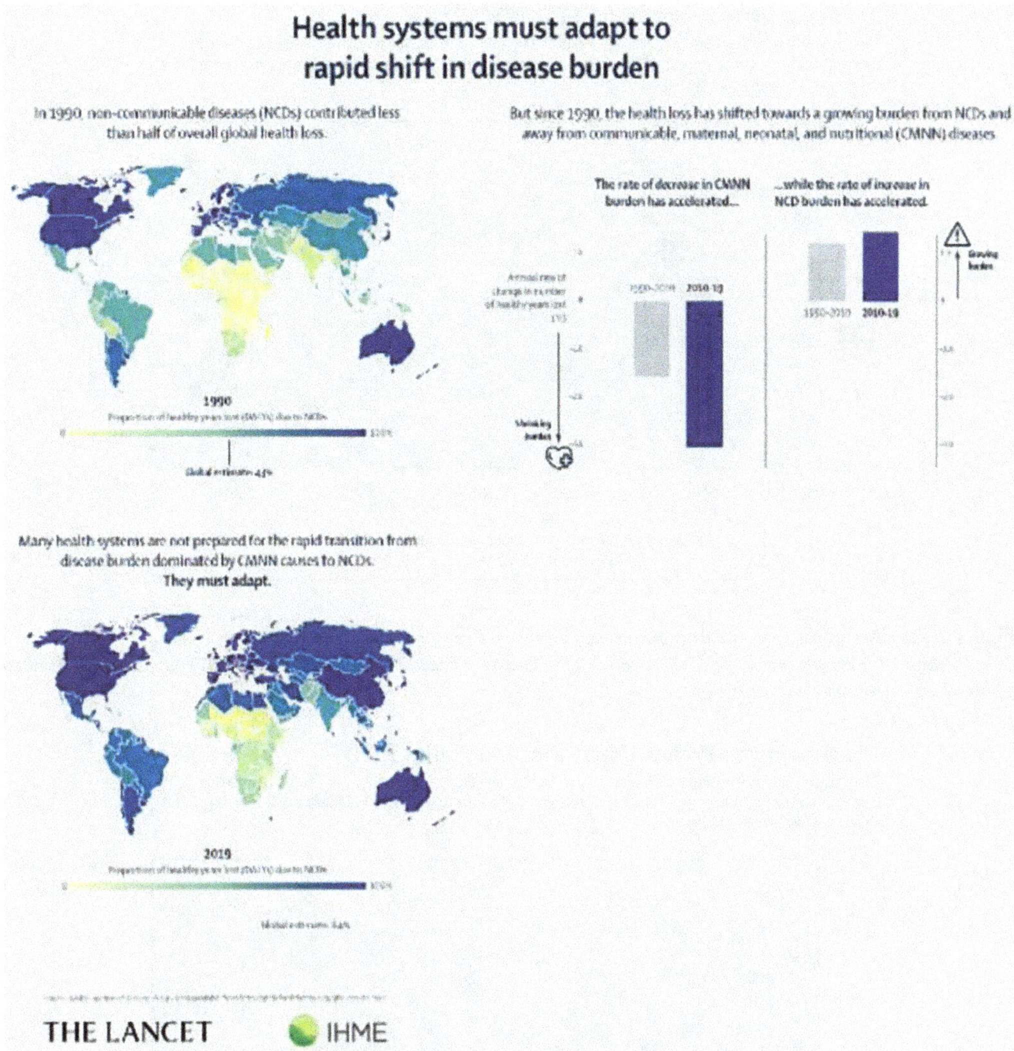

Figure 11.1. Change in global burden of chronic disease, 1990–2019.
Source: Lancet, Institute for Health Metrics and Evaluation. Global burden of disease 2019. Lancet; 2020. http://ghdx
.healthdata.org/gbd-results-tool

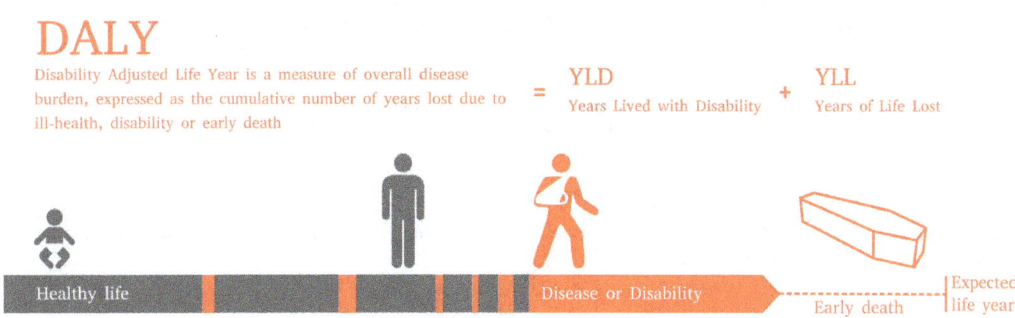

Figure 11.2. How disability-adjusted life years (DALYs) are measured.
Source: Wki Commons. https://commons.wikimedia.org/wiki/File:DALY_disability_affected_life_year_infographic.svg.
Accessed 10/17/2023.

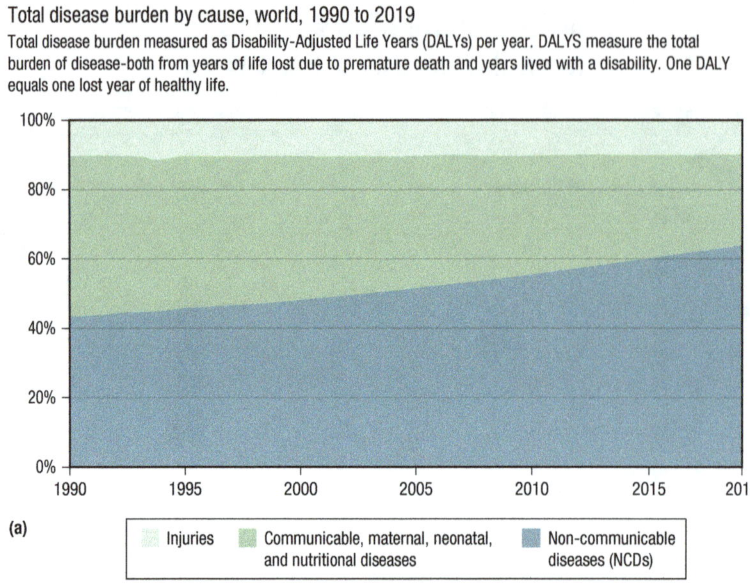

Figure 11.3a. World disease burden by cause, 1990–2019.
Source: Institute for Health Metrics and Evaluation. Global burden of disease. Our World in Data. 2019. https://ourworldindata.org/grapher/total-disease-burden-by-cause

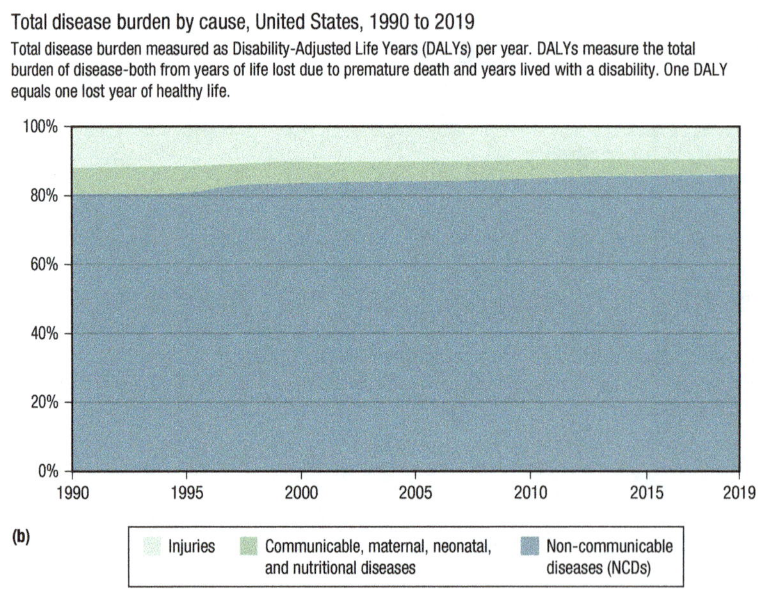

Figure 11.3b. U.S. disease burden by cause, 1990–2019.
Source: Institute for Health Metrics and Evaluation. Global burden of disease. Our World in Data.2019. https://ourworldindata.org/grapher/total-disease-burden-by-cause

from those for infectious diseases. Unlike infectious diseases that have a main causative agent (e.g., viruses, bacteria), chronic conditions do not have a single specific cause, but result from complex interactions between contextual environment factors and an individual's lifestyle behaviors.[9]

COVID-19 and Its Impacts on Chronic Disease Since 2020

The overall societal impacts of the COVID-19 pandemic since its start in early 2020 are yet to be fully understood. While the pandemic increased the world burden of infectious disease, it also appears to have adversely affected progress made in managing and treating chronic diseases. It was recognized early in the pandemic that persons with chronic diseases were at substantially greater risk of severe disease and death from COVID-19.[10]

As overall data have accumulated since the inception of the pandemic, a concept called **health debt** has emerged. While population-wide positive health behavior changes result in societal benefits, health debt is a negative concept; it can be defined as the potential adverse effects over time of populations' engagement in poor health behaviors.[11] It is known that rates of provider visits for chronic disease management and routine healthcare screenings substantially decreased during the pandemic. As a result, providers have reported faster progression of chronic diseases and instances of identifying serious diseases too late for effective treatment.[12]

Pandemic-related stay-at-home orders, job loss and subsequent loss of insurance coverage, and requests from hospitals that patients delay nonurgent care—among other factors—contributed to reduced provider visits. In addition, health behaviors that increase chronic disease risk appear to have increased during the pandemic. For example, reduced access to public spaces may have curtailed time spent in physical activity.[13] Evidence indicates that behaviors related to mental health issues such as anxiety, depression, and grief have resulted in increased emotional eating and use of substances such as alcohol and drugs.[14] Thus, the health debt resulting from the COVID-19 pandemic, and its impact on chronic disease burden has yet to be fully calculated.[11]

CHRONIC DISEASE PREVENTION

In general, strategies aimed at preventing chronic disease are categorized into three levels:

- **Primary prevention:** Prevention of a chronic condition so that it does not occur; the primary focus of interventions is healthy populations.
    - Public health nutrition practitioners should education populations on chronic disease preventive behaviors, which include good nutrition and maintaining a healthy weight, engaging in regular physical activity, never smoking, getting enough sleep, avoiding excessive alcohol intake, obtaining recommended health screenings, and sharing one's family health history with health providers.[1]
- **Secondary prevention:** Early detection (screening) to identify a chronic condition early; the primary focus of interventions is at-risk populations.
    - Public health nutrition practitioners should educate populations on the importance of regularly obtaining recommended health screenings to prevent chronic disease or identify it early.[1]
- **Tertiary prevention:** Treatment or management strategies for chronic disease; primary focus is populations diagnosed with chronic disease(s).
    - Timely screening and early disease identification can enable treatment that slows disease progression, improves disease management, and prevents or delays disease complications. Ultimately, tertiary prevention strategies are intended to promote the highest possible quality of life for persons with chronic diseases. Tertiary prevention strategies should be conducted by qualified healthcare professionals such as physicians, RNs, or registered dietitians.[1]

Evidence indicates that primary prevention is effective in reducing rates of chronic diseases. Public health and public health nutrition strategies should focus on primary prevention by addressing social and economic determinants of health which have major impacts on the development of chronic diseases.[15]

Risk Factors for Chronic Disease

Chronic diseases can often be prevented by adopting healthy lifestyle behaviors, including a healthy diet, regular physical activity, adequate sleep, stress management, social connection, and avoiding the use of risky substances. Risk factors for chronic disease fall into two major categories:

- **Nonmodifiable**: Factors that an individual cannot influence, such as age, genetics and heredity, and sex.[9]
- **Modifiable**: Factors that an individual can influence, such as time spent in physical activity, usual dietary intake, and adherence to recommendations for disease screenings.[9]

Four Major Chronic Disease Risk Factors

Four lifestyle factors—poor nutrition, physical inactivity, tobacco use, and excessive alcohol use—account for more than two thirds of the incidence of major chronic diseases combined, including cardiovascular disease, cancer, chronic respiratory disease, and diabetes.[15] A U.S. study documented the impact of adopting a healthy lifestyle on life expectancy. Researchers compared adults who adopted five low-risk lifestyle factors with those with none of these factors. The low-risk lifestyle factors included: (1) never smoking, (2) body mass index (BMI) 18.5–24.9 kg/m^2, (3) ≥30 minutes/day of moderate–vigorous physical activity, (4) moderate alcohol intake, and (5) high diet quality. The investigators found that life expectancy at age 50 was on average 14 years longer for females and 12 years longer for males who adopted a healthy lifestyle.[6] Interventions to promote healthy lifestyle behaviors in populations may have favorable impacts on chronic disease rates. The four major risk factors for chronic disease are as follows:

- Poor nutrition
  - Nutrition behaviors that may increase chronic disease risk include inadequate fruit and vegetable consumption, excessive consumption of sodium and saturated fats, and overconsumption of sugar-sweetened beverages.[16]
- Physical inactivity
  - Persons who live sedentary lifestyles will not receive the substantial benefits of physical activity in fighting chronic disease, including improved cardiorespiratory, skeletal, and muscular fitness; better weight management; more restful sleep; and mental health benefits including reduced stress and improved mood.[17]
- Tobacco use
  - The leading cause of preventable death and disability in the United States is tobacco use. Tobacco cessation interventions have a direct positive impact on chronic disease risk.[18] One study found that even with a significant weight gain—which often follows tobacco cessation—indicators of chronic disease risk and risk of death did not increase in the study population.[19]
- Harmful use of alcohol
  - According to the CDC, excessive alcohol use can reduce the life span by an average of 26 years, and includes:
    - Heavy drinking (eight or more drinks per week for females; 15 or more drinks per week for males)

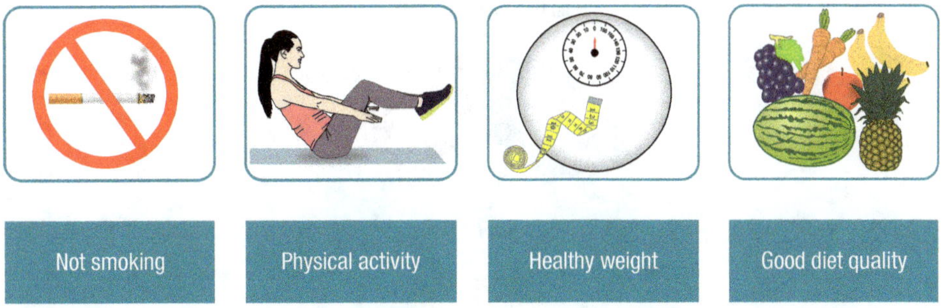

Figure 11.4. Major healthy lifestyle factors for chronic disease prevention.

- Binge drinking (four or more drinks on one occasion for females; five or more drinks on one occasion for males)
- Any alcohol use during pregnancy or by anyone under 21 years of age.[20] Note that alcohol intake in earlier life cycle phases, for example, in early adolescence, is associated with a nearly threefold increased risk of developing alcohol use disorder as an adult.[21]

One **standard drink** of alcohol is defined as the amount of a beverage that provides about 14 g of pure alcohol.[21] In terms of serving sizes, this is the approximate amount of alcohol provided by:

- 12 oz of beer
- 5 oz of wine
- 1.5 oz (1 "shot") spirits/hard liquor[21]

The 2020–2025 *Dietary Guidelines for Americans* recommend that persons in the adult life cycle phase can choose not to consume alcohol; if alcohol is consumed, *moderate intake* is recommended on days alcohol is consumed.[22] Moderate alcohol intake is defined as no more than one standard drink per day for females, and no more than two standard drinks per day for males.[22] To reiterate, alcohol should not be consumed at all during the pregnancy life cycle phase.

Figure 11.4 illustrates four major healthy lifestyle factors for chronic disease prevention.

SOCIAL DETERMINANTS OF HEALTH RELATED TO CHRONIC DISEASE PREVENTION AND MANAGEMENT

Risk factors for chronic conditions range from individual-level unhealthy behaviors (**downstream factors**) to the social and environmental factors that affect an individual's behaviors (**upstream factors**). Examples of downstream factors include but are not limited to nutrition and physical activity behaviors, smoking, and maintaining a healthy weight. Upstream factors, commonly referred to as social determinants of health, are the social and environmental factors that affect people's health.[23]

The framework for **social determinants of health** (SDOH) from the U.S. Department of Health and Human Services (DHHS) *Healthy People 2030* includes five main domains: Health Care Access and Quality, Neighborhood and **Built Environment**, Social and Community Context, Financial Stability, and Education Access and Quality. Figure 11.5 provides an illustration of the DHHS model of SDOH.[24] Each component of the model is described here:

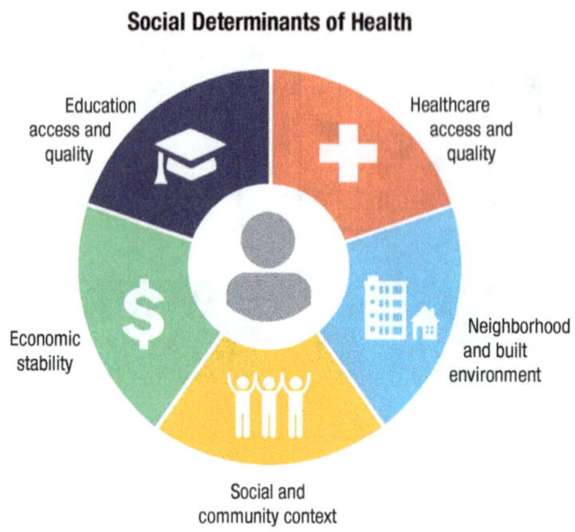

Figure 11.5. U.S. Department of Health and Human Services model of the social determinants of health.
Source: Office of Disease Prevention and Health Promotion. *Healthy People 2030*: social determinants of health. U.S. Department of Health and Human Services. 2020. https://health.gov/healthypeople/priority-areas/social-determinants-health

Health Care Access and Quality

Access to quality healthcare is crucial for prevention and management of chronic conditions.[25] Healthcare services are expensive. People with health insurance have better access to healthcare services; however, many people with low income often cannot afford health insurance. In addition, the type of health insurance as well as environmental factors play an important role in access to high-quality services. Location plays an important role in the availability of services. For example, rural residents may have less access to employment that provides insurance benefits. Due to lack of broadband internet access in some rural areas, residents may be unable to utilize telehealth services such as ongoing in-home monitoring and management of chronic disease monitoring.[26]

Neighborhood and Built Environment

The surroundings in which a person lives have a major impact on chronic disease risk. The built environment refers to human-made surroundings that influence a person's health behaviors. The environment in which one lives and works can affect opportunities for physical activity and access to healthy foods, and can influence one's risk of developing various chronic diseases. Examples include safe spaces to walk, and the distance to reach a full-service grocery store or farmers' market.[1,27]

Social and Community Context

An individual's relationships with others can affect overall health and well-being. Relationships promote a sense of purpose and belonging in one's community. The ability to connect within the community through participation in self-governance, such as voting, and community events can promote health, while discrimination or lack of support for obtaining basic needs can negatively affect health. *Healthy People 2030* focuses specifically on helping people through interventions that promote social support.[24]

Economic Stability

There is a vicious circle between a low economic status and the presence of chronic conditions. The risk of chronic conditions is higher among people who live in poverty, at least partly because of reduced access to healthful food and healthcare services. In turn, people with chronic conditions and disability have limited abilities to work, resulting in their low economic status.[28]

Education Access and Quality

Children who lack access to high-quality education are less likely to continue to higher education, and so, they are less likely to find employment in a well-paying job. People with lower education attainment are at higher risk of poverty, which in turn increases their risk of chronic conditions. Evidence indicates an inverse association between education level and chronic disease prevalence.[29]

IMPACTS OF CHRONIC DISEASES THROUGHOUT THE LIFE CYCLE

Chronic diseases are common among older adults, but can occur at different ages throughout the life cycle. The **life course theory** proposes that life occurs as a continuous progression. Each life stage flows consecutively into the next, with health behaviors of each previous stage impacting the current stage.[30] A plethora of influences including environmental, social, genetic, and behavioral factors interact with health behaviors to modulate chronic disease risk. Examples from each major life cycle stage are provided next:

Chronic Diseases and Their Impact During Pregnancy

Chronic disease concerns during pregnancy include the risks associated with the developing fetus as well as the risk for chronic disease later in life for the mother. Pregnancy is a time when potential risk factors for chronic disease may become more pronounced due to the immense physiologic and metabolic changes that occur to provide nourishment to the developing fetus. The weight status and weight gain patterns of the mother determine the birth weight of the infant, which is a key predictor of infant health.[31] Disease risk in the child, across its life course, can also be impacted by nutritional exposures during fetal life.[31]

The unique metabolic milieu during pregnancy can manifest in the development of chronic disease during pregnancy, an increased risk for fetal complications and future disease, and an increased risk for chronic disease for the mother. For example, risk of diabetes may be increased because the body favors greater blood glucose availability as the major source of energy for the fetus. Examples of chronic disease during pregnancy include overweight/obesity, diabetes, and hypertension.

Overweight/Obesity

Approximately 25% of women are overweight prior to pregnancy, and 22% are obese.[32] The rates of overweight/obesity among women of childbearing age are higher among Hispanic and non-Hispanic Black women.[32]

Overweight and obesity—particularly abdominal obesity—are associated with reduced rates of fertility and conception.[32] Overweight and obesity before and during pregnancy are linked to increased risk for the birth of **large-for-gestational-age** (LGA) newborns as well as a higher incidence of preterm delivery, cesarean delivery, gestational diabetes, and hypertensive disorders of pregnancy.[33] The metabolic disruptions caused by excess body fat produce chronic inflammation and oxidative stress that are implicated in insulin resistance, elevated blood glucose, insulin and triglyceride concentrations, and increased blood pressure.[34] Obesity during pregnancy increases lifetime risk for type 2 diabetes, cardiovascular disease, orthopedic disorders, depression, and reproductive cancers.[32]

Obesity during pregnancy impacts the health of the child, and possibly future generations. The **fetal origins of disease** hypothesis suggests that weight and nutritional status of the mother before and during pregnancy can affect the long-term health of her children, including increased risk for obesity, hypertension, cardiovascular disease, diabetes, and depression, as well as her own reproductive health.[32,35]

Diabetes

Diabetes may be a preexisting condition before pregnancy or can develop during pregnancy, when it is referred to as gestational diabetes. Either situation can impact birth outcomes and disease risk for the child later in life, as well as increasing maternal disease risk or complications. Diabetes during pregnancy increases the risk for birth defects, large-for-gestational-age infant, assisted delivery, and preterm delivery.[32,36] About 2% of women have diabetes prior to pregnancy, while gestational diabetes develops in 6% to 17% of pregnant women in direct relation to prepregnancy BMI.[32,36] Gestational diabetes carries a 13-fold risk for developing subsequent diabetes and that risk increases if the mother also experiences preeclampsia or hypertension, showing the confounding effects of multiple chronic disease states.[32,37]

Hypertension

Hypertension has a national prevalence of 10% among women of reproductive age and is one of the leading causes of maternal death.[38,39] Increased rates have paralleled the increase in maternal obesity over the past two decades.[40] Hypertension before pregnancy is associated with a higher risk of serious maternal and fetal complications, including preeclampsia, placental abruption, gestational diabetes, preterm delivery, **small-for-gestational-age** (SGA) infant, and fetal death.[39,41] Hypertension during pregnancy, gestational hypertension, increases the risk for preeclampsia, eclampsia, insulin resistance, and long-term development of diabetes.[42–44]

Chronic Diseases and Their Impact in Children and Adolescents

Chronic health conditions during childhood include physical conditions such as asthma and behavioral conditions such as attention deficit hyperactivity disorder (ADHD). In the United States, about 20% of children ages 0 to 5 years and more than 40% of children ages 6 to 17 years have at least one chronic health condition.[45]

Chronic health conditions during childhood may continue into adulthood, particularly if modifiable risk factors like diet quality are not improved, and result in significant health and economic burdens for persons, families, and society. In addition, chronic health conditions can have negative impacts on quality of life and academic outcomes, such as absenteeism. In addition to the examples discussed here, chronic and developmental conditions affecting children are discussed in Chapter 5.

Asthma

In the United States, 1 in 12 children ages 0 to 17 years (about 6 million children) have asthma.[46] This chronic condition can cause permanent lung damage over a lifetime. The rate of children with asthma varies by sociodemographic factors with asthma being twice as common in Black children than in White children. Asthma management has improved such that fewer attacks or missed school days are occurring, but one in six children with asthma are still experiencing at least one asthma attack each year. ED visits for asthma-related attacks are highest among children 0 to 4 years of age and non-Hispanic Black children. Asthma management plans help children use medications properly and avoid triggers of asthma such as pet dander, tobacco smoke and air pollution.

Diabetes

An estimated 0.3% of children have diabetes in the United States, and the rates of both type 1 and type 2 diabetes are on the rise.[47] Type 1 diabetes may be caused by an autoimmune reaction that stops insulin production, and requires insulin for treatment. Most people with diabetes (90%–95%) have type 2, which typically develops in adulthood, but rates are increasing in children secondary to the increase in childhood obesity as a major factor in the development of insulin resistance.[48] Diabetes is associated with long-term complications, such as cardiovascular disease, kidney failure, amputations, and blindness, which can be prevented by managing the disease through improving lifestyle factors such as diet, physical activity, and monitoring blood glucose.[48]

Overweight/Obesity

From 2017 to 2020, the prevalence of obesity among U.S. children and adolescents ages 2 to 19 years was 19.7%, with higher rates for older age groups, Hispanic and non-Hispanic Black children, and children coming from lower socioeconomic status families.[49] Obesity increases the risk of several health conditions, such as type 2 diabetes, cardiovascular diseases, and depression. Poor nutrition quality and low levels of physical activity are important reasons for excessive weight gain.[50]

Dental Caries

Dental caries are the most common chronic diseases in children, affecting about half of school-age children in the United States and, similar to other chronic conditions, disproportionately affecting children from lower-income households. A high intake of sugary foods and beverages are a major risk factor for the development of dental caries, as is lack of access to a fluoridated water source. Untreated cavities can cause pain and infection that may affect eating, speaking, and learning.[51]

Chronic Diseases and Their Impact in Adults and Older Adults

Chronic conditions are major public health problems among adults worldwide. Globally, one in three adults has more than one chronic condition. In the United States, six in 10 adults (60%) have at least one chronic condition, and almost two in four (42%) have more than one chronic condition.[52] Because adults with chronic diseases advance to becoming older adults who have had the condition for a longer period of time with varying degrees of disease management, these same conditions tend to become increasingly more debilitating with loss of function and quality of life.

Chronic diseases are the leading causes of death and disability in adults. Globally, chronic conditions contributed to 42 million deaths (74% of all deaths) in 2019. Of these, cardiovascular disease is the leading cause of death, accounting for 17.9 million annual deaths.[2]

Chronic diseases impose an economic burden to society and the healthcare system. In the United States, chronic diseases create an economic burden of more than $4 trillion

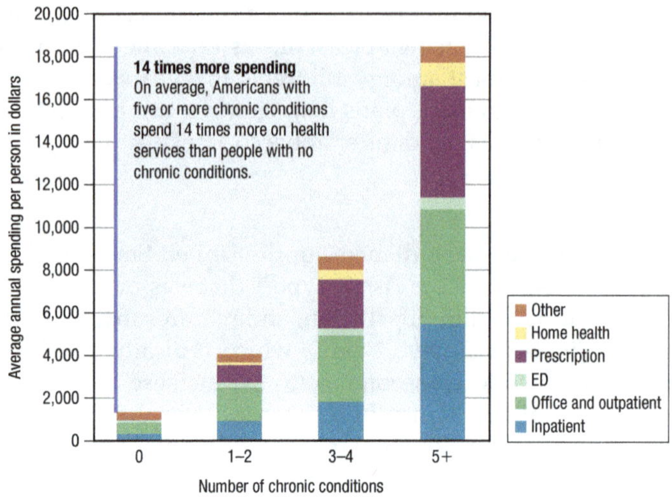

Figure 11.6. Impact of multiple chronic diseases on healthcare spending.
Source: Buttorff C, Ruder T, Bauman M. *Multiple Chronic Conditions in the United States*. RAND Corporation; 2017. https://www.rand.org/content/dam/rand/pubs/tools/TL200/TL221/RAND_TL221.pdf

annually in healthcare costs.[1] The use of the healthcare system and healthcare costs increase as the number of chronic conditions increase. For example, people with five or more chronic conditions have, on average, 20 outpatient visits per year compared to six visits per year for those with one or two chronic conditions, and two visits per year for those without chronic conditions.[52] Older adults are more likely than younger adults to live with multiple chronic conditions.

Chronic conditions negatively impact people's daily activities and cognitive functions. The limitations to functional status are greater among older adults. Chronic conditions in adulthood may often be prevented and/or delayed and managed with a balanced, healthy dietary pattern including a variety of fruits, vegetables, whole grains, lean protein, and low-fat dairy products and limited added sugars, saturated fats, and sodium.[53] Figure 11.6 illustrates the financial impact of multiple chronic diseases.

Cardiovascular Disease

Cardiovascular diseases are the leading cause of death in the United States, with more than 800,000 deaths every year (one third of annual deaths), and accounting for 32% of deaths globally in 2019.[2] High blood pressure and high cholesterol levels are the top two chronic conditions increasing the risk of heart disease and stroke, which are responsible for the majority of these deaths. The economic burden of cardiovascular disease is $363 billion per year when factoring in medical costs and lost productivity.[54]

Cancer

Cancer is the second leading cause of death in the United States with about 600,000 deaths each year.[55] Based on the number of new cases, the top five most common cancers are breast, lung, prostate, colorectal, and melanoma of the skin. There were 16 million cancer survivors in the United States in 2019, with an estimated cost of $150.8 billion for medical services and prescription drugs.[55]

Diabetes and Prediabetes

In the United States, 37.3 million people have diabetes and 96 million (one in three adults) have prediabetes.[56] Diabetes is the seventh leading cause of death in the United States. If poorly managed, diabetes can lead to complications such as cardiovascular disease, kidney disease, visual impairments, and amputations. The costs of diabetes are $327 billion yearly in medical costs and lost productivity.[56]

Arthritis

Arthritis affects 58.5 million Americans, and the incidence increases as the population gets older. While there are many different types of arthritis, the most common form is osteoarthritis, which is associated with overuse ("wear and tear") on joints, obesity, and aging.[57] Thus, arthritis is commonly found secondary to the other chronic diseases described in this chapter. Arthritis is the leading cause of work disability, costing $303.5 billion annually in medical costs and lost earnings. The Arthritis Foundation has estimated that one in four workers in the United States are dealing with some form of arthritis.[58]

POLICY PERSPECTIVES, GLOBAL ISSUES, AND CHALLENGES

Policy Perspectives

Battling chronic disease requires a comprehensive approach, as illustrated with the **social-ecological model (SEM).** The SEM holds space for the individual, interpersonal, community, and policy levels of intervention. As the focus of this chapter section is policy, it is important to note that the SEM suggests that policy determines what resources are available to connect or inhibit connection for individuals to their larger social and physical environments.[59] Figure 11.7 provides a visual representation of the SEM.

According to the CDC's Office of the Associate Director for Policy and Strategy, policy in the context of public health refers to "the advancement and implementation of public

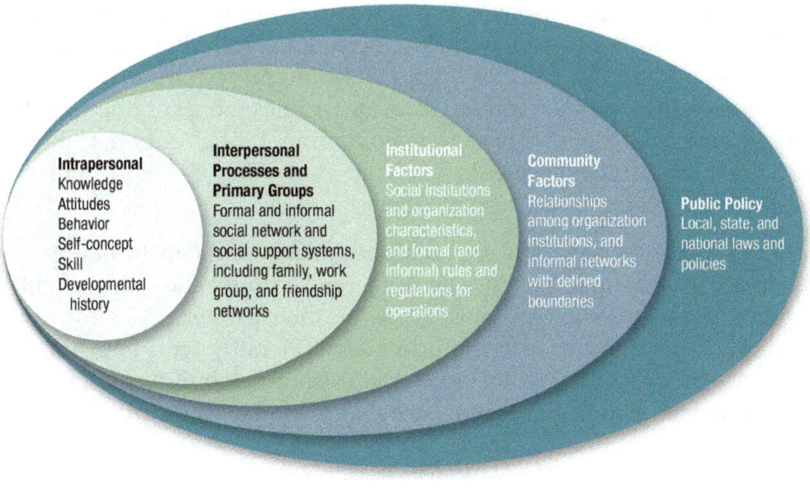

Figure 11.7. The social-ecological model.
Source: Adapted from McLeroy KR, Steckler, A. and Bibeau, D. (Eds.). The social ecology of health promotion interventions. *Health Educ Q.* 1988;15(4):351–377. https://doi.org/10.1177/109019818801500401

health law, regulations, or voluntary practices that influence systems development, organizational change, and individual behavior to promote improvements in health."[60] Policy, or the lack thereof, can enable or constrain action at the other levels of the SEM such as participation in broader community life, engagement in workplaces or other social institutions, and in family life at the interpersonal levels.

To achieve change in policies, several factors are essential. Among these are adequate and rigorous research, partnership development, and effective communications with policy makers that lead to change.[60] Policy development and adoption that impact chronic disease may be reflected at the local, state, or federal level; and budgetary documents, design codes, laws, and other aspects of policies may influence chronic disease. Public health professionals have an opportunity to stay abreast of important public health nutrition issues and strategies in order to inform and influence policy development.

Budgetary policy is a key area of focus because prevention and intervention activities cost money; funds are required for staff time and organizational infrastructure to create, implement, and evaluate programs.[60] This kind of support allows for educational efforts to be directed to both organizations and consumers on chronic diseases, risk factors, and SDOH as well as funds to begin to change the environments where people live, learn, work, play, and pray.[26,61]

Additional policy changes may focus on the built environment via design codes, laws, and other aspects of policies that influence chronic disease. Design codes at the municipal level may require property owners to install sidewalks at the time of construction; such an intervention will increasingly elevate the walkability of the community. Another example might be that new buildings must include stairs in a location that makes walkability more accessible for those occupying the building.[26]

Also notable is that not all policy development that impacts individual health outcomes must be governmental in nature. Most organizations, including businesses and nonprofits, have policies that can impact health. Many of those policies do not require action by the government. For instance, a corporation may determine that they will incentivize employees to participate in a wellness plan that includes frequent physical activity, dietary counseling, and other lifestyle changes by reducing their insurance premiums in exchange for completing the program. A different company may also comprehensively ban smoking on all of its property; and finally, another organization might require that vending machine providers only stock items with specified nutrition profiles more conducive to health. Such efforts are policy changes that do not require government intervention. Colloquially, individuals working in public health refer to governmental policy as "Big P" policy, and at the organizational level, refer to it as "little p" policy.[61]

While "Big P" policy is impactful and can both enable and constrain opportunities for individuals to achieve optimal health, one must not discount the value of "little p" policy. Organizational decisions to ban tobacco use on their property, to allow employees to engage in walking meetings, to increase prices for unhealthy food items in vending machines, providing breastfeeding or lactation spaces in office buildings, and others are all "little p" policy actions that promote or curb behaviors related to chronic disease.

Global Issues

Considering global issues in chronic disease prevention and management is essential in our increasingly connected world.[62] It is important to consider lessons learned in other contexts and how they may apply to the United States, because the intrapersonal, interpersonal, institutional, community, and policy factors at play elsewhere may be either a reflection of factors in the United States or a precursor of things to come. Exploring challenges and opportunities in global contexts can also validate the experiences of public health professionals in the United States. Consider **food swamps**, described as an oversaturation of fast food and less healthful, non-nutritious food options in a defined geographic area. The assertion that poor health outcomes in the United States and other global north settings are associated with food swamps is ubiquitous, but the concept had not been studied in the global south until Chew et al. published results of a similar challenge in the global south.[63] The global literature in chronic disease prevention and management can serve as a guidepost for development of the field in the United States or can help to validate that public health professionals are already moving in the right direction.

Challenges

Implementing policy solutions to chronic diseases across the life course is essential, as noted at length here; however, doing so is not without challenges. At a meta-level, one challenge in chronic disease prevention and management is in gaining the attention of a younger population of individuals needing attention for prevention strategies but who don't have a sense of the need for behavior change until later in life when chronic disease may strike. This challenge is actually the result of progress—that is, the epidemiologic transition wherein causes of death began to move from being primarily infectious diseases and injuries to chronic disease.

Development and deployment of more vaccines, a move to more commercial agriculture with automated technology, safer vehicles for transportation, and other advances all reduced premature death, on one hand. On the other, technologies of this sort introduced global challenges like tobacco use, increased availability of unhealthy food options, and less physical activity. With this transition, the population began living longer, resulting in the body breaking down due to lifestyle factors such as nutrition, physical activity, tobacco use, and other modifiable factors.

The globally connected nature of individuals made possible through relatively easy travel and enhanced communications technology underscores the need for addressing chronic disease prevention in a global context. These advancements create rapid exposure for people across the world to new trends and health behaviors that may be both positive or negative. Most recently, the COVID-19 pandemic, while an infectious or communicable disease, illustrates the connectedness that makes coordination in disease prevention so essential. In particular, the pandemic highlighted challenges in our network related to data and the overt need for a coordinated epidemiologic surveillance system. An optimal data system would allow for tracking and real time response to both infectious and chronic diseases. The COVID-19 pandemic underscored this need; however, scholars and practitioners have been discussing the topic for more than a decade. McKenna and Collins, in 2010, noted that improved data management is needed in the chronic disease space for three reasons:

1. To identify groups of people who are at risk of developing chronic disease or who experience fewer benefits from interventions
2. To measure the effect of program interventions
3. To identify newly emerging chronic diseases[64]

Currently, public health experts use mortality data to drive the understanding of the impact of chronic diseases. While this data may be useful, it has limitations and is not sufficient for enacting change. This is true because of the difficult nature of systems and behavior change in humans, which are at the heart of chronic disease. As noted elsewhere in this text, there are certainly genetic components to these health outcomes, but they are often facilitated by the options we have made possible through our physical and policy environments and the choices we make that are a part of those environments.

EFFECTIVE PUBLIC HEALTH NUTRITION INTERVENTIONS FOR CHRONIC DISEASE: U.S. AND GLOBAL

In the previous sections, issues at multiple levels of chronic disease prevention and management have been raised; and as such, it is essential that solutions be considered at each of those levels. A well-tested guide for interventionists in addressing these challenges is the SEM.[59] The SEM illustrates the way that individuals are nested in interpersonal relationships, which are nested in communities and are a part of broader social and policy contexts.

A key to success across each of these levels or domains is **community engagement**, a term often used among applied public health professionals and researchers. WHO has defined community engagement as "a process of developing relationships that enable stakeholders to work together to address health-related issues and promote well-being to achieve positive health impact and outcomes."[65] WHO further argues that using a community engagement framework in chronic disease prevention and management requires trust, accessibility, contextualization, equity, transparency, and autonomy.[65]

While public health nutrition professionals play a key role in facilitating community engagement, the concept places individuals, families, and communities—not healthcare providers, public health professionals, or researchers—at the center of change. WHO posits that key aspects of change include communication, collaboration or partnership, and resources.[65] In research contexts, investigators often use a **community-based participatory research** framework, which is an approach to research that "involves collective, reflective and systematic inquiry in which researchers and community stakeholders engage as equal partners in all steps of the research process with the goals of educating, improving practice or bringing about social change."[66] This is essential for developing interventions that, as noted earlier, center around the end users rather than those developing them.

WHAT WORKS: NATIONAL DIABETES PREVENTION PROGRAM

Community-engaged chronic disease prevention and management interventions at the individual and family levels are often tested, but they are not often supported across the trajectory of development to implementation and adoption in community-based settings. However, one example of a successful program of this sort is the National Diabetes Prevention Program (DPP).[67] According to the CDC, the National DPP originated in 2010 to address the increasing burden of prediabetes and type 2 diabetes in the United States. The program was built on partnerships between public and private organizations with the goal of offering evidence-based, cost-effective interventions to aid in preventing type 2 diabetes among individuals at the community level across the United States. The program is based on a robust randomized controlled trial supported by the National Institutes of Health. The original research demonstrated that participants with prediabetes who engage in a structured lifestyle change program focused on healthy eating and physical activity can cut their risk of developing type 2 diabetes by 58%.[68]

After the original research study, the DPP was adopted by the CDC for development as a curriculum that could be easily operationalized in community settings and for consistent management. It has been implemented by community organizations, private insurers, faith communities, employers, healthcare organizations, and government organizations. Led by a trained lifestyle coach, the program is implemented over the course of a year in a group-based setting. To help grow participation, public health practitioners have worked with health insurance companies and employers to incentivize participation because of the cost benefit for healthcare payers. This program is a strong illustration of the importance of considering multiple levels of intervention: (1) at the individual level, (2) at the group level encompassing the group in which the individual is situated, and, in many cases, (3) at the organizational policy level.

SUMMARY

Chronic diseases are conditions that last for a long time, significantly impact health and quality of life, and impose a high economic burden. Cardiovascular disease (a disease of the heart or blood vessels, such as stroke), cancers, chronic respiratory diseases, and diabetes are the major contributors to this global public health crisis. Many risk factors for chronic disease, particularly nutrition, are modifiable and offer preventive benefits. Public health nutrition professionals have the opportunity for advocacy in shaping policies and developing and implementing programs that can reduce the burden of chronic disease; community-engaged interventions for prevention and management offer evidence as a successful strategy.

KEY CHAPTER CONCEPTS

1. Chronic diseases are a global crisis; four major categories of chronic conditions—cardiovascular disease (a disease of the heart or blood vessels, such as stroke), cancers, chronic respiratory diseases, and diabetes—account for 80% of deaths worldwide, but also contribute to disability and economic burden.
2. These four health behaviors are major modifiable risk factors for chronic disease: poor nutrition, physical inactivity, tobacco use, and harmful use of alcohol.
3. Strategies to prevent chronic disease are categorized into three levels: primary prevention is focused on prevention in healthy populations, secondary prevention is focused on identification in at-risk populations, and tertiary prevention is focused on treatment and management strategies in those diagnosed with a chronic disease.
4. The COVID-19 pandemic significantly affected the treatment and management of chronic disease.
5. Chronic conditions can occur during any life stage; The life course theory considers how each life stage flows consecutively into the next, with health behaviors of each previous stage impacting the current stage.
6. Challenges to chronic disease prevention and management occur at multiple levels; the social-ecological model offers a comprehensive approach to chronic disease policy and interventions.
7. Exploring global challenges and opportunities can validate experiences and inform directions of public health nutrition professionals in the United States.
8. Community-engaged intervention models offer a promising solution for chronic disease prevention and management.

CASE STUDY

A public health nutrition professional (JL) works within a county health department. Recent data indicate that the prevalence of type 2 diabetes within the county has increased by about 1% over the past 5 years.[68] JL has been asked to assess SDOH in the county, with a focus on type 2 diabetes prevention. The assessment is to be structured around the five main categories of SDOH as described by the CDC: (1) Health Care Access and Quality; (2) Neighborhood and the Built Environment; (3) Social and Community Context; (4) Economic Stability; (5) Education Access and Quality. The short-term goal of the assessment is to identify feasible opportunities for intervention in the health and nutrition environment of the community. The county's long-term goal is to see a decrease in the prevalence of type 2 diabetes over the next 5 years. **Complete the following table.**

Social Determinant of Health (SDOH)	List two specific factors to assess for each SDOH; one factor must be nutrition-related	List two data sources that could be used for each assessment[25]	List and describe a feasible intervention for each factor	What is an expected outcome for each intervention?[1]
Health Care Access and Quality				
Neighborhood and Built Environment				
Social and Community Context				
Economic Stability				
Education Access and Quality				

1. Data sources may include preexisting publicly available data, gathered data such as surveys, focus groups, or other sources. For preexisting data, list the specific source (such as the **Behavioral Risk Factor Surveillance System [BRFSS]**).
2. Provide a reference for each outcome to justify your expectation.

DISCUSSION QUESTIONS

1. Describe chronic diseases you have seen in your community/work setting and strategies for prevention/management you have found successful. Do these strategies match any of the information presented in this chapter?
2. Discuss factors from each level of the social-ecological model that impact chronic disease prevalence and/or intervention strategies. Select one of the chronic diseases described in this chapter, specifically, and consider risk factors in the context of the SEM.

3. Describe three reasons the COVID-19 pandemic has incurred greater health debt.
4. Select a chronic condition described in this chapter and discuss examples of primary, secondary, and tertiary prevention efforts for that condition.
5. Select a chronic disease described in this chapter and describe how it affects persons and populations at various stages of the life cycle.
6. What components would you include in a community-engaged chronic disease prevention and management intervention model for your community?
7. What factors do you see as posing key challenges to chronic disease management in a global context?

SUGGESTED LEARNING ACTIVITIES

1. Find the prevalence of chronic diseases in general as well as specific chronic diseases in your community. What are the most common chronic conditions? Which stages of life are most impacted? What else do you find interesting about the data?
2. Design a community-engaged chronic disease prevention and management intervention for one of the most prevalent conditions described in item 1. What life stage does this target? Consider levels of primary, secondary and tertiary prevention. The SEM may help you with your approach.
3. Consider an SDOH screening tool for your facility in order to collect data to better serve your community by preventing or managing chronic disease. Include at least one question from each SDOH category descried in this chapter.
4. Interview a health professional about the effects of COVID-19 on chronic disease in your community. Design three to five questions based on the information from this chapter. What did you learn?
5. Develop an infographic targeting chronic disease prevention and management. What key information would you include about lifestyle factors based on the information in this chapter?

RESOURCES FOR FURTHER LEARNING

- American Heart Association: www.heart.org
  - Provides information and resources to improve heart health and reduce deaths from cardiovascular disease
- American Diabetes Association: www.diabetes.org
  - Presents research, community services, education, and advocacy resources for those with diabetes
- Centers for Disease Control and Prevention, National Center for Chronic Disease Prevention and Health Promotion: www.cdc.gov/chronicdisease
  - Provides chronic disease data and publications; helps people and communities prevent chronic diseases and promote health and wellness for all
- National Heart, Lung and Blood Institute: www.nhlbi.nih.gov
  - Materials for patients and health professionals on many heart, lung, blood, and sleep conditions, based on the latest scientific findings
- American Cancer Society: www.cancer.org
  - Organization combating cancer through advocacy, research, and patient support

- National Cancer Institute: www.cancer.gov
  - Comprehensive cancer information from the U.S. government's principal agency for cancer research
- World Health Organization: www.who.int
  - Information and resources from the United Nations agency working to promote international public health
- Academy of Nutrition and Dietetics: www.eatright.org
  - Information on nutrition and health that can help prevent or manage health conditions

REFERENCES

1. Centers for Disease Control and Prevention. About chronic diseases. National Center for Chronic Disease Prevention and Health Promotion. Accessed October 19, 2023. https://www.cdc.gov/chronicdisease/about/index.htm
2. World Health Organization. Noncommunicable diseases. September 16, 2023. https://www.who.int/news-room/fact-sheets/detail/noncommunicable-diseases
3. Doshi RP, Aseltine RH Jr, Sabina AB, Graham GN. Racial and ethnic disparities in preventable hospitalizations for chronic disease: prevalence and risk factors. *J Racial Ethn Health Disparities.* 2017;4(6):1100–1106. https://doi.org/10.1007/s40615-016-0315-z
4. Lancet, Institute for Health Metrics and Evaluation. Global burden of disease 2019. Lancet; 2020. http://ghdx.healthdata.org/gbd-results-tool
5. World Health Organization. Disability-adjusted life years. Global Health Observatory. Accessed October 18, 2023. https://www.who.int/data/gho/indicator-metadata-registry/imr-details/158
6. Li Y, Pan A, Wang DD, et al. Impact of healthy lifestyle factors on life expectancies in the U.S. population. *Circulation*. 2018;138(4):345–355. https://doi.org/10.1161/CIRCULATIONAHA.117.032047
7. GBD 2019 Diseases and Injuries Collaborators. Global burden of 369 diseases and injuries in 204 countries and territories, 1990–2019: a systematic analysis for the Global Burden of Disease Study 2019. *Lancet*. 2020;396(10258):1204–1222. https://doi.org/10.1016/S0140-6736(20)30925-9
8. Institute for Health Metrics and Evaluation. Global burden of disease. Our World in Data. 2019. https://ourworldindata.org/grapher/total-disease-burden-by-cause
9. Egger G. In search of a germ theory equivalent for chronic disease. *Prev Chronic Dis*. 2012;9:E95. https://doi.org/10.5888/pcd9.110301
10. Centers for Disease Control and Prevention. About COVID-19: people with certain medical conditions. Updated May 11, 2023. https://www.cdc.gov/coronavirus/2019-ncov/need-extra-precautions/people-with-medical-conditions.html
11. Ruth L, Alongi J, Robitscher J. Confronting the health debt: the impact of COVID-19 on chronic disease prevention and management. *Health Affairs Blog. September 17, 2021. https://www.healthaffairs.org/content/forefront/confronting-health-debt-impact-covid-19-chronic-disease-prevention-and-management*
12. Czeisler ME, Marynak K, Clarke KEN, et al. Delay or avoidance of medical care because of COVID-19-related concerns—United States, June 2020. *MMWR Morb Mortal Wkly Rep*. 2020;69(36):1250–1257. https://doi.org/10.15585/mmwr.mm6936a4
13. Gutierrez SB, Quispe KO. Weight gain and physical inactivity during the COVID-19 pandemic. *Rev Panam Salud Publica*. 2021;45:e136. https://doi.org/10.26633/RPSP.2021.136
14. Panchal N, Saunders H, Rudowitz R, Cox C. The implications of COVID-19 for mental health and substance use. Updated March 20, 2023. KFF. https://www.kff.org/coronavirus-covid-19/issue-brief/the-implications-of-covid-19-for-mental-health-and-substance-use

15. Beaglehole R, Bonita R, Horton R, et al. Priority actions for the non-communicable disease crisis. *Lancet*. 2011;377(9775):1438–1447. https://doi.org/10.1016/S0140-6736(11)60393-0
16. National Center for Chronic Disease Prevention and Health Promotion. Poor nutrition. Accessed October 19, 2023. https://www.cdc.gov/chronicdisease/resources/publications/factsheets/nutrition.htm
17. National Center for Chronic Disease Prevention and Health Promotion. Physical inactivity. Accessed October 19, 2023. https://www.cdc.gov/chronicdisease/resources/publications/factsheets/physical-activity.htm
18. National Center for Chronic Disease Prevention and Health Promotion. Tobacco Use. https://www.cdc.gov/chronicdisease/resources/publications/factsheets/tobacco.htm
19. Sahle BW, Chen W, Rawal LB, Renzaho AMN. Weight gain after smoking cessation and risk of major chronic diseases and mortality. *JAMA Netw Open*. 2021;4(4):e217044. https://doi.org/10.1001/jamanetworkopen.2021.7044
20. National Center for Chronic Disease Prevention and Health Promotion. Excessive alcohol use. Accessed October 19, 2023. https://www.cdc.gov/chronicdisease/resources/publications/factsheets/alcohol.htm
21. National Institute on Alcohol Abuse and Alcoholism. Alcohol's effects on health: What is a standard drink? National Institutes of Health. Accessed October 19, 2023. https://www.niaaa.nih.gov/alcohols-effects-health/overview-alcohol-consumption/what-standard-drink
22. Centers for Disease Control and Prevention. Alcohol and public health: dietary guidelines for alcohol. Accessed October 19, 2023. https://www.cdc.gov/alcohol/fact-sheets/moderate-drinking.htm
23. Merck A. The upstream-downstream parable for health equity. Salud America! UT Health; October 8, 2018. https://salud-america.org/the-upstream-downstream-parable-for-health-equity
24. Office of Disease Prevention and Health Promotion. *Healthy People 2030*: Social determinants of health. U.S. Department of Health and Human Services. 2020. https://health.gov/healthypeople/priority-areas/social-determinants-health
25. Cockerham WC, Hamby BW, Oates GR. The social determinants of chronic disease. *Am J Prev Med*. 2017;52(1 suppl 1):S5–S12. https://doi.org/10.1016/j.amepre.2016.09.010
26. Rural Health Information Hub. Social determinants of health for rural people. Accessed October 19, 2023. https://www.ruralhealthinfo.org/topics/social-determinants-of-health
27. Centers for Disease Control and Prevention. Built environment: NCCDPHP's program successes. National Center for Chronic Disease Prevention and Health Promotion. Accessed October 19, 2023. https://www.cdc.gov/chronicdisease/healthequity/sdoh-and-chronic-disease/nccdphp-and-social-determinants-of-health/built-environment.htm
28. Jayathilaka R, Joachim S, Mallikarachchi V, Perera N, Ranawaka D. Do chronic illnesses and poverty go hand in hand? *PLoS One*. 2020;15(10):e0241232. https://doi.org/10.1371/journal.pone.0241232
29. Choi AI, Weekley CC, Chen SC, et al. Association of educational attainment with chronic disease and mortality: the Kidney Early Evaluation Program (KEEP). *Am J Kidney Dis*. 2011;58(2):228–234. https://doi.org/10.1053/j.ajkd.2011.02.388
30. Florida Department of Health. The life course theory. Accessed October 19, 2023. https://www.floridahealth.gov/programs-and-services/womens-health/florida-life-course-indicator-report/life-course-theory-1.html
31. Mahumud RA, Sultana M, Sarker AR. Distribution and determinants of low birth weight in developing countries. *J Prev Med Public Health*. 2017;50(1):18–28. https://doi.org/10.3961/jpmph.16.087
32. Stang J, Huffman LG. Position of the Academy of Nutrition and Dietetics: obesity, reproduction, and pregnancy outcomes. *J Acad Nutr Diet*. 2016;116(4):677–691. https://doi.org/10.1016/j.jand.2016.01.008
33. Ferrara A, Hedderson MM, Brown SD, et al. A telehealth lifestyle intervention to reduce excess gestational weight gain in pregnant women with overweight or obesity (GLOW): a randomised, parallel-group, controlled trial. *Lancet Diabetes Endocrinol*. 2020;8(6):490–500. https://doi.org/10.1016/S2213-8587(20)30107-8
34. Manna P, Jain SK. Obesity, oxidative stress, adipose tissue dysfunction, and the associated health risks: causes and therapeutic strategies. *Metab Syndr Relat Disord*. 2015;13(10):423–444. https://doi.org/10.1089/met.2015.0095
35. Calkins K, Devaskar SU. Fetal origins of adult disease. *Curr Probl Pediatr Adolesc Health Care*. 2011;41(6):158–176. https://doi.org/10.1016/j.cppeds.2011.01.001

36. Centers for Disease Control and Prevention. Reproductive health: diabetes during pregnancy. Accessed October 19, 2023. https://www.cdc.gov/reproductivehealth/maternalinfanthealth/diabetes-during-pregnancy.htm
37. Diaz-Santana MV, O'Brien KM, Park Y-MM, Sandler DP, Weinberg CR. Persistence of risk for type 2 diabetes after gestational diabetes mellitus. *Diabetes Care*. 2022;45(4):864–870. https://doi.org/10.2337/dc21-1430
38. Robbins CL, Zapata LB, Farr SL, et al. Core state preconception health indicators—Pregnancy Risk Assessment Monitoring System and Behavioral Risk Factor Surveillance System, 2009. *MMWR Surveill Summ*. 2014;63(3):1–62. https://www.cdc.gov/mmwr/preview/mmwrhtml/ss6303a1.htm
39. Lo JO, Mission JF, Caughey AB. Hypertensive disease of pregnancy and maternal mortality. *Curr Opin Obstet Gynecol*. 2013;25(2):124–132. https://doi.org/10.1097/GCO.0b013e32835e0ef5
40. Martin JA, Hamilton BE, Ventura SJ, et al. Births: final data for 2009. *Natl Vital Stat Rep*. 2011;60(1):1–70. https://www.cdc.gov/nchs/data/nvsr/nvsr60/nvsr60_01.pdf
41. Livingston JC, Maxwell BD, Sibai BM. Chronic hypertension in pregnancy. *Minerva Ginecol*. 2003;55(1):1–13. https://doi.org/10.1016/S0889-8545(05)70213-8
42. Gaillard R, Durmuş B, Hofman A, Mackenbach JP, Steegers EA, Jaddoe VW. Risk factors and outcomes of maternal obesity and excessive weight gain during pregnancy. *Obesity (Silver Spring)*. 2013;21(5):1046–1055. https://doi.org/10.1002/oby.20088
43. Athukorala C, Rumbold AR, Willson KJ, Crowther CA. The risk of adverse pregnancy outcomes in women who are overweight or obese. *BMC Pregnancy Childbirth*. 2010;10:56. https://doi.org/10.1186/1471-2393-10-56
44. Feig DS, Shah BR, Lipscombe LL, et al. Preeclampsia as a risk factor for diabetes: a population-based cohort study. *PLoS Med*. 2013;10(4):e1001425. https://doi.org/10.1371/journal.pmed.1001425
45. Centers for Disease Control and Prevention. CDC healthy schools: managing chronic health conditions. Accessed October 19, 2023. https://www.cdc.gov/healthyschools/chronicconditions.htm
46. Centers for Disease Control and Prevention. Asthma in children. Updated August 10, 2018. https://www.cdc.gov/vitalsigns/childhood-asthma
47. Centers for Disease Control and Prevention. What is diabetes? Accessed October 19, 2023. https://www.cdc.gov/diabetes/basics/diabetes.html
48. Centers for Disease Control and Prevention. Rates of new diagnosed cases of type 1 and type 2 diabetes continue to rise among children, teens. Accessed October 19, 2023. https://www.cdc.gov/diabetes/research/reports/children-diabetes-rates-rise.html
49. Centers for Disease Control and Prevention. Childhood obesity facts. Accessed October 19, 2023. https://www.cdc.gov/obesity/data/childhood.html
50. Centers for Disease Control and Prevention. Healthy weight, nutrition, and physical activity. Accessed October 19, 2023. https://www.cdc.gov/healthyweight/index.html
51. Centers for Disease Control and Prevention. Children's oral health. Accessed October 19, 2023. https://www.cdc.gov/oralhealth/basics/childrens-oral-health/index.html
52. Buttorff C, Ruder T, Bauman M. *Multiple Chronic Conditions in the United States*. RAND Corporation; 2017. https://www.rand.org/content/dam/rand/pubs/tools/TL200/TL221/RAND_TL221.pdf
53. Centers for Disease Control and Prevention. How you can prevent chronic diseases. Accessed October 19, 2023. https://www.cdc.gov/chronicdisease/about/prevent
54. Benjamin EJ, Virani SS, Callaway CW, et al. Heart disease and stroke statistics—2018 update: a report from the American Heart Association. *Circulation*. 2018;137(12):e67–e492. https://doi.org/10.1161/CIR.0000000000000558
55. National Cancer Institute. Cancer statistics. National Institutes of Health. Updated September 25, 2020. https://www.cancer.gov/about-cancer/understanding/statistics
56. Centers for Disease Control and Prevention. Diabetes fast facts. Accessed October 19, 2023. https://www.cdc.gov/diabetes/basics/quick-facts.html
57. Centers for Disease Control and Prevention. Fast facts about arthritis. Accessed October 19, 2023. https://www.cdc.gov/arthritis/basics/arthritis-fast-facts.html.
58. Arthritis Foundation. Meet arthritis@work. Accessed October 19, 2023. https://www.arthritis.org/partnership/atwork.
59. McLeroy KR, Bibeau D, Steckler A, Glanz K. An ecological perspective on health promotion programs. *Health Educ Q*. 1988;15(4):351–377. https://doi.org/10.1177/109019818801500401
60. Centers for Disease Control and Prevention. CDC policy process. Accessed October 19, 2023. https://www.cdc.gov/policy/paeo/process/

61. Collins S. Big P, little P—a guide to policy engagement at all levels. Association of Maternal & Child Health Programs. April 2019. https://amchp.org/2019/04/15/big-p-little-p-a-guide-to-policy-engagement-at-all-levels
62. Airhihenbuwa CO, Tseng TS, Sutton VD, Price L. Global perspectives on improving chronic disease prevention and management in diverse settings. *Prev Chronic Dis*. 2021;18:E33. https://doi.org/10.5888/pcd18.210055
63. Chew A, Moran A, Barnoya J. Food swamps surrounding schools in three areas of Guatemala. *Prev Chronic Dis*. 2020;17:E75. https://doi.org/10.5888/pcd17.200029
64. McKenna M, Collins J. Current issues and challenges in chronic disease control. In: Remington PL, Brownson RC, Wegner MV, eds. *Chronic Disease Epidemiology and Control*. 3rd ed. American Public Health Association; 2010:1–26. https://webcourses.ucf.edu/courses/1373076/files/84142325/download?wrap=1
65. World Health Organization. *Community Engagement: A Health Promotion Guide for Universal Health Coverage in the Hands of the People*. World Health Organization; 2020. https://www.who.int/publications/i/item/9789240010529
66. Tremblay MC, Martin DH, McComber AM, McGregor A, Macaulay AC. Understanding community-based participatory research through a social movement framework: a case study of the Kahnawake Schools Diabetes Prevention Project. *BMC Public Health*. 2018;18(1):487. https://doi.org/10.1186/s12889-018-5412-y
67. Centers for Disease Control and Prevention. National Diabetes Prevention Program: working together to prevent type 2 diabetes. https://www.cdc.gov/diabetes/prevention/index.html
68. Centers for Disease Control and Prevention. National Diabetes Prevention Program: research behind the National DPP. Accessed September 23, 2023. https://www.cdc.gov/diabetes/prevention/what-is-dpp.htm
69. Khan MAB, Hashim MJ, King JK, Govender RD, Mustafa H, Al Kaabi J. Epidemiology of Type 2 diabetes—global burden of disease and forecasted trends. *J Epidemiol Glob Health*. 2020;10(1):107–111. https://doi.org/10.2991/jegh.k.191028.001

12

PUBLIC HEALTH NUTRITION EMERGENCY MANAGEMENT WITH A LIFE CYCLE FOCUS

Kyle L. Thompson and Natasha Johnson-Griffin

LEARNING OBJECTIVES

Upon completing this chapter students will be able to:

1. List six domains of emergency preparedness.
2. Describe a three-step strategic planning framework for emergency preparedness.
3. Align the 15 CDC-CEPR public health emergency planning capabilities with selected public health nutrition (PHN) applications.
4. Use **social vulnerability** index tools to assess a given community's social determinants of health and visualize potential impacts on **community resilience** and **recovery**.
5. Categorize food and nutrition-related emergency considerations by life cycle stage.
6. Describe the role of governmental and nongovernmental, nonprofit, and food banks and food pantries in food and nutrition emergencies.
7. Describe and explain applications of new technology to food **emergency management**.

INTRODUCTION

Natural disasters and emergency situations are a fact of human life. These events include but are not limited to hurricanes, floods, tornados, blizzards, droughts, heat waves, tsunamis, earthquakes, landslides, wildfires, environmental disasters such as oil and chemical spills, pandemics and disease outbreaks, wars, terrorism, political upheavals, infrastructure breakdowns, and severe economic disruptions.[1] Disasters affect both populations and individuals, and the impacts can be long-term and overwhelming.

Populations may experience consequences including total or partial destruction of communities and infrastructure, massive loss of resources, disruption of the activities of normal life, loss of historical sites and community context, and overwhelming challenges to rebuilding and recovering. Consequences for individuals may include the loss of loved ones, property, employment, access to resources, and savings. The lasting effects of grief, physical injury, and economic disruption on persons are lifelong, and severe and long-lasting emotional and mental health difficulties can result from losing one's sense of safety and security in the wake of a disaster.

Another fact of human life is that through natural disasters and emergency situations, people still need to eat. Food and clean water are basic survial needs for humans.[2] Access to adequate and appropriate nutrition and food and water supplies for populations and individuals during and after emergency events is a key factor in promoting **community resilience** and supporting recovery.[3] Preparation for food and nutrition disasters is an essential component of emergency preparedness. Public health and public health nutrition professionals play a crucial role in ensuring that food and nutrition considerations are an integral component of individual, community, state, local, and regional emergency and disaster planning.

OVERVIEW OF THE ROLE OF PUBLIC HEALTH NUTRITION IN EMERGENCY MANAGEMENT

Principles of Emergency Management

Six Domains of Emergency Preparedness With Food and Nutrition Implications

The Centers for Disease Control and Prevention Center for Emergency Preparedness and Response (CDC-CEPR) has defined **six major domains of emergency preparedness** that should be the focus of disaster planning.[4] Each domain of emergency preparedness has important nutrition implications:

- First, **community resilience** is enhanced by thorough planning for emergency access to crucial food and nutrition supplies. Careful consideration of the location(s) of emergency food supplies within a given community and means of access to those supplies may enhance resilience in an emergency.
- Establishment of a structure for **incident management** is required to ensure that emergency food and nutrition supplies can be deployed effectively. Effective incident management establishes a command structure to coordinate all emergency response efforts so that services and supplies, including food, are delivered when and where most needed.
- **Information management** refers to the overall communications plan designed to provide essential information to emergency responders and the public. Integration of nutrition communications within the master communications plan is crucial to educate and inform the public on food supplies and food safety updates.
- PHN professionals are involved in **countermeasures and mitigation** efforts by providing access to food and nutrition supplies such as baby formula, baby food, prenatal vitamins, and medical food supplements such as nutritional beverages to populations with special life stage needs. These measures are designed to prevent or ameliorate poor health outcomes.
- During emergencies, PHN professionals may participate in **surge management** efforts by assisting in providing food to first responders and other emergency response personnel, and by collaborating with community healthcare facilities in regard to distribution of emergency food supplies.

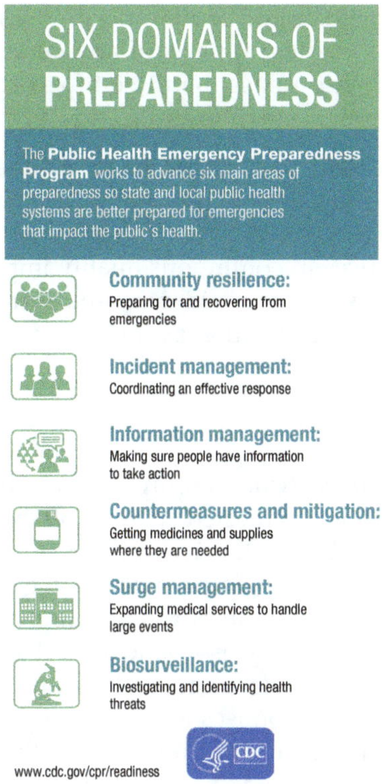

Figure 12.1. Centers for Disease Control and Prevention Center for Emergency Preparedness and Response (CDC-CEPR) six domains of emergency preparedness.
Source: Center for Disease Control and Prevention. Six domains of preparedness. Accessed September 23, 2023. https://www.cdc.gov/cpr/readiness/sixdomains.htm

- **Biosurveillance** of the safety of food and water supplies is essential to promote the well-being of the public during a disaster and especially during its aftermath. PHN professionals may be involved in the plan for testing and monitoring community food and water supplies to promote public safety and prevent food- and waterborne illness.

The six emergency preparedness domains are listed and described in Figure 12.1.

Planning for Emergency Preparedness

In 2018, the CDC-CEPR published guidelines titled *Public Health Emergency Preparedness and Response Capabilities*, providing national standards for emergency response capabilities for state, local, tribal, and territorial public health agencies.[5] These resources were updated in 2021. The standards and accompanying guidance provide a framework for assessing, planning, and implementing specific public health functions during emergency situations. The standards are designed to promote effective emergency preparedness and response.[5]

The CDC-CEPR three-part planning model for emergency response follows these three steps: (1) assess, (2) determine, and (3) plan[5]:

Assess

During the assessment phase, public health organizations should define their specific roles, responsibilities, and functions in responding to emergencies, determine and describe their available resources, and assess their current performance in regard to emergency response. Assessment of organizational roles and responsibilities may encompass collaborating public health agencies or community partners such as food pantries and resource centers that would be integral parts of any emergency food response efforts. Resource assessment should encompass the three broad components of emergency response resourcing: preparedness, skills/training, and equipment/technology.[5]

An initial assessment of current performance may include consideration of the organization's current performance indicators in providing "normal" services and achieving selected state/national benchmarks, current efforts to train personnel in emergency response procedures, and current practices in continuous quality improvement (CQI); that is, does the organization have processes in place to identify and correct deficiencies?[5] Effective implementation of CQI within an organization over time is an important indicator of ability to develop emergency management plans.

Determine

In the determination phase, *jurisdictional* resources should be considered. The term *jurisdictional* refers to matters that are connected with an official governmental organization that has designated and prescribed authority to make decisions.[6] Thus, in planning for emergency situations, information and data from official governmental organizations are crucial. Jurisdictional input may include but is not limited to existing local, state, and national emergency response capability assessments and strategic plans, information on government funding sources, and data from local, state, and national public health authorities on previous emergency responses and follow-up activities.[5] PHN practitioners should conduct their review of jurisdictional resources with a focus on food-related topics.

Following the assessment of jurisdictional resources, emergency planners should identify and prioritize specific agency priorities for improvement, and develop short- and long-term goals for emergency preparation, based on the emergency response capabilities defined by the CDC-CEPR.[5] The CDC-CEPR defines *short-term goals* as initiatives to be achieved in 1 year or less; *long-term goals* are those goals expected to be achieved in 2 to 5 years' time.[5]

Plan

In the planning phase, specific organizational activities and initiatives are implemented in order to achieve the organization's desired capability-focused emergency response short- and long-term goals. Development of collaborations and material, financial, and human resources to build and sustain emergency response capability over time should be considered. The CDC-CEPR strongly encourages the testing of plans by implementing emergency exercises and simulations/scenarios, and measuring performance in actual emergencies; **jurisdictional partners** such as the CDC-CEPR offer resources for this type of testing.[5]

Following emergency testing, identification of areas for improvement and subsequent improvement initiatives can enhance emergency response capabilities. Actual emergency situations also provide opportunities to identify and prioritize further emergency capability development needs. Figure 12.2 provides the CDC-CEPR's **Public Health Emergency Preparedness and Planning Model**.

Fifteen Public Health Capabilities for Emergency Management

Along with broad domains of emergency management functions and a framework for strategic emergency planning, the CDC has provided a list of 15 key public health capabilities related to emergency management. The list includes definitions, implementation guidance, and evaluation guidelines for each capability. A crucial overall observation of the 15 capabilities is that an effective emergency preparedness and management plan is collaborative. That is, the plan is based on cooperation and teamwork among many different agencies, organizations, and individuals. PHN emergency planning efforts are a crucial component of community preparedness, recovery, and resilience, and should be embedded within the overall community planning process. Table 12.1 lists each capability, its description, and examples of aligned public health and PHN applications.

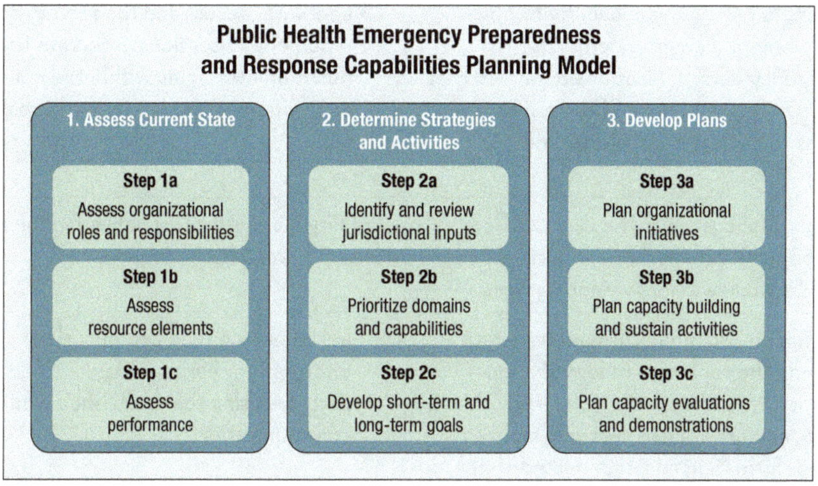

Figure 12.2. Public health emergency preparedness and response capabilities planning model.
Source: Center for Disease Control and Prevention. *Public Health Emergency Preparedness and Response Capabilities: National Standards for State, Local, Tribal, and Territorial Public Health*. U.S. Department of Health and Human Services Updated 2019. https://www.cdc.gov/orr/readiness/00_docs/cdc_preparednesresponsecapabilities_october2018_final_508.pdf

Table 12.1. CDC-CEPR Public Health Emergency Management Capabilities With PHN Applications

Capability	PHN Applications
1. *Community Preparedness*: The capability to plan and prepare for, persevere through, and recover from public health emergencies.	• Prepare a comprehensive community food and nutrition plan for emergencies, with the goals of promoting community preparedness, endurance, and recovery.
2. *Community Recovery*: The capability to identify, prioritize, and deploy crucial resources and partnerships to promote recovery from public health emergencies.	• Identify all community food and nutrition resources, assess assets and gap areas, prioritize needs, stockpile appropriate supplies, and map nutrition resource and personnel deployment.
3. *Emergency Operations Coordination*: The capability to quickly implement an emergency command center that can effectively manage and coordinate all emergency operations, and is in compliance with all applicable regulations and laws.	• Partner with jurisdictional and community partners to integrate the food and nutrition emergency response plan within the coordinated overall emergency response plan, to heighten resilience and promote community recovery.

(Continued)

Table 12.1. CDC-CEPR Public Health Emergency Management Capabilities with Examples of Aligned PHN Applications. *(Continued)*

Capability	PHN Applications
4. *Emergency Public Information and Warning:* Emergency public information and warning is having the capability to quickly implement a coordinated system of emergency communications to ensure that emergency personnel and the public have access to critical news, alerts, and information.	• Develop a plan to provide the public with critical information regarding food and water access and food safety during emergency situations; integrate food and nutrition messaging within the community's coordinated overall emergency response plan.
5. *Fatality Management:* The capability to collaborate with appropriate partners to provide fatality management services.	*Fatality management is not within the PHN scope of practice.*
6. *Information Sharing:* Information sharing is having the capability to identify and communicate effectively with jurisdictional, public, and private partners who need to share information and data related to the emergency.	• Participate in food and nutrition information sharing with identified partners using the established plan of communication.
7. *Mass Care:* The capability to collaborate with local agencies to support congregate sites providing services to those impacted by the emergency.	• Work with local agencies as needed to determine the food and nutrition support needs of congregate sites; include meeting the needs of these sites within the food and nutrition emergency plan and overall disaster planning.
8. *Medical Countermeasure Dispensing and Administration:* The capability to provide medical interventions to prevent, treat, or ameliorate negative health impacts of the emergency.	*Medical countermeasure dispensing and administration is not within the PHN scope of practice.*
9. *Medical Material Management and Distribution:* The capability to obtain and effectively distribute necessary medical supplies during a public health emergency.	*Medical material management and distribution is not within the PHN scope of practice.*
10. *Medical Surge:* The capability to handle medical care needs that exceed the usual capacity of available facilities.	• Work with local healthcare facilities (hospitals, emergency care sites, etc.) to develop a plan to meet the food and nutritional needs of staff, patients, and families during the emergency.

Table 12.1. CDC-CEPR Public Health Emergency Management Capabilities with Examples of Aligned PHN Applications. ***(Continued)***

Capability	PHN Applications
11. *Nonpharmaceutical Interventions:* The capability of community residents to implement practices that can help mitigate the impacts of public health emergencies.	• Work within the overall emergency communications plan to provide appropriate messaging regarding food safety and hygiene during emergencies, food and water access, and access to important nutritional supplies for life cycle groups, such as baby formula, baby food, prenatal vitamins, and medical food supplements.
12. *Public Health Laboratory Testing:* The capability to use appropriate and safe laboratory methods to identify and confirm threats to public health and to disseminate data to collaborators as needed.	• Assist as requested with necessary food-related laboratory testing during the emergency, such as the collection of water and food samples for safety testing.
13. *Public Health Surveillance and Epidemiological Investigation:* The capability to conduct routine assessments of public health as needed, to expand those functions as needed in an emergency, and to collect and share epidemiological data as appropriate.	• Collect and provide food- and nutrition-related data as indicated in the overall emergency plan.
14. *Responder Safety and Health:* Responder safety and health is the capability to protect emergency responders and personnel before, during, and after an emergency deployment.	• Develop a plan for providing food and beverages to emergency responders; collaborate with community partners and integrate efforts within the overall emergency plan.
15. *Volunteer Management:* The capability of emergency management personnel to collaborate and coordinate efforts to identify, train, and deploy volunteers before, during, and after an emergency deployment.	• As part of the overall food- and nutrition-related emergency plan, identify and train volunteers to assist in the delivery of food- and nutrition-related services.

CDC-CEPR, Centers for Disease Control and Prevention Center for Emergency Preparedness and Response; PHN, public health nutrition.

Source: Adapted from Center for Disease Control and Prevention. *Public Health Emergency Preparedness and Response Capabilities: National Standards for State, Local, Tribal, and Territorial Public Health*. U.S. Department of Health and Human Services. Updated 2019. https://www.cdc.gov/orr/readiness/00_docs/cdc_preparednesresponsecapabilities_october2018_final_508.pdf

SOCIAL DETERMINANTS OF HEALTH RELATED TO FOOD AND NUTRITION EMERGENCY MANAGEMENT

Social determinants of health (SDOH), according to theCDC, are "conditions in the places where people live, learn, work, and play that affect a wide range of health and quality-of life risks and outcomes."[7] SDOH that impact particular populations' disaster resilience include but are not limited to the built environment, median income level, typical housing, transportation availability and infrastructure, access to healthcare, and the availability of healthful and wholesome food.[8]

The CDC Agency for Toxic Substances and Disease Registry (CDC-ATSDR) defines **social vulnerability** as "the potential negative effects on communities caused by external stressors on human health."[9] Social vulnerability is associated with poor SDOH such as lower income levels and less access to resources. Evidence indicates that populations with fewer resources—that is, with greater social vulnerability—tend to experience more severe short- and long-term impacts from natural disasters.[8,10] The CDC-ATSDR has developed a **Social vulnerability index (SVI)** based on U.S. Census tract data.[9]

The CDC-ATSDR SVI is based on 16 factors recorded in census tract data and grouped into four thematic domains: (1) socioeconomic status; (2) household composition and disability; (3) minority status and language; and (4) housing type and transportation.[11] Vulnerability scores are stratified as low, medium, and high, with higher scores associated with greater social vulnerability.[11] The SVI is particularly useful for disaster planning since data are reported by census tract, making it possible to tailor disaster plans to specific neighborhoods.

Hahn et al. found that under nondisaster conditions, locations with medium and high social vulnerability scores experienced worse mental health outcomes (19% and 56% higher rates of poor outcomes, respectively, than low social vulnerability locations) and worse physical health outcomes as well (22% and 69% higher rates of poor outcomes, respectively, than low social vulnerability locations).[8] In disaster conditions, risks increased even more for communities with medium and high social vulnerability. Hahn et al. reported that measurable increases in mental and physical health risk worsened with each recurring natural disaster.[8] Alderman et al. found that in regard to flooding, the most common natural disaster, developing countries impacted by lack of infrastructure and overall worse health experienced more severe and long-lasting effects than developed countries.[10] PHN professionals should assess social vulnerability and SDOH when preparing emergency preparedness plans for specific communities.

The SVI is a useful tool for public health food emergency planning. The SVI tools, guidance, interactive maps, and data provided at the CDC-ATSDR website are important jurisdictional resources to aid in formulating disaster responses. SVI maps and materials can help identify areas of greater vulnerability to promote more effective targeting of food assistance resources.[11] In addition, PHN professionals may use SVI maps to determine optimal locations for emergency feeding centers, amounts of supplies required for various communities, and staffing needs.[11] Figure 12.3 provides a listing of the categorized variables used to collect data to determine the 2018 SVI benchmarks for census tracts.[12]

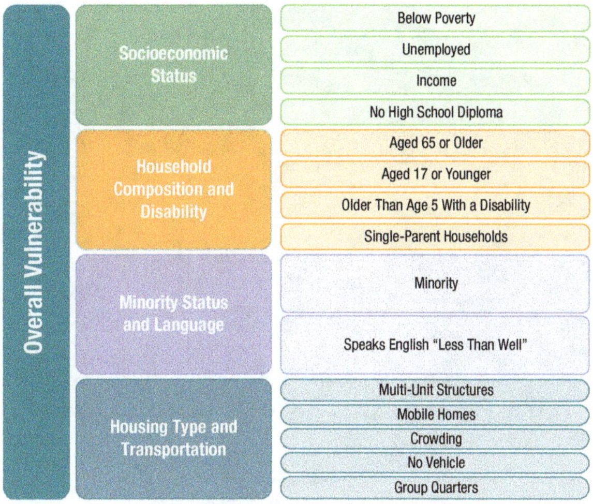

Figure 12.3. Categorized data variables used to determine 2018 social vulnerability index (SVI) benchmarks.

Source: Agency for Toxic Substances and Disease Registry. CDC SVI 2018 documentation. Centers for Disease Control and Prevention. January 31, 2020. https://www.atsdr.cdc.gov/placeandhealth/svi/documentation/SVI_documentation_2018.html

An Inclusive, Community-Centered, Strengths-Based Approach to Emergency Planning

Biedrzycki and Koltun wrote an article in 2012 for the U.S. Department of Homeland Security (DHS) that posited the importance of what they described as the "whole of community" approach to emergency planning.[3] While professional knowledge and skills are crucial in disaster management, community resilience and recovery—the overarching goals of emergency planning—are fostered by an inclusive planning process in which the community and its leaders are fully integrated as key partners from the inception of emergency preparation.[3] By respecting the community's knowledge, traditions, leaders, culture, environment, and priorities, emergency preparedness is enhanced.

A strengths-based approach to community assessment may multiply the results of effective emergency planning. Identifying and celebrating existing social networks, resources, and positive community developments is an important aspect of supporting confidence and resilience in target populations. A community-inclusive paradigm for disaster planning is likely to lead to a deeper understanding of community strengths, as well as enhancing trust, collaboration, and effective working relationships among members of the emergency response team, which includes designated community leaders. Inclusive emergency preparedness planning may especially benefit communities with higher SVI scores by identifying and leveraging previously underutilized community assets that could prove critical in maintaining resilience under stress.[13]

Michael Meit of the University of Chicago's NORC Walsh Center for Rural Health Analysis prepared a rural asset map, which may be a helpful tool for asset mapping in any community, whether rural, urban, or global.[13] A **strengths-based assessment** of community nutrition resources is an important component of nutrition emergency preparedness. The rural assets map is found in Figure 12.4.

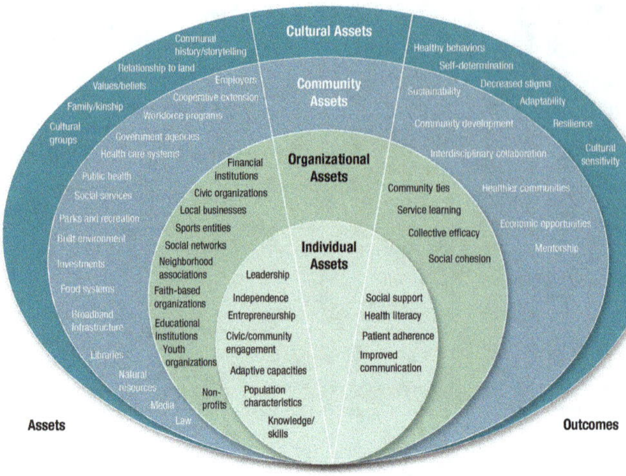

Figure 12.4. Rural asset map. This tool may be useful in conducting community-inclusive emergency preparedness activities in any setting, whether rural, urban, or global.
Source: Meit M. *Final Report: Exploring Strategies to Improve Health and Equity in Rural Communities*. NORC Walsh Center for Rural Health Analysis, University of Chicago; 2018. https://www.norc.org/PDFs/Walsh%20Center/Final%20Reports

FOOD AND NUTRITION EMERGENCIES: LIFE CYCLE NUTRITION CONSIDERATIONS

When planning for food and nutrition emergencies, public health and PHN professionals should consider special nutrition needs related to life stage, since some life stages are more vulnerable to nutritional insults than others. A lack of specific nutrients at certain life stages can result in lifelong consequences including poor health outcomes. The nutrition needs of various life stage groups provide helpful inputs for developing community- and household-level emergency resources and supplies.[14] *Note that at any life stage, special medical needs may require additional emergency planning to ensure the availability of needed foods, medications, and/or supplies and equipment.* Examples include but are not limited to diabetes and other metabolic disorders, celiac disease and food allergies, conditions for which vitamin/mineral supplements may be medically prescribed, swallowing or dental disorders requiring soft foods, conditions for which medical food supplements (such as liquid meal replacements) are recommended, and tube feeding supplies and equipment. Table 12.2 provides a list of life cycle stages in order, along with specific nutrition emergency planning considerations and suggestions.[14]

Resources for Emergency Feeding

U.S. Department of Agriculture

The U.S. Department of Agriculture Food and Nutrition Service (USDA-FNS) provides a number of resources and services to assist in disaster preparation, management, and recovery.[15] Some USDA-FNS functions are focused on life cycle groups, including infants. A

Table 12.2. Life Cycle Stages With Considerations and Suggestions for Food and Nutrition Emergency Planning

Life Cycle Stage	Considerations for Emergencies	Suggestions for Emergency Planning
Pregnancy and Lactation	Adequate calories, protein, and water to support pregnancy or lactation Prenatal vitamins	Community level: Ensure that the comprehensive community emergency plan addresses nutrition needs during pregnancy Household level: Develop an appropriate household emergency plan that includes recommended amounts of food and water, and an emergency supply of prenatal vitamins
Infancy	Infant formula Baby food	Community level: Ensure that the comprehensive community emergency plan addresses nutrition needs of babies, including infant formula and shelf-stable baby food Household level: Develop an appropriate household emergency plan that includes recommended amounts of infant formula and shelf-stable baby foods
Young Childhood (Toddlers and Preschoolers)	Adequate calories, protein, and water to support appropriate growth Appropriate food textures, avoid choking hazards Based on available food supply, determine if multivitamins are appropriate	Community level: Ensure that the comprehensive community emergency plan addresses food and nutrition needs of young children, including water, appropriately textured foods and avoidance of foods that present choking hazards, multivitamin if needed Household level: Develop an appropriate household emergency plan that includes recommended amounts of foods and water for young children, including appropriately textured foods and avoidance of foods that present choking hazards, multivitamin if needed
School Age	Adequate calories, protein, and water to support appropriate growth Based on available food supply, determine if multivitamins are appropriate	Community level: Ensure that the comprehensive community emergency plan addresses food and nutrition needs of school-age children, multivitamin if needed Household level: Develop an appropriate household emergency plan that includes recommended amounts of food and water for school-age children, multivitamin if needed

(Continued)

Table 12.2. Life Cycle Stages With Considerations and Suggestions for Food and Nutrition Emergency Planning *(Continued)*

Life Cycle Stage	Considerations for Emergencies	Suggestions for Emergency Planning
Adolescence	Adequate calories, protein, and water to support appropriate growth Based on available food supply, determine if multivitamins are appropriate	Community level: Ensure that the comprehensive community emergency plan addresses food and nutrition needs of adolescents, multivitamin if needed Household level: Develop an appropriate household emergency plan that includes recommended amounts of food and water for adolescents, multivitamin if needed
Adulthood	Adequate calories, protein, and water to support life activities Based on available food supply, determine if multivitamins are appropriate	Community level: Ensure that the comprehensive community emergency plan addresses food and nutrition needs of young and middle adults, multivitamin if needed Household level: Develop an appropriate household emergency plan that includes recommended amounts of food and water for young and middle adults, multivitamin if needed
Older Adulthood	Adequate calories, protein, and water to support life activities	Community level: Ensure that the comprehensive community emergency plan addresses food and nutrition needs of older adults, including appropriate medical food supplements if needed Household level: Develop an appropriate household emergency plan that includes recommended amounts of food and water, and medically recommended supplements as needed, such as liquid meal substitutes

Note: At any life stage, be aware that special medical needs may require additional emergency planning to ensure the availability of needed food, medication, and equipment.
Source: Centers for Disease Control and Prevention. Emergency preparedness and response. Department of Health and Human Services. Accessed November 6, 2022. https://emergency.cdc.gov

key jurisdictional partner, the USDA-FNS carries out the following functions, which may provide critical support in emergency situations:

- Maintains food stores nationwide, which can be deployed to assist states and localities.
- Administers the Disaster Supplemental Nutrition Assistance Program (D-SNAP) at state request, to provide food assistance in situations in which USDA-FNS

authorized retail food outlets are able to operate so that recipients can purchase food.

- At state or FEMA request, in some situations USDA-FNS can rapidly provide infant formula and baby food.[15]

USDA-FNS provides extensive information and resources focused on disaster planning, including but not limited to guidance for D-SNAP; other USDA food programs including the Special Supplemental Food Program for Women, Infants, and Children (WIC); emergency deployment of food supplies; mapping tools focused on building capacity for resilience and recovery by identifying local resources; and directories of contact information for USDA-FNS state and regional staff, and state emergency management offices staff.[15–19] PHN professionals in the United States should consult with the USDA-FNS when developing local, regional, and state emergency preparedness plans.

Federal Emergency Management Agency

The mission of the Federal Emergency Management Agency (FEMA) of the U.S. Department of Homeland Security is to assist people before, during, and after disasters.[20] To carry out its mission, FEMA coordinates the federal response to disasters, including providing assistance to persons, families, and businesses who have incurred property losses not covered by insurance.

Prior to an incident (for example, a hurricane) and during the immediate recovery period, FEMA provides mass care and emergency assistance services at strategically located response centers.[21] Services are available to any disaster survivor affected by the incident and include emergency feeding services—often using shelf-stable meals—and distribution of emergency supplies. Response centers also provide reunification services, services for persons with disabilities, and support for pets and service animals. FEMA provides extensive guidance for the development of mass care and emergency assistance shelters, and encourages collaboration among public health agencies and FEMA to develop and implement such plans.[22]

PHN disaster plans should include consideration of communicating the locations of mass care shelters where disaster survivors can receive services including nutrition services. Advance planning for nutrition communications can promote the FEMA computer app, which provides response center locations, or other available communication tools such as texting or websites.[21] PHN professionals should be aware of FEMA guidance for emergency feeding, and coordinate with FEMA and other jurisdictional partners throughout the disaster planning process.

United Nations

The World Food Programme (WFP) of the United Nations (UN) is the largest emergency food program—and the largest humanitarian agency overall—in the world.[23] Providing services in more than 120 countries, the WFP has delivered services to tens of millions of persons since its founding in 1961, serving nearly 128.2 million people in 2021 alone.[24] In 2020, the Norwegian Nobel Committee awarded the WFP the Nobel Peace Prize for its work.[23]

The mission of the WFP is "delivering food assistance in emergencies and working with communities to improve nutrition and build resilience."[25] To that end, the WFP provides emergency food assistance to communities and regions impacted by conflict and/or disasters, and supports initiatives to improve population-wide nutrition and enhance community and regional resilience. Examples of initiatives designed to improve disaster resilience and build resilience include promotion of maternal and child health, provision of school meals, asset creation such as reclamation of farmland, climate initiatives, gender equality, and sustainable economic and ecosystem development.[25]

To fulfill its mission, the WFP collaborates with a wide variety of international entities, including governments, nongovernmental agencies, private sector partnerships, academia, and other stakeholders. Emergency preparedness and response strategies implemented by the WFP may provide helpful models for other emergency response efforts. Emergency preparedness strategies utilized by the WFP include:

- The utilization of early warning systems, including evidence-based risk assessment tools and geospatial positioning system (GPS) technology to map the impacts of disasters
- Effective collaboration management to ensure effective delivery of services and avoid duplication of effort
- Coordination among civilian and military resources; as a UN agency, the WFP is able to utilize UN communications channels to collaborate with military leaders to enhance delivery of humanitarian services.[26]

Emergency response strategies are considered the highest priority by WFP. Basic elements include:

- Developing, building, and deploying a skilled emergency workforce
- Developing, building, and maintaining global supply chain capacity
- Maintenance and utilization of an operations management and information center in Rome, Italy, to provide overall coordination of emergency response efforts, including the coordination of multiagency collaborations
- Strong efforts to acquire and store information, knowledge, and experiences from those working in the field, in order to build a library of lessons learned to inform future emergency responses

The WFP is supported entirely by donations.[23] The organization provides a number of options for becoming involved in its work, and provides contact information for both its headquarters in Rome, Italy, as well as links to country offices.

The Role of Food Banks and Food Pantries

Food Banks

Food banks are nonprofit organizations that acquire, store, and distribute large amounts of food to community food resource centers, such as food pantries.[27] Food banks typically do not directly provide food to clients, but instead support and supply a network of constituent local food pantries, which carry out the work of direct food distribution in neighborhoods and communities.[28]

The largest private hunger relief organization in the United States is Feeding America, which operates a nationwide network of about 200 food banks serving about 60,000 constituent food pantries.[29] Feeding America leverages its resources to assist in disaster preparedness, response, and recovery efforts.[30] Initiatives include the maintenance of a nationwide network of quickly deployable food stores, warehouse facilities, and trucking capabilities. The organization engages in many collaborations with public and private partners able to provide considerable human and material support for relief efforts, and cultivates durable, long-lasting partner and community relationships to promote resilience.[30,31] PHN professionals should include a consideration of Feeding America resources when developing emergency preparedness plans.

Food Pantries

Food pantries are local organizations, usually private, that provide emergency food resources to food-insecure persons in their communities.[28] Because federal food security programs such as the Supplemental Nutrition Assistance Program (SNAP) and WIC are not intended to meet 100% of participants' nutritional needs, local food pantries play an important role in filling nutritional gaps for their clients.

Local food pantries are a critical resource for food and nutrition emergency preparedness for several reasons. Pantries are already distributed throughout and deeply embedded within communities—often for decades. Many locales have a network of food pantries, ranging from two to several. Food pantries continuously engage in the work of food acquisition, storage, and distribution. Most food pantries have trained volunteer staff available to assist in the day-to-day functions of the organization.

If affiliated with a food bank, food pantries have access to significant resources. Existing communication networks support breadth and depth in food pantries' community interactions, and pantries are often closely aligned with other community social services and organizations, including faith-based organizations. Some food pantry networks within communities maintain interpantry communications, so that use of resources can be optimized by sharing. PHN professionals should consider local food pantries in emergency preparedness planning, and food pantry representatives should be part of the emergency planning team.

Role of Public Health and PHN Professionals in Household-Level Emergency Preparedness Education

Emergency preparedness education focused on nutrition considerations is a major role of public health and PHN professionals working in communities. Community-level emergency preparedness is essential, but true resilience is undergirded by well-prepared community members who have planned for emergencies at the household level. Household planning may help to ameliorate the intitial impact of disasters, reduce demand on emergency responders and congregate facilities, and help to mitigate medical surge events. An inclusive approach to community emergency planning may enhance household-level preparation by leveraging the influence of community leaders to encourage households to engage in emergency preparation.[3]

The CDC has provided extensive emergency preparedness resources for the public.[14] Examples of food and nutrition topics that public health and PHN professionals can address in household-level emergency preparedness education include but are not limited to:

- General disaster planning principles, including the importance of advance planning and household-community collaboration during disasters[32]
- Preparation of a 72-hour emergency kit, including food, water, and essential medications[33,34]

- Importance of heeding evacuation orders from authorities; preparation of an 'evacuation kit' with adequate food, water, and essential medications for evacuation travel[35]
- Food and water safety considerations during different types of emergencies; how to maintain food and water safety at home during a disaster[36]
- Household-level emergency preparedness to meet the food and water needs of persons with special needs; the CDC lists eight populations with specific needs in disaster planning, three of which represent life stage groups: older adults, expectant and new parents, children and their caregivers, evacuees, people with chronic illnesses, people with disabilities, persons experiencing homelessness, and tribal communities.[37]

Public health and PHN professionals should coordinate and collaborate food and nutrition disaster planning education within the overall community emergency preparedness plan.

NEW FRONTIERS IN EMERGENCY MANAGEMENT: EARTH OBSERVATIONS TECHNOLOGY

Collecting information about Earth's biological, chemical, and physical systems enables us to monitor natural and human-made environments and assess changes that may be occurring in the weather, land use, management of natural resources, and more.[38] This gathering of information is known as **Earth observations** (EO), and it provides an opportunity to better understand our global environment.

Today, the ability to observe our world has advanced with the combination of remote-sensing satellites in orbit and sophisticated in situ instruments collecting data on Earth.[38] Satellites and instruments continue to evolve and the possibilities for research and applications are increasing. EO instruments can include ocean buoys, land stations, sonar and radar, environmental satellites, and GPS stations that can collect data about land and ocean temperature, air quality, seismic activity, and precipitation trends, and estimate wildlife or human populations.[38] EO data can help forecast weather, address health risks and the spread of disease, monitor crops for food and nutrition security impacts, and assist with the mitigation and response to disasters.[38]

The use of EO in PHN can help inform decision-making and support public health surveillance, sustainable agriculture, disaster resilience, and food and nutrition security.[39] Environmental observations can be integrated with public health surveillance to monitor and assess health risk to support decision-making in disease-control. Insights about the climate, crops, land use, soil, and water; data can be gleaned from EO providing context for conditions in communities and the food system that informs response and targeted nutrition interventions.[11,40] The integration of EO data and socioeconomic data can help PHN professionals better understand the impact SDOH can have on a population's health before, during, and after an emergency or disaster.[41]

In order to prepare health **hazard mitigation**, federal and state level planning often utilizes socioeconomic data to identify vulnerable populations to reduce the risk of negative health outcomes associated with a disaster.[42] Current projects aim to integrate EO data like temperature, power outages, flooding, and rainfall estimates with socioeconomic data that can enhance vulnerability indices like the CDC-ATSDR SVI to improve response time for those most at risk and inform emergency management decisions.[42]

On September 28, 2022, Hurricane Ian made two landfalls in Florida near the barrier island of Cavo Costa and again near Punta Gorda, Florida, in the United States. As a

Category 4 hurricane with sustained winds near 150 miles per hour at landfall, Ian was responsible for at least 156 confirmed deaths in the United States as well as catastrophic damage with losses over $112 billion. In a report released by the National Hurricane Center in April 2023, Hurricane Ian was upgraded to a Category 5 hurricane at its peak just hours before making landfall and weakening to a Category 4 storm.[43]

EO data from the Landsat satellites provided opportunities to view the effects of heavy rainfall and storm surges in states impacted by Hurricane Ian.[40] Landsat images are quickly released after a disaster by the U.S. Geological Survey (USGS) Earth Resources Observation and Science (EROS) Center and feed into the International Charter Space and Major Disasters' Hazard Data Distribution System to support communities and agencies with disaster monitoring, mapping, and response efforts.[43]

The CDC-ATSDR SVI uses U.S. Census data and 16 social factors that are grouped into the four themes of socioeconomic status, household characteristics, racial and ethnic minority status, and housing type and transportation to create databases and maps to determine social vulnerability.[11] Utilizing geospatial analyses and tools like a geographic information system (GIS), the CDC-ATSDR SVI interactive map helps visualize socioeconomic data for identifying and mapping communities that will most likely experience the most need for support before, during, and after a disaster event to support decision-making.[11]

Integrating EO data like Landsat imagery from Hurricane Ian and socioeconomic data from the CDC-ATSDR SVI can help identify areas that may have experienced damage and assess the health status of populations in those areas for rescue efforts and long-term recovery planning.[40,42]

Integrating EO and socioeconomic data into useful tools enhances public knowledge and can increase accessibility and reduce barriers for those with limited EO, data analysis, or GIS skills. The importance of data accessibility and availability is an ongoing discussion, and many open-source platforms exist to make socioeconomic and EO data freely available for social benefit.

In emergency response, PHN professionals can use GIS-enabled tools and downloadable data to:

- Estimate the need of supplies like food and water to prevent malnutrition and address life cycle nutrition needs of affected populations[11]
- Identify areas needed for emergency shelters and food pantries[11]
- Identify communities in need of a Disaster Recovery Center (DRC) that offers accessible mobile offices where disaster survivors can get recovery assistance and referrals from local, state, and federal officials concerning critical needs like housing, food stamp replacement, enrollment with D-SNAP, and information about loan programs and insurance to support local farmers and ranchers[41]
- Aid in evacuation planning of vulnerable people including those with disabilities, the elderly, non-English speakers, and those without vehicles[11]

For mitigation and intervention planning, PHN professionals can use data to:

- Create a map of local food banks and pantries where food insecure individuals and families can access food in preparation for a potential disaster like a forecasted hurricane or flooding event
- Identify vulnerable populations who may need food assistance and lack access to communication tools like internet, a telephone, or transportation, or have language barriers to assist with registration for PHN services like SNAP or WIC

- Identify communities where nutrition education programs may increase food and nutrition security
- Better understand factors that can influence food and nutrition security with tools like the U.S. Drought Monitor, satellite-based assessments of power outage and recovery data, and supply chain mapping

Leading organizations and agencies around the world like the United Nations Food and Agriculture Organization (FAO), Feed the Future, the WFP, and the U.S. Agency for International Development (USAID) use EO data and applications to support food security initiatives.[44,45]

WHAT WORKS: FEEDING AMERICA

On September 28, 2022, hurricane Ian hit land near Fort Myers, Florida, in the United States. A Category 5 storm with winds clocked at up to 160 miles per hour prior to landfall, Ian resulted in 149 confirmed deaths in Florida as well as catastrophic property damage with losses over $112 billion.[43]

Feeding America (FA), the largest private hunger relief organization in the United States, has developed extensive capacity for addressing disasters through its nationwide network of food banks.[30] Year-round, FA maintains emergency food supplies at strategic locations, along with extensive distribution capabilities including a fleet of over 2,000 trucks. When needed, emergency supplies can be quickly targeted and deployed to communities and regions in need of assistance. FA's disaster response is enhanced by its range of governmental and non-governmental partnerships, which include collaborations with agencies such as FEMA and the American Red Cross. FA also partners with organizations such as the Institute for Diversity and Inclusion in Emergency Management to identify and expedite delivery of supplies to underserved communities.[46]

As soon as the situation on the ground made travel possible in Florida after hurricane Ian, FA identified its constituent food banks in the disaster area's epicenter. By deploying its emergency food supplies via its established transportation network in the immediate aftermath of the disaster, FA was able to quickly deliver 78 semitruckloads of supplies and safe water to food banks in impacted areas of Florida. The food banks were then able to assess needs in their own communities and target emergency assistance appropriately. In the long-term recovery period after the disaster, FA delivered an additional 6 million pounds of donated supplies by working with national partners.[47]

SUMMARY

Disasters affect both populations and individuals, and the impacts can be long-term and overwhelming. Access to adequate and appropriate nutrition and food supplies for populations and individuals during and after emergency events is a key factor in promoting community resilience and supporting recovery. Preparation for food and nutrition disasters is an essential component of emergency preparedness. Nutrition professionals should take a holistic approach to disaster planning, recognizing that effective planning is a collaborative process that involves private and jurisdictional partners, and recognizes that those impacted by disasters represent every life cycle phase. PHN professionals play a crucial role in ensuring that food and nutrition considerations are an integral component of individual, family, community, local, state, and regional emergency and disaster planning.

KEY CHAPTER CONCEPTS

1. Access to adequate and appropriate nutrition and food supplies for populations and individuals during and after emergency events is a key factor in promoting community resilience and supporting recovery. Preparation for food and nutrition disasters is an essential component of emergency preparedness.
2. The CDC-CEPR has defined six major domains of emergency preparedness that should be the focus of disaster planning. Each domain of emergency preparedness has important nutrition implications: (1) community resilience; (2) incident management; (3) information management; (4) countermeasures and mitigation; (5) surge management; (6) biosurveillance.
3. The Public Health Emergency Preparedness and Response Capabilities Planning Model includes three major components: (1) assess current state; (2) determine strategies and activities; (3) develop plans.
4. Effective emergency preparedness and management plan is collaborative. That is, the plan is based on cooperation and teamwork among many different agencies, organizations, and individuals. PHN emergency planning efforts are a crucial component of community preparedness, recovery, and resilience, and should be embedded within the overall community planning process.
5. Social determinants of health that impact particular populations' disaster resilience include but are not limited to the built environment, median income level, typical housing, transportation availability and infrastructure, access to healthcare, and the availability of healthful and wholesome food. Social Vulnerability Index tools, guidance, interactive maps, and data provided by the CDC are important jurisdictional resources to aid in formulating disaster responses. It is recommended that public health and PHN professionals take an inclusive, community-centered, strengths-based approach to emergency planning.
6. When planning for food and nutrition emergencies, public health and PHN professionals should consider special nutrition needs related to life stage, since some life stages are more vulnerable to nutritional insults than others. A lack of specific nutrients at certain life stages can result in lifelong consequences including poor health outcomes. The nutrition needs of various life stage groups provide helpful inputs for developing community- and household-level emergency resources and supplies.
7. Governmental and nongovernmental collaborators for emergency planning and provision of emergency services include the USDA, FEMA, and the UN. Private collaborators include regional food banks, such as those affiliated with Feeding America, as well as local food pantries.
8. The gathering of information about Earth's biological, chemical, and physical systems is known as Earth observations (EO). EO instruments can include ocean buoys, land stations, sonar and radar, environmental satellites, and GPS stations that can collect data about land and ocean temperature, air quality, seismic activity, precipitation trends, and estimate wildlife or human populations. EO data can help forecast weather, address health risks and the spread of disease, monitor crops for food security impacts, and assist with the mitigation and response to disasters. The use of EO in PHN can help inform decision-making and support public health surveillance, sustainable agriculture, disaster resilience, and food and nutrition security.

CASE STUDY: STRENGTHS-BASED FOOD AND NUTRITION EMERGENCY PLANNING

As a staff member of a community health department, you are responsible for developing an emergency food and nutrition plan for your community. You decide to begin by conducting a food and nutrition strengths-based assessment of community resources. Your goals are (1) to identify strengths, capacities, and assets that can be leveraged to plan effectively for emergencies, and (2) to define potential linkages and networks that can be deployed prior to, during, and following emergencies to promote resilience and recovery.

Review Figure 12.4, the rural asset map. This model can be applied to many different community settings, including urban settings.

Note: A comprehensive strengths-based assessment usually requires an extended period of time and substantial resources to complete. The case study here is intended to provide you with an understanding of the framework and methods used to conduct a comprehensive assessment. A few examples from each asset category are sufficient to complete this assignment.

Case Study Questions

1. Define *strengths-based assessment*.
2. What are three advantages of beginning emergency planning with a strengths-based assessment?
3. The four asset categories from the rural asset map are provided here. Define each category and provide one or two food- and nutrition-related examples of each.
   a. Individual assets
   b. Organizational assets
   c. Community assets
   d. Cultural assets
4. A comprehensive strengths-based food and nutrition community assessment should be conducted by a team. In terms of roles in your community, who should be included on your team? Remember to include individual, organizational, community, and cultural leaders and influencers. For example, the child nutrition director for your local school district would be an important team contributor.
5. Read the following instructions and complete the provided table:
   a. **Select a specific community** as the focus for your asset map. *Be specific*. For example, instead of selecting a region or county, select a specific town or neighborhood. It may be helpful to choose a community that you know well.
   b. **Identify the community's assets.** Research the community and begin to *list the food and nutrition assets* within each category (individual, organizational, community, and cultural) on the asset map. Doing a walking tour on Google maps may help you identify organizations and agencies such as schools, restaurants, food retail, extension, social services, faith-based organizations, and farmers markets. Record your findings on the table.
   c. **Describe what the assets provide.** Conduct a *capacity inventory* within the community. Normally this process could take weeks or months; for the purpose of this exercise, focus on the top assets within each category on the asset map. Fill in this information on the table.
   d. **Plan how the assets will connect.** Once the assets are identified, it is helpful to consider the existing (and potential) partnerships that link the community. This method helps to identify the mutually beneficial exchange between the partners. Answer the questions about partnerships after completing Table 12.3.

Table 12.3. Strengths-Based Assessment Planning Table

	What are the community's food and nutrition assets? *List three to five assets in each.*	***What do the assets provide?*** *Describe the skills + resources.*
Cultural + Policy Assets	• *SAMPLE: The community strongly values caring for others.*	• *SAMPLE: Because this community places value on caring for others, the community is likely to value planning and preparation to provide food for those impacted by an emergency.*
Community Assets	• *SAMPLE: School district*	• *SAMPLE: A school is a center of trust and influence. It may provide meals, emergency shelter, food distribution, and other nutrition services in an emergency.*
Organizational Assets	• *SAMPLE: Boys and Girls Club*	• *SAMPLE: The local Boys and Girls Club is trusted by the community to care for children. It may provide emergency meals and food distribution to children and families.*
Individual Assets	• *SAMPLE: Strong family and friendship ties*	• *SAMPLE: Family and friendship ties are important in this community, and this asset can be leveraged to develop education and communication tools designed to enhance family and neighborhood preparedness for emergencies to promote resilience.*

6. How do the assets connect?

   Consider how the assets identified in the asset table connect with one another. Think about existing and potential cross-sector partnerships (a cross-sector partnership is a crossing over from one asset category to another. For example, are there potential partnership opportunities among the school district and the Boys and Girls Club in regard to emergency management?

   Answer the following (provide three examples each for *a* and *b*):
   a. What cross-sector partnerships might already exist within your chosen community?
   b. What new cross-sector partnerships could be formed? What opportunities and challenges exist in creating these new partnerships?
   c. What are the advantages of each partnership? What impact will these partnerships have on the health of the rural community?

7. Finally, in a paragraph or two, summarize your thoughts about the process of incorporating strengths-based assessment into emergency planning initiatives.

DISCUSSION QUESTIONS

1. Review the list of emergencies and disasters provided in the first paragraph of this chapter. Choose three or four disaster types, and discuss the possible nutritional implications of each disaster chosen.

2. What do you see as the top three principles of disaster planning? What do you think are the fundamental characteristics of an effective disaster plan?
3. Disaster resources include jurisdictional/governmental resources as well as private resources. Describe the general functions of these two types of resources in responding to disasters. What types of preplanning are needed to ensure effective coordination of public and private resources in disasters?
4. Review Table 12.1, CDC-CEPR Public Health Emergency Management Capabilities With PHN Applications. Which of the capabilities do you think is most important from a PHN perspective? Provide a rationale for your answer, and discuss with classmates.
5. Discuss the relationship(s) among social vulnerability and disaster resilience and recovery. How can PHN professionals utilize the disaster planning process to positively impact disaster resilience and recovery in communities with higher social vulnerability?
6. Review Table 12.2, Life Cycle Stages With Considerations and Suggestions for Nutrition Emergency Planning. Are there additional considerations that you would suggest adding to the table? Provide a rationale for your responses, and discuss with classmates.
7. What are some ways you think Earth observations could be used to enhance the responses of nutrition professionals to emergency and disaster situations?

SUGGESTED LEARNING ACTIVITIES

1. Review a chosen locality's disaster preparedness plan. You may choose your own locality if a plan is available. An example of such a plan for Myrtle Beach, South Carolina, is found at cms6.revize.com/revize/myrtlebeachsc/DisasterRecoveryPlan.pdf. Review the plan you have identified, then answer the following questions:
   a. When was the plan last updated?
   b. Who participated in preparing the plan?
   c. Under what authority was the plan created?
   d. Which agencies are responsible for implementing the plan?
   e. What are the major sections of the plan?
   f. What food and nutrition topics are included in the plan? In your opinion, are food and nutrition topics adequately addressed?
2. Interview the director or other leader of a local food pantry or food bank to learn about the food pantry/bank's emergency preparedness plan. Sample interview questions could include:
   a. Describe your emergency preparedness plan.
   b. How many days' supply of food do you maintain for emergency situations?
   c. What is your plan for dealing with a lack of volunteer staff?
   d. What is your plan for food acquisition in an emergency situation?
   e. Do you collaborate with other community organizations in regard to your disaster plan? How do community organizations support your emergency preparedness plan?
   f. If you are a food bank constituent pantry, how does your food bank support emergency preparedness?
3. Describe the CDC-CEPR's definitions of *short-term* and *long-term* goals. List three emergency management goals you think could be accomplished in the short term, and provide a rationale for each. Then, list three long-term emergency management goals, and provide a rationale for each.

4. Choose one of the emergency management capabilities from Table 12.1. For the capability you've chosen, develop a one- to two-page plan summary presenting nutrition implications of the capability and your recommendations for addressing them. Prepare your summary as though you are going to present it to your local or regional emergency planning board. If possible, present your summary to your classmates.
5. Learn more about the World Food Programme. Review the WFP website at www.wfp.org. Choose one of the four main website topic areas: (1) Who We Are; (2) Our Work; (3) Where We Work; (4) Get Involved. Review your chosen website area, and write a two- to three-page report describing your findings.
6. Review the Colorado State University Extension's publication "Three-Day Emergency Supply of Shelf-Stable Food for One Person" at extension.colostate.edu/disaster-web-sites/three-day-emergency-supply-of-shelf-stable-food-for-one-person. Based on the publication, design a 3-day menu for a person from a life cycle group of your choice (excluding infants) using shelf-stable foods. For each day's menu, include breakfast, lunch, dinner, and one or two snacks.
7. Visit the NASA ARSET (Applied Remote Sensing Training) website, and complete the Fundamentals of Remote Sensing Training Webinar (appliedsciences.nasa.gov/join-mission/training/english/arset-fundamentals-remote-sensing). A variety of webinars are provided and can be viewed at any time. To access a webinar, click on its "Take This Online Training" button and register by providing the requested information.

RESOURCES FOR FURTHER LEARNING

- Mass Care/Emergency Assistance Pandemic Planning Considerations: www.fema.gov/sites/default/files/202006/mcea_pandemic_planning_considerations_guide.pdf
  - FEMA guidelines for planning mass care and emergency assistance responses; includes pandemic considerations
- World Food Programme (United Nations): www.wfp.org
  - Information and resources on the world's largest humanitarian assistance organization, which provided emergency food assistance to over 120 million people in 2021
- Feeding America Disaster Response and Relief: www.feedingamerica.org/our-work/disaster-response
  - Information on how the largest private food assistance organization in the United States responds to disasters
- Centers for Disease Control and Prevention Emergency Preparedness and Response: https://emergency.cdc.gov
  - Extensive and comprehensive information and resources regarding emergency preparedness planning and response in public health settings; provides much useful information on nutrition implications of emergencies and disasters, including life-stage specific information
- CDC Crisis and Emergency Risk Communication Course: https://emergency.cdc.gov/cerc/ppt/CERC_Introduction.pdf
  - Provides training and a manual on communication with the public during emergency situations; basic communication principles are presented that will be useful in communicating nutrition information in emergencies.

- Colorado State University Extension: Three-day emergency supply of shelf-stable food for one person: https://extension.colostate.edu/disaster-web-sites/three-day-emergency-supply-of-shelf-stable-food-for-one-person
  - Example of a shelf-stable food plan for household-level nutrition education on emergency planning
- NASA ARSET (Applied Remote Sensing Training) Training Modules: https://appliedsciences.nasa.gov/join-mission/training/english/arset-fundamentals-remote-sensing
  - Provides training in using Earth observation data in a variety of contexts, including emergency and disaster management, agriculture, health and air quality, and more
- NASA Harvest: https://nasaharvest.org
  - NASA global consortium to promote food security, agriculture, and human/environmental resiliency

SPRINGER PUBLISHING CONNECT™

A robust set of instructor resources designed to supplement this text is located at http://connect.springerpub.com/content/book/978-0-8261-8623-2. Qualifying instructors may request access by emailing textbook@springerpub.com.

REFERENCES

1. Centers for Disease Control and Prevention. Natural disasters and severe weather. Accessed November 6, 2022. https://www.cdc.gov/disasters/index.html
2. Taormina RJ, Gao JH. Maslow and the motivation hierarchy: measuring satisfaction of the needs. *Am J Psychol*. 2013;126(2):155–177. https://doi.org/10.5406/amerjpsyc.126.2.0155
3. Biedrzycki PA, Koltun R. Integration of social determinants of community preparedness and resiliency in 21st century emergency management planning. *Homel Secur Aff*. 2012;8:14. https://www.hsaj.org/resources/uploads/2022/05/8.1.14.pdf
4. Centers for Disease Control and Prevention. Six domains of preparedness. Accessed September 23, 2023. https://www.cdc.gov/cpr/readiness/sixdomains.htm
5. Centers for Disease Control and Prevention. Public Health Emergency Preparedness and Response Capabilities: National Standards for State, Local, Tribal, and Territorial Public Health. State and Local Readiness. U.S. Department of Health and Human Services. Updated 2019. https://www.cdc.gov/orr/readiness/00_docs/cdc_preparednesresponsecapabilities_october2018_final_508.pdf
6. Jurisdictional. In: *Cambridge Dictionary*. Cambridge University Press; 2022. https://dictionary.cambridge.org/us/dictionary/english/jurisdictional
7. Centers for Disease Control and Prevention. Social determinants of health at CDC. Accessed November 3, 2022. https://www.cdc.gov/socialdeterminants/index.htm
8. Hahn MB, Van Wyck R, Lessard L, Fried R. Compounding effects of social vulnerability and recurring natural disasters on mental and physical health. *Disaster Med Public Health Prep*. 2022;16:1013–1021. https://doi.org/10.1017/dmp.2020.476
9. Agency for Toxic Substances and Disease Registry. CDC/ATSDR social vulnerability index. Centers for Disease Control and Prevention. Accessed April 20, 2023. https://www.atsdr.cdc.gov/placeandhealth/svi/index.html
10. Alderman K, Turner LR, Tong S. Floods and human health: a systematic review. *Environ Int*. 2012;47:37–47. https://doi.org/10.1016/j.envint.2012.06.003
11. Agency for Toxic Substances and Disease Registry. CDC/ATSDR SVI fact sheet. Centers for Disease Control and Prevention. Accessed November 3, 2022. https://www.atsdr.cdc.gov/placeandhealth/svi/fact_sheet/fact_sheet.html
12. Agency for Toxic Substances and Disease Registry. CDC SVI 2018 documentation. Centers for Disease Control and Prevention. January 31, 2020. https://www.atsdr.cdc.gov/placeandhealth/svi/documentation/SVI_documentation_2018.html

13. Meit M. *Final Report: Exploring Strategies to Improve Health and Equity in Rural Communities*. NORC Walsh Center for Rural Health Analysis, University of Chicago; 2018. https://www.norc.org/PDFs/Walsh%20Center/Final%20Reports
14. Centers for Disease Control and Prevention. Emergency preparedness and response. Accessed November 6, 2022. https://emergency.cdc.gov
15. U.S. Department of Agriculture Food and Nutrition Service. FNS disaster assistance. Accessed November 7, 2022. https://www.fns.usda.gov/disaster/disaster-assistance
16. U.S. Department of Agriculture Food and Nutrition Service. *Disaster SNAP Guidance: Policy Guidance, Lessons Learned, and Toolkits to Operate a Successful D-SNAP.* U.S. Department of Agriculture; 2014. https://fns-prod.azureedge.us/sites/default/files/resource-files/D-SNAP_handbook.pdf
17. U.S. Department of Agriculture Food and Nutrition Service. *USDA Foods in Disasters Manual June 2021.* U.S. Department of Agriculture; 2021. https://www.fns.usda.gov/usda-foods/program-disaster-manual
18. U.S. Department of Agriculture Food and Nutrition Service. *Guide to Coordinating Special Supplemental Nutrition Program for Women, Infants, and Children (WIC) Services When Regular Operations Are Disrupted.* U.S. Department of Agriculture; 2021. https://www.fns.usda.gov/wic/guide-coordinating-wic-service-during-disasters
19. U.S. Department of Agriculture Food and Nutrition Service. FNS resilience and recovery tool. ArcGIS. Accessed April 20, 2023. https://experience.arcgis.com/experience/9005f4c02a19469d9ccc26add2ce1777
20. U.S. Department of Homeland Security. Federal Emergency Management Agency (FEMA). Updated February 3, 2023. https://www.dhs.gov/employee-resources/federal-emergency-management-agency-fema
21. Federal Emergency Management Agency. Programs to support disaster survivors. U.S. Department of Homeland Security. Updated August 1, 2023. https://www.fema.gov/assistance/individual/disaster-survivors#households
22. Federal Emergency Management Agency. *Mass Care/Emergency Assistance Pandemic Planning Considerations for State, Local, Tribal, Territorial and Non-Government Organizational Planners, Providers and Support Agencies*. U.S. Department of Homeland Security; 2020. https://www.fema.gov/sites/default/files/2020-06/mcea_pandemic_planning_considerations_guide.pdf
23. World Food Programme. Who we are. United Nations. Accessed April 10, 2023. https://www.wfp.org/who-we-are
24. World Food Programme. *Annual Performance Report for 2021*. World Food Programme; 2022. https://executiveboard.wfp.org/document_download/WFP-0000138079
25. World Food Programme. Mission. United Nations. Accessed April 10, 2023. https://www.wfp.org/overview
26. World Food Programme. Emergency preparedness and response. United Nations. https://www.wfp.org/emergency-preparedness-and-response
27. Feeding America. What is a food bank? Accessed November 7, 2022. https://www.feedingamerica.org/our-work/food-bank-network
28. Thompson KL, Sugg M, Barth MM. The North Carolina Food Pantry Organizational Capability and Mapping Study: research brief and pilot study. *J Agric Food Syst Community Dev.* 2019;9(1):75–87. https://doi.org/10.5304/jafscd.2019.091.031
29. Feeding America. Working together to end hunger. Accessed November 7, 2022. https://www.feedingamerica.org/our-work
30. Feeding America. Our work: how we respond to disasters. Accessed November 6, 2022. https://www.feedingamerica.org/our-work/disaster-food-assistance
31. Feeding America. Disaster relief partners. Accessed November 6, 2022. https://www.feedingamerica.org/about-us/partners/disaster-relief-partners
32. Centers for Disease Control and Prevention. Protect yourself and your loved ones Accessed November 6, 2022. https://emergency.cdc.gov/protect.asp
33. Centers for Disease Control and Prevention. Take action. Accessed November 6, 2022. https://www.cdc.gov/prepyourhealth/takeaction/index.htm
34. Centers for Disease Control and Prevention. Personal needs. Accessed November 6, 2022. https://www.cdc.gov/prepyourhealth/takeaction/personalneeds/index.htm
35. Centers for Disease Control and Prevention. Preparing for a hurricane or other tropical storm. https://www.cdc.gov/disasters/hurricanes/before.html

36. Centers for Disease Control and Prevention. Food, water, sanitation, and hygiene information for use before and after a disaster or emergency. Accessed November 6, 2022. https://www.cdc.gov/disasters/foodwater/index.html
37. Centers for Disease Control and Prevention. Emergency preparedness and response: information for specific groups. Accessed November 6, 2022. https://emergency.cdc.gov/groups.asp
38. Group on Earth Observations. Frequently Asked Questions. Accessed November 13, 2022. https://www.earthobservations.org/g_faq.html
39. National Aeronautics and Space Administration. *Earth Observations for Health (EO4HEALTH) Initiative: 2020–2022 Implementation Plan.* National Oceanic and Atmospheric Administration; 2019. https://earthobservations.org/documents/gwp20_22/EO4HEALTH.pdf
40. Earth Resources Observation and Science Center. Landsat 9 captures swirling hurricane Ian. U.S. Geological Survey; September 28, 2022. https://www.usgs.gov/centers/eros/news/landsat-9-captures-swirling-hurricane-ian
41. Florida Division of Emergency Management. Disaster recovery centers purpose. Accessed November 28, 2022. https://www.floridadisaster.org/dem/recovery/individual-assistance/disaster-recovery-centers/purpose
42. Poteet LN. Connecting human, animal and environmental health: NASA's role in One Health Day 2021. NASA Earth Applied Sciences Program. November 4, 2021. http://appliedsciences.nasa.gov/our-impact/news/connecting-human-animal-and-environmental-health-nasas-role-one-health-day-2021
43. Bucci L, Alaka L, Hagen A, Delgado S, Beven J. *National Hurricane Center Tropical Cyclone Report: Hurricane Ian.* National Hurricane Center; 2023. https://www.nhc.noaa.gov/data/tcr/AL092022_Ian.pdf
44. European Space Agency. ESA and FAO unite to tackle food security and more. April 20, 2021. https://www.esa.int/Applications/Observing_the_Earth/ESA_and_FAO_unite_to_tackle_food_security_and_more
45. Food and Agriculture Organization of the United Nations. Focus: FAO response to global food security challenges. Accessed November 28, 2022. https://www.fao.org/in-focus/en
46. I-DIEM. Institute for Diversity and Inclusion in Emergency Management. https://i-diem.org
47. Morello P. Updated: Food banks and Feeding America responding to Hurricane Ian. *Hunger Blog.* Updated October 7, 2022. https://www.feedingamerica.org/hunger-blog/updated-food-banks-and-feeding-america-responding-hurricane-ian

13

PUBLIC HEALTH NUTRITION COMMUNICATIONS AND EDUCATION: DEMONSTRATING CULTURAL COMPETENCE THROUGHOUT THE LIFE CYCLE

Sonja Stetzler

LEARNING OBJECTIVES

At the end of this chapter, students will be able to:

1. Define the terms *communication* and *public health nutrition communication* and describe their relationship to nutrition education and health literacy.
2. List patient and provider contributions to nutrition and health discussions.
3. Explain the Iceberg Model of Culture.
4. Summarize **Molinsky's Six Dimensions of Culture**, and explain how it relates to the Iceberg Model.
5. Describe three ways to develop and improve one's own cultural competence.
6. Explain how social determinants of health can impact **nutrition communications**, nutrition education, and health literacy.
7. Describe the *who, why, what, and how* model for preparing nutrition communications for a variety of audiences.
8. Evaluate advantages and disadvantages of using technology to disseminate nutrition communications.
9. Describe four strategies for effectively using **social media** for nutrition communications.
10. Summarize and explain best practices for social media and mass media nutrition communications, with consideration for ethical issues.

INTRODUCTION

Communication is a universal skill that is learned from the time of our birth to express our wants, needs, and emotions and to receive information from others. Communication not only entails our verbal skills, it includes our nonverbal skills such as body language, facial expressions, and tone of voice. The basic communication model includes a sender of a message, the receiver of the message, the message itself, the channel through which the message is sent, and feedback to signify that the message was received.[1] Sometimes interference, otherwise known as "noise," interferes with the reception of the message. This chapter looks at and considers best practices for effective nutrition communication from several perspectives.

COMMUNICATING NUTRITION MESSAGES

Nutrition Communications

Nutrition communication has been defined by Mayfield as "communication about food and nutrition for the purpose of developing a platform for the inquiry and exchange of ideas or to influence knowledge, understanding, attitudes, decision-making processes, or behaviors."(p. 8)[2] Both eating and health are universal experiences, and as nutrition professionals our focus centers on maximizing messages to diverse audiences so that health can be optimized through food.

Health Literacy

Nutrition communication and education fit under the umbrella of **health literacy**, which is the capacity of persons to access, understand, and apply health information to make their own health choices and decisions.[3] Based on this definition, effective nutrition communication is strategic in that it is designed to reach a specific targeted audience through a channel in which the audience prefers to receive and understand the messaging. The reception of the messaging impacts the degree to which it influences its intended audience to make changes. We look at potential obstacles that may impede or mediate the impact of the messaging later in this chapter.

Nutrition information is communicated through many different channels. **Channels** are mediums through which messages are transmitted.[1] Channels can be visual, auditory, or both. Some examples of channels are as follows:

- Live speeches or presentations, including nonverbal expressions
- Written communication such as books, articles, handouts
- Electronic or digital media such as websites, webinars, social media posts, television
- Visuals such as illustrations, photographs, props, billboards
- Auditory such as radio broadcasts, podcasts, audiobooks

Choosing the right channel for a targeted audience can greatly impact decision-making processes and lead to successful health outcomes, which is the ultimate goal of health literacy.

Health literacy is a key consideration for public health nutrition professionals because:

- Patients typically have less face-to-face time with their providers to ask questions and process health-related information essential to their health and well-being.

- Patients, along with their caregivers, are expected to carry out a wide array of health-related tasks that may be complex or unfamiliar.
- Patients are expected to be active consumers and advocates for their own health, and need to be empowered to make key health decisions for themselves and those for whom they care.[3]

In 2010, The U.S. Department of Health and Human Services launched its initiative, *National Action Plan to Improve Health Literacy,* with the stated intention to provide accessible, high-quality, safe, cost-effective healthcare to enhance health and quality of life in the United States.[4]

Health literacy is a collaborative effort between providers and patients and/or caregivers that can result in sustainable long-term solutions and successful outcomes in populations. Healthcare communication is a two-way conversation. Patients need to be able to describe their symptoms, ask pertinent questions, and express their thoughts on how well they can maintain recommended dietary and nutrition interventions. On the other hand, practitioners need to be able to assess the patient using the verbal information that is presented, provide education in a way that the patient understands, and thoughtfully communicate nutrition interventions within what is often a time-limited encounter. Effective communication starts with empathy, or the ability to recognize how we, ourselves, might feel if in the situation of another.[5] How clients hear and perceive provider messages often matters more than the exact words providers may use.

CULTURALLY TAILORING NUTRITION COMMUNICATIONS AND EDUCATION

Culture shapes nearly all aspects of our lives—our behavior, lifestyle, choices, and beliefs. Culture can be thought of as those characteristics that are shared by members of a group or population, including but not limited to their beliefs, practices, and behaviors, that are

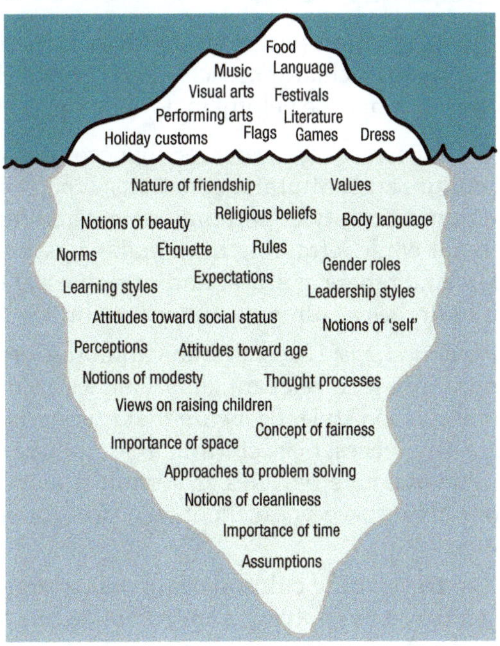

Figure 13.1. The Iceberg Model of culture.

inculcated generationally and distinguish that group from other groups.[6] The **Iceberg Model of Culture**, developed in the mid-1970s by anthropologist Edward T. Hall, is often used as an analogy for the cultural code that exists in any society and helps to depict the complexity of one's culture in order to gain insights into one's culture.[7] According to Hall, approximately 10% of a culture is visible and includes tangible items such as food, clothing, artifacts, and language. The other 90% of culture is invisible and includes intangibles such as values, beliefs, attitudes, communication style, and so forth that are generally more difficult to know or understand by those who are not familiar with the culture.[8] The iceberg model depicts the challenges in evaluating food or health behaviors by what is seen on the surface (above the water line). Often, misunderstandings and conflicts arise from what is hidden (below the water line).[8] The Iceberg Model of Culture is shown in Figure 13.1.

From Cultural Knowledge to Cultural Competence

From working on a team to working individually with people from different cultures, regions within one's own country, or even different parts of the world, skills in **cultural competence** are increasingly important. Cultural competence is more encompassing than just having cultural knowledge and can be defined as the ability to interact and work effectively with others who come from cultures that are different from one's own.[9]

Dr. Andy Molinsky, associate professor and specialist in cross-cultural interactions and adaptations, developed a six-dimensional approach for diagnosing the cultural code of a culture. These six dimensions represent key aspects of communication across cultures and can be used in identifying key differences and similarities between cultural styles.[10] The degree to which the dimensions apply to specific cultures can be helpful when tailoring messages to achieve professional outcomes with peers, colleagues, and patients/clients. The six dimensions along with determinative questions are found in **Table 13.1**:

Strategies for Cultural Competence

Becoming culturally competent requires an open mind, awareness and understanding of cultural differences, and a nonjudgmental approach working toward a successful health outcome. The following suggestions may be helpful in developing cultural competence skills:

- *Take steps to develop and improve self-awareness*: By becoming aware and knowledgeable of one's own culture and cultural inclinations, it becomes easier to recognize differences in communication styles and preferences among other cultures. Be mindful and observant while refraining from making assumptions about others. Be curious to understand others' cultural norms, values, and beliefs. Remember that much of what underlies a culture is under the surface in most interactions.
- *Adapt and tailor communications*: Use communication resources to craft messaging that is culturally appropriate, is relevant, and matches your client or audience's learning and communication style. Be aware that miscommunication can be caused by language differences, bias, cultural assumptions, and misunderstood cultural interpretation of nonverbal cues. Community agencies and community health organizations often serve as excellent resources for culturally appropriate nutrition information.
- *Evaluate one's success*: Developing cultural competence requires acquiring knowledge of the target culture and applying mindfulness while adapting behaviors. Experimentation and reflection on interactions with others from different cultures can be helpful in adapting new behaviors that produce successful outcomes.

Table 13.1. Molinsky's Six Dimensions of Culture

Cultural Dimension	Determinative Questions
1. Directness: Degree of straightforward-ness in particular situations	Does one say exactly what they mean? Or do they "hint" at what they are trying to convey in an indirect manner?
2. Enthusiasm: Amount of energy or expressions demonstrated when commu-nicating	Does one communicate with a high degree of emotion (even positive emotions), or is emotion held back during communication?
3. Formality: Degree of deference and respect expressed when communicating	Is there deference and respect given to those who have more status or hierarchy in their role, such as a manager or leader? Are people with higher status addressed with titles? Or, is there more informality in communications with others who have more status?
4. Assertiveness:	Is there an expectation that you can strongly assert one's voice, point of view, or contribution in discussions or in situations in this culture? Or are thoughts and opinions kept hidden and not disclosed?
5. Self-promotion	Can one freely and openly speak about their achievements and success without retribution? Or is self-promotion frowned upon by others?
6. Self-disclosure	Is it appropriate to disclose personal information and details about oneself? Or is it not appropri-ate to not share or express personal information?

Source: Molinski A. *Global Dexterity: How to Adapt Your Behavior Across Cultures Without Losing Yourself in the Process.* Harvard Business Review Press; 2013.

Developing Self-Awareness

The survey found in **Table 13.2,** known as the **Short Form Cultural Intelligence Assessment (SFCIA),** may be helpful in assessing one's own cultural intelligence. This instrument was developed by Thomas et al. and is the result of over a decade of academic research. The SFCIA was created and validated in response to the need for an easy-to-administer assessment of individual differences in cultural intelligence.[6,11]

SOCIAL DETERMINANTS OF HEALTH RELATED TO NUTRITION COMMUNICATIONS AND EDUCATION THROUGHOUT THE LIFE CYCLE

A healthy diet is considered one of the key components that can positively impact the effects of chronic diseases such as diabetes, cardiovascular disease, hypertension, and cancer. In our current media and information environment, relevant topics on nutrition

Table 13.2. Short Form Cultural Intelligence Assessment

Statement*	Not at All	A Little	Somewhat	A Lot	Extremely Well
1. I know the ways in which cultures around the world are different.	1	2	3	4	5
2. I can give examples of cultural differences from my personal experience, reading, and so on.	1	2	3	4	5
3. I enjoy talking with people from different cultures.	1	2	3	4	5
4. I have the ability to accurately understand the feelings of people from other cultures.	1	2	3	4	5
5. I sometimes try to understand people from another culture by imagining how something looks from their perspective.	1	2	3	4	5
6. I can change my behavior to suit different cultural situations and people.	1	2	3	4	5
7. I accept delays without becoming upset when in different cultural situations and with culturally different people.	1	2	3	4	5
8. I am aware of the cultural knowledge I use when interacting with someone from another culture.	1	2	3	4	5
9. I think a lot about the influence that culture has on my behavior and that of others who are culturally different.	1	2	3	4	5
10. I am aware that I need to plan my course of action when in different cultural situations and with culturally different people.	1	2	3	4	5

*Ten statements about one's experience when interacting with people from other cultures. Please indicate to what extent each of the following statements describes you.

Scoring: Your score is the average value for the 10 items. In a sample of more than 3,500 individuals from around the world, the average score was 3.51 with a standard deviation of .63. If you answer the questions honestly, the this assessment is a good indicator of your present level of CQ (cultural intelligence).

Source: Thomas D, Inkson K. *Cultural Intelligence: Surviving and Thriving in the Global Village*. 3rd ed. Berrett-Koehler Publishers; 2017. Used with permission.

and diet combined with food marketing messaging can be complex and confusing to the public. The research into the role of social determinants suggests that there are multiple factors and varying levels of influence of social determinants that impact health behaviors. Although evidence suggests that public health campaigns can influence healthy behaviors and reduce risks for disease, factors such as social class, race, ethnicity, and neighborhood can influence food choices and therefore impact health.[12]

There are three reasons to focus on social determinants, also known as social drivers, and their relevance to diet and nutrition communication: (1) one's social environment influences an individual's behaviors that can impact their health, (2) social determinants contribute to inequalities related to access to healthcare, and (3) health communication is mediated by access to and use of information regarding diet and nutrition. The following discussion considers some of the major social determinants that are related to nutrition communications and education.

Socioeconomic Status and Its Components

Socioeconomic status (SES) is the term used to characterize social position and social class. Research has shown that a higher SES is associated with better health outcomes due to completion of higher levels of education, higher incomes, more autonomy at work, more access to grocery stores, health resources, knowledge, skills, and the capacity to act on health recommendations. Four major factors related to SES that influence health outcomes are education, income, occupation, and occupational settings.[12]

Education

Persons with higher education levels tend to use a variety of media and pay attention to health content in the media. Additionally, education develops the critical thinking, quantitative, and reasoning skills that are needed to evaluate and apply nutrition information.[13]

Income Levels

Those with higher incomes tend to use their discretionary income to purchase more communication resources, which provides more opportunities to access nutrition messaging. Additionally, with more discretionary resources, individuals can then act on the nutrition messages they have consumed by purchasing products or services they have heard about. Persons with fewer financial resources are less likely to hear healthful promotional messaging, and thus are much less likely to access accompanying products or services.[14]

Occupation and Occupational Settings

Occupation can be a subtle contributor to nutrition education in that it may provide access and opportunities that would otherwise be prohibitive in cost. The influence of social norms at the workplace and of coworkers can be either a positive or negative influence over food choices and healthful behaviors. Occupational settings have been used with success to shift dietary and nutritional changes within a workplace when combined with mass media campaigns.[15] For example, workplace interventions have included programs that increased nutrition awareness and engagement strategies that have resulted in consumption of fruit and vegetables.

EFFECTIVE NUTRITION COMMUNICATIONS AND EDUCATION

For any public health or public health nutrition communication to have impact, there must be a process in place to ensure its effectiveness. Effective nutrition communication is strategic and is created to produce a specific outcome for its intended audience. An effective nutrition communication strategy has three components: the audience, the message, and the channel.[1] Practitioners must consider the *who*, *why*, *what*, and *how* for their communications:

Who: Audience

For communication to occur, there must be a sender and a receiver. The recipient of the sender's message is the audience. Before any message is created, a nutrition communicator needs to think about the receiver/audience and what the receiver/audience wants and needs. Demographic information is often a good starting point for identifying information about an audience's perceived wants and needs. A deeper analysis of an audience reveals **psychographic information** which includes an audiences' values, attitudes, and beliefs.[16] Knowing and understanding one's audience is essential in crafting nutrition messaging that will resonate with the target audience. An audience who perceives that a communicator understands their challenges and concerns is going to be more receptive to hearing the information they are receiving.

An often-overlooked step in learning about an audience is conducting a **needs assessment**. A needs assessment is the collection of data and the analysis process that provides information about an audience in order to direct all aspects of communication planning and implementation. This includes discovering gaps in knowledge, identifying accessible resources, defining outcomes, and determining the most optimal delivery channels.[17] Advantages of conducting a needs assessment include identifying gaps in what an audience knows and what the nutrition communicator assumes the audience knows, determining the type of the nutrition messaging to create, and deciding the most appropriate channel for the target audience. A well-constructed needs assessment can inform a nutrition communicator of their target audience's current behaviors or practices, motivators and barriers to change, as well as readiness to make changes. All of this increases the likelihood of successful reception of the messaging.[17]

Why: Purpose

Once the target audience is assessed and their needs are known, the next step is to identify the purpose of the communication. There are generally two purposes for messaging: (1) to inform or educate, or (2) to persuade or influence.[18] To determine the purpose of the message, consider the desired outcome of the message. When the outcome for the messaging is clear, the purpose also becomes clear.

What: Messaging

Once an audience's needs have been assessed and the purpose of the message is clear, the messaging to meet the target audience's needs can commence. Effective communication starts with empathy for the intended audience, and effective messaging answers an unspoken question that most audiences will ask: What's in it for me? Crafting messages that resonate with an audience will include these attributes:

- *Clarity:* The messaging is simple and contains words that the audience is familiar with and understands. Abstract concepts are made clear through analogies or concrete examples. The words are short and sentences are simple. The speaker avoids jargon or terminology the audience does not recognize.
- *Accuracy:* Messaging is accurate and evidence-based. A natural consequence of research is that as new findings are uncovered, it is increasingly difficult to find credible, reliable sources of information. It is essential that nutrition messaging is sourced from trustworthy resources to maintain the trust and confidence of one's audiences. For examples of trustworthy nutrition messaging resources, see Chapter 1, Tables 1.2 and 1.3 in this textbook.
- *Connection:* Effective nutrition messaging is tailored to meet the needs of its intended audience. Effective messaging is based in fact and evidence, and it also connects with an audience on an emotional level. Visual representations of the ideas and concepts that are conveyed as well as stories make an emotional connection with an audience as well as making the messaging more memorable.

How: Channel

As previously mentioned, the channel is the medium through which a message is delivered.

- *Channel:* The most effective choice of a channel is determined by the audience, the message, and the availability of the channel. In best use cases, several channels are used to optimize the reach and receptivity of the targeted audience. For example, when presenting nutrition information, visual aids and handouts that accompany what is heard audibly can enhance retention of the information that is delivered. A public health nutrition campaign may include radio public service announcements, billboards and social media posts to extend the campaign's outreach potential. Using several communication channels simultaneously can enhance a message's reach and impact.

Tailoring Nutrition Education and Communications Across the Life Span

Life cycle stage of the intended audience is one of the many attributes nutrition communicators must consider when crafting effective nutrition communications and education messages. Because different developmental tasks and concerns are common to specific life stages, communications tailored to reach the audience become more important. Table 13.3 provides cultural considerations for tailoring nutrition communications to various stages of the life cycle.

USING TECHNOLOGY TO PROMOTE HEALTHFUL EATING

The use of technology has proliferated the exchange of information in the lives of most people. Technology includes the use of personal computers, laptops, tablets, personal cell

Table 13.3. Cultural Considerations for Nutrition Messaging Throughout the Life Cycle

Life Cycle Stage	Examples: Suggested Public Health Nutrition Messaging Topics	Life Cycle Stage Concerns	Examples: Cultural Considerations When Preparing Nutrition Communications/Education
Pregnancy	• Healthful diet in pregnancy • Appropriate weight gain • Association of good nutrition with reduced risk of preterm birth	• Optimal maternal and infant pregnancy outcomes • Desirable weight gain	• Beliefs about weight gain in pregnancy • Perceptions of a healthful pregnancy diet and specific foods thought to be beneficial during pregnancy • Cultural practices during pregnancy • Roles of family members in food and meal management during pregnancy • Cultural foods
Infancy (messaging to parents and caregivers)	• Feeding practices to promote appropriate growth and development	• Optimal growth and development	• Cultural practices and norms for infant feeding • Roles of family members in infant feeding • Beliefs about healthy infancy
Young and school-age childhood (messaging to parents and caregivers)	• Optimal growth and development • Prevention of overweight and obesity • Ongoing development of feeding skills	• Optimal growth and development • Prevention of overweight and obesity • Ongoing development of self-feeding skills	• Cultural practices and norms for feeding young children • Cultural practices in regard to family meals • Roles of family members in child feeding • Cultural foods • Beliefs about healthy childhood

Adolescence (parents, caregivers, mentors)	• The role of nutrition in healthy adolescence • Prevention of overweight and obesity in adolescents • Helping adolescents develop a positive relationship with food • Mentoring adolescents in the acquisition of food management and self-nourishment skills for adulthood	• Optimal growth and development • Prevention of overweight and obesity • Ongoing development of skills in food management and self-nourishment • Ongoing development of a healthy relationship with food	• Cultural practices and norms for food and meals in adolescence • Cultural practices for recognizing increased independence in self-nourishment • Cultural foods in relationship to acculturated eating practices • Roles of family members in relationship to peers in relationship to food • Beliefs regarding health in adolescence
Young and middle adulthood	• Nutrition and the prevention of chronic disease • Healthy weight management in adulthood • Developing and maintaining a positive relationship with food and eating	• Healthful weight management • Preventing chronic disease • Maintaining a healthy attitude toward food and eating • Effectively managing one's own self-nourishment	• Cultural practices and norms for food and meals including family meals • Cultural norms and practices in regards to food and parenting • Cultural foods in relationship to acculturated eating practices • Beliefs regarding health in adulthood
Older adulthood	• Healthful diet • Benefits of physical activity • Accessing healthful food • Maintenance of healthful weight • Healthy aging • Nutrition and quality of life	• Maintaining independence • Maintaining quality of life • Maintaining optimal nutrition status	• Cultural practices and norms regarding aging • Cultural practices and norms regarding nutrition for older adults • Roles of family members in older adult nutrition • Cultural foods • Beliefs regarding health in older adulthood

phones, and other electronic devices. These devices are used for emails, text messaging, video chats, viewing videos, viewing or posting on social media, taking notes, researching information, and many other tasks related to receiving and delivering information.

The many advantages to using technology in public health and public health nutrition communications and education include convenience, time-savings, and timeliness. One can send and receive messages at the time best suited to their schedule. Provider and patient interactions can occur without the need for travel. Information can be sent and received almost instantly, rather than in a matter of days or longer. Patients and clients can read and review information at their convenience.

There are disadvantages to using technology as well. Some patients and clients lack access to technology; for example, inadequate broadband infrastructure in some rural areas may prevent access to telehealth and other important services.[19] Other persons may be unfamiliar with available technology and not understand how to use it. Some individuals prefer in-person communication. Nutrition professionals must maintain an open and flexible attitude surrounding the use of technology with their patients and clients to determine what kind of technology will best serve the needs and interests of the population served in order to achieve the best health outcomes.

Nutrition Communications and Social Media Platforms

Social media is a collective term for websites and applications that focus on communication, community-based input, interaction, content-sharing, and collaboration.[20] Increasingly, **digital literacy** is an essential skill for all healthcare practitioners. Cornell University defines digital literacy as "the ability to find, evaluate, utilize, share, and create content using information technologies and the Internet."[21]

Social media has become a dominant source for health information for the public and has vastly changed the way most of our population consumes health information as social media channels efficiently and effectively reach and influence large audiences. It is estimated that one in three U.S. adults use the internet to diagnose or learn about a health concern.[22] One perspective of social media has been its ability to "democratize" the flow of information and allow anyone to become an author or publisher of information.[23] While there are advantages and disadvantages of informational democratization, one result has been a proliferation of inaccurate information. Therefore, it has become increasingly important for nutrition professionals to incorporate and utilize social media channels within their communication strategies to promote accurate and credible health information.

Social media is not only used by healthcare professionals to engage with consumers in general, but also with their patients and clients on an individual basis. Educators are using social media to engage with students, collaborate with colleagues, and network with other professionals. Social media has been used to advocate for health, start movements, and impact health campaigns such as programs for weight loss, chronic disease management, increased physical activity, and smoking cessation.

Strategies for Effective Use of Social Media

The unlimited potential of social media to promote health and well-being is an exciting channel for practitioners seeking improved outcomes for patients and clients. Here are effective strategies for integrating social media into public health nutrition practice:

- *Identify goals:* Begin by identifying desired outcomes from the use of social media. Is the aim to build one's business? Attract clients? Establish oneself as an expert? Knowing what one is looking to achieve will help with subsequent decisions such as identifying which social media platform to utilize, where to find the target audience, and what kinds of content to post.
- *Focus on the audience:* Having clarity on who the audience is allows the practitioner to serve them better by becoming equipped with knowledge of what the audience needs and wants. By serving a specific audience, a practitioner sets the stage for attaining a reputation for expertise in a specific practice area.
- *Commit to engaging:* Frequent and consistent engagement on social media has been shown to be the best way to build and grow an audience. According to Becky Robinson, author of "Reach: Create the Biggest Possible Audience for Your Message, Book, or Cause" there are four commitments one must make to expand one's audience and create an impact[24]:
  - *Value*: Offer knowledge, expertise, point of view, and approaches toward the topic.
  - *Consistency*: Be consistent with sharing value with the audience, as consistency promotes memorability, reliability, trust.
  - *Longevity*: The longer one maintains a presence on social media, the more credibility is built and impact is created.
  - *Generosity*: Audience-centered sharing of information contributes to the expansion of social media's reach.
  - *Collaborate and share:* When utilizing social media, one must also respond and engage with others about content, and share content from other credible sources. Collaborative efforts with other health professionals can increase social media's reach to impact audiences and meet social media goals.[24]
- *Measure results*: Because of the time and resources devoted to developing one's social media presence, one must measure the return on investment. Are the goals initially set for utilizing social media being met? Tools are available to monitor and track the reach of social media posts in order to compare results to original goals and determine if a particular message or platform needs to be changed.[25] Following the process of identifying goals, engaging regularly, and measuring results can build reach for one's message and audience.

Best Practices for Communicating via Social Media

Best practices for communicating via social media include:

- *Maintain professional and ethical standards.* Communication delivered through social media should adhere to the code of ethics for one's individual health profession. For example, a code of ethics has been established by the Academy of Nutrition and Dietetics and guides all areas of dietetics practice. The Code of Ethics for the Profession of Nutrition and Dietetics provides standards for practice including competence, integrity, professionalism, and social responsibility.[26] Another example is the American Public Health Association's Code of Conduct, which describes attributes of APHA members including respect, responsibility, fairness, and honesty, and sets forth guidelines for conduct for public health practitioners.[27]

- *Promote civility.* Maintaining high standards is essential to professionalism, and social media is not a forum for attacking others and their points of view. Content posted by nutrition professionals is expected to be science-based; however, there is room for personal opinions on all platforms. As an example, the Academy of Nutrition and Dietetics *Food and Nutrition Magazine* developed a Pledge of Civility that provides guiding principles for positive social media engagement.[28]
- *Stay informed about social media platform updates, changes, and services.* Social media and its platforms continually evolve to meet the needs of its users and adhere to ever-changing regulations. Successfully utilizing social media as a means for promotion entails staying abreast of changes and policies to ensure a positive experience for your audience.

NUTRITION WRITING AND COMMUNICATIONS FOR THE POPULAR MARKET

Writing for the popular market—sometimes called the *mass market*—enables nutrition professionals to gain further reach to deliver their nutrition messages to impact health. Each media channel has the potential to reach thousands, even millions, of readers. Although traditional print media (newspapers, magazines) have shown decline over the past years, many publishers have replaced traditional print media with online content as readers have moved from physical publications to consuming online content.[22] Blog posts and scripts for video and television are examples of other forms of written communication and are highly effective for optimizing nutrition messaging to various audiences. As with all other forms of communication, the key to success in the written communication market is knowing and tailoring the messaging to fit the needs of the target audience to the specific publication.

There are a variety of strategies for public health nutrition professionals who wish to utilize mass media. Editors and producers look for stories and information that are unique and can engage their audience. For freelance writing for print or web, as well as TV and radio, professionals can pitch ideas to editors and producers by suggesting a compelling idea or angle on a nutrition topic. In addition to providing ideas, it is helpful to include examples of one's work—whether it's writing, audio, or video—so that an editor or producer can see the strength and quality of one's work.

Another strategy for building one's presence in written media is to be quoted in an article. One effective way to connect with reporters is through a service called *Help a Reporter Out* (HARO).[29] The service provides a free basic option. Registrants receive a digest of daily media opportunities soliciting replies. Working with media in this way requires perseverance; however, an advantage is that reporters have already chosen the idea they are planning to write about and are looking for experts to add credibility and accurate content for their story.

Social media also offers opportunities to connect with reporters. One may wish to join Facebook or other social media groups that are targeted toward media opportunities for reporters. Media Mastery for Dietitians & Health Professionals is one such group that features weekly opportunities from reporters from a plethora of outlets who are looking for registered dietitians and health professionals to interview.

If a public health nutrition professional networks with reporters over time, the chances are greatly improved that reporters will reach out to that professional when up-to-date, accurate content is needed. When participating in interviews, always include a credit line. One can also include a link back to a personal website in the credit line so that if published, more traffic will be directed to the personal website, which can lead to more recognition and more potential clients.

Best Practices for Public Health and Public Health Nutrition Writing and Communications

- *Always adhere to deadlines.* Missed deadlines have negative consequences for both nutrition professionals and reporters and others with whom the nutrition professional is working. Answers to a reporter's questions provided after a deadline result in wasted work, since the reporter may not be able to use what you have offered. Additionally, one's reputation as a reliable source is damaged.
- *Keep in mind ethics and disclosure when working with the media.* Current or potential conflicts of interest must be disclosed. For example, if one is working as a spokesperson, brand ambassador, nutrition partner, or consultant for a particular entity or entities—essentially, if there is a paid relationship with a brand, for example, to an editor, reporter, or producer—this must be disclosed when discussing the brand's products. Appropriate confidentiality must always be maintained when providing nutrition communications. Specific legal requirements for one's profession and jurisdictions should be ascertained prior to engaging in nutrition communications.

WHAT WORKS: THE GUIDING STAR PROGRAM

Although there is strong evidence that links a healthy diet with the reduction of chronic diseases, many Americans need help in following the *Dietary Guidelines for Americans* (DGA). In efforts to help consumers make better food choices and to quickly identify foods and beverages with the highest nutrition profiles, a supermarket retailer collaborated with a panel of nutritionists and public health professionals to create the Guiding Star program, a front-of-package food labeling system.[30] The goal of the program is to quickly and clearly communicate nutrition information so that consumers can choose foods and beverages with the highest nutritional values and can better align their choices with the recommendations of the DGA. The Guiding Star program evaluates foods with a proprietary algorithmic scoring system, which examines both positive and negative attributes of the food and assigns points. The Guiding Star ratings of one, two, or three stars are then assigned to the particular food based on the results of that food's score (see Figure 13.2).

The Guiding Star program, which has been in existence since 2006, has shown in several studies that it has positively impacted consumer choices. Research published in the *American Journal of Clinical Nutrition* showed that Guiding Stars positively influenced food purchases and confirmed that consumers preferred rating systems that used a simple icon and a tiered approach rather than rating systems that were more complicated.[31] Another study published in the journal *Food Policy* supports the claim that nutrition programs whereby nutrition information is easy to find and easy to understand such as the Guiding Star program, helped consumers select products that were more nutritious. Additionally, the *Food Policy* study noted that the Guiding Star program ratings significantly increased demand for products that were rated more nutritious, at the expense of those that were not.[32]

According to Lori Kaley, MS, RDN, LD, MSB, a member of the Guiding Stars advisory panel who was interviewed in 2022, "This program is a public health intervention and was in response to consumer requests for a quick and easy way to identify healthier and more nutritious foods in the grocery store. Working in public health, we know we can't do this alone. We know we need to collaborate with other sectors to move the needle in helping consumers make healthier choices for themselves and their families."

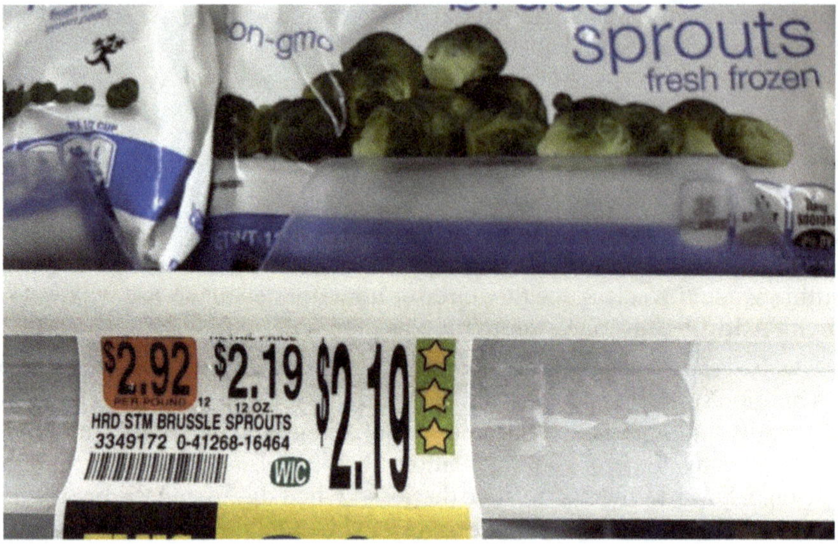

Figure 13.2. Guiding Star rating example.
Image used with permission of Kaley LA. Maine SNAP-Ed | University of New England.

SUMMARY

This chapter considers best practices for effective public health and public health nutrition communication through the life cycle from several perspectives. Good nutrition communications are the basis of health literacy. Effective nutrition messages are delivered with cultural competence, using evidence-based strategies and best practices. Social determinants of health impact every aspect of communication—the sender, the receiver, the message, the communication channel, and the impact of the message received—and should be considered when developing nutrition messaging. Opportunities for nutrition communicators include but are not limited to social media, print, and broadcast communications. Nutrition communications are an essential component of delivering effective nutrition messages throughout the life cycle.

KEY CHAPTER CONCEPTS

1. The basic communication model consists of a sender of a message, the receiver of the message, the message itself, the channel through which the message is sent, and feedback to signify that the message was received.
2. Nutrition communication has been defined by Mayfield as "communication about food and nutrition for the purpose of developing a platform for the inquiry and exchange of ideas or to influence knowledge, understanding, attitudes, decision-making processes, or behaviors. (p. 8)"[2]
3. Health literacy is a collaborative effort between providers and patients and/or caregivers that can result in sustainable long-term solutions and successful outcomes in populations.
4. The Iceberg Model of Culture, developed by anthropologist Edward T. Hall, is often used as an analogy for the cultural code that exists an any society and helps to depict the complexity of

culture. According to Hall, approximately 10% of a culture is visible and the other 90% of culture is invisible.

5. Molinsky's six dimensions of communication across cultures are directness, enthusiasm, formality, assertiveness, self-promotion, and self-disclosure.
6. The SFCIA may be helpful in assessing one's own cultural intelligence.
7. Three reasons to focus on social determinants of health and their relevance to diet and nutrition communication are as follows: (1) one's social environment influences behaviors that can impact health, (2) social determinants contribute to inequalities related to access to healthcare, and (3) health communication is mediated by access to and use of information regarding diet and nutrition.
8. Effective public health nutrition communication is strategic and is created to produce a specific outcome for its intended audience. An effective nutrition communication strategy has three components: the audience, the message, and the channel. Practitioners must consider the who, why, what, and how for their communications.
9. Among the advantages to using technology in nutrition communications and education are convenience, time-savings, and timeliness. Disadvantages include the problem that some clients may lack access to technology or may be unfamiliar with technology and how to use it.
10. Social media has become a dominant source for health information for the public and has vastly changed the way most of our population consumes health information. It has become increasingly important for public health nutrition professionals to incorporate and utilize social media channels within their communication strategies.

CASE STUDY

Amy Gorin, MS, is a registered dietitian nutritionist (RDN), and before she became a dietitian, she was a magazine editor at *Prevention*, *Health*, *Parents*, *American Baby*, and *Weight Watchers* magazines. While working as an editor, she returned to school to become a RDN. After becoming an RDN, she combined her love of the media with her love of nutrition.

In reestablishing her relationship with print media, Ms. Gorin pitched herself to reporters through HARO and to reporters with whom she had made connections with through her magazine work. She also connected with editors she had met over the years. Within a matter of weeks, she began writing for publications such as *Everyday Health* and for the Food Network and was being interviewed in outlets including *U.S. News*, *The Washington Post*, *Women's Health*, and *Men's Health*.

Through word of mouth, TV producers began reaching out to her for segments. Ms. Gorin was featured on Associated Press segments and beyond. Additionally, brands began to reach out to represent them as a nutrition spokesperson. In addition to writing freelance articles, being quoted by major media, and being featured on TV, she started working with brands to host media events, create recipes for them, and help make their products healthier. Ms. Gorin started small, with compelling stories for reporters, and her career as a media dietitian grew from there.

Case Study Questions

1. What are some transferable skills Ms. Gorin used in her career as a magazine editor that she also applied to her career as a nutrition professional?

2. While still working as a magazine editor, Ms. Gorin returned to school to become an RDN. What are some of the challenges of returning to school as a working professional, and how do you think these challenges can be successfully addressed?
3. What were some of the strategies Ms. Gorin used to establish herself as a nutrition communications expert once she completed her dietetics education?
4. How would you describe the progression of Ms. Gorin's career in media?
5. If Ms. Gorin were providing you with career advice, what do you think are three things she would say to you?

DISCUSSION QUESTIONS

1. What is health literacy? How is it related to delivering optimal services to clients?
2. How does health literacy apply to different stages of the life cycle (e.g., children, young adults, older adults)?
3. What is cultural competence, and what are the six dimensions of communication across cultures? Can you provide examples of situations in which knowledge of the six dimensions could be helpful in nutrition communications?
4. What are three social determinants that are relevant to nutrition communications across the life cycle?
5. What are three considerations practitioners must consider in preparing for nutrition education for their clients? (Who is the audience? What is the purpose or desired outcome of the communication? What channel best serves the audience and the message?)

SUGGESTED LEARNING ACTIVITIES

1. You are a program director for a local federal Nutrition Programs for Older Adults Congregate Meal Program. You have been asked to create a nutrition message promoting improved fruit and vegetable consumption. Design a public health nutrition message for your audience, targeted toward the desired outcome. Consider your audience, the desired outcome of the message, and the best channel to deliver the message.
2. Design a social media strategy to reduce consumption of sugary beverages among adolescents. Refer to the section of this chapter titled "Nutrition Communications and Social Media platforms" for guidelines and suggestions.
3. Using the Iceberg Model, research and describe the visible and tangible aspects and the *in*visible and *in*tangible aspects of your own culture. Include nutritional aspects of your culture in your description. Present your information using some type of media as your chosen communication channel.
4. Select a particular life cycle stage (pregnancy, infant, toddler and preschooler, school-age, adolescent, young adult, middle adult, older adult). Create a presentation on at least three specific communication strategies for your chosen life cycle stage. Include examples showing application of your listed strategies.
5. Locate a nutrition communications article. Your article could be found in a social media post, a newspaper or magazine (print or digital), or some other communication venue. Critique your article from a communications viewpoint:

a. What message is being conveyed?
b. What is the purpose of the article?
c. Is the content accurate?
d. Is the communication channel appropriate for the message? Why or why not?
e. Will the message be effective for the intended audience? Provide a rationale for your answer.
f. How does the visual presentation of the message interact with the content? For example, a message can be visual even without illustrations: Does the message appear cluttered? Is the text dense? Is there adequate clear space on the page?
g. What does the article do well? What suggestions for improvement can you provide?

6. Look at the "Social Media Resources" section at the end of the following "Resources for Further Learning" section. Choose one of the resources suggested, either for patient social media or website management. Review the website and resources. Prepare a short visual report summarizing your findings using presentation slides, digital video, or some other medium of your choice.

RESOURCES FOR FURTHER LEARNING

- Peace Corps, Culture Is Like an Iceberg: www.peacecorps.gov/educators/resources/culture-iceberg
  - Provides a lesson plan and helpful teaching resources on the Iceberg Model of Culture; while the lesson is designed for middle and high school students, it is a clear and thorough introduction to the Iceberg Model for anyone interested in the concept.
- Food and Nutrition: Professional Civility: https://foodandnutrition.org/professionalcivility
  - Provides the Pledge of Professional Civility, along with Pledge guidelines and Frequently Asked Questions
- Google Analytics: www.google.com/analytics
  - Tools to help online nutrition communicators understand their clients, analyze data on website performance, plan marketing outreach, and much more
- Guiding Stars: https://guidingstars.com
  - Information about the Guiding Stars front-of-package food labeling system
- HARO.com: www.helpareporter.com
  - Facilitates communication between journalists seeking expertise and persons who have that expertise
- Health Information Translations website: www.healthinfotranslations.org
  - Easy-to-read health education information in more than 15 languages
- How to evaluate health information on the internet: https://ods.od.nih.gov/HealthInformation/How_To_Evaluate_Health_Information_on_the_Internet_Questions_and_Answers.aspx
  - Tips and hints for assessing online health information
- Master the Media: https://masterthemedia.co/about
  - The business website of Amy Gorin, MS, RDN, nutrition communications expert; offers free tools for enhancing nutrition communications and entrepreneurial skills

- National Action Plan to Improve Health Literacy: https://health.gov/our-work/national-health-initiatives/health-literacy/national-action-plan-improve-health-literacy
    - Information and resources for promoting health literacy; includes the Health Literacy Online tool to help in developing health materials for a wide range of population groups including persons with lower literacy
- U.S. Department of Health and Human Services: Think cultural health: https://thinkculturalhealth.hhs.gov
    - Provides resources, training, and continuing education on providing Culturally and Linguistically Appropriate Services (CLAS) in healthcare
- Utilization Review Accreditation Commission: www.urac.org/accreditations-certifications/accreditation-faqs
    - Provides accreditations and certifications for various aspects of healthcare delivery, including health content provider certification and health website accreditation

Social Media Resources

- Consumers can engage and share health information with one another through social sites such as PatientsLikeMe.com (www.patientslikeme.com/?format=html), Smart Patients (www.smartpatients.com), and The Mighty (https://themighty.com).
- Participating on social media platforms can be time-consuming, and there are tools available to help automate posting such as Buffer (https://buffer.com), CoSchedule (https://coschedule.com), Hootsuite (www.hootsuite.com), HubSpot (www.hubspot.com), to name a few.

SPRINGER PUBLISHING CONNECT™ | **A robust set of instructor resources designed to supplement this text is located at http://connect.springerpub.com/content/book/978-0-8261-8623-2. Qualifying instructors may request access by emailing textbook@springerpub.com.**

REFERENCES

1. Usera D, Appignani T, DeBord S, et al. Basic process models of communication. Libretext. Accessed April 14, 2023. https://socialsci.libretexts.org/Bookshelves/Communication/Introduction_to_Communication/Communicating_to_Connect_-_Interpersonal_Communication_for_Today_(Usera)/01%3A_Fundamentals_of_Interpersonal_Communication/1.02%3A_Basic_Process_Models_of_Communication
2. Mayfield BJ, ed. *Communicating Nutrition: The Authoritative Guide*. Academy of Nutrition and Dietetics; 2020.
3. Osborne H. *Health Literacy From A to Z: Practical Ways to Communicate Your Health Message.* 2nd ed. Aviva Publishing; 2018.
4. Office of Disease Prevention and Health Promotion. *National Action Plan to Improve Health Literacy.* U.S. Department of Health and Human Services. 2010. https://health.gov/our-work/national-health-initiatives/health-literacy/national-action-plan-improve-health-literacy
5. Thompson KL, Stetzler SK. Medical improvisation training as a vehicle to improve empathetic communication skills in nutrition and dietetics students. *Top Clin Nutr*. 2019;34(2):114–124. https://doi.org/10.1097/TIN.0000000000000175
6. Thomas DC, Inkson K. *Cultural Intelligence: Surviving and Thriving in the Global Village.* 3rd ed. Berrett-Koehler Publishers; 2017.
7. Hall ET. *Beyond Culture.* Anchor Books; 1977.

8. Peace Corps. Culture is like an iceberg. Accessed April 16, 2023. https://www.peacecorps.gov/educators/resources/culture-iceberg
9. National Prevention Information Network. Cultural competence in health and human services. Centers for Disease Control and Prevention. September 10, 2021. https://npin.cdc.gov/pages/cultural-competence
10. Molinsky A. *Global Dexterity: How to Adapt Your Behavior Across Cultures Without Losing Yourself in the Process.* Harvard Business Review Press; 2013.
11. Thomas DC, Liao Y, Aycan Z, et al. Cultural intelligence: a theory-based, short form measure. *J Int Bus Stud.* 2015;46(9):1099–1118. https://doi.org/10.1057/jibs.2014.67
12. Braveman P, Gottlieb L. The social determinants of health: it's time to consider the causes of the causes. *Public Health Rep.* 2014;129(suppl 2):19–31. https://doi.org/10.1177/00333549141291S206
13. Viswanath K, Breen N, Meissner H, et al. Cancer knowledge and disparities in the information age. *JHealth Commun.* 2006;11(suppl 1):1–17. https://doi.org/10.1080/10810730600637426
14. Rogers EM. A prospective and retrospective look at the diffusion model. *JHealth Commun.* 2004;9(suppl 1):13–19. https://doi.org/10.1080/10810730490271449
15. Hunt MK, Lederman R, Stoddard A, Potter S, Phillips J, Sorensen G. Process tracking results from the Treatwell 5-a-Day Worksite Study. *Am J Health Promot.* 2000;14(3):179–187. https://doi.org/10.4278/0890-1171-14.3.179
16. Psychographics. In: *Merriam-Webster.com Dictionary*. Merriam-Webster; 2023. https://www.merriam-webster.com/dictionary/psychographics
17. Community Tool Box. Section 7: conducting needs assessment surveys. University of Kansas. Accessed April 27, 2023. https://ctb.ku.edu/en/table-of-contents/assessment/assessing-community-needs-and-resources/conducting-needs-assessment-surveys/main
18. West J. Strategic communication to inform or persuade. University of Virginia Darden School of Business. February 12, 2015. https://ideas.darden.virginia.edu/strategic-communication-to-inform-or-persuade
19. U.S. Department of Agriculture. Broadband: e-connectivity for all rural Americans is a modern-day necessity. Accessed April 18, 2023. https://www.usda.gov/broadband
20. Lutkevich B, Wigmore I. Social media. TechTarget. Updated September 2021. https://www.techtarget.com/whatis/definition/social-media
21. Lynch M. What is digital literacy? The Tech Edvocate. October 23, 2017. https://www.thetechedvocate.org/what-is-digital-literacy
22. Jacobs W, Amuta AO, Jeon KC. Health information seeking in the digital age: an analysis of health information seeking behavior among US adults. *Cogent Soc Sci.* 2017;3(1):1302785. https://doi.org/10.1080/23311886.2017.1302785
23. Baym NK. *Personal Connections in the Digital Age.* 2nd ed. Polity Press; 2015.
24. Robinson B. *Reach: Create the Biggest Possible Audience for Your Message, Book, or Cause.* Berrett-Koehler Publishers; 2022.
25. Google. Welcome to Google Analytics. Google; 2023. www.google.com/analytics
26. Academy of Nutrition and Dietetics. Code of ethics for the nutrition and dietetics profession. June 1, 2018. https://www.eatrightpro.org/about-us/our-members/code-of-ethics
27. American Public Health Association. APHA Code of Conduct. Accessed November 1, 2023. https://apha.org/Membership/Code-of-Conduct
28. Academy of Nutrition and Dietetics. The pledge of professional civility. *Food and Nutrition Magazine.* Accessed October 16, 2023. https://foodandnutrition.org/professionalcivility/
29. HAROt. A source for every story. Cision. Accessed February 13, 2023. https://www.helpareporter.com
30. Fischer LM, Sutherland LA, Kaley LA, et al. Development and implementation of the Guiding Stars nutrition guidance program. *Am J Health Promot.* 2011;26(2):e55–e63. https://doi.org/10.4278/ajhp.100709-QUAL-238
31. Sutherland LA, Kaley LA, Fischer L. Guiding stars: the effect of a nutrition navigation program on consumer purchases at the supermarket. *Am J Clin Nutr.* 2010;91(4):1090s–1094s. https://doi.org/10.3945/ajcn.2010.28450C
32. Rahkovsky I, Lin B-H, Lin C-TJ, Lee J-Y. Effects of the Guiding Stars Program on purchases of ready-to-eat cereals with different nutritional attributes. *Food Policy.* 2013;43(C):100–107. https://doi.org/10.1016/j.foodpol.2013.08.013

14

ECONOMIC ASPECTS OF PUBLIC HEALTH NUTRITION ACROSS THE LIFE CYCLE

Janani Rajbhandari-Thapa, Onyedikachi Emmanuel Chike, and Conrad Lyford

LEARNING OBJECTIVES

At the end of this chapter, students will be able to:

1. Understand key theoretical models of the costs and trade-offs of nutrition choices.
2. Be aware of the economic consequences of public health and nutrition across the life cycle.
3. Be able to evaluate society's current efforts toward improving nutrition and addressing the obesity epidemic.
4. Consider using behavioral economics to address the obesity epidemic and other related chronic diseases.

INTRODUCTION

Diet and nutrition are one of the key determinants of health—that is, a state of complete physical, mental, and social well-being and not merely the absence of disease or infirmity, as defined by the World Health Organization (WHO).[1] The consumption of proper nutrition is vital in maintaining healthy living and avoiding major chronic disease risk factors, such as obesity. This chapter focuses on the economic impact of nutrition across the life cycle and goes on to consider societal efforts to improve nutrition and food security of communities while addressing the obesity epidemic.

Notwithstanding various substantial efforts to create more nutrition awareness, the overwhelming number of chronic diseases that obesity is a risk factor for has continued to inflict substantial and increasing health and financial burdens on individuals and society. The relative risk of mortality associated with obesity has continued to rise. In the year 2000, over 111,909 excess deaths were associated with the obesity epidemic.[2] In more recent years that number has increased to 186,000 excess deaths.[3] Furthermore, it is well known that obesity substantially increases the risk of diabetes, cardiovascular disease (CVD), and cancer, accounting for the substantial mortality risk associated with obesity[4] as well as societal costs including increased medical costs.

This chapter outlines the healthcare costs and economic consequences among communities and populations of nutrition across the life cycle. We begin the chapter with a perspective on obesity leading into a discussion of the economic consequences of poor nutrition—obesity and other chronic diseases—which affect health status among communities and populations across different life stages. In recent decades, there has been a trend of continuously increasing rates of obesity accompanied by ever-alarming increasing rates of chronic diseases, together leading to global economic costs and consequences.

A PERSPECTIVE ON OBESITY: THE ENERGY BALANCE MODEL

A high-calorie, low-nutrition diet accompanied with low levels of physical activity is known to lead to obesity and generates substantial economic burden.[5,6] This public health perspective on obesity states that obesity is caused by an imbalance between energy intake and energy used. Obesity can be attributed to increased intake of high-energy food without a balancing level of physical activity. We discuss this first under the energy balance model (EBM) and then discuss a more conceptual perspective on health and obesity.

The dominant EBM built its foundation on the law of thermodynamics and argues that obesity is a result of a mismatch between energy consumption and energy expenditure and is an outcome when energy consumption is higher than expenditure. Energy intake is through the consumption of food and drink and spent through the resting metabolic rate (RMR) and physical activities.[7]

Furthermore, many who use the EBM indicate that the current obesity epidemic is caused by changes in food choices due to the rise in the consumption of cheap, accessible, high-energy, highly processed foods with an exuberant amount of fat and sugar accompanied with low protein and fiber.[8] Generally, we consume energy from the intake of energy-based macronutrients such as protein, carbohydrate, and fat; excess consumption of any of these nutrients is stored as fat cells in the body. A single plate of a "good" meal (food from a sit-down restaurant) typically contains an average of 2,000 to 3,500 calories. This is the amount a healthy adult may need for an entire day to maintain a healthy weight.[9] The exact amount of calorie requirement for a specific person is a factor of their basal metabolic rate, gender, age, activity levels, and muscle mass.[10]

More recently, the EBM has been challenged by a model based on human physiology—the carbohydrate-insulin model. This model focuses on the physiology of energy balance and fat storage and proposes a reversal of causal direction wherein the fat deposition is a result of hormonal responses to a diet high in glycemic load.[11] Both perspectives are based on diet, and thus, the perspective of obesity that we follow in this chapter considers the state of being obese as a function of nutrition/calorie intake and levels of physical activity.

AN ECONOMIC FRAMEWORK FOR PUBLIC HEALTH AND ROLE OF NUTRITION

In this section we apply the concepts of economics in considering health and nutrition. In general, health is defined a state of physical, mental, and social well-being and the absence of disease or other abnormal condition; however, to an economist health can also be considered to be a durable good and a type of capital that can be invested to yield return. As a durable good, we consume health, we receive satisfaction by utilizing healthy days, and our health provides a service. For example, our ability to go to work or enjoy a day off is a service provided by health. We therefore have an intrinsic motivation to stay healthy so that we have abundance of health as a durable good.

Now let's switch to discussing health as an investment good, that is, public health. Every individual during conception receives the genetic coding for their "health stock." Over time, health inputs such as maternal healthcare, maternal diet, diet after birth, infant healthcare, childhood development, and access to healthy lifestyle options such as sleep conditions provide the impetus for health investment. Adolescent health choices are similarly important and future lifestyle choices determine the health stock over time, and the combination of these inputs also entails an optimal point and rate of decline. That is, as we invest in health at all stages of life, we are increasing the number of healthy days available for communities to use. In health economics, this has been conceptualized in the health investment model (HIM).

In this model, healthcare, diet, exercise, and time spent in other health-generating activities are inputs to produce health and in return be able to consume health as reflected by the number of healthy days. The health stock begins in the womb from maternal nutrition and prenatal care and continues to death where the stock dwindles to zero. Because nutrition and lifestyle choices can increase and lengthen the life span, we invest in health. This health stock is durable and depreciates with age but its value over a course of life can be improved by diligent investment in health. Folland, Goodman, and Stano[12] had earlier emphasized that there is a positive and diminishing relationship between healthy days and health stock. The diminishing rate is a function of the individual's health behavior such as food choice and activities. The return to health of investing in health is diminishing and eventually health stock begins to decline, primarily as a function of age. Most relevant to the context of nutrition and health, the rate of decline and the point of inflection when health begins to deteriorate with time is largely under our control and nutrition plays a key role—as has been explained throughout this book.

It is also important to discuss individual time preference and health. Because we invest in health, that is, we make a current contribution to health for a future gain and expected return, our current choices affect future health. So, our time preferences and view of the value of future benefits matter. In terms of decisions made to invest in health, such as skipping a sweet treat, reduced current satisfaction can result in future benefit at the individual and population levels. In decisions related to investing in health, current consumption does not always lead to current satisfaction. Therefore, for an individual investing in health, it is important to consider future potentially positive health outcomes rather than only current immediate satisfaction. This is depicted in many day-to-day consumption decisions (or investment decisions as conceptualized by this model), for example a donut versus an apple for a snack, steak versus salad for dinner, an hour spent watching television versus an hour at the gym.

ECONOMIC FACTORS ASSOCIATED WITH POOR NUTRITION AND OBESITY

Obesity is among the most complex and complicated public health challenges with a plethora of influencing factors. Various economic factors contribute to the changes in personal and community nutrition patterns, which in turn affect our health outcomes. In this section, we discuss the economic causes and consequences of obesity.

Food prices. To an economist, demand of an item is a function of it's price. The inverse relationship between price and quantity demanded entails that variation in food prices alter consumption pattern and nutritional behavior. In recent decades, we have seen a general surge in food prices.[13] Increases in food prices have a crucial effect on general health status. More visible is the drastic fall in real prices of high-calorie foods relative to healthy nourishing food.[14] Specifically, Christian and Rashad[15] studied the trend in food prices in the United States from 1950 to 2007. They found 34.9% and 17.2% decrease in real prices of a 2-L bottle of soda and a 12-inch pizza, respectively. On the other hand, vegetable and fruit prices increased at a faster rate than inflation.[16] Provided that foods in both healthy and unhealthy categories are normal goods, consumers will likely neglect the nourishing food and shift their consumption toward high-calorie energy-dense foods because they are relatively cheaper. This diversion in choice and demand due to relative prices is one factor that leads to excess energy consumption. Again, with absence of constant expenditure of the energy consumed, it may result in weight gain, obesity, and other associated chronic health complications.

Income. Another economic factor that plays an important role in nutrition choices is income. Household income is a key determinant of purchasing power. The continuous rise in real prices of healthy food relative to real income has made food cost a key barrier for many low-income households.[13] The U.S. Bureau of Labor Statistics revealed that real average hourly earnings decreased by 3.0% between July 2021 and July 2022.[16] To understand the effect of changes in income on food demand we treat foods in all categories as normal goods. In this case, decrease in real income leads to a decrease in consumption of normal goods. A rational consumer will seek a low-cost food option among the options available to maximize utility and this may lead to higher consumption of unhealthy high-calorie food as they tend to be relatively cheaper than the healthy food option.[17]

Food insecurity. The access to healthy food plays a key role in the health and well-being of individuals. The problem of food insecurity has created disparity in access to nutritious foods. In 2017, WHO identified access to healthy food as a fundamental human right.[18] However, this right has been threatened by food insecurity across the world, including developed economies. The economic concept of food insecurity is dominated by the lack of available food and the problem of unaffordability. These concepts are tied to financial factors[19] and location.[20] The U.S. Department of Agriculture found that in 2020 about 35.3% of U.S. households with incomes below the Federal poverty line were battling with food insecurity.[21] Variations in food supply, rise in eating out, rise in unhealthy food advertising and fall in healthy food advertising, reduction in healthy eating promotion and education, and food pricing, among others, influence dietary behavior. Similarly, for individuals located in a place where available food options are constrained to fast foods, their nutrition behavior is distorted, and they are forced to live with food insecurity. Such food deserts have disproportionately low food access and often low incomes. Leonard et al.[22] found that location (especially, black resident locations) and presence of poverty highly worsen food insecurity, and a higher proportion of black residents is associated with a higher likelihood of lying within overlapping clusters of food insecurity and poor health, such as obesity. Again, the prohibitively high travel cost to obtain food in neighboring locations worsens the chances of healthy food access/security. Meanwhile, it has been observed that decreasing the driving distance to Fruit and Vegetable (FV) outlets would increase FV consumption in the community.[23] This study found that a 1-mile decrease in the driving distance to FV stores would increase

FV consumption by 8.9%. In some of these localities, the only accessible food is nutrient-poor. Many of these easily accessible foods are ultraprocessed foods that contribute to obesity. Continuous consumption of such unhealthy meals contributes to unhealthy eating habits over time.[24]

ECONOMIC COST OF POOR NUTRITION AND OBESITY

In this section, we focus on the economic costs of poor nutrition and obesity. We dissect the economic costs of poor nutrition and obesity from not just the healthcare perspective but a societal perspective as this perspective considers opportunity costs (i.e., alternative uses of scarce resources) as well as costs across sectors to include welfare of a society in general and not just a limited view of maximizing benefit for one sector. Specifically, this section discusses the global perspective on poor nutrition and obesity, costs to the healthcare system, and costs due to loss in human capital, followed by economic cost of poor nutrition and obesity at different life stages.

Malnutrition or Obesity: Global Perspective on Cost of Poor Nutrition and Obesity

The World Bank[25] noted that poor nutrition is among "the world's most serious but least-addressed" problems, with its largest impacts on the poor masses, children, and women across various ages. Evidence shows that countries are struggling with and trying to address either one of the nutrition-related crises: malnutrition or obesity. Transition economies that have seen massive economic growth in the recent decade, such as India and China, are facing a double-edged sword. For example, although the prevalence of obesity in China is close to 7%, compared to a global prevalence of 13%, the rate of increase in China is among the highest, with a 20-year increase rate of 400%.[26] Vast improvements in economic conditions have led to an increase in obesity. Moreover, worldwide public health is tackling high rates of chronic noncommunicable disease compared to the past of high rates of communicable diseases. More recently, communicable disease such as COVID-19 has rung a loud alarm in that obesity and poor nutrition are associated with worst outcomes from COVID-19 infection. Post-COVID-19, obesity and poor nutrition are recognized to play a role in the outcomes of communicable diseases in addition to chronic diseases.

There are economic consequences of malnutrition and obesity as these adversely affect the nation's human capital and public health. With over 12.5% of the world population suffering with nutrition-related problems, findings show that poor nutrition has a global cost of about $500 per individual per year resulting in over $3.5 trillion annually.[27] According to the study, the direct costs associated with overweight or obesity and malnutrition conditions such as stunting, wasting and micronutrient deficiencies have added extra financial burden, thus exacerbating the cost of excess weight-related chronic diseases. Also, about 45% of preventable deaths among children are attributed to undernutrition, notwithstanding the high cost of health insurance.[26]

Direct and Indirect Costs of Poor Nutrition and Obesity

Obesity involves both direct and indirect costs[28] with some significant influence emerging from obesity-related physical exertion. It has been identified that diet-related behaviors have huge effects on morbidity, mortality, and productivity. For example, about 3.58% indirect cost on gross national product (GNP) in 2000 was due to obesity and obesity-related dietary diseases in China and this is expected to rise to about 8.73% by

2025.[6] Similarly, the direct health costs associated with obesity, especially in the United States include increased utilization of office visits, hospitalizations, nursing home care, treatments, and medications.[29]

A summary of healthcare costs across the Organisation for Economic Co-operation and Development (OECD) countries found that U.S. healthcare is spending twice as much as other high-income countries. The U.S. government in 2018 spent 17.7% of gross domestic product (GDP) on servicing healthcare costs and this has been projected to rise to 19.7% by 2028.[30] This high cost is accompanied by highest rates of chronic disease burden in the United States among all OECD countries[31,32] and the complications of the chronic disease have been attributed to a rise in risky behaviors—11.4% of U.S. population age 15 years and older smoke daily, and 70.1% are either obese or overweight.[32] This is in contrast to the strong downward trend in smoking in the United States along with an upward trend in obesity rates.

Persons with obesity incur 30% more in medical costs than their normal weight peers.[33] The obesity rate is two times higher in the United States than the OECD average.[31] Furthermore, hospitalizations from preventable causes and avoidable deaths are highest in the United States compared to peer OECD countries.[31] Finkelstein et al.[34] estimated that about a $40 billion increase in total medical spending and $7 billion cost of Medicare prescription drugs were associated with obesity. More Americans are killed by heart disease and stroke than any other cause, and these diseases cost the U.S. healthcare system $216 billion per year.[35] Also, among the complications of obesity is Type 2 diabetes. In 2017, the estimated cost of diabetes was $327 billion, which includes $237 billion in direct medical costs and $90 billion in estimated costs for reduced productivity.[36]

The costs and consequences of obesity are also increasing globally. Among some Asian countries, obesity and overweight have acquired epidemic dimensions with a high number of obesity-related disorders such as diabetes, hypertension, and cardiovascular diseases, which develop at a younger age than in Western populations.[37] Economic development and advances in technology globally are associated with obesity. In Africa, the tremendous rise in obesity has been attributed to the adoption of Western lifestyle and lack of proper management.[38] In Ghana, about 19% of children are either obese or overweight.[39] Additionally, the pervasiveness of maternal obesity within the African region has risen to a high 50.7%, with older and multiparous mothers more likely to be obese.[40] The cost of obesity includes labor market costs. Poor nutritional behavior drains the human capital of a nation. In the words of Beaudreault,[41] obesity complications "rob countries of human capital," which is "the foundation of economic development and resilience." Obesity and chronic diseases decrease the opportunity to work and significantly increase job **absenteeism**. Absenteeism and **presenteeism** contribute to high indirect costs.[42] A 2018 study reported that heart disease and stroke cause $147 billion in lost job productivity per year.[35]

Furthermore, in the United States, the majority of the population is covered by private insurance, that is, employer-sponsored insurance. As of 2021, private insurance coverage is being utilized by 53.8% of children and 66.6% of adults ages 18 to 64 years.[43] Employees with obesity tend to incur a greater financial burden for their employer through increased medical bills. Studies have found discrimination in job hiring and pay scale based on weight status.[44,45] Individuals with obesity may not be able to undertake some jobs. Obesity and disability contribute to employment discrimination with disabled people at higher risk of being discriminated against and not securing a job compared with nondisabled persons.[46] Additionally, individuals with obesity cannot undertake some government jobs such as serving in the military due to physical demands required for military service.

Economic Costs Associated With Obesity and Chronic Diseases at Different Life Stages

Obesity and associated chronic diseases create a substantial burden on both developed and developing economies.[46] However, nutrition is an important health investment whose return on investment (ROI) has multiplier implications on all tiers of economic factors —household, firms, government, and the rest of the world.[48]

Early nutrition, the environment in which newborns are raised, and maternal lifestyle during pregnancy are all thought to be important factors in the prevention of childhood obesity.[49] Maternal obesity is among the key contributors to adiposity of infants. Also, both high pregnancy weight gain and gestational diabetes increase the likelihood of excess adiposity in the progeny.[50] In addition, sometimes pregnant women develop eating disorders, such as binge eating, which further contributes to the weight gain of both mother and infant. Infant obesity contributes to difficulties in childbirths and cesarean section complications, and cesarean-section delivery has consequently been associated with early childhood obesity.[51]

The individual economic costs associated with obesity and chronic disease consist of the cost of medication and healthcare spending, job absenteeism, lost income, morbidity, comorbidity, and mortality. Ward et al.[52] used data from Medical Expenditure Panel Survey (MEPS) 2011–2016 to estimate the healthcare expenditure related to Body Mass Index (BMI). The study found that medical expenditure by BMI was higher for females relative to males. Specifically, they discovered that for every individual with observed obesity, each unit of BMI increase was associated with an additional $253 per person and adult obesity was associated with $1,861 excess annual medical cost.

The economic cost of obesity was impactful among children, and severe childhood obesity was found to be associated with an additional $310 cost per child and $1.32 billion in medical spending.[52] Though recent evidence has found expansion of Medicaid and establishment of the Children's Health Insurance Program (CHIP) have increased high rates of coverage and healthcare access for children, especially those in low-income families,[53] it has been found that a $1 increase in the per-child premium is associated with a slight increase in a typical child's monthly probability of increasing coverage from 7.70% to 7.83%.[54] Therefore, increasing healthcare cost and its reflection on insurance premium could impact access and utilization of healthcare services via insurance coverage.

Among young adults, the decline in physical activity, poor nutrition, and an increase in busy work schedules have added to the trend in young adult health decline. Many young adults are battling with strokes, hypertension, and other chronic diseases that were usually attributed to older people.[55,56] Low physical activity and hypertension have been identified as the most important risk factors among young adults, accounting for 59% and 21.1%, respectively, of all strokes among young adults.[57]

Among the older adult population obesity, overweight, and chronic diseases inflict financial burdens. Studies have found up to 13% more lifetime healthcare spending for obese and overweight older adult men with overweight and obesity at age 65 than those with normal weight, and up to 17% more spending for older women.[58] Because most older adults in the United States utilize Medicare, a federal healthcare coverage program, obesity in the United States is not just an individual problem but also a societal problem. And the story is similar with other economies with social health insurance system.

Obesity has also been observed as an important determinant of quality of life and life expectancy. A study by Abdelaal et al.[4] examined the morbidity and comorbidity of obesity and various chronic diseases and revealed that each obese individual has an elevated risk of chronic diseases, such as cardiovascular disease and cancer, thus increasing their mortality risk. Also, the incidence of arthritis, especially, rheumatoid arthritis (RA), is increasing among the older adult population in the United States. RA is among the leading causes of work disability among the older adult population with about 58.5 million older adults suffering some form of chronic arthritis, resulting in $303.5 billion in medical costs and lost earnings in 2013.[59] RA has been identified to worsen the complication of various chronic diseases like cancer[60] and cardiovascular disease.[61] The impediments arising from RA increases the risk of mortality by 40% to 50% among the older population.[60] Due to these complications, obesity has been regarded by the American Medical Association as not just weight gain but a complex chronic disease with major health implications[62,63]

Obesity and Chronic Disease Prevention Versus Treatment

earlier in this chapter, we cover the economic causes, cost, and consequences of obesity. This section focuses on examining the cost of prevention relative to the cost of treatment of obesity. Many techniques and pharmaceutical drugs are on the market to treat obesity. Among these medications and treatment techniques, there are basically two categories of Food and Drug Administration regulated devices: four intended for weight loss (gastric band, electrical stimulation systems, gastric balloon systems, and gastric emptying systems) and two for weight management (oral removable palatal space-occupying device, ingested transient space-occupying device).[64] In addition, antiobesity drugs such as orlistat (Xenical), lorcaserin (Belviq and Belviq XR), phentermine/topiramate (Qsymia), naltrexone/bupropion (Contrave), and liraglutide (Saxenda) have enabled the potential of achieving clinically significant weight loss.[65] While treatment is available, there are unintended consequences of these interventions that have implications for the healthcare system and are individual-centric rather than being population health–centric.

However, treatment of obesity can be cost intensive with some level of risk depending on weight level. The first treatment approach for obesity is behavioral interventions that focus on physical activity, diet, behavior modifications, and pharmacotherapy regimens.[66] If this approach is unsuccessful, surgical procedures (bariatric surgery) may be adopted. The sum of national cost of bariatric surgeries increased from $147 million in 1998 to $1.26 billion in 2004.[67] A 2020 study has shown an increasing trend in the rate of in-patient obesity diagnosis as well as a rise in the number of diagnosed cases receiving bariatric surgery among adult patients age 18 or older.[66]

Meanwhile, preventive measures have no risk exposure, but are mainly a function of behavior, lifestyle, and dietary patterns. Applying precautionary actions such as approaching nutrition as a health investment and applying all necessary measures needed to obtain a positive ROI is a very important preventive technique with zero risk. Prevention costs less, and the benefit outweighs the cost, yielding a positive ROI.[68]

It is important to add that the results of most surgical procedures are dependent on age, weight prior to surgery, the exact surgical procedure and expertise of the medical personnel, and dietary pattern and physical activities after surgery.[69] This implies that the success rate of surgical treatment is dependent on the implementation of preventive techniques such as an active lifestyle and healthful diet, following surgery.

EXISTING PROGRAMS AND POLICIES TO ADDRESS OBESITY

In this section, we outline the ROI of investing in health early in life. We then outline examples of programs in place at the federal level to address obesity. It is important to note that many programs and policies are also available at the state level.

As noted earlier, obesity is a complex chronic disease involving high healthcare, societal, and other economic costs. However, continuous investment in solving this health problem will yield a positive ROI. For instance, there is a $16 ROI for every $1 invested in children's nutrition.[41] Also, another necessary investment is implementation of preventive measures. A 3-year randomized, controlled study by Cao et al.[70] found that there are significant and reliable long-term effects from preventing childhood obesity, particularly among girls. Investing in techniques that can prevent the health challenges that obesity brings has been associated with substantial economic gains due to improved health and productivity.[68]

Meanwhile, investing in early life nutrition and applying preventive measures requires a collective effort both as a group and individually. This starts with healthy nutrition habits in childhood and continues with an active lifestyle in adulthood. Some government policies have been introduced to encourage and facilitate healthy nutritional investment both for children and adults. We discuss some of these policies next.

Supplemental Nutrition Assistance Program and Supplemental Nutrition Assistance Program Education

This program began post World War II as a food assistance program in an effort to support the country's agriculture sector and enhance nutrition among low-income households.[71] The electronic benefit transfer (EBT) cards that eligible households now receive each month allow them to make purchases at participating supermarkets and grocery stores. Unfortunately, the Supplemental Nutrition Assistance Program (SNAP) participants face challenges to meet the dietary guidelines despite the programs' effectiveness on reducing food insecurity.[72] Since the affordable food that was available was not necessarily nutritious for eligible low-income families in the SNAP and did not improve their health as planned, in 2008 the program was remodeled with its present focus to encourage health nutrition.[73]

In 2020, the Pandemic EBT (P-EBT), which is very similar to SNAP benefits, was introduced by the U.S. government in response to the COVID-19 pandemic to assist children who would have received free or reduced-price school meals, if not for COVID-related school closures and/or COVID-related reductions in school hours or attendance.[21]

In the United States, a related and key effort is the Supplemental Nutrition Assistance Program Education (SNAP-Ed). The goal of the program is to encourage and foster good nutrition, living physically active lifestyles, and engaging partners to build healthier communities. This is among the biggest and most diverse nutrition programs with hundreds of implementation partner agencies reaching millions of Americans. In assessing the effectiveness of this nutritional intervention program, Molitor et al.[74] examined the external validity of SNAP–Ed interventions as implemented by various organizations with diverse populations in California for various age groups. They found a positive impact on adults, teenagers, and children within the intervention areas. They observed an increase in vegetable and fruit consumption as well as an increase in active lifestyle for those in intervention areas. However, there were variations in impact level; some localities were barely reached. The success of SNAP-Ed has been constrained by limited numbers of sites, educator readiness, and capacity in some regions; communication breakdowns; and prioritization of nutrition education over policy, systems, and environmental (PSE) change strategies.[75]

National School Lunch Program

Another nutrition program in the United States is the school lunch program. The aim is to provide children with quality healthy food during their lunch. The success of this program will help to reduce childhood obesity and chronic diseases caused by lack of nutrition among children. An experimental study on this program revealed that despite substantial food waste by children and servings with significantly high levels of fruits and fiber, the program is cost-effective.[76] In addition to the school lunch program, the smart snack was introduced in 2014 to reduce unhealthy snacking among students. However, within the first year of the program it was discovered that 87% of high school students nationwide still had access to sugar-sweetened beverages through snack venues.[77]

In China, the cost and cost-effectiveness of a comprehensive intervention program for childhood obesity was evaluated using a randomized controlled trial in six Chinese cities.[78] The experiment assessed the outcome of nutrition education, physical activity (PA), and a combination of both and found that school-based integrated obesity intervention programs were cost-effective for children in urban China.[79]

Worksite Wellness Program

The Centers for Disease Control and Prevention's (CDC) workplace health program is targeted to creating a healthier working-class American. Most Americans who work full-time jobs spend more than a third of their day at work, 5 days a week. Effective workplace regulations and programs can lower health hazards and raise the standard of living for American employees. This initiative focuses on creating healthy environments in companies, schools, early learning centers, and the neighborhood. It also emphasizes collaborating with communities and health systems to lessen the effects of various chronic diseases like diabetes, heart disease, and stroke. Making healthy living simpler for all Americans is the aim.[80] The program has been embraced by different corporate entities. Some companies now have gyms at their workplace while others provide external gym cards for their employees. Worksite wellness programs have contributed to an 8.3% increase in employees' participation in regular exercise and an additional 13.6% higher likelihood of employees maintaining their weight.[81]

Patient Protection and Affordable Care Act and Obesity

One recent change in addressing the obesity epidemic is through Medicaid expansion associated with the Affordable Care Act (ACA). Medicaid expansion has helped to increase access to healthcare to millions of Americans. With the constant rising cost of medical treatment, many low-income households are constrained by what they can spend on healthcare. Also, people who have underlying health conditions like obesity and chronic diseases can now more easily get proper healthcare.[81] Again, the ACA eradicated 44% of the healthcare coverage gap across income groups, with the Medicaid expansion accounting for the total decline.[54]

In practice, there are other nonfederal policies and practices that have been evaluated. One such approach is the taxation of sugar-sweetened beverages to regulate high sugar intake while increasing tax revenues that could in turn be invested to promote healthy eating and physical activity. Sometimes called "soda taxes," this approach has significantly increased the prices of sweetened beverages and is associated with a decline in sales volume due to a fall in demand.[82] Soda taxation can be an effective policy tool for reducing the purchase of sweetened drinks. A similar soda tax was also passed in France in 2012 and after 6 months of implementation, the tax burden was entirely shifted to the final consumer in the form of an increase in price.[83] This tax burden has the effect of deterring consumers from the consumption of these products per the **law of demand on normal goods**.

BEHAVIORAL ECONOMICS BASED INTERVENTION

In this section, we focus on the "why" behind food choices. Economics is a study of human behavior. Economists often assume humans are rational decision-makers; that is, we are able to consistently weigh costs and benefits of each possible action or decision. In practice, this assumption is unrealistic and ignores the behavior studied by cognitive and social psychologists. To a psychologist, decisions are based on emotions and habits. Day-to-day decisions—both healthy and unhealthy choices, including food choices— are a product of our thought system. The marriage of economics and psychology is the field of **behavioral economics**. According to Rice[84] enumerated behavioral economics accepts that people frequently act irrationally from an economic standpoint. For example, some bad choices like unhealthy eating, overeating, and other risky behaviors have posed more danger to human health. Orthodox economics does not offer adequate insights into human behaviors. Consequently, behavioral economics provides a potentially richer range of tools than previous methods by using economic theory and psychology methods to understand behavior.

Food choices are a result of both economic factors, such as price and supply, and psychological factors, such as habit and emotional triggers. Hence, one of the very important and positive means of influencing healthy consumption is by infusing behavioral change and providing nudges toward healthy food choices. Nudging is a systematic process of influencing choices through provision of triggers that alter a behavioral response. Low-cost nudges are expected to trigger changes in behavior. These efforts are expected to focus on enhancing health, wealth, and happiness decisions.[85] This behavioral economic strategy helps to alter human decisions with the aim of improving health and economic well-being.

Individuals, irrespective of age, may have aligned with the taste of certain unhealthy foods such that the taste of healthy food is not appetizing. For example, nutritious foods, like fruits and vegetables, are regularly not preferred by children and frequently not eaten even when served.[86] Also, some rural communities in the United States have been identified to consume fewer amounts of fruits and vegetables than those in the urban area.[23] It has been found that it is possible to increase choices for healthy food by changing food behavior through nudging.[86]

Making small changes in the decision setting, also referred to as choice architecture interventions, has been found to promote behavioral change toward healthy eating.[87] For example, choice architecture changes in the school lunchrooms were found to be effective in improving food choices. Different studies have examined the role of nudging and various nudging techniques in influencing children's consumption choices.[23,78,87,88] While studying how to make healthier food more convenient for consumption, Hanks et al.[88] prepared a lunch line that portrayed healthier food to look more convenient and this increased the sales of healthier foods by 18% with consumption of nutritious food increasing from 33% to 36%. Also, Thapa and Lyford[89] incentivized vegetable and fruit consumption in the school lunch program by using stickers of images that are appealing and friendly and gifts of toys; this inexpensive strategic process increased the number of servings of fruit and vegetables consumed from 1.77 at baseline to 6.08 at end of intervention. In another experimental study by Miller et al.,[90] the investigators examined the effects of preordering and nudging on school lunch item selection for students in Florida. The study found that nudging significantly increased orders for fruit by 51.4%, vegetables by 29.7%, and low-fat milk by 37.3%.[90] Generally, various experimental studies have demonstrated a strong significant effect of behavioral intervention programs on consumption decisions.

WHAT WORKS: THE MIDDLE FORK GREENWAY

A growing body of research indicates that the *built environments* in which people live have substantial impacts on population health.[91-94] Built environments are the human-made infrastructure, surroundings, and buildings that make up the neighborhoods and localities in which people live their lives. The built environment is considered an important social determinant of health (SDOH). Some neighborhoods are impacted by adverse SDOHs such as increased rates of violent crime, impaired ability to access community resources due to transportation and/or safety concerns, and a lack of safe and accessible amenities, such as parks and sidewalks, to promote physical activity.[93] It follows that community efforts to provide safe opportunities for physical activity such as walking and biking can have positive effects on population health including obesity rates.

The Blue Ridge Conservancy is a private, nonprofit organization chartered in North Carolina that is focused on protecting and preserving lands in the beautiful Blue Ridge Mountain region of northwest North Carolina.[95] Since 1995, the Conservancy has protected over 23,000 acres including farmland and other areas of ecological, cultural, recreational, and scenic interest.

One of the Blue Ridge Conservancy's current projects is the Middle Fork Greenway (MFG).[96] The MFG will eventually join two northwest North Carolina communities, the towns of Boone and Blowing Rock, and will be about 6.5 miles in length. At this writing, 1.75 miles are completed and in use by the public, and another 2.3 miles are under construction. The MFG is a recreational trail serving its surrounding communities, and is designed for accessible, flexible usage including walking, jogging, hiking, and biking, with no motorized vehicles other than wheelchairs allowed. Along the trail, visitors will be able to enjoy beautiful natural vistas of the Blue Ridge, three small parks, and a variety of recreational destinations.

Development of the MFG has been underway since it was first envisioned in the late 1990s. At that time, some older adult residents recalled times when walking was the main mode of transportation among the surrounding communities, and expressed a desire to revitalize this aspect of Appalachian culture. In 2000, the Middle Fork Greenway Trail Association was incorporated under North Carolina law. In subsequent decades, and especially since 2013, development of the trail has involved extensive long-term planning and forward progress through collaborations with state, regional, and local jurisdictional entities and private partnerships. Many private businesses and local supporters have participated in the project.[96]

In 2017, an economic impact report on the project used the World Health Organization's Health Economic Assessment Tool (HEAT) to assess the potential benefits of walking and cycling.[97] In 2017 dollars, it was estimated that the combined benefit of reduced health risks to regular trail users would be about $10 million over 10 years of increased life expectancy.[98] Tourist visits to the completed trail are expected to generate about $6 million annually for the local economy. Because a healthy local economy is associated with improved public health in general, the MFG's overall health impact could be substantially greater than direct estimations of benefits. Endeavors such as the MFG require substantial investments in relationship-building, planning, logistics, and funding, but can have large and long-term impacts on populations' physical and economic quality of life in a particular region.

SUMMARY

The economics of nutrition over the life cycle is the focus of this chapter. The chapter summarizes the key theories in the area, covers the economic cost of obesity, and then goes over efforts primarily in the United States to improve nutrition, reduce the obesity epidemic, and develop effective solutions in terms of improving eating behaviors. Addressing the obesity epidemic is one of the essential challenges to the public health of society, and it is not clear that we have found the solution to this problem. As healthcare workers, nutritionists, and other professional readers, we have the challenge and opportunity to look for, test, and develop solutions.

KEY CHAPTER CONCEPTS

- Economic cost is the financial and opportunity cost of public health and health choices.
- Health is an investment good, or stock, and the value of that stock is influenced by health investment choices, such as medical care, nutrition, and exercise.
- Time preference concerns delayed gratification for some future benefit. For an individual investing in health, it is important to consider future potentially positive health outcomes rather than only current immediate satisfaction.
- Economic costs of obesity and poor nutrition are increasing globally.
- Societal efforts to improve nutrition include several government programs as well as the work of many nongovernmental groups.
- Behavioral economics can be used as an approach to modify behavior by using economic theory and psychology methods to understand behavior in regard to nutrition choices.

CASE STUDY

It is likely, as a member of the workforce in a public health-related profession, you will be asked to provide your expert advice, develop ideas, and implement targeted strategies. As the obesity epidemic has grown, many businesses in food, health, government, and other areas have worked on methods to do their part in seeking to address it. It would make sense that supermarkets and other food providers would play a key role in improving health. Let's consider the statement provided by the Kroger Company (a retail company that operates across the United States) relative to their efforts in this areas (bolding added by the authors):

> As America's leading grocer, The Kroger Co. understands the **importance** of **simplifying** complex nutrition science to equip shoppers to make **informed** grocery choices. To accomplish this, nutrition education must be affordable, easy to access, and widely available. Kroger Health, the healthcare arm of Kroger, aims to help shoppers **see the grocery store as a healthcare destination** by providing practical and **personalized nutrition education**. Kroger Health values registered dietitians as the foremost experts in nutrition, which is why Kroger has provided retail registered dietitian services through multiple modalities since 2016. Kroger Health's registered dietitians are specially trained to bridge the gap between healthcare guidance and the foods and beverages people choose at the grocery store. From in-aisle personalized nutrition care to nationwide virtual appointments via two-way video chat, Kroger Health registered dietitians balance a variety of factors to deliver **personalized care, including health conditions, food budget, household food**

preferences, culinary abilities, and access to transportation. Kroger Health's registered dietitians bring their clinical, food, and grocery expertise to shoppers to provide personalized, practical guidance in a non-judgmental way. – Kroger Company

It is likely that your supermarket has a similar program to Kroger or that you shop at Kroger.

Case Study Questions

1. Were you aware that these public health and nutrition resources were available to you? If so, have you used them?
2. How can the grocery store serve as a healthcare destination?
3. Now, imagine that you have started a role at Kroger to help customers live healthier and you wish to address the following questions:
    a. What nutrition programs does the U.S. government have that you could recommend for low-income customers to utilize?
    b. How can you improve the number of people using the provided nutrition education and counseling?
    c. What principles of behavioral economics could you use to help improve how customers are being successful in this program?

DISCUSSION QUESTIONS

1. What economic theory do you think best describes why the obesity epidemic is happening?
2. Do you think the current efforts in the United States will be successful in reducing the obesity epidemic? Why or why not?
3. What are the overall costs and consequences of the obesity epidemic? Do you see these impacts growing over time if they are not addressed?
4. What are the key efforts that are being done that you think are having the greatest impact on improving nutrition across the life cycle?

SUGGESTED LEARNING ACTIVITIES

1. Consider a public health organization you might like to work for or your current workplace; using a web search, identify the behavioral or nutrition health statement of this organization. Write a one-page essay comparing their statement with Kroger's statement in the case study.
2. Break the class into small groups of three or four students. Have each group develop an action plan for applying the principles of nudging and behavioral economics.
3. Consider the U.S. policies toward public health nutrition education. Write an essay making recommendations for improving this system.

RESOURCES FOR FURTHER LEARNING

- Centers for Disease Control and Prevention Division of Nutrition, Physical Activity, and Obesity Policy Resources: www.cdc.gov/nccdphp/dnpao/division-information/policy/index.htm
  - Resources for those engaging in health policy and advocacy, including information on health surveillance tools, nutrition and physical activity resources, breastfeeding resources, and more
- The Expanded Food and Nutrition Education Program (EFNEP): www.nifa.usda.gov/grants/programs/capacity-grants/efnep/expanded-food-nutrition-education-program
  - A federal extension program, EFNEP is the first nutrition education program in the United States for populations with low income; it provides nutrition education and hands-on cooking instruction to adults and youth to teach food management skills and ameliorate nutrition insecurity.
- The State of Childhood Obesity: https://stateofchildhoodobesity.org
  - A project of the Robert Woods Johnson Foundation, the State of Childhood Obesity collects, synthesizes, and analyzes childhood obesity data in the United States, and makes recommendations on policy to address childhood obesity issues.
- The State of Childhood Obesity: Explore Data by States: https://stateofchildhoodobesity.org/state-policy
  - An interactive map of the United States that provides quick access to individual state data on childhood obesity.
- The U.S. Department of Agriculture Economic Research Service (USDA ERS): www.ers.usda.gov
  - A service of the USDA, the ERS provides data, information, and research results on agriculture and economics in the United States; provides many nutrition resources including information on food safety, food assistance, food markets in the United States, and food and health.

SPRINGER PUBLISHING CONNECT™ | **A robust set of instructor resources designed to supplement this text is located at http://connect.springerpub.com/content/book/978-0-8261-8623-2. Qualifying instructors may request access by emailing textbook@springerpub.com.**

REFERENCES

1. World Health Organization. Constitution. Accessed September 20, 2023. https://www.who.int/about/governance/constitution
2. Flegal KM, Graubard BI, Williamson DF, Gail MH. Excess deaths associated with underweight, overweight and obesity. *JAMA*. 2005;293(15):1861–1867. https://doi.org/10.1001/jama.293.15.1861
3. Preston SH, Vierboom Y, Stokes A. The role of obesity in exceptionally slow US mortality improvement. *Proc Natl Acad Sci U S A*. 2018;115(5):957–961. https://doi.org/10.1073/pnas.1716802115
4. Abdelaal M, le Roux CW, Docherty NG. Morbidity and mortality associated with obesity. *Ann Transl Med*. 2017;5(7):161. https://doi.org/10.21037/atm.2017.03.107
5. Ding D, Lawson KD, Kolbe-Alexander TL, et al. The economic burden of physical inactivity: a global analysis of major non-communicable diseases. *Lancet*. 2016;388(10051):1311–1324. https://doi.org/10.1016/S0140-6736(16)30383-X

6. Popkin BM, Kim S, Rusev ER, Du S, Zizza C. Measuring the full economic costs of diet, physical activity and obesity-related chronic diseases. *Obes Rev*. 2006;7(3):271–293. https://doi.org/10.1111/j.1467-789X.2006.00230.x
7. Hill JO, Wyatt HR, Peters JC. The importance of energy balance. *Eur Endocrinol*. 2013;9(2):111–115. https://doi.org/10.17925/EE.2013.09.02.111
8. Hall KD, Farooqi IS, Friedman JM, et al. The energy balance model of obesity: beyond calories in, calories out. *Am J Clin Nutr*. 2022;115(5):1243–1254. https://doi.org/10.1093/ajcn/nqac031
9. Osilla EV, Safadi AO, Sharma S. Calories. In: *StatPearls*. StatPearls Publishing; 2021. https://www.ncbi.nlm.nih.gov/books/NBK499909
10. Douglas CC, Lawrence JC, Bush NC, Oster RA, Gower BA, Darnell BE. Ability of the Harris Benedict formula to predict energy requirements differs with weight history and ethnicity. *Nutr Res*. 2007;27(4):194–199. https://doi.org/10.1016/j.nutres.2007.01.016
11. Ludwig DS, Aronne LJ, Astrup A, et al. The carbohydrate-insulin model: a physiological perspective on the obesity pandemic. *Am J Clin Nutr*. 2021;114(6):1873–1885. https://doi.org/10.1093/ajcn/nqab270
12. Folland S, Goodman A, Stano M. *The Economics of Health and Health Care*. Pearson Education; 2013.
13. Lo Y-T, Chang Y-H, Lee M-S, Wahlqvist ML. Health and nutrition economics: diet costs are associated with diet quality. *Asia Pac J Clin Nutr*. 2009;18:598–604.
14. Cawley J. An economy of scales: A selective review of obesity's economic. *J Health Econ*. 2015;43:244–268. https://doi.org/10.1016/j.jhealeco.2015.03.001
15. Christian T, Rashad I. Trends in U.S. food prices, 1950–2007. *Econ Hum Biol*. 2009;7(1):113–120. https://doi.org/10.1016/j.ehb.2008.10.002
16. U.S. Bureau of Labor Statistics. Real earnings summary. Economic News Release. September 13, 2023. https://www.bls.gov/news.release/realer.nr0.htm
17. Levy A. *A Theoretical Analysis of Rational Diet of Healthy and Junk Foods*. Department of Economics, University of Wollongong; 2007. https://ro.uow.edu.au/cgi/viewcontent.cgi?article=1167&context=commwkpapers
18. World Health Organization. Health is a fundamental human right. World Health Organization. December 10, 2017. https://www.who.int/news-room/commentaries/detail/health-is-a-fundamental-human-right
19. Gaines A, Robb CA, Knol LL, Sickler S. Examining the role of financial factors, resources and skills in predicting food security status among college students. *Int J Consum Stud*. 2014;38(4):374–384. https://doi.org/10.1111/ijcs.12110
20. Ejaz REA, Azid T, Toseef MU. Determinants of food security in rural areas of Pakistan. *Int J Soc Econ*. 2012;39(12):951–964. https://doi.org/10.1108/03068291211269082
21. U.S. Department of Agriculture Economic Research Service. Food security and nutrition assistance. Updated July 19, 2023.
22. Leonard T, Hughes AE, Donegan C, Santillan A, Pruitt SL. Overlapping geographic clusters of food security and health: where do social determinants and health outcomes converge in the U.S? *SSM Popul Health*. 2018;5:160–170. https://doi.org/10.1016/j.ssmph.2018.06.006
23. Katapodis ND, Zhang D, Giabbanelli PJ, Li Y, Lyford CP, Rajbhandari-Thapa J. Evaluating the impact of improving access on consumption of fruits and vegetables in a rural community in Texas: a modeling study. *Health Equity*. 2019;3(1):382–389. https://doi.org/10.1089/heq.2018.0090
24. Naughton P, McCarthy M, McCarthy S. Acting to self-regulate unhealthy eating habits. An investigation into the effects of habit, hedonic hunger and self-regulation on sugar consumption from confectionery foods. *Food Qual Preference*. 2015;46:173–183. https://doi.org/10.1016/j.foodqual.2015.08.001
25. World Bank. The World Bank and nutrition: overview. Updated June 29, 2023. https://www.worldbank.org/en/topic/nutrition/overview
26. Asia Pacific Cohort Studies Collaboration. The burden of overweight and obesity in the Asia-Pacific region. *Obes Rev*. 2007;8(3):191–196. https://doi.org/10.1111/j.1467-789X.2006.00292.x
27. Food and Agriculture Organization of the United Nations. *The State of Food and Agriculture: Food Systems for Better Nutrition*. Food and Agriculture Organization of the United Nations; 2013. https://www.fao.org/3/i3300e/i3300e.pdf
28. Shi J, Wang Y, Cheng W, Shao H, Shi L. Direct health care costs associated with obesity in Chinese population in 2011. *J Diabetes Complications*. 2017;31(3):523–528. https://doi.org/10.1016/j.jdiacomp.2016.11.007

29. Colditz GA, Stein C. Costs of obesity. In: Kumanyika S, Brownson R, eds. *Handbook of Obesity Prevention: A Resource for Health Professionals*. Springer; 2007:73–84.
30. Centers for Medicare & Medicaid Services. National health expenditure data. Accessed October 19, 2022. https://www.cms.gov/Research-Statistics-Data-and-Systems/Statistics-Trends-and-Reports/NationalHealthExpendData/NHE-Fact-Sheet
31. Tikkanen R, Abrams M. *U.S. Health Care from a Global Perspective, 2019: Higher Spending, Worse Outcomes?* Commonwealth Fund; 2020. https://doi.org/10.26099/7avy-fc29
32. Papanicolas I, Woskie L, Jha A. Health care spending in the United States and other high-income countries. *JAMA*. 2018;319(10):1024-1039. https://doi.org/10.1001/jama.2018.1150
33. Withrow D, Alter DA. The economic burden of obesity worldwide: a systematic review of the direct costs of obesity. *Obes Rev*. 2011;12(2):131–141. https://doi.org/10.1111/j.1467-789X.2009.00712.x
34. Finkelstein E, Trogdon J, Cohen J, Dietz W. Annual medical spending attributable to obesity: payer- and service-specific estimates. *Health Aff*. 2009;28(5):822–831. https://doi.org/10.1377/hlthaff.28.5.w822
35. Benjamin EJ, Virani SS, Callaway CW, et al. Heart disease and stroke statistics-2018 update: a report from the American Heart Association. *Circulation*. 2018;137(12):e67–e492. https://doi.org/10.1161/CIR.0000000000000558
36. American Diabetes Association. Economic costs of diabetes in the U.S. in 2017. *Diabetes Care*. 2018; 41(5):917–928. https://doi.org/10.2337/dci18-0007
37. Ramachandran A, Snehalatha C. Rising burden of obesity in Asia. *J Obes*. 2010;2010:1–8. https://doi.org/10.1155/2010/868573
38. Azeez TA. Obesity in Africa: the challenges of a rising epidemic in the midst of dwindling resources. *Obes Med*. 2022;31(1):100397. https://doi.org/10.1016/j.obmed.2022.100397
39. Akowuah PK, Kobia-Acquah E. Childhood obesity and overweight in Ghana: a systematic review and meta-analysis. *J Nutr Metab*. 2020;2020:1–11. https://doi.org/10.1155/2020/1907416
40. Onubi OJ, Marais D, Aucott L, Okonofua F, Poobalan AS. Maternal obesity in Africa: a systematic review and meta-analysis. *J Public Health*. 2016;38(3):e218–e231. https://doi.org/10.1093/pubmed/fdv138
41. Beaudreault A. Nutrition and prosperity. Center for Strategic and International Studies. March 25, 2019. https://www.csis.org/features/nutrition-prosperity
42. Goettler A, Grosse A, Sonntag D. Productivity loss due to overweight and obesity: a systematic review of indirect costs. *BMJ Open*. 2017;7(10):e014632. https://doi.org/10.1136/bmjopen-2016-014632
43. Centers for Disease Control and Prevention. Health insurance coverage. Accessed October 19, 2022. https://www.cdc.gov/nchs/fastats/health-insurance.htm
44. Kungu K, Melius J, Cannonier C, Wanga V. Obesity, chronic job discrimination and social support. *Manag Res Rev*. 2019;42:586–604. https://doi.org/10.1108/MRR-02-2018-0060
45. Spahlholz J, Baer N, Konig H, Riedel-Heller SG, Luck-Sikorski C. Obesity and discrimination—a systematic review and meta-analysis of observational studies. *Obes Rev*. 2016;17(1):43–55. https://doi.org/10.1111/obr.12343
46. Keramat SA, Alam K, Rana RH, et al. Age and gender differences in the relationship between obesity and disability with self-perceived employment discrimination: results from a retrospective study of an Australian national sample. *SSM Popul Health*. 2021;16:100923. https://doi.org/10.1016/j.ssmph.2021.100923
47. Tremmel M, Gerdtham UG, Nilsson PM, Saha S. Economic burden of obesity: a systematic literature review. *Int J Environ Res Public Health*. 2017;14(4):435. https://doi.org/10.3390/ijerph14040435
48. Global Panel. *The Cost of Malnutrition. Why Policy Action is Urgent*. Global Panel on Agriculture and Food Systems for Nutrition; 2016. https://glopan.org/sites/default/files/pictures/CostOfMalnutrition.pdf
49. Larqué E, Labayen I, Flodmark CE, et al. From conception to infancy—early risk factors for childhood obesity. *Nat Rev Endocrinol*. 2019;15:456–478. https://doi.org/10.1038/s41574-019-0219-1
50. Saravanan P, Diabetes in Pregnancy Working Group, Maternal Medicine Clinical Study Group, Royal College of Obstetricians and Gynaecologists, UK. Gestational diabetes: opportunities for improving maternal and child health. *Lancet Diabetes Endocrinol. 2020* Sep;8(9):793–800. https://doi.org/10.1016/S2213-8587(20)30161-3. Epub 2020 Aug 18. PMID: 32822601.
51. Mueller NT, Zhang M, Hoyo C, Østbye T, Benjamin-Neelon SE. Does cesarean delivery impact infant weight gain and adiposity over the first year of life? *Int J Obes* (Lond). 2019 Aug;43(8):1549–1555.

https://doi.org/10.1038/s41366-018-0239-2. Epub 2018 Oct 22. PMID: 30349009; PMCID :PMC6476694.

52. Ward ZJ, Bleich SN, Long MW, Gortmaker SL. Association of body mass index with health care expenditures in the United States by age and sex. *PloS One*. 2021;16(3):e0247307. https://doi.org/10.1371/journal.pone.0247307
53. Alker JC, Kenney GM, Rosenbaum S. Children's health insurance coverage: progress, problems, and priorities for 2021 and beyond. *Health Aff*. 2020;39(10):1743–1751. https://doi.org/10.1377/hlthaff.2020.00785
54. Courtemanche CJ, Marton J, Ukert BD, Yelowitz A, Zapata D, Fazlul I. The three-year impact of the Affordable Care Act on disparities in insurance coverage. *Health Serv Res*. 2019;54(suppl 1):307–316. https://doi.org/10.1111/1475-6773.13077
55. George MG, Tong X, Bowman BA. Prevalence of cardiovascular risk factors and strokes in younger adults. *JAMA Neurol*. 2017 Jun 1;74(6):695–703. https://doi.org/10.1001/jamaneurol.2017.0020. PMID: 28395017; PMCID: PMC5559660.
56. Smajlović D. Strokes in young adults: epidemiology and prevention. *Vasc Health Risk Manag*. 2015 Feb 24;11:157–64. https://doi.org/10.2147/VHRM.S53203. PMID: 25750539; PMCID: PMC4348138.
57. Aigner A, Grittner U, Rolfs A, Norrving B, Siegerink B, Busch MA. Contribution of established stroke risk factors to the burden of stroke in young adults. *Stroke*. 2017;48:1744–1751. https://doi.org/10.1161/STROKEAHA.117.016599
58. Yang Z, Hall A. The financial burden of overweight and obesity among elderly Americans: the dynamics of weight, longevity, and health care cost. *Health Serv Res*. 2008;43(3):849–868. https://doi.org/10.1111/j.1475-6773.2007.00801.x
59. Centers for Disease Control and Prevention. Nutrition, physical activity, and obesity: data, trends and maps. Accessed October 19, 2022. https://www.cdc.gov/nccdphp/dnpao/data-trends-maps/index.html
60. Nayak P, Luo R, Elting L, Zhao H, Suarez-Almazor ME. Impact of rheumatoid arthritis on the mortality of elderly patients who develop cancer: a population-based study. *Arthritis Care Res*. 2017;69(1):75–83. https://doi.org/10.1002/acr.22997
61. Ajeganova S, Andersson ML, Frostegård J, Hafström I. Disease factors in early rheumatoid arthritis are associated with differential risks for cardiovascular events and mortality depending on age at onset: a 10-year observational cohort study. *J Rheumatol*. 2013;40(12):1958–1966. https://doi.org/10.3899/jrheum.130365
62. Funk LM, Jolles SA, Voils CI. Obesity as a disease: has the AMA resolution had an impact on how physicians view obesity? *Surg Obes Relat Dis*. 2016;12(7):1431–1435. https://doi.org/10.1016/j.soard.2016.05.009
63. Kyle TK, Dhurandhar E, Allison D. Regarding obesity as a disease: evolving policies and their implications. *Endocrinol Metab Clin North Am*. 2016;45(3):511–520. https://doi.org/10.1016/j.ecl.2016.04.004
64. U.S. Food and Drug Administration. Weight-loss and weight-management devices. Updated September 15, 2023. https://www.fda.gov/medical-devices/products-and-medical-procedures/weight-loss-and-weight-management-devices
65. Tak YJ, Lee SY. Long-term efficacy and safety of anti-obesity treatment: where do we stand? *Curr Obes Rep*. 2021 Mar;10(1):14–30. https://doi.org/10.1007/s13679-020-00422-w. Epub 2021 Jan 6. PMID: 33410104; PMCID: PMC7787121.
66. Rajbhandari-Thapa J, Ingels JB, Chung SR, Thapa K, Chen Z, Zhang D. In-patient obesity diagnosis, use of surgical treatment and associated costs by payer type in the United States: analysis of the National Inpatient Sample, 2011 through 2014. *Clin Obes*. 2020;10(5):e12385. https://doi.org/10.1111/cob.12385
67. Zhao Y, Encinosa W. *Bariatric Surgery Utilization and Outcomes in 1998 and 2004. Statistical Brief #23*. Agency for Healthcare Research and Quality; 2007. https://hcup-us.ahrq.gov/reports/statbriefs/sb23.pdf
68. Menon K, de Courten B, Ademi Z, Owen AJ, Liew D, Zomer E. Estimating the benefits of obesity prevention on productivity: an Australian perspective. *Int J Obes*. 2022;46(8):1463–1469. https://doi.org/10.1038/s41366-022-01133-z
69. Mundi MS, Lorentz PA, Swain J, Grothe K, Collazo-Clavell M. Moderate physical activity as predictor of weight loss after bariatric surgery. *Obes Surg*. 2013 Oct;23(10):1645–9. https://doi.org/10.1007/s11695-013-0979-y. PMID: 23636999.

70. Cao Z, Hua J, Zhang D, Thapa JR, Wang S, A cohort study assessing the sustainable long-term effectiveness of a childhood-obesity intervention in China. *International Journal of Epidemiology*. 2019 Feb;48(1):108–115, https://doi.org/10.1093/ije/dyy145
71. U.S. Department of Agriculture Food and Nutrition Service. A short history of SNAP. Accessed November 21, 2023. https://www.fns.usda.gov/snap/short-history-snap
72. Andreyeva T, Tripp A, Schwartz MB. Dietary quality of Americans by Supplemental Nutrition Assistance Program participation status: a systematic review. *Am J Prev Med*. 2015 Oct;49(4):594–604. https://doi.org/10.1016/j.amepre.2015.04.035.
73. U.S. Department of Agriculture Food and Nutrition Service. Supplemental Nutrition Assistance Program (SNAP). Accessed October 19, 2022. https://www.fns.usda.gov/snap/supplemental-nutrition-assistance-program
74. Molitor F, Sugerman S, Yu H, et al. Reach of Supplemental Nutrition Assistance Program–Education (SNAP–Ed) interventions and nutrition and physical activity-related outcomes, California, 2011–2012. *Prev Chronic Dis*. 2015;12:E33. https://doi.org/10.5888/pcd12.140449
75. Pope HC, Draper C, Younginer N, Whitt O, Paget C. Use of decision cases for building SNAP-Ed implementers' capacities to realize policy, systems, and environmental strategies. *J Nutr Educ Behav*. 2020;52(5):512–521. https://doi.org/10.1016/j.jneb.2019.09.020
76. Buscemi J, Clark Withington MH, Loiacono B, et al. A pilot study of a school lunchroom intervention in a predominantly Latinx sample. *Contemp Clin Trials*. 2021;111:106599. https://doi.org/10.1016/j.cct.2021.106599
77. Johnston L, O'Malley PM, Terry-McElrath YM, Colabianchi N. *School Policies and Practices to Improve Health and Prevent Obesity: National Secondary School Survey Results*. Volume 2. Robert Wood Johnson Foundation; 2012. https://eric.ed.gov/?id=ED541170 .
78. Meng L, Xu H, Liu A, et al. The costs and cost-effectiveness of a school-based comprehensive intervention study on childhood obesity in China. *PloS ONE*. 2013;8(10):e77971. https://doi.org/10.1371/journal.pone.0077971
79. Centers for Disease Control and Prevention. CDC Workplace Health Resource Center. https://www.cdc.gov/workplacehealthpromotion/initiatives/resource-center/index.html
80. Song A, Baicker K. Effect of a workplace wellness program on employee health and economic outcomes. *JAMA*. 2019;321(15):1491–1501. https://doi.org/10.1001/jama.2019.3307
81. Rajbhandari-Thapa J, Zhang D, MacLeod KE, Thapa K. Impact of Medicaid expansion on insurance coverage rates among adult populations with low income and by obesity status. *Obesity*. 2020;28(7):1219–1223. https://doi.org/10.1002/oby.22793
82. Roberto CA, Lawman HG, LeVasseur MT, et al. Association of a beverage tax on sugar-sweetened and artificially sweetened beverages with changes in beverage prices and sales at chain retailers in a large urban setting. *JAMA*. 2019;321(18):1799–1810. https://doi.org/10.1001/jama.2019.4249
83. Berardi N, Sevestre P, Tépaut M, Vigneron A. The impact of a 'soda tax' on prices: evidence from French micro data. *Appl Econ*. 2016;48(41):3976–3994. https://doi.org/10.1080/00036846.2016.1150946
84. Rice T. The behavioral economics of health and health care. *Annu Rev Public Health*. 2013;34:431–447. https://doi.org/10.1146/annurev-publhealth-031912-114353. Epub 2013 Jan 7. PMID: 23297657.
85. Vlaev I, King D, Dolan P, Darzi A. The theory and practice of "Nudging": changing health behaviors. *Public Admin Rev*. 2016;76:550–561. https://doi.org/10.1111/puar.12564
86. Thapa JR, Lyford CP. Behavioral economics in the school lunchroom: can it affect food supplier decisions? A systematic review. *Int Food Agribus Manag Rev*. 2014;17:187–208.
87. Mertens S, Herberz M, Hahnel UJJ, Brosch T. The effectiveness of nudging: a meta-analysis of choice architecture interventions across behavioral domains. *Proc Natl Acad Sci U S A*. 2022;119(1):e2107346118. https://doi.org/10.1073/pnas.2107346118
88. Hanks AS, Just DR, Smith LE, Wansink B. Healthy convenience: nudging students toward healthier choices in the lunchroom. *J Public Health*. 2012;34(3):370–376. https://doi.org/10.1093/pubmed/fds003
89. Thapa JR, Lyford CP. Nudges to increase fruits and vegetables consumption: results from a field experiment. *Journal of Child Nutrition & Management*, 2018 Spr;42(1).
90. Miller GF, Gupta S, Kropp JD, Grogan KA, Mathews A. The effects of pre-ordering and behavioral nudges on National School Lunch Program participants' food item selection. *J Econ Psychol*. 2016;55:4–16. https://doi.org/10.1016/j.joep.2016.02.010
91. Kim B, Thomsen MR, Nayga RM Jr, Fang D, Goudie A. Move more, gain less: effect of a recreational trail system on childhood BMI. *Contemp Econ Policy*. 2020;38(2):270–288. https://doi.org/10.1111/coep.12448

92. Active Living Research. *The Power of Trails for Promoting Physical Activity in Communities*. American Trails; 2011. https://www.americantrails.org/resources/the-power-of-trails-for-promoting-physical-activity-in-communities
93. Office of Disease Prevention and Health Promotion. *Healthy People 2030:* neighborhood and built environment. U.S. Department of Health and Human Services. Accessed October 19, 2022. https://health.gov/healthypeople/objectives-and-data/browse-objectives/neighborhood-and-built-environment
94. Howell NA, Booth GL. The weight of place: built environment correlates of obesity and diabetes. *Endocr Rev*. 2022;43(6):966–983. https://doi.org/10.1210/endrev/bnac005
95. Blue Ridge Conservancy. Our mission. Accessed October 19, 2022. https://blueridgeconservancy.org
96. Middle Fork Greenway. What is the Middle Fork Greenway? Accessed October 19, 2022. https://www.middle forkgreenway.org
97. World Health Organization. Health Economic Assessment Tool (HEAT) for w*alking and cycling*. https://www.who.int/tools/heat-for-walking-and-cycling
98. Middle Fork Greenway. Middle Fork new river restoration prioritization plan complete. Accessed October 19, 2022. https://www.middleforkgreenway.org/progress

15

PUBLIC HEALTH NUTRITION THROUGH THE LIFE CYCLE: FUTURE TRENDS

Karen L. Probert

LEARNING OBJECTIVES

At the end of this chapter, students will be able to:

1. Identify the four almost-certain future public health nutrition issues and concerns.
2. Identify factors that help forecast future public health nutrition issues.
3. Describe how one social or societal trend can impact the nutrition status of a community or population.
4. Describe one example of national or state policy and one example of local or organizational policy that reflect current public health nutrition priorities.
5. Identify two issues impacting the current public health nutrition workforce, and four training topics that remain constant over time.

INTRODUCTION

This chapter on future trends should begin with a crystal ball that with a page turn or finger tap would display a list of predictions for the future of public health nutrition. Although it lacks the special effects, this chapter starts with a list of four predictions. The remainder of the chapter explains the list and the implications of the list.

The use of a crystal ball to predict the future is based on the ancient belief that one needs a reflective or translucent object to foresee future possibilities; and, not ironically, reflection is exactly what is covered in the first two sections of the chapter.

Four Predictions

- *Food and nutrition security*. Food and nutrition insecurity will remain a top concern for communities across the globe.

- *Fruits, vegetables, and whole grains.* Eating the recommended intake of fruits, vegetables, and whole grains will remain the public health nutrition holy grail.
- *People.* Equitably addressing differences in social determinants of health (SDOH) to reduce **health disparities** among different population groups will be a goal for many, many years.
- *Communities.* Creating policies, systems, and environments that guarantee every community has access to healthy and sustainable foods will be the constant opportunity for ensuring good nutrition at all life cycle stages.

FUTURE FOOD AND NUTRITION ISSUES AND CONCERNS FOR LIFE CYCLE STAGES: U.S. AND GLOBAL

Perhaps more important than the list of predictions is understanding how the list was developed. An initial response to reading the predictions is to question the choice of items; in other words, to ask, "Why these topics? Why not microbiome, breastfeeding, new weight loss drugs, chronic disease, local foods, endocrine disruptors, omega-3 fatty acid supplementation in pregnancy, or added sugars?" The aforementioned topics are legitimate nutrition issues now and into the future. However, to help professionals think on their own about future issues and concerns or to understand these kinds of lists, it is valuable to understand the reasons why items are selected for such a list. The four key factors to consider when reading this list, and others like it, are:

1. The perspective of the person or entity creating the list
2. Relevant history for the topic
3. Current domestic and world matters
4. Relevant reports about the future

Each of these factors is discussed in greater detail in the following sections.

Perspective

The influence of perspective is probably the most significant for any list created. The four predictions listed earlier are based on the perspective of a public health nutritionist. Imagine the list created by a nutritionist working in the food industry—that perspective would generate different issues and concerns. As noted, a public health nutritionist created the Four Predictions list of future nutrition issues and concerns for life cycle stages. The Academy of Nutrition and Dietetics defines a public health dietitian nutritionist as a professional trained in both nutrition and the core competency areas of public health (including biostatistics, epidemiology, health behavior, health **policy** and management, and environmental science). The professional has advanced didactic and experiential training in public health and nutrition practice, or holds advanced degree(s) in public health nutrition or nutrition science.[1]

Public health nutritionists think about issues and concerns of large segments of the population and among vulnerable populations and marginalized communities, and they prioritize issues that are underlying to or upstream from top health concerns. Through this lens comes food insecurity and low fruit, vegetable, and whole grain consumption—all root causes underlying so many health concerns, and they are issues of concern across every life cycle stage according to the **life course theory**.[2] Predicting that health disparities and SDOH will remain top issues for years comes from a public health perspective that focuses on equity for people and underserved populations. And, finally, because policy, system, and environmental (PSE) changes are systemic solutions with a positive impact on all life cycle stages, the item about creating PSE changes so every community has access to healthy and sustainable foods is on the list of predicted future nutrition issues.

History

When forecasting or thinking about the future, review relevant history and note the constant, ever-present issues. Since 1943, top concerns of public health nutritionists have included nutrition for the vulnerable, hunger, and malnutrition.[3] To address these concerns, in the past 50 years, public health nutrition advocates created the two largest food and nutrition programs now known as the Special Supplemental Nutrition Program for Women, Infants, and Children (WIC) and the Supplemental Nutrition Assistance Program Education (SNAP-Ed). In 1972, WIC started as a pilot program and by the end of 1974 was operating in nearly every state.[4] It is one of the most successful and cost-effective public health nutrition programs in the nation. SNAP-Ed, first available in seven states in 1992 and available in all states by 2004, is the largest domestic public health nutrition program and effective at improving food security.[5] Even with these powerful food and nutrition programs in place, in 2022 a White House Conference on Hunger, Nutrition, and Health was held to highlight and focus the nation on the eternal issue of food insecurity.[6] Because food and nutrition insecurity has been and still is a top concern for the nation, the ongoing need for programs and conferences demonstrates the challenges and complexity of the challenge, which means that food security will continue to be a nutrition issue for many years.

Now reflect on the history of our dietary guidance and dietary intake. Year after year we see the data for every life stage—people do not eat the recommended amount of fruits, vegetables, and whole grains.[7] Americans have not been eating the recommended amount of fruits and vegetables for years, and consumption has essentially not changed in 30 years! Low fruit and vegetable consumption is a worldwide concern; the Food and Agriculture Organization of the United Nations declared 2021 as the International Year of Fruits and Vegetables in order to raise international awareness of the benefits of consuming more fruits and vegetables.[8] Interestingly, several programs and policy changes have shown evidence of increasing fruit and vegetable consumption, such as the Fresh Fruit and Vegetable Program, **produce prescriptions**, and WIC's Cash-Value Voucher/Benefit for fruit and vegetable purchases, but population-wide increases in consumption are still not realized.[9–11] Again, this decades-long gap between recommended intake and actual intake will keep fruit, vegetable, and whole grain consumption on the list of future nutrition issues and concerns for a long time.

World and Domestic Events

Consider domestic and world matters and their impact on the future of food, nutrition, and health. The four issues with global, systemic, and long-lasting impacts that, if not addressed, will worsen the nutrition and health status of communities all over the world are climate change, conflicts, crises (e.g., COVID-19), and racism. These issues are examined more closely in the next section, but all four issues threaten access to healthy food and will exacerbate disparities. In addition to these global matters there are additional considerations unique to the United States including income and wealth inequality, large segments of the population not trusting government or science, and U.S. agriculture policy and practices.

Relevant Reports About the Future

The most relevant report on future nutrition issues and concerns across all life stages is the Biden-Harris National Strategy on Hunger, Nutrition, and Health.[12] This document is a tremendous gift to the field of public health nutrition. The national strategy was produced after several months of input from thousands of people including individuals with lived experience and governmental, public, and private organizations.

The goal of the national strategy is to end hunger and increase healthy eating and physical activity. This plan recognizes the complexity of these issues and calls on our collective and sustained action across every segment of society. Given the title of the document and the 8-year timeline to achieving the goals, some might see the national strategy as merely a political document. However, the content of this document should not be discounted. The national strategy is solid. It lays out a strong plan for the future and given the breadth of input it should be embraced as the best blueprint we have to help Americans achieve **food and nutrition security** and achieve healthy eating and physical activity.[12]

Reviewing reports about the future of public health can also provide guidance to predicting public health nutrition issues and concerns. Given the enormous strain on the public health system from COVID-19, there have been several close inspections and subsequent reports about the needs and future of public health. Here we consider three available reports at the time this chapter was written. One report is prepandemic, and two others were produced after the start of the pandemic. Table 15.1 provides a summary of the three reports.[13–15]

Considering the *Biden-Harris National Strategy on Hunger, Nutrition and Health* and the three reports in Table 15.1 plus many other assessments on the future of public health,

Table 15.1. Three Relevant Reports on the Needs and Future of Public Health

Report	Summary of Recommendations
Public Health 3.0: A Call to Action for Public Health to Meet the Challenges of the 21st Century, September 2017[13]	1. Public health leaders should embrace the role of Chief Health Strategist for their communities—working with all relevant partners so that they can drive initiatives including those that explicitly address *upstream* social determinants of health. Specialized Public Health 3.0 training should be available for the public health workforce and public health students. 2. Public health departments should engage with community stakeholders from both the public and private sectors to form vibrant, structured, cross-sector partnerships designed to develop and guide Public Health 3.0–style initiatives and to foster shared funding, services, governance, and collective action. 3. Public Health Accreditation Board (PHAB) criteria and processes for department accreditation should be enhanced and supported to best foster Public Health 3.0 principles, as we strive to ensure that every person in the United States is served by nationally accredited health departments.

Table 15.1. Three Relevant Reports on the Needs and Future of Public Health (*continued*)

Report	Summary of Recommendations
	4. Timely, reliable, granular-level (i.e., subcounty), and actionable data should be made accessible to communities throughout the country, and clear metrics to document success in public health practice should be developed to guide, focus, and assess the impact of prevention initiatives, including those targeting the social determinants of health and enhancing equity. 5. Funding for public health should be enhanced and substantially modified, and innovative funding models should be explored to expand financial support for Public Health 3.0–style leadership and prevention initiatives. Blending and braiding of funds from multiple sources should be encouraged and allowed, including the recapturing and reinvesting of generated revenue. Funding should be identified to support core infrastructure as well as community-level work to address the social determinants of health.
The Future of Public Health from the Public Health Institute, May 2021[14]	1. Trust communities. 2. Build tomorrow's public health workforce today. 3. Rapidly respond to unexpected needs. 4. Believe in data and listen to communities. 5. Break down silos and build partnerships.
Meeting America's Public Health Challenge from The Commonwealth Fund, 2022[15]	1. The federal government should lead a strong and capable national public health system. 2. Congress should provide stable support matched with expectations for states, localities, tribes, and territories to protect the health of their populations. 3. The healthcare system should work closely with public health agencies in normal times and during emergencies. 4. Public health agencies should work to earn the public's trust.

there are three action words that capture themes across the recommendations: trust, listen, and build. Each of these words has multiple meanings. For example, the action word *trust* is applicable to the fact that public health professionals need to trust communities to identify and implement solutions to public health nutrition concerns. However, trust also applies to the fact that many segments of the United States, particularly those people and communities who have been marginalized, do not trust the government nor people who work for government agencies; and a different segment of the U.S. population does not trust science or experts. In this regard, active, engaged, and reciprocal *listening* to others is crucial to building trust. Similarly, *build* is the action word to apply to a range of ideas about future nutrition issues and concerns such as data systems, partnerships, resilient food systems, workforce capacity, and stable funding.

SOCIAL AND SOCIETAL TRENDS AND THEIR IMPACT ON PUBLIC HEALTH NUTRITION

The definition of social and societal trends varies depending on the source. Some sources do not distinguish between social and societal while others do, and the list of social and/or societal trends and issues has even greater variety depending on the source. Rather than identifying a new list of social and societal trends and assessing their impact on public health nutrition, here we consider the issues relevant to the public health nutrition field that are listed in the previous section under World and Domestic Events plus the three key take-away actions from the reports examining the future of public health. Table 15.2 lists those social and societal issues along with a brief description of their potential impact.[16–24] After considering the information in that table, it should be possible to take other social and societal issues not on this list, such as aging population or unaffordable housing, and have a sense of the potential impact on public health nutrition.

An interesting point about these trends and their effects on public health nutrition is that the trend often highlights or gives emphasis to an issue that was already present but just

Table 15.2. Selected Social and Societal Issues and Potential Impacts on Public Health Nutrition

Social and Societal Issue	Potential Impact
Climate change[16,17]	• Less food available (reduced crop yield and livestock production and decline in fisheries and agroforestry) • Reduced food quality (less diversity in crops that will grow, lower nutrient density, and food safety) • Food prices (volatility and continued increases) Specific example: Climate change has drastically reduced available water from the Colorado River. This river provides water to farmers and people in seven Western states. The reduction in available water has pitted agriculture against people. The climate-induced water shortage has created significant tension among the three highest water users: crops grown for livestock feed, fruit and vegetable crops, and drinking water and electricity for people in Southwest states, including large American cities such as Los Angeles, Las Vegas, and Phoenix.
Conflicts/political violence[18]	• Migration of people resulting in new populations in conflict-free areas needing housing, familiar foods, healthcare, and other basic services • Less food available (less farming, destroyed crops and livestock, and destroyed infrastructure, which disrupts delivery of needed supplies to farms and transportation to storage and distribution centers), and given the global food system, the effects on the food supply by conflicts and political violence go beyond the country directly experiencing the conflict.

Table 15.2. Selected Social and Societal Trends and Potential Impacts on Public Health Nutrition (*continued*)

Social and Societal Trend	Potential Impact
Racism[19]	• Less access to healthy food (lower access to full service grocery stores, saturation of stores with low quality and unhealthy foods, and limited financial means to purchase healthy foods) • Health effects of immense and chronic stress on people and populations
Income and wealth inequality[20]	• More food and nutrition insecurity in the future • Greater call to address social determinants of health (economic stability, healthcare access and quality, education access and quality, neighborhood and built environment, and social and community context)
Lack of trust of the government, experts, and science[21]	• Messaging needs to be tailored to intended recipients. • Messengers should be trusted by the intended recipients. For example, the National Medical Association, a national organization representing African American physicians, or the Office of Minority Health might be more effective messengers to an audience of African Americans.
Trust communities to find and implement solutions and/or listen to those with lived experience[14]	• People with lived experience can provide perspective and insight that is often not available from the commonly used sources by public health professionals. Authentic engagement of people who have lived in the communities with the conditions being addressed can help make sure programs are tailored to the specific needs of the community and increase the likelihood of effectiveness.
Build resilience in the food system[22]	• Given the food supply chain disruptions from COVID-19, many communities started building or accelerating efforts to build a more resilient food system of local foods. Even the U.S. Department of Agriculture now has guidance on how to develop a food system that prioritizes consumers and small and mid-size producers. With a locally based food supply chain, producers can communicate directly with consumers, which allows for a quick adaptation to changing needs. For local food supply chains to remain viable post COVID-19, some regulations will need to permanently change in order to support the local systems.
Build the workforce[23,24]	• Building the workforce is much more than having more public health nutrition positions. It also includes increasing diversity of the workforce, offering competitive salaries, developing clear paths for professional development and advancement, building leadership skills, and making available competency-based training. Investing in the public health nutrition workforce is a key element to having more successful interventions, which results in better health outcomes and improved quality of life for people in communities.

not well known. For example, in 2020 when the COVID-19 pandemic hit the United States, adequate access to food became a foremost topic of mind for many. Although food insecurity had been an issue in the United States for generations, it took the global pandemic to elevate the issue and make it a priority for people who had not, previously, been aware of the need. Another example is the 2022 infant formula shortage. Some public health professionals and market industry experts had long understood the vulnerabilities of the concentrated market for infant formula, in that nearly all infant formula was produced by only three companies. But until a facility that manufactured a very high percentage of infant formula had to stop production, which sparked a nationwide and months-long infant formula shortage, most people knew nothing about the fragility of the infant formula supply chain.[25]

Policy Trends in Public Health Nutrition

In the public health nutrition field, the term *policy* is used frequently and somewhat nonspecifically, so before jumping into a list of public health nutrition policy trends, let's first clarify what public health nutrition policy is. Here, we consider policy as broader than a bill that members of the U.S. Congress are debating. Policy has a vast meaning with several issues to consider including whether the discussion is about national, state, or local government level or an organization; legislation or regulation; authorization bills or appropriation bills; policy documents; or policy action. For example, the word *policy* describes each of the following items:

- A letter to parents with children at an in-home, family child care provider that describes the provider's priority to purchase and serve local, seasonal foods from Black and brown farmers as part of the child care provider's new farm to preschool program
- The federal Fiscal Year 2023 Omnibus Appropriations bill allocating $1.7 trillion for defense and nondefense federal programs signed into law on December 29, 2022. (And just for context and curiosity, here is the funding level for three of the many federal public health nutrition-relevant programs within this bill: WIC funding was $6.7 billion, Title V Maternal and Child Health Block Grant Program was $882.7 million, and CDC's High Obesity Rate Counties program was $16.5 million.[26])
- The State of the State: Annual Mississippi Health Disparities and Inequalities Report in 2015 that, for the first time, publicly reported health disparity data for the state and called people to action[27]
- A private breastfeeding room in an onsite construction trailer that allows new mothers to successfully pump breast milk or feed their baby while at work
- Healthy, Hunger Free Kids Act of 2010. A national bill signed into law December 2010 that authorized funding for federal school meal and child nutrition programs and increased access to healthy food for low-income children. The bill reauthorized child nutrition programs, such as school breakfast and lunch, summer food, Child and Adult Care Food Program, and WIC for 5 years and included $4.5 billion in new funding for these programs. The bill also had several elements that would improve nutrition for children such as giving the U.S. Department of Agriculture (USDA) authority to set new standards for food sold in schools other than school breakfast and lunch; providing resources to increase the nutritional quality of food provided by USDA programs; and mandate a minimum on fruit, vegetable, and whole grain servings.[28]
- New York State Assembly Bill A5107, introduced in March 2023, to impose a tax on sugary drinks and establish a health equity fund with the tax revenue[29]

- The local school wellness policy for Melba School District in Idaho that addresses foods sold at school during the school day, fundraising food sales, food at classroom celebrations, plus several other measures to promote nutrition and physical activity[30]
- November 21, 2022, *Federal Register* notice of proposed revised WIC food packages including a proposed increase in money for families enrolled in WIC to buy fruits and vegetables[31]
- A 2018 maternal and child health nutrition policy brief on supporting breastfeeding in homeless shelters, "Shelters are Home to Breastfeeding Moms and Babies"[32]
- The proclamation by the Board of Curry County Commissioners in New Mexico to designate February 2023 as Heart Awareness Month and encourage all citizens to participate in preventive health screenings[33]
- A document published by Illinois Hospital Association with best practices and innovative strategies to help small and rural hospitals in the state implement sodium reduction strategies in the hospital setting[34]
- Any of the following publications are key public health nutrition policy documents: *Dietary Guidelines for Americans, 2020–2025*; *Healthy People 2030*; The Community Guide; and Biden-Harris Administration National Strategy on Hunger, Nutrition, and Health[12,35–37]

This list could continue and fill a whole book, which is why *policy* is a common word and common practice in public health nutrition. Policy work is fun, it is essential, and it covers action that affects a few children in a family day-care provider's home or the billions of dollars of federal government funding for every single health, food, and nutrition program available to Americans.

Again, key ideas to understand when discussing policy include:

- Whether the policy applies to the national, state, or local government level or to an organization
- Whether the issue is legislation (provides the overarching guidance) or regulation (provides the details on implementation)
- If legislative, whether the legislative bill is authorization (permitting, continuing, and/or changing an agency or program) or appropriation (how much money will be awarded)
- Whether the content is from a document that provides foundational direction to programs, initiatives, or other interventions
- Whether the issue is an action resulting from government or organizations' policy, e.g., a list of healthy vending machine snacks or medically tailored, home-delivered meals

Given the scope of public health nutrition policy, the trends listed below are high-level. Notice how closely the trends align with the four predictions of future public health nutrition issues covered at the start of this chapter. There are also two tips to help the reader predict or track other future policy trends.

- *More government policy*. The momentum continues for federal, state, and local government interest and ability to address nutrition and healthy eating through policy. Government agencies will focus on reducing barriers and creating opportunities to access healthy foods.[12]
- *Food security and nutritional quality*. For years, antihunger advocates and nutrition advocates worked independently from each other and at times in conflict with each other. That is changing and both groups are focused on increasing access to

healthy foods. This trend is even evident in terminology, with a shift from *hunger* (antihunger, end hunger, hunger prevention, etc.) to the phrase *food and nutrition security*. Terminology in this area of public health nutrition is rapidly changing.[38]

- *Food processing, ingredients, packaging, and marketing*. As pressure builds to provide more healthful options, the food industry will respond. Industry can change how food is processed, packaged, marketed, and what ingredients are used in products. As a result there will be ongoing policy attention in these four areas. For example, the nutrition and health field is highly interested in added sugars; one response by industry is to find new alternative sweeteners, which then triggers federal agencies to provide guidance on labeling and safety.
- *Disparities*. Given the social and societal trends described in the previous section plus the growing interest in underlying causes of poor health by politicians and health professionals, policy efforts to reduce disparities and address social determinants of health will increase.
- *Politics*. Although not yet stated, politics is an obvious trend affecting public health nutrition policy. There is a constant push/pull on public health nutrition issues, depending on the political party in charge. The push/pull happens within and across all levels of government—federal, state, and local.

Tips for Predicting and Tracking Policy Trends

Tip: Watch for the national and state policy issues that the food industry supports and challenges, as those issues can be markers of policy matters ahead. Industry tends to prefer policy that puts the responsibility of healthy choice on the individual such as providing education and information to consumers. Groups to watch include the Consumer Brands Association (since 2020, formerly the Grocery Manufacturers Association),[39] Food Marketing Institute,[40] and specific industry trade associations, such as American Egg Board, International Fresh Produce Association, National Cattlemen's Beef Association, and the Peanut Institute.

Tip: Watch the programs and interventions that are being piloted or permitted in federal or state program waivers. Permanent food and nutrition programs always started out as a pilot or existed through a waiver. For example, these programs started out in just a handful of states and are now permanent and available nationwide: WIC, SNAP-Ed, and Fresh Fruit and Vegetable Program. At the time of this publication, two examples of pilot programs are produce prescriptions and **food as medicine**. One specific, federally funded initiative launched in 2023 is $2.5 million in government funding for the Produce Prescription Pilot Program in Native communities.[41] Another example pilot program that could eventually become a permanent benefit of Medicaid and/or Medicare is California's Medi-Cal Medically Tailored Meals Pilot Program, which provides medically tailored meals and medical nutrition therapy to people living with congestive heart failure.[42]

TRAINING AND PREPARATION OF THE PUBLIC HEALTH NUTRITION WORKFORCE

In public health nutrition, some issues seem eternal: workforce training, including populations of students, interns, and practitioners; data surveillance and program evaluation; and advocacy for issues and for the profession. The need for workforce development is heightened by the increased emphasis placed on nutrition interventions by major public health organizations, such as the World Health Organization (WHO), and the need for qualified professionals to implement these initiatives.[23] Serious workforce shortages have been identified, especially in lower-resource countries, although workforce gaps have been identified in higher-resource countries as well.[23,43] This section of the chapter focuses on future trends in training the public health nutrition workforce.

Existing and Emerging Workforce Characteristics

Conditions and environments in which public health nutrition professionals work are always changing. The last 5 years or so have brought enormous societal shifts, just a few of which include the rise of social media, aging populations, and the massive impacts of a global pandemic.

The current situation of the existing public health workforce includes pandemic fatigue, with extreme fatigue among professionals working in governmental public health agencies and healthcare facilities.[44,45] Public health position turnover tends to be high and attrition is substantial, leaving vacancies and subsequent gaps in ability to address issues. Turnover and attrition may be related in part to pandemic burnout, as well as an aging workforce and an increasing number of retirements.[46] Exacerbated by the COVID-19 pandemic, constant crisis management reduces available time to address chronic, underlying nutrition issues, which have major impacts on health, such as populations' inadequate whole grain and fruit and vegetable consumption.

The emerging public health nutrition workforce encompasses members of Generation Z (Gen Z), including those born between 1997 and 2012.[47] Top issues for Gen Z include racial equity and inclusion, and mental health. Many are passionate advocates for social change, and are initiating strong challenges to the norms of previous generations.[48] Members of Gen Z are also financially astute, and the traditionally lower salaries for governmental public health nutrition positions may be a barrier to entering the workforce.[46]

Education and Training Needs

General areas for ongoing education and training needs for public health nutrition professionals include:

- Data accumulation and management, with emphasis on population surveillance and program evaluation
- Training in effective advocacy for both specific nutrition issues and the nutrition profession
- Training in networking to develop effective partnerships and collaborations, and to identify opportunities for professional development and career advancement
- Training in developing effective collaborations among nutrition practitioners and public health nutrition faculty to enhance workforce development

Education and Training Trends

While this text does not provide a comprehensive list of academic programs in public health and public health nutrition, this information is readily available through internet searches. A number of academic programs provide training in public health, public health nutrition, and nutrition and dietetics (for those who wish to obtain a registered dietitian nutritionist credential).

In January 2024, a master's degree will be required to become eligible to sit for the Registration Examination for Registered Dietitian Nutritionists. The impacts of this change, which requires a larger investment of time and money prior to entering the profession, are as yet unknown. In 2021 El-Kour et al. proposed that although the new requirement may be a net positive for the profession, ongoing monitoring is needed to determine the effects on the racial and ethnic diversity of the profession as well as impacts on the number of dietitians entering public health-related positions.[24]

Extensive continuing education and training opportunities are offered by organizations such as the Association of State Public Health Nutritionists (ASPHN; asphn.org), the Academy of Nutrition and Dietetics (AND; www.eatrightpro.org), and the American Public Health Association (APHA; www.apha.org), among many others, and this trend is expected to continue. Public health agencies and programs such as the Supplemental Nutrition Assistance Program (SNAP), the Special Supplemental Nutrition Program for Women, Infants, and Children (WIC), and others in both governmental and nongovernmental settings also provide opportunities for ongoing professional development.[4,5]

Training Guidance for the Future

To stay abreast of current and anticipated workforce training needs, it is recommended that nutrition professionals participate in their professional organizations, such as the APHA, AND, and ASPHN. These organizations offer ongoing continuing education and training opportunities including annual conferences, mentoring programs, leadership opportunities, educational webinars, job listings, practice interest groups, and many other venues for professional growth.

Workforce development may also be guided by standards documents and resources provided by professional organizations. The AND has developed *Revised 2022 Standards of Practice and Standards of Professional Performance for Registered Dietitian Nutritionists (Competent, Proficient, and Expert) in Public Health and Community Nutrition.*[49] These standards can be used for self-evaluation, goal-setting, and a variety of other purposes. The ASPHN provides an extensive array of professional development resources at https://publichealthnutrition.org. Professional organizations typically make these types of resources available to their members.

WHAT WORKS: CDC POLICY PROCESS

This chapter provides numerous examples of effective public health nutrition policies and programs. The Centers for Disease Control and Prevention (CDC) provides the systematic CDC policy process, which may be helpful in guiding the initiation, implementation, management, and evaluation of effective public health policies and programs, including nutrition policy and programming.[50]

At the center of policy development are stakeholders, or those who will be affected and impacted by the policy and who should be engaged in every step of the policy process. The CDC policy process has five steps: (1) identification of a problem at the root cause level; (2) policy analysis, which involves choosing among options; (3) strategy and policy development, which determines how policy goals will be achieved; (4) policy enactment, which addresses any legislative, regulatory, and/or legal requirements prior to (5) policy implementation, or putting the policy into practice.[50] A final essential component of the policy process is program/policy evaluation to determine effectiveness, efficiency, and needs for improvement.[51]

The CDC's Office of Policy, Performance, and Evaluation provides a number of policy/programming professional development resources at www.cdc.gov/policy/polaris/policyprocess/index.html. Figure 15.1 illustrates the CDC policy process.

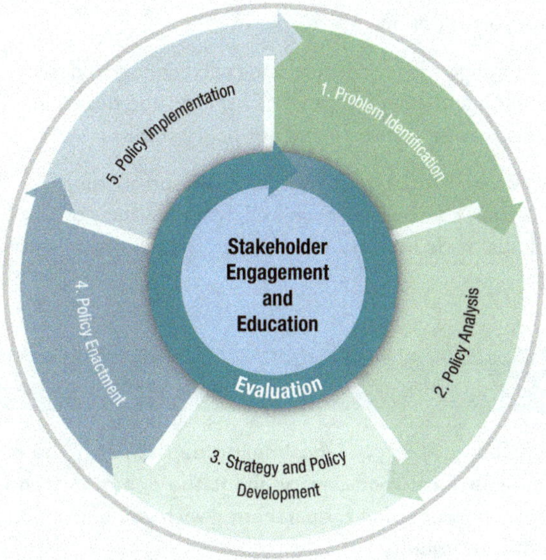

Figure 15.1. The Centers for Disease Control and Prevention (CDC) policy process.

Source: Centers for Disease Control and Prevention. *The CDC policy process.* Office of Policy, Performance, and Evaluation. Accessed June 12, 2023. https://www.cdc.gov/policy/polaris/policyprocess/index.html

SUMMARY

Four key predictions for the future of public health nutrition are (1) an emphasis on food and nutrition security rather than food security only, (2) the promotion of fruits, vegetables, and whole grains as a means of health promotion and chronic disease prevention, (3) equitably addressing SDOH to reduce health disparities, and (4) focusing on the development of policies, systems, and environments to ensure all communities have access to healthy and sustainable food. These trends are based on the perspectives of individuals and groups, the history of nutrition intervention and dietary guidance, world and domestic events, and relevant reports about the future. This chapter reviews a number of social and societal trends impacting future public health nutrition practice and the development of public health nutrition policy. Examples of successful nutrition programs are discussed. Finally, issues affecting the future and development of the public health nutrition workforce are discussed. The future of nutrition and public health is likely to be focused on food systems and policy to promote the accessibility of adequate, nutritious, and health-promoting food for all.

KEY CHAPTER CONCEPTS

1. The four almost-certain future public health nutrition issues and concerns are described in this chapter: food and nutrition security; fruit, vegetable, and whole grain consumption; addressing the social determinants of health that will reduce health disparities; and driving policy, systems, and environmental changes that enhance healthy food access.
2. The factors that help forecast future public health nutrition issues include perspective, history, world and domestic events, and relevant future reports.
3. Societal trends, such as crises, conflict, structural racism, and climate change, can impact the nutrition status of a community or population in multiple ways, and a trend often highlights an issue that was already present but just not well known.

4. Policy has a vast meaning with several issues to consider, including whether the discussion is about national, state, or local government level or an organization.
5. High-level public health nutrition policy trends align with the future issues and concerns described in this chapter by considering government health and nutrition regulations, food and nutrition security, food processing directions, health disparities, and the impact of political shifts.
6. Initiatives to develop the public health nutrition workforce must address issues surrounding burnout and high turnover. Public health nutrition careers may align well with the values of members of Generation Z, and efforts should be made to remove barriers to the education and training needed to pursue these careers.

CASE STUDY

You are working as a public health nutrition professional at your local health department. You have been approached by the executive director of your local food pantry about the common trend in health disparities seen among your shared clients and her vision for partnering with you in developing a solution to increase healthy food access for the community.

Case Study Questions

1. Based on the information presented in this chapter, where might you begin?
2. Who are the stakeholders you would want to involve in such an initiative?
3. What research or data would you need to consider collecting and from who?

Now, review the National Produce Prescription Program and Food Is Medicine Collaborative/Initiatives (links provided under Resources for Further Learning later in this chapter).

4. Which future trend(s) from the chapter do these programs address (food and nutrition security, fruit, vegetable and whole grain consumption, people/social determinants of health, communities/policies), and how?
5. Does one of these program sound like a better fit for your partnership and current resources? Keep in mind at least one of these programs, maybe both, as you answer the following questions.
6. Does this information change any of your preceding answers? What additional information do you need or additional key players might you want to involve now that you've taken a deeper dive into some program models?
   a. How would you identify eligible clients?
   b. How would you source the additional healthy food or make it more accessible for clients?
   c. Would you need to offer nutrition education to supplement the foods offered? What might this look like?
   d. How does your program support the needs of each life cycle stage?
   e. What are the workforce development and training needs to implement this program successfully?
7. What are some policies that would need to be put in place at the organizational, systems, and environmental levels to make this program possible? For example, the food pantry relies on donations, which are commonly shelf-stable, processed foods. How would you obtain more fresh foods, whole grains, and lower sodium options?

8. What are the challenges or barriers you might encounter when implementing this program? Consider at least two challenges or barriers and describe how you would overcome them.

Fast forward to successful implementation of this program in your community.

9. What does success look like for individuals, your community, healthcare system, and organizations?
10. What do you need to think about to sustain this program and keep up with future public health nutrition trends? How might the program evolve or expand over time?

DISCUSSION QUESTIONS

1. Of the future public health nutrition issues and concerns described in this chapter, which one can you relate to the most, based on your experiences, opinions, or the information provided here? Comment on how it relates to your community, programs or policies, or place of employment.
2. Considering your perspective, history, worldview, and relevant future reports, are there any significant public health nutrition issues that you would add to this list? Please describe the issue and justify your rationale.
3. Select one of the societal trends described in this chapter and describe its impact on your community or population of interest (e.g., life stage).
4. Choose a public health nutrition policy described in this chapter or one with which you have experience. Do you feel this policy has been effective? Why or why not?
5. Consider one of the high-level public health nutrition policy trends from this chapter and describe how it impacts your work now or future career goals as a public health nutrition professional.
6. Describe your role in the development of a competent and effective public health nutrition workforce based on the information provided in this chapter.

SUGGESTED LEARNING ACTIVITIES

1. Select one of the reports in Table 15.1 to review in more detail. Visit the source cited in the table. How can you work to meet the recommendations in the report?
2. Choose one of the societal issues in Table 15.2 that you feel relates to your work or future career goal. Use the reference cited to extend your learning about this trend and consider how it does or will impact your work in the public health nutrition field.
3. Review one of the organizations or federal/state waiver programs described in the *Tips for Predicting and Tracking Policy Trends* section of this chapter. How do the policies fit within the strategic directions proposed by the White House Conference on Hunger, Nutrition, and Health.
4. Create an infographic that educates your community about the four future public health nutrition trends described in this chapter. Include an explanation, example, and resource for each trend.
5. Research food and nutrition policies in your local area. You may search for a food policy council in your county, state, or region. Describe how you would implement this policy within your current role or future career.
6. Think about the type of career in public health and nutrition that would most appeal to you. Then use a standard template to write a job description for that position. Include criteria such as the job

title, a summary of the position including job responsibilities and duties, educational requirements, and skills required. Once you have created your job description, do an internet search to see if you are able to find any similar positions.

RESOURCES FOR FURTHER LEARNING

- USDA SNAP-Ed Connection, Policy, Systems, and Environmental Change Resource Guide: Strategies for Increased Access to Healthy Foods, Beverages, and Physical Activity: https://snaped.fns.usda.gov/library/materials/policy-systems-environmental-change-resource-guide-strategies-increased-access
  - Provides samples of regional and national evidence-based, practice-based, and emerging tools and resources to achieve policy, systems, and environmental change to advance obesity prevention efforts in a variety of settings.
- Comprehensive Cancer Control National Partnership, Policy, Systems, and Environmental Change Resource Guide: www.acs4ccc.org/wp-content/uploads/2020/06/PSE_Resource_Guide_FINAL_05.15.15.pdf
  - Provides models and tools to assist with the planning and implementation of policy, systems, and environmental (PSE) agendas. It teaches how to use a PSE approach, build strategic capacity, wield tactical experience, and more.
- Office of Disease Prevention and Health Promotion, White House Conference on Hunger, Nutrition, and Health: https://health.gov/our-work/nutrition-physical-activity/white-house-conference-hunger-nutrition-and-health
  - Resources and conference recordings regarding a coordinated strategy to accelerate progress and drive transformative change in the United States to end hunger, improve nutrition and physical activity, and close the disparities surrounding them.
- USDA, Food and Nutrition Services, Center for Nutrition Policy and Promotion (CNPP): www.fns.usda.gov/cnpp
  - Resources and reports related to CNPP's work to improve the health and well-being of Americans by developing and promoting dietary guidance that links scientific research to the nutrition needs of consumers.
- Rural Health Information Hub, Rural Health Promotion and Disease Prevention Toolkit: www.ruralhealthinfo.org
  - Provides several modules for developing rural community health promotion and disease prevention policies and programs.
- National Produce Prescription Collaborative: https://nppc.health
  - Provides comprehensive information about this program that supports produce prescriptions by healthcare providers as prevention and treatment for diet-related disease.
- Food Is Medicine Coalition: www.fimcoalition.org
  - Describes the program model, policy work, research, and advocacy of this organization of nonprofit medically tailored food and nutrition service providers.
- Academy of Nutrition and Dietetics *Revised 2022 Standards of Practice and Standards of Professional Performance for Registered Dietitian Nutritionists (Competent, Proficient, and Expert) in Public Health and Community Nutrition*: www.jandonline.org/article/S2212-2672(22)00201-5/fulltext

  - Provides standards for professional performance that can be used for self-evaluation, goal setting, and other workforce development purposes.
- Association of State Public Health Nutritionists (ASPHN): https://asphn.org
  - Provides a plethora of resources for public health nutrition professionals, including networking, professional development opportunities, and career development opportunities. Educational resources are provided at ASPHN's resource page: https://publichealthnutrition.org.

SPRINGER PUBLISHING CONNECT™ | **A robust set of instructor resources designed to supplement this text is located at http://connect.springerpub.com/content/book/978-0-8261-8623-2. Qualifying instructors may request access by emailing textbook@springerpub.com.**

REFERENCES

1. Academy of Nutrition and Dietetics. *Definition of Terms List.* Commission on Dietetic Registration; 2021. https://www.eatrightpro.org/-/media/files/eatrightpro/practice/academy-definition-of-terms-list-feb-2021.pdf
2. Herman DR, Taylor Baer M, Adams E, et al. Life course perspective: evidence for the role of nutrition. *Matern Child Health J.* 2014;18(2):450–461. https://doi.org/10.1007/s10995-013-1280-3
3. Shahid SM, Bishop KS. Comprehensive approaches to improving nutrition: future prospects. *Nutrients.* 2019;11(8):1760. https://doi.org/10.3390/nu11081760
4. National WIC Association. WIC program overview and history. Accessed June 12, 2023. https://www.nwica.org/overview-and-history
5. U.S. Department of Agriculture Food and Nutrition Service. A short history of SNAP. Updated September 11, 2018. https://www.fns.usda.gov/snap/short-history-snap
6. White House Briefing Room. White House announces conference on hunger, nutrition and health in September. Statements and Releases. May 4, 2022. https://www.whitehouse.gov/briefing-room/statements-releases/2022/05/04/white-house-announces-conference-on-hunger-nutrition-and-health-in-september
7. Dietary Guidelines Advisory Committee. *Scientific Report of the 2020 Dietary Guidelines Advisory Committee: Advisory Report to the Secretary of Agriculture and the Secretary of Health and Human Services.* U.S. Department of Agriculture, Agricultural Research Service; 2020. https://www.dietaryguidelines.gov/2020-advisory-committee-report
8. Food and Agriculture Organization of the United Nations. *Fruits and Vegetables—Your Dietary Essentials: The International Year of Fruits and Vegetables 2021.* Food and Agriculture Organization of the United Nations; 2020. https://www.fao.org/3/cb2395en/cb2395en.pdf
9. U.S. Department of Agriculture Food and Nutrition Service. Fresh Fruit and Vegetable Program. Accessed March 7, 2023. https://www.fns.usda.gov/ffvp/fresh-fruit-and-vegetable-program
10. Auvinen A, Simock M, Moran A. Integrating produce prescriptions into the healthcare system: perspectives from key stakeholders. *Int J Environ Res Public Health.* 2022;19(17):11010. https://doi.org/10.3390/ijerph191711010
11. U.S. Department of Agriculture Food and Nutrition Service. Policy memorandum: monthly cash-value voucher/benefit for FY 2023 fruit and vegetable purchases. Updated August 30, 2022. https://www.fns.usda.gov/wic/monthly-cash-value-voucherbenefit-2023-fruit-vegetable
12. White House Domestic Policy Council. *Biden-Harris Administration National Strategy on Hunger, Nutrition, and Health.* The White House; 2022. https://www.whitehouse.gov/wp-content/uploads/2022/09/White-House-National-Strategy-on-Hunger-Nutrition-and-Health-FINAL.pdf
13. DeSalvo KB, Wang YC, Harris A, Auerbach J, Koo D, O'Carroll P. Public health 3.0: a call to action for public health to meet the challenges of the 21st century. *Prev Chronic Dis.* 2017;14:E78. https://doi.org/10.5888/pcd14.170017
14. Public Health Institute. *The Future of Public Health.* Public Health Institute; 2021. https://www.phi.org/wp-content/uploads/2022/05/The-Future-of-Public-Health_-PHI-2021-Annual-Report-1.pdf
15. Hamburg MA, Cohen M, DeSalvo K, et al. *Meeting America's Public Health Challenge: Recommendations for Building a National Public Health System That Addresses Ongoing and Future Health*

Crises, Advances Equity, and Earns Trust. Commonwealth Fund. June 2022. https://www.commonwealthfund.org/sites/default/files/2022-07/TCF-002

16. Partlow J. The Colorado River drought crisis: how did this happen? Can it be fixed? *The Washington Post.* February 5, 2023. https://www.washingtonpost.com/climate-environment/2023/02/05/colorado-river-drought-explained
17. Hendriks SL, Montgomery H, Benton T, et al. Global environmental climate change, covid-19, and conflict threaten food security and nutrition. *BMJ.* 2022;378:e071534. https://doi.org/10.1136/bmj-2022-071534
18. International Committee of the American Red Cross. Policy brief: food security and armed conflict. October 24, 2022. https://www.icrc.org/en/document/food-security-and-armed-conflict
19. Odoms-Young AM, Bruce MA. Examining the impact of structural racism on food insecurity: implications for addressing racial/ethnic disparities. *Fam Community Health.* 2018;41(suppl 2):S3–S6. https://doi.org/10.1097/FCH.0000000000000183
20. National Institute on Minority Health and Health Disparities. Food accessibility, insecurity and health outcomes. U.S. Department of Health and Human Services. Updated April 26, 2023. https://www.nimhd.nih.gov/resources/understanding-health-disparities/food-accessibility-insecurity-and-health-outcomes.html
21. Hostetter M, Klein S. Transforming care: understanding and ameliorating medical mistrust among Black Americans. Commonwealth Fund. January 24, 2021. https://www.commonwealthfund.org/publications/newsletter-article/2021/jan/medical-mistrust-among-black-americans
22. U.S. Department of Agriculture. Food supply chain fact sheet: USDA programs in the local food supply chain. Updated February 2021. https://www.ams.usda.gov/sites/default/files/media/FoodSupplyChainFactSheet.pdf
23. Delisle H, Shrimpton R, Blaney S, et al. Capacity-building for a strong public health nutrition workforce in low-resource countries. *Bull World Health Organ.* 2017;95(5):385–388. https://doi.org/10.2471/BLT.16.174912
24. El-Kour TY, Kelley K, Bruening M, et al. Dietetic workforce capacity assessment for public health nutrition and community nutrition. *J Acad Nutr Diet.* 2021;121(7):1379–1391.e21. https://doi.org/10.1016/j.jand.2020.08.078
25. Kalaitzandonakes M, Ellison B, Coppess J. Coping with the 2022 infant formula shortage. *Prev Med Rep.* 2023;32:102123. https://doi.org/10.1016/j.pmedr.2023.102123
26. U.S. Senate Committee on Appropriations. Fiscal Year 2023 Omnibus Appropriations Bill: Highlights. https://www.appropriations.senate.gov/imo/media/doc/HIGHLIGHTS%20DOCUMENT%20FY%2023.pdf
27. El-sadek L, Zhang L, Vargas R, Funchess T, Green C. *State of the State: Annual Mississippi Health Disparities and Inequalities Report.* Mississippi State Department of Health; 2015.
28. Fact sheet: Child Nutrition Reauthorization—Healthy, Hunger-free Kids Act of 2010. December 2010. https://obamawhitehouse.archives.gov/sites/default/files/Child_Nutrition_Fact_Sheet_12_10_10.pdf
29. New York State Senate. Assembly Bill A5107: Imposes an excise tax on sugary drinks. 2023–2024 Legislative Session. March 2, 2023. https://www.nysenate.gov/legislation/bills/2023/A5107
30. Melba Idaho School District. Noninstructional operations: Melba School District No. 136. August 14, 2018. https://msd136.org/wp-content/uploads/2019/06/Local-School-Wellness.pdf
31. U.S. Department of Agriculture Food and Nutrition Service. Special Supplemental Nutrition Program for Women, Infants, and Children (WIC): revisions in the WIC food packages. *Fed Regist.* 2022;87(223):71090–71162. https://www.federalregister.gov/documents/2022/11/21/2022-24705/special-supplemental-nutrition-program-for-women-infants-and-children-wic-revisions-in-the-wic-food
32. Fisher T, Gross M, Hebert S, Rios-Avila J. Policy brief: shelters are homes to breastfeeding moms and babies. Association of State Public Health Nutritionists. May 1, 2018. https://asphn.org/wp-content/uploads/2017/10/2018-Supporting-Breastfeeding-in-Homeless-Shelters.pdf
33. Board of Curry County Commissioners. News and proclamations: February 2023 declared as Heart Awareness Month. January 31, 2023. https://www.currycounty.org/Home/Components/News/News/967/16
34. Illinois Hospital Association. *Small and Rural Hospitals Constituency Section Sodium Reduction Initiative Best Practices/Innovative Strategies.* Association of State Public Health Nutritionists. 2013. https://asphn.org/wp-content/uploads/2017/12/Illinois-Small-Rural-Hospitals-Best-Practices.pdf

35. U.S. Department of Agriculture, U.S. Department of Health and Human Services. *Dietary Guidelines for Americans 2020–2025*. 9th ed. U.S. Department of Health and Human Services; 2020.
36. Office of Disease Prevention and Health Promotion. *Healthy People 2030*: building a healthier future for all. U.S. Department of Health and Human Services. Accessed May 25, 2023. https://health.gov/healthypeople
37. The Community Guide. About the Community Preventive Services Task Force. Updated June 22, 2023. https://www.thecommunityguide.org/pages/about-community-preventive-services-task-force.html
38. Association of State Public Health Nutritionists. Food and nutrition security primer: introduction. Updated July 24, 2022. https://asphn.org/food-and-nutrition-security-primer
39. Consumer Brands Association. About the Consumer Brands Association. 2023. https://consumerbrandsassociation.org/about-us/#timeline__year-2000s
40. Food Marketing Institute. FMI: The Food Industry Association. 2023. https://www.fmi.org/
41. U.S. Department of Health and Human Services. News: HHS announces $2.5 million for produce prescription programs in Indian country. April 26, 2023. https://www.hhs.gov/about/news/2023/04/26/hhs-announces-25-million-produce-prescription-programs-indian-country.html
42. California Department of Health Care Services. Medically Tailored Meals Pilot Program. Accessed May 25, 2023. https://www.dhcs.ca.gov/services/ltc/Pages/Medically-Tailored-Meals-Pilot-Program.aspx
43. Davis AM, Vogelzang JL, Affenito SG. The shortage of registered dietitians or nutritionists with a terminal degree: a call to action for the profession. *J Acad Nutr Diet*. 2023;123(4):569–575. https://doi.org/10.1016/j.jand.2023.01.003
44. Novilla MLB, Moxley VBA, Hanson CL, et al. COVID-19 and psychosocial well-being: did COVID-19 worsen U.S. frontline healthcare workers' burnout, anxiety, and depression? *Int J Environ Res Public Health*. 2023;20(5):4414. https://doi.org/10.3390/ijerph20054414
45. Søvold LE, Naslund JA, Kousoulis AA, et al. Prioritizing the mental health and well-being of healthcare workers: an urgent global public health priority. *Front Public Health*. 2021;9:679397. https://doi.org/10.3389/fpubh.2021.679397
46. Sellers K, Leider JP, Gould E, et al. The state of the U.S. governmental public health workforce, 2014–2017. *Am J Public Health*. 2019;109(5):674–680. https://doi.org/10.2105/AJPH.2019.305011
47. Dimock M. Defining generations: where millennials end and Generation Z begins. Pew Research Center. January 17, 2019. https://www.pewresearch.org/short-reads/2019/01/17/where-millennials-end-and-generation-z-begins
48. Annie E. Casey Foundation. What are the core characteristics of Generation Z? Updated February 14, 2023. https://www.aecf.org/blog/what-are-the-core-characteristics-of-generation-z
49. Bruening M, Perkins S, Udarbe A. Academy of Nutrition and Dietetics: Revised 2022 Standards of Practice and Standards of Professional Performance for Registered Dietitian Nutritionists (Competent, Proficient, and Expert) in Public Health and Community Nutrition. *J Acad Nutr Diet*. 2022;122(9):1744–1763.e49. https://doi.org/10.1016/j.jand.2022.04.005
50. Centers for Disease Control and Prevention. The CDC policy process. Office of Policy, Performance, and Evaluation. Accessed June 12, 2023. https://www.cdc.gov/policy/polaris/policyprocess/index.html
51. Centers for Disease Control and Prevention.Program evaluation. Office of Policy, Performance, and Evaluation. Accessed June 12, 2023. https://www.cdc.gov/evaluation/index.htm

APPENDICES

APPENDIX A: BRIEF REVIEW: BASIC PRINCIPLES OF NUTRITION AND DIETARY GUIDANCE TOOLS

PART I: BASIC PRINCIPLES OF NUTRITION

SECTION A: DEFINITIONS AND FOUNDATIONS

1. What is nutrition?

The Academy of Nutrition and Dietetics has adopted the following definition of *nutrition*, which is the definition used in this textbook: "the science of food, the nutrients and other substances therein, their action, interaction and balance in relation to health and disease, and the process by which the organism ingests, absorbs, transports, utilizes and excretes food substances."[1,2]

a. Nutrition is a relatively new science.

Ancient civilizations in Africa, eastern and western Asia, and Europe recognized that there is a connection between food and health, and throughout recorded history, people have recognized this link.[3] Humans have been aware for thousands of years that food is necessary for maintaining life, and that certain foods are more associated with health than others. Beginning in the early 1800s, there began to be a recognition that certain constituents of food are associated with health, but it was not until the late 1800s through the mid-1900s that scientists recognized and defined vitamins as specific nutrients.[3,4]

b. Nutrition recommendations are updated as nutrition knowledge is gained.

It's important to remember that nutrition as a science is still a very young field of study compared to many other sciences. Much has been learned about nutrition in the past 200 years, but there is still a great deal of nutrition knowledge that is poorly understood. The knowledge base underlying nutrition recommendations is constantly expanding, and recommendations are updated over time as evidence accumulates.

2. What are three foundational nutrition concepts?

a. First, nutrition affects EVERYONE and EVERYTHING.

Everyone eats; everyone must be nourished to survive. Food systems are inextricably interwoven into all our lives, activities, and environments, throughout our lives, from birth to death.

b. Second, healthy people all need the same nutrients, but not always in the same amounts and proportions.

During specific life cycle phases, the same nutrients are needed in differing amounts and proportions. Levels of physical activity and special medical conditions also affect needs for nutrients.

c. Third, the life course theory states that each life cycle phase affects its subsequent life cycle phases, and this can be applied to nutrition as well.[5]

So, we can expect that nutritional status as a child will impact adolescent nutritional status and health, which will impact young adult nutritional status and health, and so on through older adulthood.

Review Questions

1. After reviewing the Academy of Nutrition and Dietetics definition of nutrition, write a definition of nutrition in your own words.
2. When was the idea that there are specific substances considered nutrients in food first proposed?
3. During what period of time did the identification and definition of the various vitamins take place?
4. Why are nutritional recommendations updated from time to time?
5. What are three foundational nutritional concepts?

SECTION B: DIGESTION

Digestion is the process of breaking down food so its nutrients can be absorbed and utilized by the body. The digestive system is made up of the gastrointestinal (GI) tract and its accessory organs.6 Each part of the digestive system helps to move food and liquid through the GI tract, breaks it down into smaller particles for digestion via physical or chemical means, or both.[6] Food can be broken down into smaller particles through physical digestion, chewing, for example, or by chemical digestion by the acid in the stomach. The hollow organs that make up the GI tract are the mouth, esophagus, stomach, small intestine, large intestine, and anus.[6] The solid organs of the digestive system are the liver, pancreas, and gallbladder.[6]

The digestive process begins when food enters the mouth and teeth begin breaking it down by chewing. Saliva helps moisten chewed food to make it easier to swallow, and enzymes in the saliva begin breaking down the starches in food. After swallowing, food is transported through the esophagus into the stomach via muscle contractions called peristalsis. Powerful stomach muscles churn food; in the process, food becomes liquified and mixed with gastric acid and enzymes that further break down food particles.[6] Food travels next to the small intestine, where a variety of enzymes—including pancreatic juices and bile from the liver—continue food breakdown into molecules of protein,

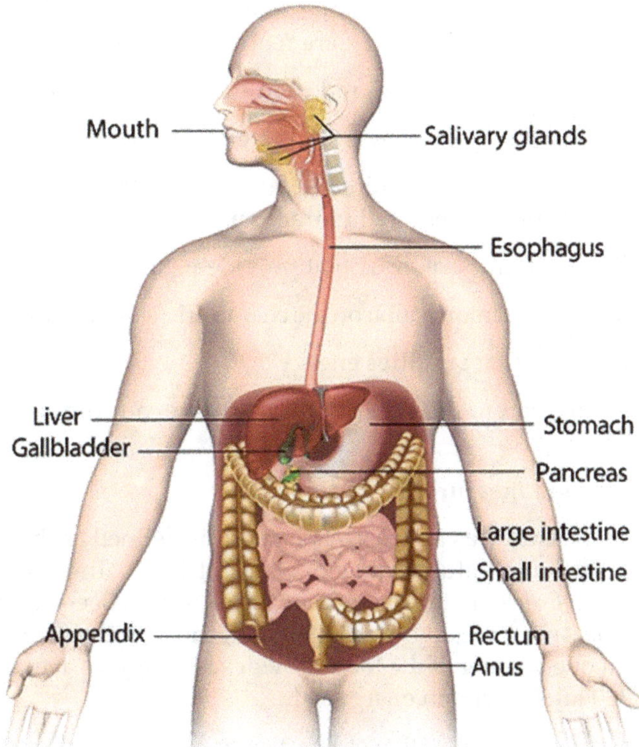

Figure A.1. The digestive system.
Source: National Institute of Diabetes and Digestive and Kidney Diseases. Your digestive system & how it works. Accessed October 27, 2023. https://www.niddk.nih.gov/health-information/digestive-diseases/digestive-system-how-it-works

carbohydrate, and fat, as well as vitamins, minerals, and water. Via peristalsis, the products of digestion move from the small to the large intestine.

Most absorption of nutrients takes place in the small intestine, as nutrient molecules are transported through the small intestine's walls to be absorbed into lymph and the bloodstream. Absorbed nutrients are delivered to body cells to be utilized as energy, raw materials for body growth and repair, and necessary substrates for chemical reactions in the body. From the small intestine, digested food moves into the large intestine. In the large intestine, water is reabsorbed from the digestive tract, and bacteria help break down remaining nutrients. The waste products of digestion become stool in the large intestine and are excreted from the body through the anus.[6]

Figure A.1 provides a diagram of the major parts of the digestive system.

SECTION C: INTRODUCTION TO FOOD AND NUTRIENTS

1. What is food?

Food is an essential need of humans. Food has been defined as "anything that, when taken into the body, serves to nourish, build, and repair tissues, supply energy, or regulate body processes."[2] Food provides energy, nutrients, and other substances (such as phytochemicals and fiber) that are required for human survival and health.

2. **What are the six classes of nutrients and their basic characteristics?**

   The six classes of nutrients are carbohydrate, protein, fat, vitamins, minerals, and water.

   Macronutrients are nutrients required in large amounts when compared to micronutrients. Micronutrients are required in trace amounts.[7]

   Energy-yielding nutrients are those that provide measurable energy to the body.

   Table A.1 provides basic information on the characteristics of the six classes of nutrients.

3. **What is a non-nutrient that supplies energy?**

   Alcohol is not considered to provide nutritional value, but provides 7 calories in energy per gram.

4. **How is energy in food measured?**

   Energy in food is measured as calories. A *kilocalorie* is defined as the amount of energy required to raise the temperature of 1 kg of water, at 1 atm atmospheric pressure, by 1 degree Celsius.[7] A *calorie* is 1/1,000 of a kilocalorie. In practice—for example, on food labels—the term *calorie* is usually used interchangeably with *kilocalorie*. So, a food label reporting that one serving of the food provides 300 calories actually means that the food provides 300 kilocalories in energy value.

   To calculate the calories in a serving of a particular food, multiply the grams of each energy-yielding nutrient in the food by that nutrient's per-gram calorie value. For example:

   One serving of a food is composed of 15 g carbohydrate, 4 g protein, and 7 g fat. The calorie value is: (15 g x 4 calories/g) + (4 g x 4 calories/g) + (7 g x 9 calories/g) = 60 + 16 + 63 = 139 calories/serving.

Table A.1. The Six Classes of Nutrients and Their Basic Characteristics

Nutrient Class	Macro- or Micronutrient?	Energy-yielding?*
1. Carbohydrate	Macro	Yes: 4 calories per gram
2. Protein	Macro	Yes: 4 calories per gram
3. Fat	Macro	Yes: 9 calories per gram
4. Vitamins	Micro	No
5. Minerals	Micro	No
6. Water	Macro[7]	No

*In this table and throughout this text, the term *calorie* is used in its common sense to mean *kilocalorie*.
Source: U.S. Department of Agriculture. Macronutrients. National Agricultural Library. Accessed May 29, 2023. https://www.nal.usda.gov/human-nutrition-and-food-safety/food-composition/macronutrients; U.S. Department of Agriculture, U.S. Department of Health and Human Services. *Dietary Guidelines for Americans 2020–2025*. 9th ed. U.S. Department of Health and Human Services; 2020. https://www.dietaryguidelines.gov

5. What are essential and nonessential nutrients?

Essential nutrients are those that our bodies cannot synthesize for ourselves; we *must* obtain them from food. Essential nutrients are vital for survival. Essential nutrients include several amino acids (the building blocks of proteins); the fatty acids linoleic acid and α-linolenic acid; carbohydrates; vitamins; minerals; and water. Nonessential nutrients are those we can synthesize for ourselves given the necessary raw materials; an example is nonessential amino acids, which our bodies can synthesize.[8]

An example of the concept of essential nutrients is that dogs can synthesize their own vitamin C. So, vitamin C is not an essential nutrient for dogs. Vitamin C is essential for humans, who are unable to synthesize the nutrient.[9]

It should be noted that vitamin D, and to a lesser extent, vitamin K, can be made in the human body. Technically, these substances do not meet the official definition of vitamins, which must be obtained from food. However, in common usage nutrition professionals refer to them as vitamins.

Review Questions

1. Define *food* in your own words.
2. What is the difference between macronutrients and micronutrients?
3. What are the six classes of nutrients?
4. Which of the six classes of nutrients are energy-yielding, and how many calories does each supply?
5. What is a calorie? The term *calorie* is usually used interchangeably with which term?
6. A particular food has 20 g carbohydrate, 15 g protein, and 7 g fat per serving. How many calories are provided by a serving of the food?
7. How many calories per gram are provided by alcohol?
8. Explain the difference between essential and nonessential nutrients.

SECTION D: A CLOSER LOOK AT THE SIX CLASSES OF NUTRIENTS: MACRONUTRIENTS

1. Carbohydrates

a. What are carbohydrates and how do we obtain them?

Carbohydrates are the body's main energy source, and are composed of chains of sugar molecules that the body converts into energy sources such as glucose and glycogen. Carbohydrates are obtained through the diet, and come mostly from plant foods. Plant foods providing carbohydrates include fruits, vegetables, grains, beans, and legumes. Beans and legumes provide both carbohydrates and protein. The only animal source of carbohydrates is dairy milk, which provides both carbohydrates and protein.[10]

Carbohydrates in plants occur as long strings of sugar molecules bonded together as sugars and starches.

b. What are the three different classifications of carbohydrates?

There are three main carbohydrate classifications:

1. Monosaccharides (*mono* = 1): These consist of one sugar molecule, and are known as *simple sugars*. There are three monosaccharides: (1) glucose; (2) fructose; and (3) galactose. Examples of foods providing monosaccharides are fresh, canned, and dried fruits, and honey.
2. Disaccharides (*di* = 2): These consist of two simple sugars joined together. There are three disaccharides: (1) sucrose (also known as table sugar), which consists of glucose + fructose; (2) lactose (occurs in dairy milk), which consists of glucose + galactose; and (3) maltose, which consists of two molecules of glucose joined together. Examples of foods providing disaccharides include table sugar and foods containing table sugar, carrots, molasses, dairy milk, and yogurt.[10]
3. Polysaccharides (*poly* = many), also known as complex carbohydrates: These are composed of long chains of many glucose molecules. The three types of polysaccharides are:
   (a) Starches. Examples of starchy foods are potatoes, breads, rice, and pasta.
   (b) Fiber, which is formed by carbohydrate chains that cannot be digested by the human body. Fiber has many important health-promoting functions in the body, aiding with digestive function, weight management, blood sugar metabolism, and heart health. Fiber-containing foods include whole grains, beans and legumes, fruits, and vegetables.[10] Animal foods do not contain fiber.
   (c) Glycogen, which is the storage form of carbohydrate in the body. Excess glucose from dietary consumption is converted to glycogen and stored in the liver, skeletal muscles, and brain (a very small amount) for future use. The healthy body maintains tight control over blood sugar levels, and glycogen is converted back to glucose for the body's use when blood sugar levels threaten to become too low, or when additional energy is needed to meet physiologic needs (for example, during athletic competition).[11]

d. How much carbohydrate do we need each day?

Recommended intake of carbohydrates is measured in grams per day and is calculated as 45% to 65% of total calories.[12] So, for a person consuming a 2,000-calorie per day diet, the appropriate amount of carbohydrates would be 225 to 325 g carbohydrate per day. The minimum amount of carbohydrate required to promote good health is 130 g/day.[13]

2. Proteins

a. What are proteins and how are they synthesized in the body?

Proteins can be thought of as the building blocks and raw materials of the body; they are necessary for the maintenance and repair of body cells and tissues, as well as the physiologic functions of the body, since they serve as enzymes. Proteins are built within the body's cells, with construction (coding) directed by each cell's genetic material. Thousands of different types of proteins in the body are composed of varying combinations of 20 different amino acids.

In a very simplified analogy, one could think of the assembly of strings of amino acids as similar to beading a necklace in a particular pattern. Once assembled,

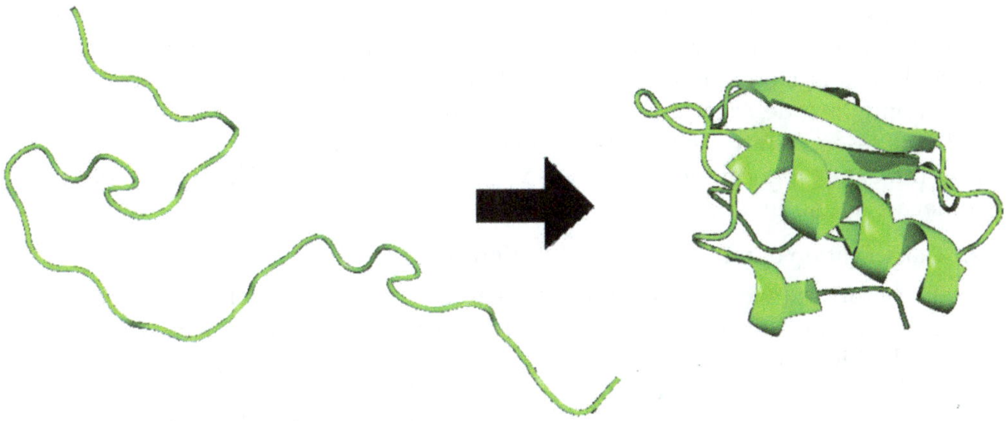

Figure A.2. Formation of a protein from amino acid chain to folded, functional shape.
Source: Courtesy of Magnus Kjaergaard, PhD.

the amino acid chain folds, bends, and twists into a distinctive shape based on the chemical and electrical characteristics of the component amino acids (**see Figure A.2**). The function of the protein molecule is highly dependent on its shape.

Denaturation of a protein occurs when a folded protein unfolds and becomes nonfunctional due to factors such as heat or chemicals. A common example of protein denaturation is the process of scrambling an egg. The proteins in the egg, when exposed to heat, unfold and assume a solid rather than liquid form. Denaturation of a protein is often, but not always, irreversible.

b. What are essential and nonessential amino acids?

The 20 amino acids can be broken down into two groups, essential amino acids and nonessential amino acids. Essential amino acids are those that humans can only obtain from the diet. Nonessential amino acids are those we can manufacture for ourselves given the appropriate raw materials in protein foods.[14]

c. What are complete proteins?

A *complete protein* source provides all the essential amino acids. Animal foods such as meat, fish and seafood, poultry, eggs, and dairy provide complete proteins, as does the plant food soy. While plant foods provide protein, they are often missing one or more amino acids. By combining plant foods that have complementary proteins, plant-based meals can provide all essential amino acids. Two examples of such meals include: (1) corn tortillas with beans; and (2) a sandwich of whole grain bread and peanut butter.[14]

d. How much protein do we need each day?

The Dietary Reference Intakes (DRIs) recommend daily consumption of 10% to 35% of total calories as proteins.[14]

3. Fats

There is a common misconception that fats are "bad." However, fats support many vital physiologic functions and are essential for life. Fat protects body structures and organs, provides a concentrated energy source, is a component of hormones and nerve/brain tissue, and aids in body temperature control.

Fats are lipids. The lipid family has been described as "fatty or waxy substances your body makes that don't dissolve in water."[15] Lipids include triglycerides, fatty acids, bile salts, steroid hormones, phospholipids, and cholesterol.[15] Dietary fats most commonly include triglycerides, essential fatty acids, phospholipids, and cholesterol.[16] The essential fatty acids, which can only be obtained from food, include linoleic acid (omega-6, found in foods such as vegetable oil, nuts, seeds) and α-linolenic acid (omega-3, found in foods such as walnuts, canola oil, and flaxseed oil).

a. Classification of fats based on saturation state

The term *saturation* refers to the chemical structures of fats, which are organic molecules formed of carbon, hydrogen, and oxygen. *Saturated fat* means that there are no double bonds in the molecular structure of a fat; the fat is completely saturated with hydrogen atoms. A simplified analogy could be to think of the fat's carbon chain as a parking lot with every space filled. Saturated fats are usually solid at room temperature. Examples include the fat found in meats (as marbling), full-fat dairy products including cheese, coconut oil, and many processed foods. The Dietary Guidelines for Americans (DGAs) recommend that saturated fat intake in healthy people be limited to no more than 10% of total daily calories.[13]

Unsaturated means that a fat has at least one double bond in its molecular structure. These can be monounsaturated (one double bond) or polyunsaturated (more than one double bond). A simplified analogy could be to think of the fat's carbon chain as a parking lot with one or more spaces empty. Because of the double bonds, or open parking spaces, unsaturated fat molecules have shapes that allow them to be more fluid than saturated fats. Thus, unsaturated fats are usually liquid at room temperature. Examples of foods providing unsaturated fats include olive oil, canola oil, peanut oil, peanut butter, avocados, many seeds and nuts, corn oil, safflower oil, walnuts, sunflower seeds, and fish.

b. Trans-fats: a public health nutrition policy story

Trans-fats are artificially created fats manufactured by hydrogenating, or saturating, oils such as corn oil or safflower oil to transform them into solid fats. Trans-fats in the diet are almost all artificial, although very small amounts of naturally occurring trans-fats occur in full-fat dairy products and meats. First developed in the late 1800s, trans-fats gradually became ubiquitous within processed foods in America, as they impart desirable flavor and texture characteristics to food as well as greatly extending the shelf life of processed foods.

A large body of research evidence accumulated since the 1990s strongly links trans-fats with heart disease, diabetes, and other chronic diseases.[17] Trans-fats became enmeshed in the U.S. food system before the bad health effects were known. Based on the evidence, in 2003 the Food and Drug Administration (FDA) required that trans-fat content be included on the Nutrition Facts label, and in 2015 trans-fats were declared to be "not generally recognized as safe" to include in foods. The FDA ordered that trans-fats be eliminated from the U.S. food supply by 2018. With a few additional phase-outs allowed by the FDA, by 2021 trans-fats were nearly eliminated from the U.S. food supply.[17] It has been estimated that nearly one of five heart attacks could be prevented by this public health initiative, and early data have been promising.[17]

The DGAs recommend that trans-fat consumption be limited to "as low as possible."[13]

d. Fats: Recommendations

Make most of your fats healthy fats (unsaturated). Remember that these fats are found in nuts, seeds, olive oil, peanut butter, fish, avocados, etc. Humans can handle saturated fat in moderation (less than 10% total calories per day). Use small amounts of saturated fat where the fat will be most enjoyed. Example: A teaspoon of butter on toast or melted over vegetables. Keep trans-fat intake as low as possible.

The DRIs recommend daily consumption of 20% to 35% of total calories as fats.[14]

4. Water

Water is essential for life; humans can survive only a short time without water. All body processes require water. Adult humans are about 60% to 70% water. Water is supplied by liquids and foods. Recommended average daily intake for menis about 15.5 cups (from water, other liquids, and food); for women it is about 11.5 cups (from water, other liquids, and food). Food provides about 20% of our daily water intake. The best advice for most people is to drink to thirst, and to adjust fluid intake based on activity levels.

Review Questions

1. What is the main function of carbohydrates?
2. What is the basic molecular structure of carbohydrates?
3. Which foods contain carbohydrates?
4. What is recommendation for carbohydrate consumption as a percentage of total calories? What is the minimum intake of carbohydrate, in grams, required to meet basic physiologic needs?
5. What is the main function of proteins?
6. Proteins are made up of ____________ ____________.
7. The function of a protein is highly dependent on its ____________.
8. Which foods provide proteins?
9. What is the recommendation for protein consumption as a percentage of total calories?
10. What is the main function of dietary fat?
11. What is the basic molecular structure of fat?
12. Explain the difference between saturated and unsaturated fats in terms of molecular structure. Describe a rule of thumb for determining whether or not a fat is saturated or unsaturated.
13. Which foods provide fat? Which fats are considered to provide health benefits?
14. What is the recommendation for fat consumption as a percentage of total calories?
15. What are daily recommendations for water intake for males and females?

SECTION E: A CLOSER LOOK AT THE SIX CLASSES OF NUTRIENTS: MICRONUTRIENTS, AND NON-NUTRIENT PHYTOCHEMICALS

1. **Vitamins**

Vitamins are essential organic nutrients that we must obtain from foods, and that are necessary to carry out the physiologic functions of the body. They act as coenzymes that are necessary for the action of enzymes that facilitate body processes, as antioxidants that stop the action of the damaging substances—free radicals—in the body, and in many other ways. Specific recommendations for vitamin intake for the various age and gender groups are found in the DRIs.

The vitamins are divided into two major classes: water soluble and fat soluble. Water-soluble vitamins include thiamine, riboflavin, niacin, vitamin B_6, folate, vitamin B_{12}, biotin, pantothenic acid, choline, and vitamin C. The four fat-soluble vitamins are vitamins A, E, D, and K.

The DRIs provide recommended values for vitamin intake based on age and gender group.

2. **Minerals**

Minerals are essential inorganic nutrients that we must obtain from food, and they are necessary to carry out the physiologic functions of the body. Calcium, chromium, copper, fluoride, iodine, iron, magnesium, manganese, molybdenum, phosphorus, selenium, zinc, potassium, sodium, and chloride are all minerals that have widely varying functions within the body.

The DRIs provide recommended values for mineral intake based on age and gender group.

3. **Vitamins and minerals: be aware**

The best source of vitamins and minerals is a healthful diet rich in fruits, vegetables, whole grains, beans, legumes, and dairy products. Most healthy people do not need vitamin and mineral supplements if they consume an adequate and healthful diet. Some people with specific health conditions, or in some life cycle phases, may benefit from certain supplements. For example, infants should begin receiving a supplement of 400 IU vitamin D within the first few days of life.[18] Consultation with a healthcare provider such as a physician or registered dietitian nutritionist is recommended prior to using nutritional supplements.

More is not necessarily better: symptoms of toxicity can result from excessive intake of some vitamins and minerals. Nutrient toxicity from chronic overconsumption can be serious. When working with a healthcare provider, it is important to provide information on any nutritional supplements being used so that potential nutrient–medication interactions can be assessed.

4. **Dietary supplements**

In the United States, regulation of nutritional supplements is less rigorous than regulation of pharmaceuticals or over-the-counter medications. While pharmaceuticals/

over-the-counter medications must be determined to be safe by the FDA prior to selling the products to the public, by law the FDA cannot take action to protect consumers until nutritional supplements are already on the market and adverse effects are reported.[19] Reliable information on dietary supplements is available from the National Institutes of Health Office of Dietary Supplements at https://ods.od.nih.gov.[20]

5. **Phytochemicals**

   Phytochemicals are not nutrients in the sense that they are not essential for life; rather, they are chemicals found in foods that have health effects in the body—and it is thought that many of these effects may be positive. Knowledge of phytochemicals and their effects is still emerging, and research is ongoing. One reason to eat recommended amounts of brightly colored produce is to consume their pigments, which are rich sources of phytochemicals that may confer some of the health benefits of fruit and vegetable consumption.

SECTION F: ABOUT MALNUTRITION

1. **What is malnutrition?**

"Mal" means "bad" in Latin. The Cleveland Clinic defines malnutrition as "an imbalance between the nutrients your body needs to function and the nutrients it gets."[21] Malnutrition can result from both over- and undernutrition. So, malnutrition can occur in persons with obesity. Malnutrition is a key contributor to the development of chronic diseases. Population-level health promotion and prevention of chronic diseases by facilitating good nutrition and preventing malnutrition is the specific field of practice of the public health nutrition professional.

2. **Who is at nutritional risk?**

   Certain groups of people at different life cycle phases may be at greater risk of becoming malnourished, including during pregnancy, infants and children, older adults—especially those who are frail, people with chronic health conditions, and persons living in environments presenting adverse social determinants of health.[22]

Review Questions

1. What is the definition of a *vitamin*?
2. What are the two classes of vitamins and minerals?
3. What is the definition of a *mineral*?
4. What are phytochemicals?
5. What is the ideal way to obtain recommended amounts of vitamins and minerals?
6. What is the difference between the way pharmaceuticals and nutritional supplements are regulated in the United States?
7. Define *malnutrition* and describe two ways an individual can become malnourished.
8. Which groups are most likely to be at nutritional risk?

PART II: NUTRITION GUIDANCE TOOLS

1. **About official nutrition guidelines**

   a. Official nutrition guidelines, such as the Dietary Guidelines for Americans, are based on the best scientific evidence available at the time of guideline revision and development, and provide accurate advice for the populations for whom the guidelines are intended.

   Official guidance may seem at times to lag somewhat behind current popular diets often found online or on social media, and that is because it takes time to accumulate research knowledge to address the safety and effectiveness of new interventions. Guidelines are updated at regular intervals (in the United States, every 5 years), and the body of new evidence is used to revise the older recommendations.

   b. Many countries around the world develop and publish their own nutrition guidelines; see Chapter 1 of this text for more information.

   c. Guidelines are considered standards that can be used to plan and evaluate population-based public health nutrition interventions. A *standard* provides a basis for comparison. For example, a ruler is a standard for length measurement. Likewise, official nutrition guidance tools such as the Dietary Reference Intakes or the Dietary Guidelines for Americans provide a standard against which the adequacy of population or individual nutrient or dietary intake can be measured.

2. **Examples of official nutrition standards and guidelines**

   Examples of nutrition standards and guidelines include the Dietary Reference Intakes, the Dietary Guidelines for Americans, MyPlate, and Food Labeling/Daily Values.

   Public health nutrition practitioners should be familiar with these tools, as they are used frequently in population nutrition interventions and research.

   a. Dietary Reference Intakes (DRIs)

   The DRIs provide recommendations for consumption of the various nutrients by age group, gender group, and life cycle stage. DRIs are a set of values used to describe acceptable intake ranges for nutrients. The DRIs apply to healthy persons ages 2 and up.

   The DRIs are established by the Food and Nutrition Board, Institute of Medicine, and National Academy of Sciences, Engineering, and Medicine.[23] To use DRIs, determine the age group, gender group, and/or life cycle stage (e.g., pregnancy) for which you'd like information. Then, locate the corresponding nutrient in the appropriate DRI document to determine the DRI value. Links to DRI documents are found at this web page: https://health.gov/our-work/nutrition-physical-activity/dietary-guidelines/dietary-reference-intakes/applying-dietary-reference-intakes-professional-settings.[12]

   1. Dietary Reference Intakes values
      (a) Estimated Average Requirement (EAR)
      (b) Recommended Dietary Allowance (RDA)
      (c) Adequate Intake (AI)
      (d) Tolerable Upper Intake Level (UL)
      (e) Estimated Energy Requirement (EER)

(f) Acceptable Macronutrient Distribution Range (AMDR)

(g) Chronic Disease Risk Reduction Intake

(a) Estimated Average Requirement (EAR)
Purpose: Meeting nutrient requirements

The EAR is defined as "The average daily nutrient intake estimated to meet the requirement of half the individuals in a particular sex and life-stage group" (p. 23)."[23] An EAR is required for the calculation of an RDA; without an EAR, an RDA cannot be determined. EARs are based on research evidence.

(b) Recommended Dietary Allowance (RDA)
Purpose: Meeting nutrient requirements

The RDA is defined as "The average daily dietary nutrient intake sufficient to meet the nutrient requirements of nearly all (97–98%) individuals in a particular sex and life-stage group" (p. 23)."[23] If data are normally distributed and a standard deviation (SD) can be calculated, the RDA is set at 2 SD above the EAR: RDA = EAR + 2 SD EAR.

From 1941 to 1991, the only DRI value available was the RDA. Because it was recognized that there was a need to develop a range of values for each nutrient, the additional DRIs were developed.

(c) Adequate Intake (AI)
Purpose: Meeting nutrient requirements

"The recommended average daily intake based on observed or experimentally determined approximations or estimates of nutrient intake by a group (or groups) of individuals that are assumed to be adequate—used when an RDA cannot be determined" (p. 23)."[23] An AI is set if insufficient research data are available to calculate an EAR and thus an RDA.

AIs are more common for pregnancy, and for infant nutrition, as there may be insufficient research evidence to establish EARs. The AI can be thought of as a well-educated guess.

(d) Tolerable Upper Intake Level (UL)
Purpose: Preventing excessive intake of nutrients

"The highest average daily nutrient intake that is likely to pose no risk of adverse health effects to almost all individuals in the general population; as intake increases above the UL, the potential risk of adverse effects may increase."[23] In regard to nutrients, it is not necessarily true that more is better, and excessive intakes can cause toxic effects. Some nutrients are of more concern than others. An intake level at the UL is unlikely to pose a risk for most individuals. Between the RDA and the UL is a safe range of intake; however, an intake greater than the RDA does not necessarily mean greater benefit. The UL does not apply to persons receiving dietary supplements under medical supervision.

Populations most likely to benefit from the use of the UL include older adults, who tend to use more dietary supplements than other age groups in addition to consuming fortified foods. In addition, athletes tend to use more supplements than the general population and may benefit from reviewing the UL values.

(e) Estimated Energy Requirement (EER)
Purpose: Meeting nutrient requirements

"The average dietary energy intake that is predicted to maintain energy balance in an adult of a defined age, sex, weight, height, and level of physical activity" (p. 23). The EER may be used in determining whether population or individual energy (calorie) intake exceeds or fails to meet recommended needs.

(f) Acceptable Macronutrient Distribution Ranges (AMDRs)
Purpose: Reducing risk of chronic disease

"A range of usual intakes for a macronutrient that is associated with a reduced risk of chronic disease while providing adequate intakes of essential nutrients; an AMDR is expressed as a percentage of total energy intake" (p. 23).[23] The AMDRs help to promote balanced intake of macronutrients and ensure that adequate amounts of macronutrients are consumed to meet physiologic needs.

For adults the AMDRs are:

- Fat: 20% to 35% of total calories
- Carbohydrate: 45% to 65% of total calories
- Protein: 10% to 35% of total calories

(g) Chronic Disease Risk Reduction Intake (CDRR)
Purpose: Reducing risk of chronic disease

"Characterizes nutrient intakes that are expected to reduce the risk of developing chronic disease" (para. 4)."[25] Until 2017, no DRI was focused on chronic disease risk reduction as the RDAs are focused on adequacy. It 2017, the nutrients sodium and potassium were prioritized for development of the first CDRRs. In 2019, a news release from the National Academies of Science, Engineering, and Medicine announced the establishment of the first CDRR, for sodium. Insufficient evidence was found to establish a CDRR for potassium.

b. Dietary Guidelines for Americans (DGAs)

The current 2020–2025 DGAs provide science-based advice on diet and physical activity for healthy Americans ages 2 years and older. The 2020–2025 DGAs, for the first time, provide dietary guidance specific to each major life cycle phase.

The DGAs are used as the basis of recommendations for the nutrition programming and policy of the U.S. Department of Agriculture (USDA) and the Department of Health and Human Services (DHHS).[13]

Information on the DGAs, and a link to the DGAs document, are available at www.dietaryguidelines.gov.

c. MyPlate

The USDA's consumer-focused food guidance system is called MyPlate. Housed within the USDA Center for Nutrition Policy and Promotion, MyPlate was released in 2011 to provide actionable, practical, and easy-to-implement dietary guidance in a consumer-friendly format. The centerpiece of the MyPlate system is the MyPlate graphic, found in **Appendix B**.

Aligned with the DGAs, MyPlate now provides specific recommendations for the various life cycle stages. Public health nutrition professionals should be aware of the many nutrition education resources available at www.myplate.gov.[26]

d. Nutrition Facts Labeling

The Nutrition Labeling and Education Act was passed by the U.S. Congress in 1990 to provide the FDA with authority to regulate food labels and health claims on food labels. The information on food labels in the United States is calculated from the FDA's Daily Values (DVs), which are suggested guidelines for nutrient intake based on sample 2,000-calorie and 2,500-calorie diets.

Remember that while the DVs provide values similar to the DGAs and DRIs, they are not the same; rather, they are a specific set of values housed within the FDA and used for food labeling purposes. The DVs are more general than the DRIs and DGAs since only one value is provided for each nutrient listed on the label. Food labels would quickly become unreadable if values were listed for each age and gender group, as is done by the DRIs.[27] **Appendix G** provides an infographic with a consumer-friendly explanation of food labels based on the DVs.

Public health nutrition professionals should be prepared to educate populations on the use of food labels to make optimal nutritional choices. Two key points to remember about the Nutrition Facts Label are:

- The most important piece of information on the food label is the portion size. All of the other numbers on the label refer to one portion. Thus, if there are two servings per container, and you consume the whole container, you should multiply all the other numbers on the label by 2.
- Remember this rule of thumb: 5% or less = low, 6% to 19% = moderate, and 20% or greater = high. So, a product providing 3% of the DV for sodium would be low in sodium, while a product providing 38% of the DV for sodium would be high in sodium.

e. Nutrient density

Nutrient density is not an official dietary guidance term used to direct nutrition policy. The term, however, can be a helpful concept for understanding which foods are most healthful and for providing nutrition education to the public.

Nutrient density can be thought of as the relationship between the nutrient content of a food and the energy (calories) it provides. Some foods, such as fruits and vegetables, provide very high nutrient content along with low energy content.

The concept of nutrient density can be thought of as analogous to purchasing a product; that is, consumers want to obtain the most value for each dollar. Similarly, consumption of recommended amounts of fruits and vegetables provides excellent nutrient value for fewer calories.

So, we want to base our diets on high-nutrient, low-calorie foods, *but* it is crucial to remember that some high-calorie foods are also very nutrient-dense, and are key components of a healthful diet. Examples of such foods include nuts, seeds, healthful oils and fats, nut butters, avocados, and the like. The concept of getting the most value for one's calories applies to these foods, too. The key to getting the most health value from nutrient-dense, high-calorie foods is to exercise portion control.

Review Questions

1. In your own words, list and describe each DRI.
2. Review the Executive Summary of the DGAs found at https://www.dietaryguidelines.gov/sites/default/files/2020-12/DGA_2020-2025_ExecutiveSummary_English.pdf. Then, list the four major Dietary Guidelines.
3. Review the MyPlate website at www.myplate.gov. List and describe two resources you find interesting.
4. What is considered the most important piece of information on the Nutrition Facts label, and why?
5. Explain why both low- and high-calorie foods can be nutrient-dense.

REFERENCES

1. Academy of Nutrition and Dietetics. *Definition of Terms List.* Commission on Dietetic Registration; 2021. https://www.eatrightpro.org/-/media/files/eatrightpro/practice/academy-definition-of-terms-list-feb-2021.pdf
2. Lagua RT, Claudio VS. *Nutrition and Diet Therapy Reference Dictionary.* 5th ed. Blackwell Publishing; 2004.
3. Cannon G. The rise and fall of dietetics and of nutrition science, 4000 BCE–2000 CE. *Public Health Nutr.* 2005;8(6a):701–705. https://doi.org/10.1079/phn2005766
4. Semba RD. The discovery of the vitamins. *Int J Vitam Nutr Res.* 2012;82(5):310–315. https://doi.org/10.1024/0300-9831/a000124
5. Florida Department of Health. The Life Course Theory. Florida Health: Maternal and Child Health Section. Updated March 9, 2021. https://www.floridahealth.gov/programs-and-services/womens-health/florida-life-course-indicator-report/life-course-theory-1.html
6. National Institute of Diabetes and Digestive and Kidney Diseases. Your digestive system & how it works. Accessed October 27, 2023. https://www.niddk.nih.gov/health-information/digestive-diseases/digestive-system-how-it-works
7. U.S. Department of Agriculture. Macronutrients. National Agricultural Library. Accessed May 29, 2023. https://www.nal.usda.gov/human-nutrition-and-food-safety/food-composition/macronutrients
8. Merrill AL, Watt BK. *Energy Value of Foods: Basis and Derivation.* U.S. Department of Agriculture; 1973.
9. Weininger J. Essential nutrients. In: *Britannica.* The Britannica Group; 2023.
10. Hishiyama N, Kayanuma H, Matsui T, et al. Plasma concentration of vitamin C in dogs with a portosystemic shunt. *Can J Vet Res.* 2006;70(4):305–307.
11. Hermann J. Carbohydrates in the diet. Oklahoma State University; 2021. https://extension.okstate.edu/fact-sheets/carbohydrates-in-the-diet.html
12. Cleveland Clinic. Glycogen. Accessed May 29, 2023. https://my.clevelandclinic.org/health/articles/23509-glycogen
13. Office of Disease Prevention and Health Promotion. Applying Dietary Reference Intakes in professional settings. U.S. Department of Health and Human Services. Updated January 18, 2023. https://health.gov/our-work/nutrition-physical-activity/dietary-guidelines/dietary-reference-intakes/applying-dietary-reference-intakes-professional-settings
14. U.S. Department of Agriculture, U.S. Department of Health and Human Services. *Dietary Guidelines for Americans 2020–2025.* 9th ed. U.S. Department of Health and Human Services; 2020. https://www.dietaryguidelines.gov

15. Food and Drug Administration. Interactive nutrition facts label: protein. U.S. Department of Health and Human Services; October 2021. https://www.accessdata.fda.gov/scripts/InteractiveNutritionFactsLabel/assets/InteractiveNFL_Protein_October2021.pdf
16. Cleveland Clinic. Lipids. Accessed June 1, 2023. https://my.clevelandclinic.org/health/body/24425-lipids
17. Field CJ, Robinson L. Dietary fats. *Adv Nutr*. 2019;10(4):722–724. https://doi.org/10.1093/advances/nmz052
18. Harvard T.H. Chan School of Public Health. The nutrition source: shining the spotlight on trans fats. Harvard University. Accessed June 1, 2023. https://www.hsph.harvard.edu/nutritionsource/what-should-you-eat/fats-and-cholesterol/types-of-fat/transfats
19. Centers for Disease Control and Prevention. Vitamin D. Infant and toddler nutrition. Accessed May 31, 2023. https://www.cdc.gov/nutrition/infantandtoddlernutrition/vitamins-minerals/vitamin-d.html
20. National Center for Complementary and Integrative Health. Using dietary supplements wisely. U.S. Department of Health and Human Services. Updated September 25, 2023. https://www.nccih.nih.gov/health/using-dietary-supplements-wisely
21. Office of Dietary Supplements. Strengthening knowledge and understanding of dietary supplements. National Institutes of Health. Accessed May 31, 2023. https://ods.od.nih.gov
22. Cleveland Clinic. Malnutrition. Accessed May 30, 2023. https://my.clevelandclinic.org/health/diseases/22987-malnutrition
23. Devine A, Lawlis T. Nutrition and vulnerable groups. *Nutrients*. 2019;11(5):1066. https://doi.org/10.3390/nu11051066
24. National Academies of Sciences, Engineering, and Medicine. *Dietary reference Intakes for energy*. The National Academies Press, p. 23. 2023. https://doi.org/10.17226/26818
25. The National Academies of Sciences, Engineering, and Medicine. Infographic: expansion of the dietary reference intake model. 2023. https://nap.nationalacademies.org/resource/25353/interactive/
26. U.S. Department of Agriculture. MyPlate. Accessed May 31, 2023. https://www.myplate.gov
27. Callahan A, Leonard H, Powell T. Understanding food labeling. In: *Nutrition: Science and Everyday Application*. Open Oregon Educational Resources; 2020. https://openoregon.pressbooks.pub/nutritionscience/chapter/1e-understanding-food-labels

APPENDIX B: MYPLATE GRAPHIC

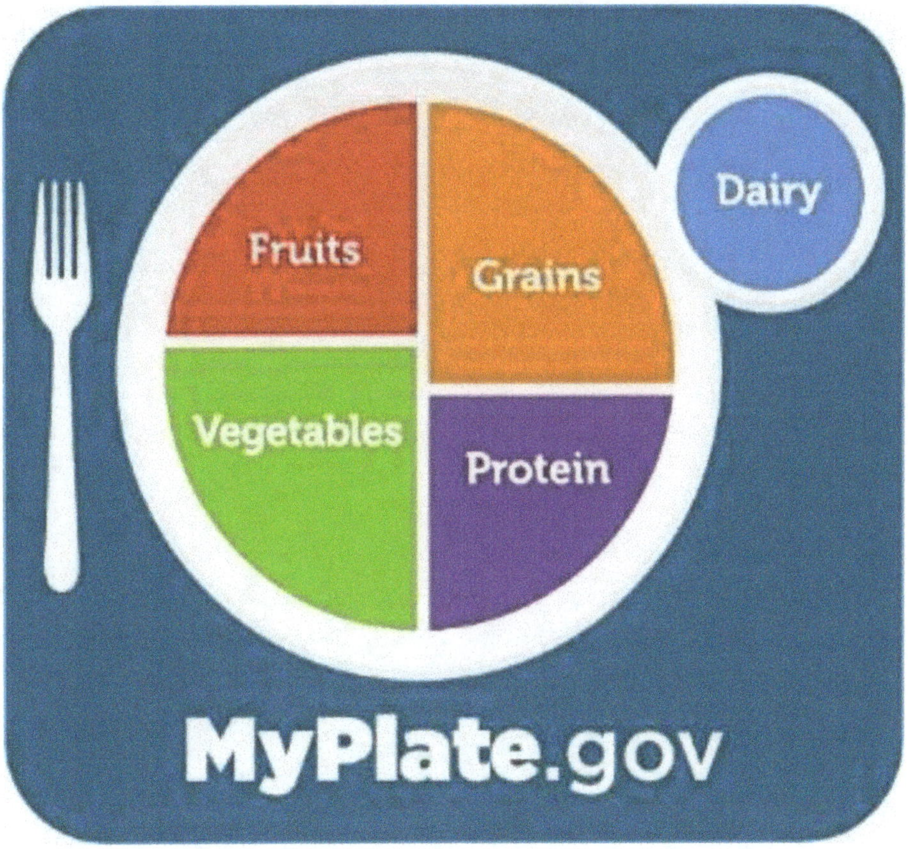

Source: Courtesy of the U.S. Department of Agriculture.

APPENDIX C: DIETARY REFERENCE INTAKES

Types of Dietary Reference Intakes (DRI) Values		
DRI Reference Value	**Definition**	**Purpose**
Acceptable Macronutrient Distribution Range (AMDR)	"A range of usual intakes for a macronutrient that is associated with a reduced risk of chronic disease while providing adequate intakes of essential nutrients; an AMDR is expressed as a percentage of total energy intake"	Preventing chronic disease
Adequate Intake (AI)	"The recommended average daily intake based on observed or experimentally determined approximations or estimates of nutrient intake by a group (or groups) of individuals that are assumed to be adequate—used when an RDA cannot be determined"	Meeting nutrient requirements
Chronic Disease Risk Reduction Intake (CDRR)	"Characterizes nutrient intakes that are expected to reduce the risk of developing chronic disease."	Preventing chronic disease
Estimated Average Requirement (EAR)	"The average daily nutrient intake estimated to meet the requirement of half the individuals in a particular sex and life-stage group"	Meeting nutrient requirements
Estimated Energy Requirement (EER)	"The average dietary energy intake that is predicted to maintain energy balance in an adult of a defined age, sex, weight, height, and level of physical activity"	Meeting nutrient requirements
Recommended Dietary Allowance (RDA)	"The average daily dietary nutrient intake sufficient to meet the nutrient requirements of nearly all (97–98%) individuals in a particular sex and life-stage group."	Meeting nutrient requirements

Types of Dietary Reference Intakes (DRI) Values		
DRI Reference Value	**Definition**	**Purpose**
Tolerable Upper Intake Level (UI)	"The highest average daily nutrient intake that is likely to pose no risk of adverse health effects to almost all individuals in the general population; as intake increases above the UL, the potential risk of adverse effects may increase."	Preventing excessive intake

Source: Adapted from National Academies of Sciences, Engineering, and Medicine. *Dietary reference intakes for energy*. 2023. The National Academies Press. p. 23. https://doi.org/10.17226/26818. All quotations except CDRR are from this source; CDRR quote is from The National Academies of Sciences, Engineering, and Medicine. Infographic: expansion of the dietary reference intake model. 2023. https://nap.nationalacademies.org/resource/25353/interactive/
Dietary reference intakes: the essential guide to nutrient requirements is available to read online or as a PDF download at https://nap.nationalacademies.org/catalog/11537/dietary-reference-intakes-the-essential-guide-to-nutrient-requirements
Links to many DRI documents for many specific nutrients are available at: https://health.gov/our-work/nutrition-physical-activity/dietary-guidelines/dietary-reference-intakes/applying-dietary-reference-intakes-professional-settingsi

APPENDIX D: MAJOR U.S. DOMESTIC POLICIES AND PROGRAMS FOR PUBLIC HEALTH NUTRITION, ORGANIZED BY LIFE COURSE STAGE

Life Course Stage	Program	Eligibility	Major Provisions
Across the Lifespan	Supplemental Nutrition Assistance Program (SNAP)[1]	Income, assets, and work status State Eligibility[2]	Monthly benefits to purchase food through certified retail locations (excludes alcohol and tobacco products)
Across the Lifespan	SNAP Nutrition Education (SNAP-Ed)[3]	States with Broad-Based Categorical Eligibility (BBCE) policies with gross income limits up to 200% of the federal poverty level. SNAP-Ed eligibility limits should not exceed the State threshold for BBCE, as listed at www.fns.usda.gov/snap/broad-based-categorical-eligibility.	Direct nutrition education, social marketing campaigns, and policy systems and environmental strategies Nutrition education and obesity prevention promoting healthy food choices and physical activity consistent with the most recent Dietary Guidelines for Americans
Across the Lifespan	The Gus Schumacher Nutrition Incentive Program (GusNIP)[4]	Nonprofit organizations and government agencies are eligible to apply for the GusNIP Nutrition Incentive Program and the GusNIP Produce Prescription Program.	Competitive grant program Provides financial incentives to participants at nutritional risk, to increase fruit and vegetable consumption

Life Course Stage	Program	Eligibility	Major Provisions
Across the Lifespan	The Expanded Food and Nutrition Education Program (EFNEP)[5]	Federal Extension (community outreach) program operating in every state, the District of Columbia, and the six U.S. territories by the 1862 and 1890 Land-Grant Universities	Nutrition education via hands-on learning and applied science, to support participants' efforts toward self-sufficiency, nutritional health, and well-being Collection of program data to measure and ensure program effectiveness, efficiency, and accountability
Across the Lifespan	The Emergency Food Assistance Program (TEFAP)[6]	Income eligibility, set by states Recipients of prepared meals are considered low-income and eligible.	Through TEFAP, the U.S. Department of Agriculture (USDA) purchases nutritious, high-quality USDA Foods, which are then available for distribution by states. Local agencies can either distribute the USDA Foods to eligible recipients for household consumption or use them to prepare and serve meals in a congregate setting.
Across the Lifespan	Food Distribution Program on Indian Reservations (FDPIR)[7]	Income-eligible American Indian and non-Indian households that reside on a reservation and households living in approved areas near a reservation or in Oklahoma that contain at least one person who is a member of a Federally recognized tribe are eligible to participate in FDPIR. Households are certified based on income standards set by the Federal government Households may not participate in FDPIR and SNAP in the same month.	Many households participate in FDPIR as an alternative to SNAP because they do not have easy access to SNAP offices or authorized food stores. Each month, participating households receive a food package to help them maintain a nutritionally balanced diet. Participants may select from over 100 products.

Life Course Stage	Program	Eligibility	Major Provisions
Maternal and Infant Health	Special Supplemental Nutrition Program for Women, Infants and Children (WIC)[8]	Categorical—pregnant, postpartum, breastfeeding women, infant, or child to age 5 Residential—must live within the state in which they apply Income—eligibility guidelines[9] Nutritional risk—medical-based or dietary-based conditions	Federal grants to states, territories, and Indian Tribal Organizations for supplemental food prescription; healthcare referrals; and nutrition education
Maternal and Infant Health	Breastfeeding Peer Counselors	Must be a WIC participant	Breastfeeding support is a standard component of WIC. The Peer Counselor program has specific funding from Congress. Address the barriers to breastfeeding through breastfeeding education, support, and role modeling
Maternal and Infant Health	WIC Farmers Market Nutrition Program	Must be a WIC participant Women, infants over 4 months old, children 1 to 5 years of age	Federal grants to states, territories, and Indian Tribal Organizations In addition to their regular WIC benefits, eligible participants are issued Farmers Market Nutrition Program coupons, which can then be used to purchase eligible foods from specific vendor types (farmers, farmers markets, or roadside stands).

Life Course Stage	Program	Eligibility	Major Provisions
Infant and Child Health	WIC/WIC Breastfeeding Peer Counselors/WIC Farmers Market Nutrition Program	See preceding entry	
Infant and Child Health	Child and Adult Care Food Program (CACFP)[10]	Children and adults enrolled in participating child care centers, day-care homes, and adult day-care centers Children and youth participating in afterschool care programs, children residing in emergency shelters, and adults over the age of 60 or living with a disability and enrolled in day-care facilities	Provides reimbursements for nutritious meals and snacks to eligible children and adults Nutrition standards for meals and snacks based on age of participant
Child and Adolescent Health	School Breakfast[11]	Families with children may be determined "categorically eligible" for free meals through participation in certain Federal Assistance Programs, or based on their status as a homeless, migrant, runaway, or foster child. Families with children can also qualify for free or reduced-price school meals based on household income and family size. Children from families with incomes at or below 130% of the Federal poverty level are eligible for free meals. Those with incomes between 130% and 185% of the Federal poverty level are eligible for reduced-price meals.	Federally assisted meal program operating in public and nonprofit private schools and residential child care institutions Nutrition standards are based on age of participating child. Meals can be served in the cafeteria, in the classroom, or "on the go."

Life Course Stage	Program	Eligibility	Major Provisions
Child and Adolescent Health	Special Milk Program[12]	Participating schools and institutions receive reimbursement from the USDA for each half pint of milk served. Any child at a participating school or half-day prekindergarten program can get milk through the Special Milk Program. Children may buy milk or receive it free, depending on the school's choice of program options. Same income guidelines as the NSLP for families with children eligible for free or reduced-price milk.	Provides milk to children in schools, child care institutions, and eligible camps that do not participate in other federal child nutrition meal service programs. Schools or institutions must offer only pasteurized fluid types of fat-free or low-fat (1%) milk.
Child and Adolescent Health	National School Lunch Program (NSLP)[13]	Children may be determined "categorically eligible" for free meals through participation in certain Federal Assistance Programs, or based on their status as a homeless, migrant, runaway, or foster child. Children can also qualify for free or reduced-price school meals based on household income and family size. Children from families with incomes at or below 130% of the Federal poverty level are eligible for free meals. Those with incomes between 130% and 185% of the Federal poverty level are eligible for reduced price meals.	Federally assisted meal program operating in public and nonprofit private schools and residential child care institutions. NSLP institutions must serve lunches that meet Federal meal pattern requirements. States receive cash reimbursement and can select USDA Foods for their schools from a list of foods purchased by USDA and provided through the NSLP.

Life Course Stage	Program	Eligibility	Major Provisions
Child and Adolescent Health	Fresh Fruit and Vegetable Program (FFVP)[14]	Elementary schools in all 50 States, the District of Columbia, and the territories of Guam, Puerto Rico, and the Virgin Islands are eligible to participate. Schools must operate the NSLP Program prioritizes schools with the highest percentage of children certified as eligible for free and reduced-price meals.	Federally assisted program providing free fresh fruits and vegetables to children at eligible elementary schools during the school day The goals of the FFVP: Introduce children to fresh fruits and vegetables. Increase overall acceptance and consumption of fresh, unprocessed produce among children. Provide nutrition education and thus encourage healthier school environments.
Child and Adolescent Health	Farm to School[15]	Schools and districts, Indian Tribal Organizations, agricultural producers or groups of agricultural producers, nonprofit entities, and State and local agencies	Increase the amount of local foods served in school meals Improve nutrition education to support local foods in schools
Adult Health	Senior Farmers Market Nutrition Program[16]	Income <185% of federal poverty income guidelines	Provide low-income seniors with access to locally grown fruits, vegetables, honey, and herbs Grants to states, the District of Columbia, U.S. Territories, and federally recognized Indian tribal governments
Adult Health	Child and Adult Care Food Program (CACFP)	See preceding entry	

Life Course Stage	Program	Eligibility	Major Provisions
Adult Health	Senior Nutrition Programs (Older Americans Act)[17]	Includes Congregate Nutrition Program and the Home Delivered Nutrition Program 60 years of age or older to be eligible for the nutrition programs While there is no income/means test, services are targeted to older individuals who have the greatest economic or social need.	Provide grants to states to help support nutrition services for older people Meals provide at least one-third of the recommended Dietary Reference Intakes established by the Food and Nutrition Board of the Institute of Medicine of the National Academy of Sciences, and adhere to the current Dietary Guidelines for Americans. The purposes of these programs are to (1) reduce hunger and food insecurity, (2) promote socialization, (3) promote health and well-being, and (4) delay adverse health conditions. Overall, these programs increase the ability of older adults who are at risk of losing their independence to stay in their community by providing nutrition services.
Adult Health	Commodity Supplemental Food Package (CSFP)[18]	Must be a resident of a state, territory or Indian Tribal Organization that administers the program States/jurisdictions establish income limits for persons 60 years of age or older and who are at or below 130% of the Federal Poverty Income Guidelines. Children who were certified and receiving CSFP benefits as of February 6, 2014, can continue to receive assistance until they are no longer eligible. States determine eligibility.	USDA distributes both food and administrative funds to participating states and Indian Tribal Organizations (ITOs).

REFERENCES

1. U.S. Department of Agriculture Food and Nutrition Service. Supplemental Nutrition Assistance Program. Accessed August 30, 2022. https://www.fns.usda.gov/snap/supplemental-nutrition-assistance-program
2. U.S. Department of Agriculture Food and Nutrition Service. SNAP state directory of resources. Accessed August 30, 2022. https://www.fns.usda.gov/snap/state-directory
3. U.S. Department of Agriculture SNAP-Ed Connection. About. Accessed August 30, 2022. https://snaped.fns.usda.gov/about
4. U.S. Department of Agriculture National Institute of Food and Agriculture. Gus Schumacher Nutrition Incentive Program. Accessed August 30, 2022. http://www.nifa.usda.gov/grants/programs/hunger-food-security-programs/gus-schumacher-nutrition-incentive-program
5. U.S. Department of Agriculture National Institute of Food and Agriculture. Expanded Food and Nutrition Education Program (EFNEP). Accessed August 30, 2022. http://www.nifa.usda.gov/grants/programs/capacity-grants/expanded-food-nutrition-education-program-efnep
6. U.S. Department of Agriculture. The Emergency Food Assistance Program. Published January 2020. https://fns-prod.azureedge.us/sites/default/files/resource-files/tefap-program-fact-sheet-2019_1.6.20.pdf
7. U.S. Department of Agriculture. Food distribution program on Indian reservations. Accessed August 30, 2022. https://www.fns.usda.gov/fdpir/food-distribution-program-indian-reservations
8. U.S. Department of Agriculture Food and Nutrition Service. Special Supplemental Nutrition Program for Women, Infants, and Children (WIC). Accessed August 30, 2022. https://www.fns.usda.gov/wic
9. U.S. Department of Agriculture Food and Nutrition Service. Publication of the 2022–2023 WIC Income Eligibility Guidelines. Published April 19, 2022. https://www.fns.usda.gov/wic/ieg-2022-2023
10. U.S. Department of Agriculture Food and Nutrition Service. Child and Adult Care Food Program. Accessed August 30, 2022. https://www.fns.usda.gov/cacfp
11. U.S. Department of Agriculture. The School Breakfast Program. Updated November 2017. https://fns-prod.azureedge.us/sites/default/files/resource-files/SBPfactsheet.pdf
12. U.S. Department of Agriculture. Special Milk Program. Published August 2012 https://fns-prod.azureedge.us/sites/default/files/resource-files/SMPFactSheet.pdf
13. U.S. Department of Agriculture. The National School Lunch Program. Updated November 2017. https://fns-prod.azureedge.us/sites/default/files/resource-files/NSLPFactSheet.pdf
14. U.S. Department of Agriculture. The Fresh Fruit and Vegetable Program. Updated December 2017. https://fns-prod.azureedge.us/sites/default/files/resource-files/FFVPFactSheet.pdf
15. U.S. Department of Agriculture Food and Nutrition Service. Farm to School Grant Program. PublishedJuly 25, 2022. https://www.fns.usda.gov/f2s/farm-school-grant-program
16. U.S. Department of Agriculture. Seniors Farmers' Market Nutrition Program. Published May 2023. https://www.fns.usda.gov/sfmnp/fact-sheet
17. U.S. Department of Health and Human Services. Older Americans Act Nutrition Programs. Modified July 5, 2016. https://acl.gov/sites/default/files/news%202017-03/OAA-Nutrition_Programs_Fact_Sheet.pdf
18. U.S. Department of Agriculture Food and Nutrition Service. Commodity Supplemental Food Program. Accessed August 30, 2022. https://www.fns.usda.gov/csfp/commodity-supplemental-food-program

APPENDIX E: PEDIATRIC GROWTH CHARTS: SELECTED EXAMPLES

For a complete set of growth charts, please see the links below:

World Health Organization (WHO) Growth Charts: www.cdc.gov/growthcharts/who_charts.htm

Centers for Disease Control and Prevention (CDC) Growth Charts: www.cdc.gov/growthcharts/who_charts.htm

CDC Extended BMI-for-age Growth Charts: www.cdc.gov/growthcharts/who_charts.htm

Birth to 24 months: Boys
Head circumference-for-age and
Weight-for-length percentiles

NAME ______________________

RECORD # __________

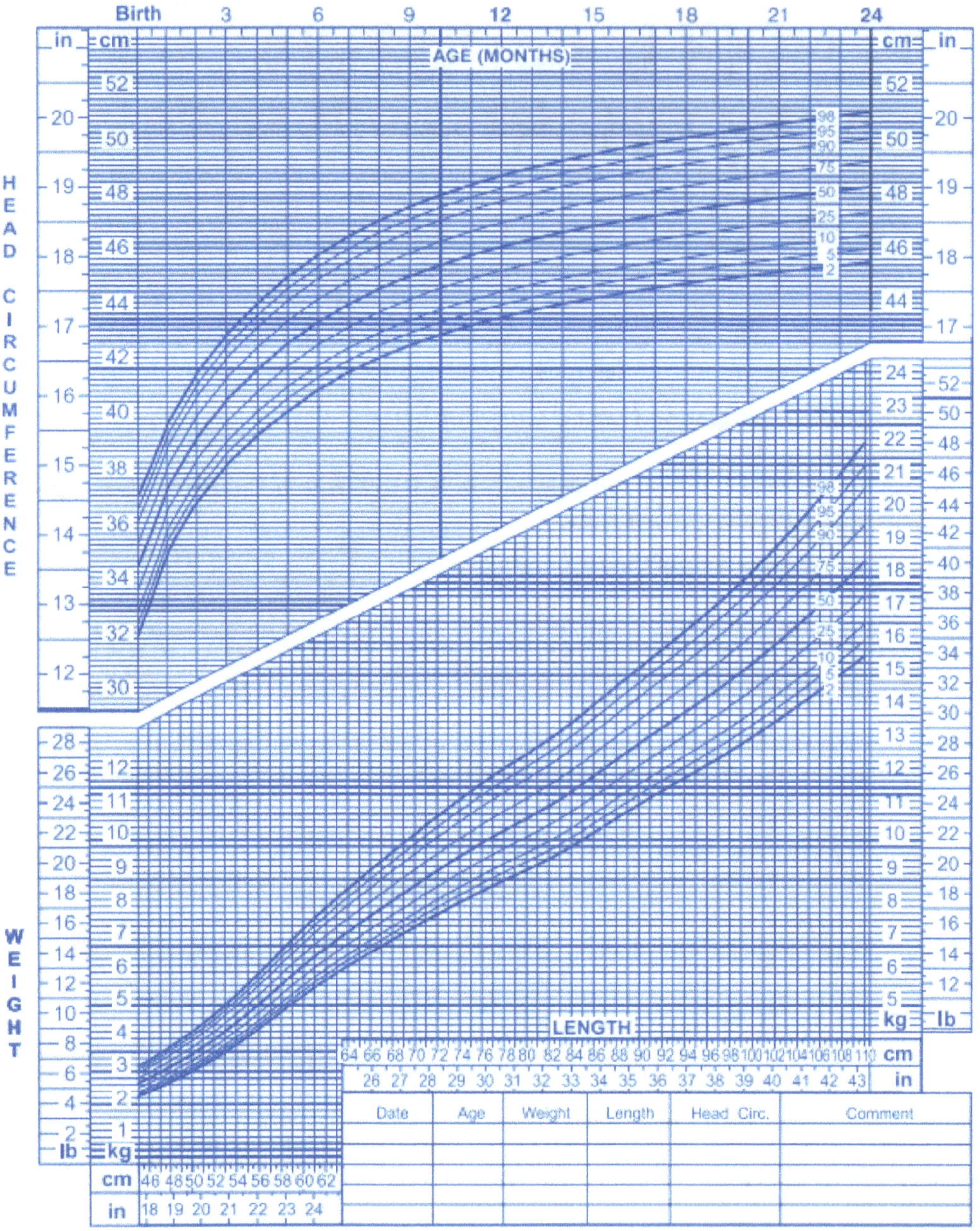

Published by the Centers for Disease Control and Prevention, November 1, 2009
SOURCE: WHO Child Growth Standards (http://www.who.int/childgrowth/en)

Birth to 24 months: Girls
Head circumference-for-age and Weight-for-length percentiles

NAME ______________________

RECORD # ____________

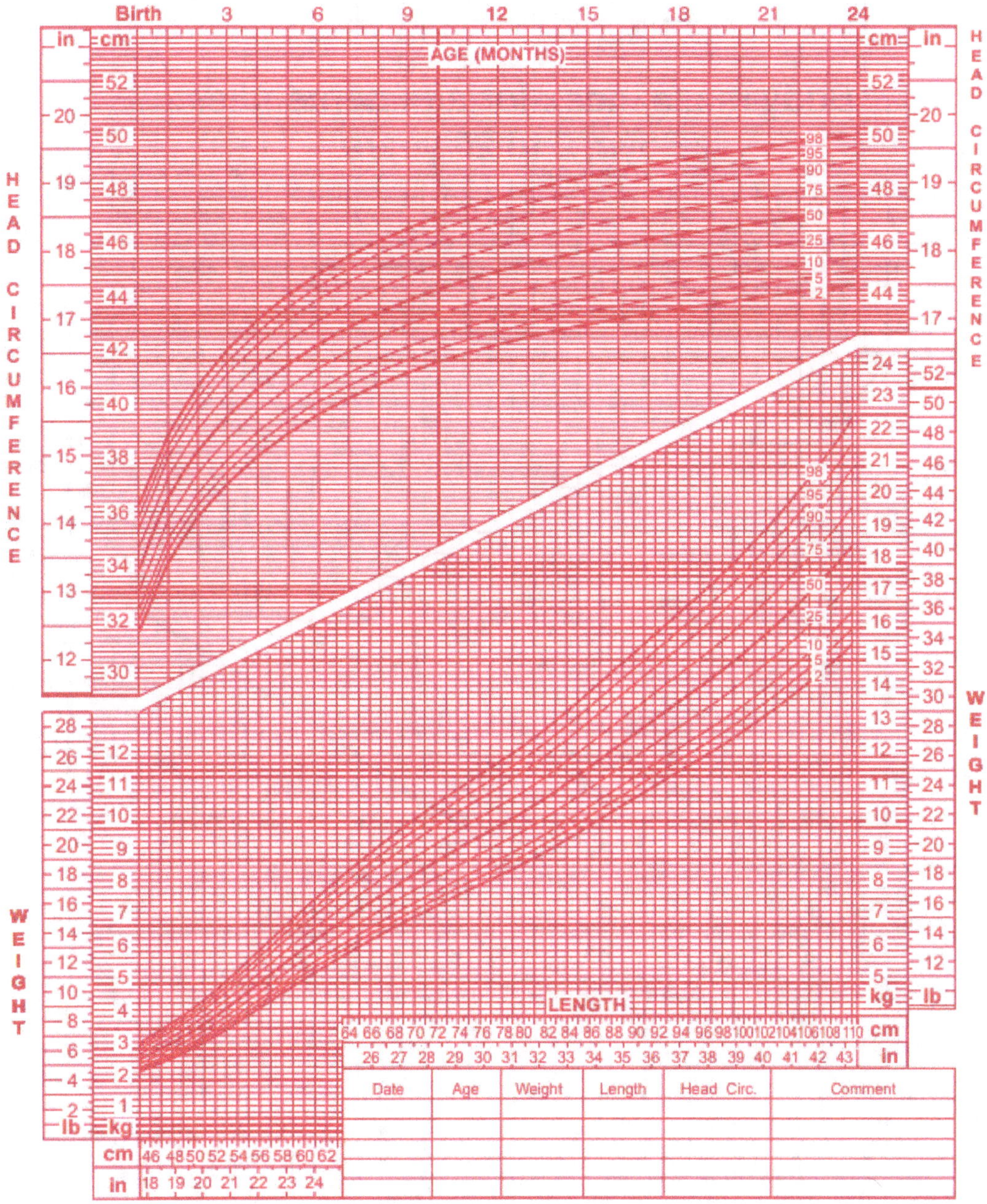

Date	Age	Weight	Length	Head Circ.	Comment

Published by the Centers for Disease Control and Prevention, November 1, 2009
SOURCE: WHO Child Growth Standards (http://www.who.int/childgrowth/en)

CDC Growth Charts: United States

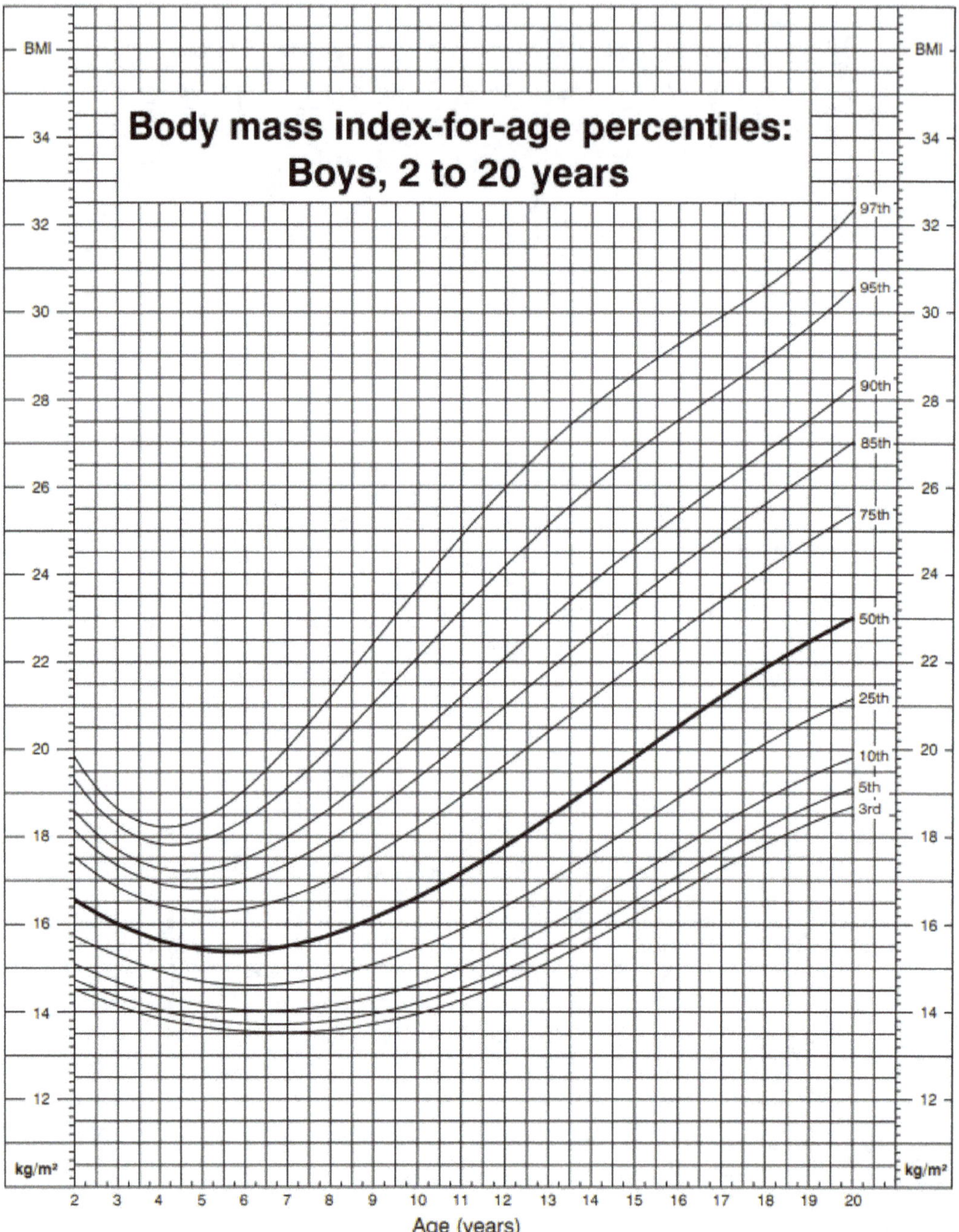

Published May 30, 2000.
SOURCE: Developed by the National Center for Health Statistics in collaboration with the National Center for Chronic Disease Prevention and Health Promotion (2000).

SAFER · HEALTHIER · PEOPLE™

2 to 20 years: Girls
Body mass index-for-age percentiles

NAME ________________

RECORD # ________

Date	Age	Weight	Stature	BMI*	Comments

***To Calculate BMI**: Weight (kg) ÷ Stature (cm) ÷ Stature (cm) x 10,000
or Weight (lb) ÷ Stature (in) ÷ Stature (in) x 703

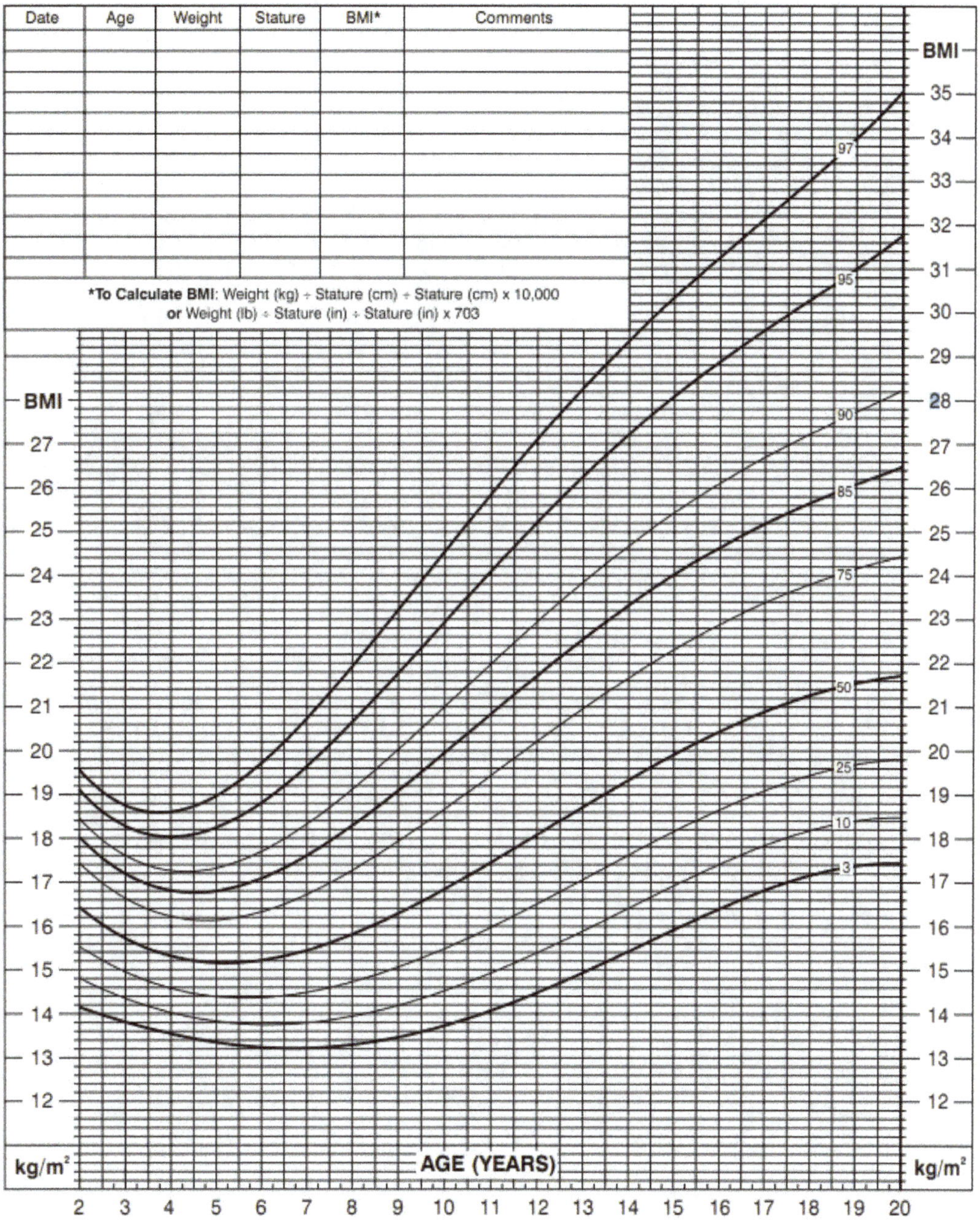

Published May 30, 2000 (modified 10/16/00).
SOURCE: Developed by the National Center for Health Statistics in collaboration with the National Center for Chronic Disease Prevention and Health Promotion (2000).
http://www.cdc.gov/growthcharts

CDC
SAFER • HEALTHIER • PEOPLE™

APPENDIX F: BODY MASS INDEX (BMI) CHART (ADULTS)

Body Mass Index Table

	Normal						Overweight					Obese										Extreme Obesity														
BMI	19	20	21	22	23	24	25	26	27	28	29	30	31	32	33	34	35	36	37	38	39	40	41	42	43	44	45	46	47	48	49	50	51	52	53	54
Height (inches)																	Body Weight (pounds)																			
58	91	96	100	105	110	115	119	124	129	134	138	143	148	153	158	162	167	172	177	181	186	191	196	201	205	210	215	220	224	229	234	239	244	248	253	258
59	94	99	104	109	114	119	124	128	133	138	143	148	153	158	163	168	173	178	183	188	193	198	203	208	212	217	222	227	232	237	242	247	252	257	262	267
60	97	102	107	112	118	123	128	133	138	143	148	153	158	163	168	174	179	184	189	194	199	204	209	215	220	225	230	235	240	245	250	255	261	266	271	276
61	100	106	111	116	122	127	132	137	143	148	153	158	164	169	174	180	185	190	195	201	206	211	217	222	227	232	238	243	248	254	259	264	269	275	280	285
62	104	109	115	120	126	131	136	142	147	153	158	164	169	175	180	186	191	196	202	207	213	218	224	229	235	240	246	251	256	262	267	273	278	284	289	295
63	107	113	118	124	130	135	141	146	152	158	163	169	175	180	186	191	197	203	208	214	220	225	231	237	242	248	254	259	265	270	278	282	287	293	299	304
64	110	116	122	128	134	140	145	151	157	163	169	174	180	186	192	197	204	209	215	221	227	232	238	244	250	256	262	267	273	279	285	291	296	302	308	314
65	114	120	126	132	138	144	150	156	162	168	174	180	186	192	198	204	210	216	222	228	234	240	246	252	258	264	270	276	282	288	294	300	306	312	318	324
66	118	124	130	136	142	148	155	161	167	173	179	186	192	198	204	210	216	223	229	235	241	247	253	260	266	272	278	284	291	297	303	309	315	322	328	334
67	121	127	134	140	146	153	159	166	172	178	185	191	198	204	211	217	223	230	236	242	249	255	261	268	274	280	287	293	299	306	312	319	325	331	338	344
68	125	131	138	144	151	158	164	171	177	184	190	197	203	210	216	223	230	236	243	249	256	262	269	276	282	289	295	302	308	315	322	328	335	341	348	354
69	128	135	142	149	155	162	169	176	182	189	196	203	209	216	223	230	236	243	250	257	263	270	277	284	291	297	304	311	318	324	331	338	345	351	358	365
70	132	139	146	153	160	167	174	181	188	195	202	209	216	222	229	236	243	250	257	264	271	278	285	292	299	306	313	320	327	334	341	348	355	362	369	376
71	136	143	150	157	165	172	179	186	193	200	208	215	222	229	236	243	250	257	265	272	279	286	293	301	308	315	322	329	338	343	351	358	365	372	379	386
72	140	147	154	162	169	177	184	191	199	206	213	221	228	235	242	250	258	265	272	279	287	294	302	309	316	324	331	338	346	353	361	368	375	383	390	397
73	144	151	159	166	174	182	189	197	204	212	219	227	235	242	250	257	265	272	280	288	295	302	310	318	325	333	340	348	355	363	371	378	386	393	401	408
74	148	155	163	171	179	186	194	202	210	218	225	233	241	249	256	264	272	280	287	295	303	311	319	326	334	342	350	358	365	373	381	389	396	404	412	420
75	152	160	168	176	184	192	200	208	216	224	232	240	248	256	264	272	279	287	295	303	311	319	327	335	343	351	359	367	375	383	391	399	407	415	423	431
76	156	164	172	180	189	197	205	213	221	230	238	246	254	263	271	279	287	295	304	312	320	328	336	344	353	361	369	377	385	394	402	410	418	426	435	443

Source: National Heart, Lung, and Blood Institute. Aim for a healthy weight: body mass index table (PDF version). Accessed October 31, 2023. https://www.nhlbi.nih.gov/health/educational/lose_wt/BMI/bmi_tbl.htm

APPENDIX G: NUTRITION FACTS LABEL

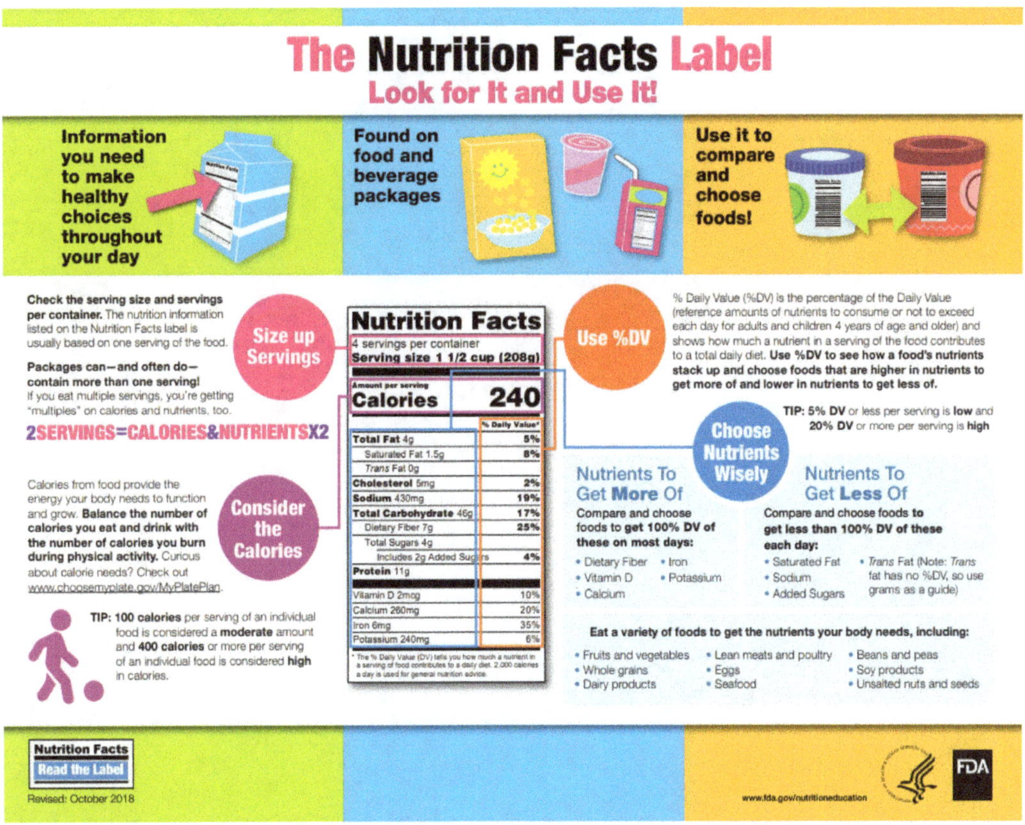

Source: U.S. Food and Drug Administration. Read the label outreach materials: read the label infographic. Accessed October 31, 2023. https://www.fda.gov/media/89314/download?attachment

GLOSSARY

Absenteeism: The absence of an employee from work for lengths of time that exceed expected guidelines and employer provisions such as paid time off, family leave, medical time off, and scheduled vacations. Health conditions such as chronic disease may be associated with absenteeism.

Adiposity rebound: Second rise in body mass index (BMI) that occurs between ages 3 and 7 years.

Adolescence: The life cycle phase during the transition from childhood to adulthood; considered to extend, with some individual variation, from about 10 to 11 years to about 18 to 21 years.

Adverse childhood experiences (ACEs): Traumatic events that occur during childhood that can have lifelong lasting effects. According to the Centers for Disease Control and Prevention, ACEs are traumatic events or ongoing situations that occur in childhood (0–17 years) such as neglect, abuse, exposure to violence, exposure to substance abuse, incarceration of a family member, and/or the mental illness of a family member. ACEs are often associated with social determinants of health such as unstable housing or poverty. The commonality among ACEs is that they impair the normal development of a child's sense of safety and stability in the world, and create barriers to healthy bonding with caring adults. ACEs are associated with higher lifetime risk of a number of difficulties including physical and mental health problems and food insecurity.

Affordable Care Act (ACA): A comprehensive healthcare reform law that was passed in 2010. Medicaid expansion associated with the ACA expanded access to healthcare for many low-income individuals in the United States; the act also made treatment for chronic diseases associated with obesity more available to many persons.

Anemia: Condition in which the body does not have enough healthy red blood cells to transport oxygen to body tissues, or there are enough red blood cells but they are impaired in their ability to transport oxygen.

Arteriosclerosis: Stiffening of the blood vessels that occurs with age.

Baby-led weaning: Infant feeding method that promotes self-feeding from the start when initiating complementary foods.

Behavioral economics: The theory that assumes people do not always approach economic decisions from a rational perspective, but often apply emotions and habits to everyday economic choices in an irrational manner. To truly understand human economic decisions, it is necessary to apply human psychology. Thus, behavioral economics is described as the marriage of economics and psychology.

Behavioral Risk Factor Surveillance System (BRFSS): A health surveillance system used to monitor trends in health-related risk behaviors, chronic health conditions, and use of preventive services (www.cdc.gov/brfss/index.html).

Bilirubin: Yellow pigment found in bile; by-product of the degradation of fetal red blood cells after birth.

Bioavailability of nutrients: Expressed as a percentage, bioavailability of a particular nutrient is the amount of that nutrient that can be utilized by the body through usual metabolic processes. It is impacted by many factors, including but not limited to dietary, culinary, genetic, and physiologic influences.

Bioavailable: The proportion of a nutrient that is absorbed and utilized by the body.

Biosurveillance: Testing for the safety of food and water supplies is essential to promote the well-being of the public during a disaster and especially during its aftermath. Public health professionals may be involved in testing and monitoring community food and water supplies to promote public safety and prevent food- and waterborne illness.

Body mass index (BMI): An individual's weight in kilograms (or pounds) divided by height in meters squared (or inches squared). The metric equation for calculating BMI is: weight (kg)/height (m^2). In English measurements, the equation is: weight (pounds)/height (inches^2) x 703 (conversion factor). BMI is most often used as a screening tool to check for degrees of body fatness (inadequate or excessive) that may increase risk for adverse health conditions. BMI results may be used as one indicator in an overall health and/or nutrition assessment performed by a qualified professional but should not be used in themselves to diagnose degree of body fatness or disease/health conditions.

Built environment: The human-made surroundings, including the human-made infrastructure and buildings that make up the neighborhoods in which people live their lives, that influence a person's health behaviors. The environment in which one lives and works can affect opportunities for physical activity and access to healthy foods, as well as one's risk for developing chronic diseases. Examples include safe spaces to walk, and the distance to reach a full-service grocery store or farmers market.

Centenarian: A person 100 years of age or older. In the past two decades, the number of centenarians in the world has approximately doubled.

Center for a Livable Future's Food Policy Networks (FPN): An organization affiliated with the Johns Hopkins Bloomberg School of Public Health that aims to help build a healthy, equitable, and resilient food system by working with policy makers, advocacy organizations, researchers, students, and community members.

Centers for Disease Control and Prevention (CDC): The primary U.S. federal agency responsible for protecting the health of the public by preventing and controlling disease, injury, and disability .

Channels: The mediums or pathways through which messages are transmitted. Communication channels include but are not limited to the spoken word, the written word, media. and the use of technology to convey messages.

Chronic condition: A condition that lasts for at least 1 year and is associated with the need for ongoing medical care and/or limitations in activities of daily living.

Clostridium botulinum: A species of bacteria that produces the toxin causing botulism.

Colic: Episodes of crying in an otherwise healthy baby, who cries for a very long time for no apparent reason without consolation.

Colostrum: The first form of breast milk following birth; it is nutrient-dense and high in antibodies.

Community engagement: According to the World Health Organization, the process of promoting well-being for positive health impacts and outcomes through relationship building with community stakeholders.

Community recovery: The process of a community's rebuilding after experiencing a disaster. Disaster recovery periods are often very difficult, and occur under substantial physical, emotional, and financial stress; however, the recovery period also offers opportunities to implement positive changes and enhance future disaster resilience.

Community resilience: The ability of a community to withstand, adjust to, and recover from disaster situations. Community resilience is enhanced by ongoing development of community resources, including nutrition resources, to enhance social determinants of health and well-being.

Community supported agriculture (CSA): A program in which individuals pledge their support to a farm operation to share the risks and benefits of food production.

Community-based participatory research: A research approach that includes community stakeholders as partners in the research process for the purpose of improving practices or promoting social change.

Complementary foods: Solid foods and fluids other than breast milk and formula.

Confounders: Factors that may impact the ability of investigators to draw conclusions from particular research studies. When confounding occurs, the effect of a specific measured factor on the outcome of interest may be blended with other, uncontrolled factors, making it difficult to determine the true impact of the measured factor.

Congregate nutrition program: A nutrition program for older adults in the United States, initiated in 1972 as a result of the federal Older Americans Act (OAA). It provides a nutritious meal served in a group setting most weekdays; contributes one third of the daily nutrient needs of older adults per the Dietary Reference Intakes (DRIs); and provides opportunities for socialization and group activities.

Countermeasures and mitigation: The provision of appropriate assistance to target populations in order to prevent, alleviate, or directly address the impacts of a disaster. In public health nutrition, countermeasures and mitigation can include access to nutrition supplies such as regular and specialized baby formula, baby food, prenatal vitamins, and medical food supplements such as nutritional beverages to populations with special life stage needs—for example, infants and older adults.

Critical period: A fixed time period when certain behaviors emerge, for example, feeding skills

Critical periods of childhood development: Specific time periods—with a well-defined beginning and ending—when the brain and body are ideally aligned for crucial developmental advancements to occur.

Cultural competence: The ability to interact and work effectively with others who come from cultures that are different from one's own.

Delayed puberty: The initiation of puberty after the age of 12 years in females, and after the age of 14 years in males. A medical evaluation is indicated.

Dental caries: Damage to a tooth that can happen when decay-causing bacteria in the mouth make acids that attack the tooth's surface, or enamel.

Diet culture: A set of social expectations (also known as wellness culture) related to how individuals should look and how they should eat, often linked to morality or worthiness, driven by systemic and structural factors.

Dietary diversity: The variety or the number of different food groups people eat over a given time

Dietary Guidelines: A set of recommendations that provides advice on what to eat and drink to meet nutrient needs, promote health, and prevent disease.

Dietary Guidelines for Americans (DGA): Nutritional advice for health promotion and disease prevention in the United States, written for policy makers, healthcare providers, and nutrition educators to provide guidance on federal, state, and local nutrition policies and programs .

Dietary Reference Intakes (DRIs): A set of reference values used to assess and plan the nutrient intakes of healthy people. With financial support from the governments of the United States and Canada, the DRIs are established jointly by the National Academies of Science, Engineering, and Medicine and Health Canada. The set of reference values includes: Recommended Daily Allowances (RDA), Estimated Average Requirements (EAR), Adequate Intakes (AI), Tolerable Upper Intake Levels (UL), Estimated Energy Requirements (EER), Acceptable Macronutrient Distribution Ranges (AMDR), and Chronic Disease Risk Reduction Intake. (CDRR). Appendix D provides further information.

Digestion: The biological process by which the nutrients in food become available to the human body. During digestion, food is ingested, broken down into its molecular components by both physical and chemical processes, and absorbed and utilized by the body. In the final stages of digestion, the waste products of nutrient breakdown are excreted.

Digital literacy: The ability to use information technologies and the Internet to find, evaluate, utilize, share, and create content.

Disability-adjusted life years (DALYs): Expected years of life after accounting for loss of health and presence of disabilities. A higher DALY value represents a greater disease burden. One DALY is equivalent to 1 year of health lost, and the total value of an individual's DALY is calculated as: (Expected years of life) – (Years of disability + Years of life lost). DALY data can be gathered for populations, analyzed, and used to develop policy.

Disparities: In public health, these aredifferences between the general population, or between/among population groups in factors including but not limited to race and ethnicity, sex, age, socioeconomic indicators, access to healthcare and nutrition services, access to education, and unfavorable environmental exposures.

Division of responsibility: Feeding principle developed by Ellyn Satter to guide the parent and child feeding dynamic at mealtime.

Downstream factors: Risk factors from individual-level unhealthy behaviors. For example, eating an unhealthful diet and smoking by an individual would be considered downstream health factors. Negative downstream factors may best be ameliorated by addressing upstream factors.

Early adolescence: While there is substantial developmental variation among individuals, early adolescence usually encompasses the ages of 10 to 11 years for girls and 13 to 14 years for boys. Early adolescence typically begins with the onset of puberty.

Early childhood caries: Dental caries in the primary teeth of young children (up to 5 years of age).

Early pregnancy loss: A pregnancy that ends on its own during the first 20 weeks of gestation, also called miscarriage. It is thought that as many as 10% to 20% of all known pregnancies end in miscarriage, and these usually occur as a result of fetal anomalies that are incompatible with life.

Early term: Described by the American College of Obstetricians and Gynecologists (ACOG) as the completion of pregnancy. Early term delivery is considered to occur at 37 to 38 weeks and 6 days of gestation. Until 2013, *full term* was considered delivery at any time between 37 and 42 weeks' gestation. However, more recent research indicates that important development of the lungs, liver, and brain occurs during gestational weeks 37 to 38. In addition, the risk of respiratory and other problems following birth is lowest when birth occurs at 39 to 40 weeks' gestation.

Earth observation (EO): The collection of information about Earth's biological, chemical, and physical systems to enable monitoring of natural and human-made environments and assess changes that may be occurring in the weather, land use, management of natural resources, and more. EO instruments can include ocean buoys, land stations, sonar and radar, environmental satellites, and global positioning system (GPS) stations that can collect data about land and ocean temperature, air quality, seismic activity, and precipitation trends, and estimate wildlife or human populations. EO data can help forecast weather, address health risks and the spread of disease, monitor crops for food security impacts, and assist with the mitigation and response to disasters.

Eating disorders: Serious mental and physical illnesses that involve complex and damaging relationships with food, eating, exercise, and body image.

Economic cost: Both the accounting or explicit cost *and* the opportunity or implicit cost of an action. For example, the explicit cost of an item might be $5.00; the implicit cost of the item is loss of the ability to spend that $5.00 on another item or opportunity.

Economic Research Service (ERS): A federal statistical agency that aims to conduct economic research on food, agriculture, and the environment to inform policy making.

Economic stability: A state in which people earn steady incomes that allow them to meet their health needs. Increasing employment and reducing poverty are two examples of economic stability objectives from *Healthy People 2030*.

Effectiveness: Results of an intervention (including nutrition interventions) in real-world settings.

Efficacy: Results of an intervention (including nutrition interventions) in ideal conditions, such as a laboratory or highly controlled environment.

Embryo: A newly developing offspring during weeks 4 to 8 of gestation. Developmentally, during this extremely important and delicate period, all the body's future systems are becoming differentiated and are in the first stages of development. Maternal nutritional status impacts embryonic growth and development; for example, adequate maternal folate status is associated with reduced risk of neural tube defects.

Emergency management: A management specialization that focuses on establishing systems by which communities and populations can mitigate risks of disasters and respond effectively to disasters.

Emotional intelligence: The use of perceived emotions to understand, regulate and use such perceptions in appropriate and productive ways.

Energy balance model (EBM): A model that posits that the difference in energy consumption and energy expenditure is the cause of weight changes.

Energy-yielding nutrients: Nutrients that provide calories. The energy-yielding nutrients are carbohydrates (4 calories per gram), protein (4 calories per gram), and fat (9 calories per gram). Alcohol also provides calories (7 calories per gram), but is not a nutrient.

Enteral feeding: The use of a tube to deliver feedings directly to the stomach or small intestine.

Environment: The places where people live, including their homes, communities, and societies. Environment interacts with the intrinsic capacities of older adults to impact the ability to age successfully.

Epigenetics: The study of heritable changes in gene expression that are not caused by changes in the DNA sequence.

Epiphyseal plate: A layer of cartilage within a bone that is responsible for bone growth. A long bone of the body is typically composed of three major areas: (1) the epiphyses, or the ends; (2) the diaphysis, or the shaft; and (3) the metaphysis, the area between the ends and the shaft of the bone. In children, the metaphyses encompass the epiphyseal plates. In adolescence, the cartilage cells of the epiphyseal plates continue growing, but are gradually replaced by bone cells until the bones are ossified and growth is complete—a process that is normally completed by early adulthood.

Evidence-based practice: Evidence-based practice (EBP) is an approach to decision-making in health care settings. EBP can be described as a process by which practitioners use the best quality evidence available, as well as consideration of patient/client/population values and preferences, to inform decision-making.

Extremely low birth weight: Birth weight <1,000 g (<2 lb 4 oz).

Farm bill: A package of legislation that encompasses policies on farming, healthy food access, and food systems. It expires approximately every 5 years, at which point it goes through extensive review processes and must be passed by Congress and signed by the President.

Farmers Market Nutrition Program (FMNP): A program that provides WIC participants with coupons to buy eligible foods from farmers, farmers markets, or roadside stands.

Feeding America: A hunger-relief organization that aims to ensure equitable access to nutritious food for all, in partnership with food banks, policy makers, supporters, and the communities they serve.

Fetal alcohol spectrum disorders (FASDs): A range of disorders that result from fetal alcohol exposure. Alcohol consumed during pregnancy crosses the placental barrier and results in fetal alcohol exposure. Disabilities resulting from FASDs are lifelong and can be severe, including but not limited to facial abnormalities, shorter-than-expected height, problems with internal organs such as the heart and kidneys, poor coordination, learning problems, intellectual disabilities, behavioral problems such as poor concentration and hyperactivity, speech delays, and sensory issues such as poor hearing and/or vision. For this reason, alcohol should not be consumed during pregnancy.

Fetal origins of disease hypothesis: The concept that events during very early development have an impact on disease risk in adulthood.

Fetus: An offspring in the stages of prenatal development that follow the embryo stage. The fetal period of pregnancy starts at about 9 weeks and continues until birth. By the beginning of the fetal period, most of the body's systems and organs are in place; during the remainder of the pregnancy, these continue to grow, develop, and mature in preparation for encountering the outside world.

Fine motor skills: Abilities *d*eveloped through the use and coordination of smaller muscle groups in the hands and wrists, demonstrated by stacking objects and scribbling.

First 1,000 Days: The time from conception to 24 months of a child's life.

Five Basics of Parenting Adolescents: Guidelines presented in the work of Dr. A. Rae Simpson, at the Raising Teens website, Massachusetts Institute of Technology MIT Work-Life Center. The *Five Basics* provide guidelines for parents and guardians of adolescents and may also be useful to persons who work with adolescents. The guidelines are focused on effective practices for adults to help adolescents make a successful transition into adulthood.

Fluorosis: White or brown staining of the teeth caused by excessive ingestion of fluoride before the teeth have erupted.

Folate status: Folate is a vitamin that is plentiful in green leafy vegetables and fruits and serves as a cofactor for many crucial physiologic pathways. Adequate folate status prior to and during pregnancy has been associated with a lower incidence of neural tube defects in the fetus. Inadequate folate status may also heighten the risk for inadequate fetal growth, preterm birth, and malformations such as heart anomalies and cleft palate. It is recommended that those planning to become pregnant consume a supplement providing 400 mcg of folate per day. Those who are pregnant should consume a supplement providing 600 mcg of folate per day, in addition to consuming foods that are good sources of folate.

Food: Ingestible material consisting mainly of water, protein, carbohydrate, and fat, and also including vitamins and minerals, used in the body of an organism to sustain growth, repair, and vital processes and to furnish energy.

Food allergy: An unpleasant or dangerous immune system reaction after a certain food is eaten.

Food and nutrition security: Food security is the concept of having enough food to meet physiologicl needs; nutrition security is the concept of having enough nutritious food to meet physiologic needs and promote disease prevention and optimum health. Public health nutrition professionals seek to meet populations' food and nutrition security needs.

Food as medicine: The idea that food can be used to optimize health, prevent disease, and help manage disease.

Food bank: A nonprofit organization that collects and distributes food to local frontline hunger-relief organizations, such as food pantries.

Foodborne illness: Illness caused by food contaminated with bacteria, viruses, parasites, or toxins.

Food deserts: Geographic regions with limited access to healthy and affordable food.

Food insecurity: Household-level economic and social condition of limited or uncertain access to adequate food; lack of consistent access to enough food to fuel a healthy lifestyle, typically due to lack of financial resources. The inability to reliably access and benefit from safe, nutritious, and preferred foods in culturally and socially acceptable means.

Food insufficiency: Not having enough to eat often or sometimes.

Food jag: When a child wants to repeatedly eat the same foods or foods prepared or presented in one way.

Food justice: The struggle against racism, exploitation, and oppression taking place within the food system that addresses the root causes of inequalities.

Food pantry: Food pantries are non-profit organizations that serve their local communities by providing emergency food resources to persons and households experiencing food insecurity within those communities. Food pantries are often supplied and supported by a large, regional food bank.

Food swamp: An oversaturation of fast food and less healthful, non-nutritious food options in a defined geographic area.

Food system: The entire range of people and processes involved in the chain of activities consisting of food production, gathering, processing, distribution and acquisition, consumption, and disposal of food waste; includes the physical, economic, and social environments in which these activities take place.

Food voucher programs: Nutrition incentive programs that provide coupons to use at various types of food outlets, usually with the goal of improving access to healthy foods, such as fruits and vegetables.

Frailty: Increasing weakness with aging; malnutrition is often a contributing factor to frailty.

Full term pregnancy: Defined by ACOG as the desired time frame for completion of pregnancy in which delivery occurs at 39 weeks to 40 weeks and 6 days of gestation. Until 2013, *full term* was considered delivery at any time between 37 and 42 weeks' gestation. However, more recent research indicates that important development of the lungs, liver, and brain occurs during gestational weeks 37 to 38. The risk of respiratory and other problems following birth is lowest when birth occurs at 39 to 40 weeks' gestation.

Functional ability: The capacity for a person to do what they want to do; encompasses abilities such as being able to meet one's own basic needs including food access and preparation, to continue learning and growing as a person, to make one's own decisions, to be mobile, to participate in relationships, and to contribute to society.

Gastroesophageal reflux (GER): A condition in which stomach acid repeatedly flows back into the esophagus.

Global population aging: In 2004, the global population of adults older than 65 years was about 461 million; by 2050 it is projected that those over 65 years will number 2 billion. The implications of global population aging for healthcare systems and society as a whole are enormous; some have called global population aging the single most important medical challenge the world currently faces.

Grazing: An expression describing the continual ingestion of calories throughout the day.

Gross motor skills: Abilities gained from the development and use of large muscle groups, demonstrated by walking, running, and riding a bicycle.

Growth mindset: An attitude and/or belief on the part of an individual that qualities such as one's intelligence and skills can be changed, and are not fixed and unchangeable. A growth mindset is demonstrated when individuals see failure or less-than-optimal results as an opportunity to learn, identify opportunities to improve, and find new paths and directions for moving forward.

Growth spurt: The period of the adolescent life cycle when rapid growth in height and weight occurs. In males, the growth spurt typically occurs between 12 and 16 years of age, with mean peak height velocity of 9.5 cm/year achieved on average at around 13 to 14 years. In females, the growth spurt typically occurs between 9½ and 13½ years, with mean peak height velocity of 8.3 cm/year achieved on average at around 11 to 12½ years. There is substantial individual variation in timing of the growth spurt.

Growth velocity: The rate of growth from one specific time point forward to another, usually measured in units of height and/or weight, or as a ratio of height and weight called BMI. For example, when using a standard pediatric growth chart to monitor growth at well-child visits, growth velocity would be described as the rate of growth from one practitioner visit to the next.

Gus Schumacher Nutrition Incentive Program (GusNIP): A grant program that funds projects to provide incentives to income-eligible individuals to purchase fruits and vegetables .

Hazard mitigation: Planning that often takes place on the federal and state level, utilizing socioeconomic data to identify vulnerable populations and take preemptive action to reduce the risk of negative health outcomes associated with a disaster.

Health: A state of complete physical, mental, and social well-being and not merely the absence of disease or infirmity.

Health debt: The potential adverse effects over time of populations' engagement in poor health behaviors. Some health professionals have suggested that the COvid-19 pandemic resulted in a rapid and substantial accumulation of health debt related not only to direct effects of COvid-19 but also to indirect effects such as the postponement of routine health checkups, vaccinations, and elective surgeries, mental health problems, loss of employment and health insurance, and the like.

Health disparities: Inequities in the opportunity to achieve optimal health that are linked to social, economic, ethnic, or environmental disadvantages.

Health equity: The concept in which every person has the opportunity to achieve their highest possible health potential, with no social determinants preventing the achievement of that potential.

Health inequities: Differences in health status that are caused by systemic differences in social determinants of health.

Health investment model: A health theory that perceives health as an investment good, or stock, and posits that individuals receive an initial health stock that is durable but depreciates with age and is influenced by health investment choices, such as medical care, nutrition, and exercise.

Health literacy: The ability of individuals to use basic health information and services to make health-related decisions.

Health span: The period of life during which one is able to enjoy good health and participate fully in one's desired life's activities.

Health stock: A concept in which health is seen as an investment good. Each individual receives a genetic contribution to health, which is affected throughout life by health inputs such as diet, physical activity, and social determinants of health. To a large extent, lifestyle choices determine the health stock over time and the combination of these inputs also entails an optimal point and rate of decline with age.

Health-related quality of life (HRQOL): A group or individual's perception(s) of their physical and mental health over a given period of time. The CDC measures HRQOL by utilizing a population survey to determine a measure called Healthy Days, which can be used within the *h*ealth *investment m*odel for monitoring and surveillance of overall population health, including the identification of health disparities as well as progress over time.

Healthy aging: Maintaining functional ability and well-being in older age. The concept is also referred to as successful aging.

Healthy People 2030: The fifth iteration of a nationwide program to track progress on public health priorities in 10-year increments to help individuals, organizations, and communities to improve health and well-being.

Healthy weight: A weight that is >5th percentile to <85th percentile on the CDC Growth Charts for children and adolescents.

Hierarchy of needs: An idea proposed by Abraham Maslow in 1943 that posits that there are multiple factors that motivate humans; it organizes motivations into five suggested levels, and theorizes that people prioritize motivations, with basic survival needs typically prioritized first. In Maslow's hierarchy, nutrition is considered a basic survival need.

Home-delivered Meals Program: A nutrition program for older adults in the United States; initiated in 1972 as a result of the federal Older Americans Act (OAA). Nutritious meals are delivered to homebound older adults most weekdays; the program contributes one third of the daily nutrient needs of older adults per the Dietary Reference Intakes (DRIs).

Human milk substitutes: Infant formulas that are a substitute for the preferred nutritional fluid for infants, human milk.

Hunger: Physiologic sensation of discomfort that may result from a lack of food.

Hyperemesis gravidarum: Severe nausea and vomiting during pregnancy that is ongoing and persistent, likely related to hormones released by the placenta. The condition can result in significant weight loss, debilitation, and the need for hospitalization to treat dehydration and electrolyte imbalances. It usually resolves by gestational weeks 16 to 18. Compared to the very common pregnancy condition of morning sickness, the symptoms of hyperemesis gravidarum are much more severe.

Hypertensive disorders of pregnancy: Disorders of high blood pressure during pregnancy that include prepregnancy (chronic) hypertension, gestational hypertension, and preeclampsia/eclampsia. Hypertension, also known as high blood pressure, is a major risk factor for maternal death and occurs in about 5% to 10% of pregnancies. Risk factors for hypertensive disorders of pregnancy include older maternal age (>40 years), preexisting obesity, excessive weight gain during pregnancy, and gestational diabetes.

Hypothalamic–pituitary–gonadal (HPG) axis: The relationships among the hypothalamus gland, the pituitary gland and its secreted hormones, and the gonads (ovaries in females, testes in males). The HPG axis is active in the fetus during the gestational period, but activity subsides early in infancy and enters a period of dormancy that lasts throughout childhood. The exact factor(s) that trigger the initiation of puberty are not well understood; however, it is known that renewed HPG axis activity, including the pituitary's resuming secretion of gonadotropin-releasing hormone (GnRH) in early adolescence, indicates that puberty has begun.

Iceberg Model of Culture: An idea developed in the mid-1970s by anthropologist Edward T. Hall as an analogy for the hidden culture code that exists an any society. This model helps to depict the complexity of one's culture in order to gain insights into one's culture. According to Hall, approximately 10% of a culture is visible and includes tangible items such as food, clothing, artifacts, and language. The other 90% of culture is invisible and includes intangibles such as values, beliefs, attitudes, communication style, and so forth that are generally more difficult to know or understand by those who are not familiar with the culture.

In utero: Being in the uterus; the period of development that takes place prior to birth.

Incident management: The establishment of a command structure to coordinate all emergency response efforts so that services and supplies, including food, are delivered when and where most needed.

Infant: A very young child from the period of time from birth to 1 year of age.

Infant mortality: Death of an infant before 1 year of age.

Infant mortality rate: The number of infant deaths for every 1,000 live births.

Information management: The overall communications plan designed to provide essential information to emergency responders and the public. Integration of nutrition communications within the master communications plan is crucial to inform the public of food supply and food safety updates.

Innate: Inborn; used to describe traits that are present from birth.

Intrinsic capacity: The personal capacities and resources a person can draw on during the aging process, including physical abilities, the senses including vision and hearing, energy level, and psychological functioning including mental health.

Iron deficiency: A condition of too little iron in the body.

Jurisdictional partners: Jurisdictions are defined and often incorporated areas, usually with political boundaries. Examples of jurisdictions include towns, cities, counties, townships, and others. An example of a jurisdictional partnership could be a regional food bank working with a county government's emergency management team to identify locations for emergency food delivery in a disaster situation.

Late adolescence: While there is substantial developmental variation among individuals, late adolescence encompasses the ages of 18 to 21+ years. During this life cycle stage, the shift into young adulthood is completed. Especially for males, some growth in height may continue during this period. Neurologic development continues as adult-level thinking skills (judgment, abstract thinking, evaluating consequences of actions, etc.) reach maturity.

Late term pregnancy: According to ACOG, the time frame for completion of pregnancy. Late term delivery is considered to occur between 41 weeks and 41 weeks and 6 days. Late term delivery is associated with a higher risk of poor infant outcomes such as macrosomia, breathing problems, and meconium in the lungs. While further research is needed, at least one recent study has found that maternal risks are similar to those for full-term deliveries.

Law of Demand on Normal Goods: Changes in food prices and consumer income impact the demand for food. Thus, food is a normal good, or one for which income directly and positively affects demand; that is, as income increases, demand increases. According to the Law of Demand on Normal Goods, there is a direct relationship between consumer income, food prices, and demand for food.

Large for gestational age (LGA): A birth weight exceeding the 90th percentile for gestational age. LGA status is associated with heightened maternal and infant risk for delivery complications and other poor outcomes including infant respiratory and metabolic problems. Excessive maternal weight gain increases the risk of a large-for-gestational-age birth.

Length of pregnancy: The time from the first day of the last menstrual period to the day of delivery. A normal full-term pregnancy lasts about 40 weeks or 9 months.

Life course theory: A theory that health outcomes occur due to a "complex interplay" of social and environmental factors mixed with biological, behavioral, and psychological factors across the course of a person's life. Each life stage exerts influence on the next stage and exposures accumulate over time to affect health.

Life cycle: The normal progression of developmental stages through which an organism passes during its life span. While there is no recognized standard timetable for the developmental stages through which humans progress, the stages of the human life cycle are typically understood to be the gestational period, infancy, early childhood, later childhood, adolescence, young adulthood, middle adulthood, and older adulthood.

Life cycle nutrition in public health: The application of public health principles to population nutrition issues and problems at each stage of the human life cycle.

Life span: The length of time between a person's birth and death.

Low birth weight: Birth weight <2,500 g (<5 lb 8 oz).

Macronutrients: Nutrients that are needed in large amounts to provide energy; these include fat, carbohydrates, and protein.

Macrosomia: Macrosomia is diagnosed at any gestational age if the fetus weighs more than 4,000 g (8 lb, 13 oz), and risk of poor outcomes substantially increases once fetal weight reaches 4,500 g (9 lb, 15 oz). Macrosomia is associated with heightened maternal and infant risk for delivery complications and infant respiratory and metabolic problems. Excessive maternal weight gain increases the risk of macrosomia.

Malnutrition: A condition resulting from either inadequate or excessive intake of nutrients, imbalance of nutrients consumed (e.g., very high consumption of carbohydrates but little intake of protein), or physiologic inability to utilize nutrients consumed.

Maternity care deserts: Any county lacking a hospital or birthing center providing obstetric services, or lacking a provider of obstetric care.

Mentorship: The process in which a more experienced person works with a less experienced person to share knowledge, skills, attitudes, and values to support success. While mentorship is often associated with career advancement, it is also valuable in promoting personal growth and development. Mentorship programs for adolescents have been shown to result in improved health, behavioral, and academic outcomes.

Micronutrients: Nutrients needed in smaller amounts that are vital to healthy development, disease prevention, and well-being.

Middle adolescence: While there is substantial developmental variation among individuals, middle adolescence encompasses the ages of 14 to 17 years. During this life cycle stage, adolescents usually complete most of their physical growth into adulthood.

Miscarriage: See *Early pregnancy loss.*

Moderation in alcohol consumption: Consuming no more than one standard drink per day for females, and no more than two standard drinks per day for males. Adults may choose not to drink alcoholic beverages. For adults ages 21 years and older who choose to consume alcoholic beverages, on days when alcohol is consumed, moderation at the level described here is recommended. See *Standard drink.*

Molinsky's six dimensions of culture: A six-dimensional approach for understanding the cultural code of a culture. These six dimensions represent key aspects of communication across cultures and can be used in identifying key differences and similarities between cultural styles. Developed by Dr. Andy Molinsky, the six dimensions are directness, enthusiasm, formality, assertiveness, self-promotion, and self-disclosure.

Morning sickness: Nausea and vomiting in the early months of gestation, usually resolving by the early second trimester. Morning sickness is very common in pregnancy. The symptoms are typically intermittent, allowing for adequate consumption of foods and beverages to meet nutritional needs.

MyPlate: An educational program that provides a visual framework for healthy eating for Americans, focusing on small changes that focus on increasing fruit, vegetable, and whole grain consumption.

National Center for Health Statistics (NCHS): A CDC agency that is responsible for collecting, analyzing, and disseminating health data to inform public health policy decisions.

National Health and Nutrition Examination Survey (NHANES): A series of studies that includes demographic, socioeconomic, dietary, and health-related questions to assess the health and nutritional status of U.S. adults .

Needs assessment: The collection of data and the analysis process that provides information about an audience in order to direct all aspects of communication planning and implementation. This includes discovering gaps in knowledge, identifying accessible resources, defining outcomes, and determining the most optimal delivery channels.

Neonatal jaundice: Elevated serum bilirubin manifesting as yellowish discoloration of the skin, sclerae, and mucous membranes.

Neonatal period: The first 4 weeks, or 28 days, of a baby's life. An infant in this stage of life is medically considered a neonate. The neonatal period is a time of rapid growth and development. It is a crucial time for the establishment of human bonds and attachments with parents and/or caregivers. Many other milestones take place, including development of the baby's first feeding patterns.

Neophobia: Fear of something new, such as new foods.

Nutrient-dense: Having a high vitamin and mineral content for the weight of a food; a high amount of nutrients for the calories consumed.

Nutrients: Substances in food that promote growth, proper function and overall health. The major classes of nutrients are fats, carbohydrates, proteins, vitamins, minerals, and water.

Nutrition communication: Using communication processes to convey and/or exchange nutrition information and messages among individuals and audiences for the purpose of building nutrition knowledge and/or influencing nutrition perspectives and behaviors.

Nutrition security: Equitable and dependable access to affordable, safe, and nutritious foods that support health and well-being and prevent chronic disease. Compared to food security, which seeks the provision of *enough food to meet calorie needs*, nutrition security seeks the provision of *enough of the right kind of food to meet calorie needs and promote optimal health.*

Nutrition surveillance: A system designed to gather data and information about a geographical area's nutrition-related factors so that data and information can be used to formulate and promulgate nutrition policy. Geographical areas are usually political entities such as countries, states, provinces, and the like.

Nutrition: The science of food and its nutrients as they pertain to supporting the biochemical and physiological process that maintain life.

Obesity: Weight >95th percentile on the CDC Growth Charts for children and adolescents.

Obesigenic environment: The degree to which the surrounding environment impacts rates of overweight and obesity in persons and populations. For example, poor walkability may be a factor that contributes to a community's obesigenic environment.

Old: Between ages 75 and 84 years, within the three stratifications of age.

Older adulthood: Final life cycle stage when the health and nutrition behaviors and practices of earlier life cycle stages are likely to have their greatest impact.

Older Americans Act (OAA): A U.S. law enacted in 1965 as the result of a perceived need to improve resources and social services available to older adults. The OAA established grants to states to provide services, conduct research, and train personnel with a focus on aging. The Administration on Aging was established by the OAA, housed within what was then the Department of Health, Education, and Welfare (now the Department of Health and Human Services), and was charged with administering the state grant programs.

Old-old: Ages 85 years and above, within the three stratifications of age.

Osteoarthritis: The most common form of arthritis involving degenerative damage to the joints over time.

Osteomalacia: Softening of bones that can occur in adults as a result of a lack of vitamin D.

Osteoporosis: Bone disease that develops when bone mineral density and bone mass decrease, or when the quality or structure of bone changes.

Overweight: Weight >85th percentile but <95th percentile on the CDC Growth Charts for children and adolescents.

Parenteral feeding: Providing nutrition intravenously (through a vein).

Patient Protection and Affordable Care Act. See *Affordable Care Act (ACA).*

Peak height velocity: The period of the growth spurt during which height is increasing at its fastest rate: typically about 9.5 cm/year for males and 8.3 cm/year for females.

Peak weight velocity: The period of adolescent growth during which weight is increasing at its fastest rate: in males, the growth spurt and peak weight gain velocity are roughly concurrent, averaging about 9 kg (~20 lb) per year; in females, peak weight gain tends to occur about 6 months after peak height velocity and averages around 8.3 kg (~18 lb) per year.

Perceived discrimination: A type of psychosocial stressor experienced by stigmatized racial groups directed at them by social institutions and individuals.

Physical activity: Body movements produced by skeletal muscles that contribute to an increase in energy expenditure.

Pincer grasp: the ability to hold something between the thumb and first finger.

Policy: A plan for making decisions. Policies are based on consideration of existing systems, environments, resources, and desired outcomes, among other factors. Informal policies may be called guidelines. Policies may be formalized as official regulations or as law.

Polypharmacy: Literally meaning "many medications," polypharmacy is common among older adults who consume a variety of prescribed and unprescribed pharmaceuticals on a daily basis. Older adults with polypharmacy take on average five to nine different prescription drugs per day. Many commonly used drugs have possible nutrition-related side effects that can discourage eating, including but not limited to nausea, diarrhea, stomach discomfort, *xerostomia* or dry mouth, taste changes such as metallic tastes or "off" tastes, and decreased appetite.

Population health: The health outcomes of a group of individuals, including the distribution of such outcomes within the group.

Post term: Designated by ACOG as a pregnancy with gestation extending 42 weeks and beyond. Post-term pregnancy is associated with a number of heightened maternal and infant risks, including the risk of stillbirth, macrosomia, infant breathing problems, and cesarean deliveries.

Precocious puberty: The initiation of puberty prior to the age of 8 years in females, and prior to the age of 9 years in males. A medical evaluation is indicated.

Preload study: A study used to investigate the satiating effects of foods.

Prematurity: See *Preterm birth.*

Prenatal vitamin: Vitamins designed for use during pregnancy and lactation. They can be helpful in meeting the increased nutrient needs of pregnancy and in compensating for any nutritional gaps. Prenatal vitamins should be taken only as directed by one's health provider.

Prenatal: Prior to birth; used to describe the period of development that occurs in the womb.

Preschooler: Child between the age of 3 and 5 years.

Presenteeism: The presence of an employee who comes to work when ill, injured, or otherwise unable to be as productive as usual. Presenteeism may be prompted by fear of financial loss, losing one's job, or losing opportunities. Effects of presenteeism include but are not limited to poor job performance, impaired productivity, slower recovery from the accompanying health condition, and possibly spreading communicable illnesses to other employees.

Preterm birth: A baby born alive prior to 37 weeks' gestation (from World Health Organization). Prematurity is categorized by gestational age: (1) extremely preterm, prior to 28 weeks' gestation; (2) very preterm, 28 to 32 weeks' gestation; (3) moderate to late preterm, 32 to 37 weeks. Preterm birth is a major public health nutrition issue because it is the leading global cause of death in children under 5 years of age, and because nutrition is a key factor in its prevention. Death rates from prematurity are much higher in low-income countries due to a lack of availability and access to appropriate medical care.

Preterm/premature: Refers to an infant born before 37 weeks of pregnancy are completed.

Prevalence: The proportion of the number of individuals within a population with a certain characteristic during a certain time period, compared with the number of individuals within the entire population; usually expressed as a percentage. For example, if 82 out of 100 people in a population like to eat carrots on a given day, the prevalence of persons who like to eat carrots in the population on that day is 82/100, or 82%.

Primary prevention: Actions to prevent a disease from occurring; the main focus of interventions is healthy populations.

Produce prescriptions: A program to assist people in obtaining adequate amounts of fresh fruits and vegetables to promote health and manage chronic disease, by providing a prescription for these items from a healthcare provider. The prescription provides a voucher, EBT (electronic benefits transfer) card, or cash incentive to purchase the prescribed produce. Usually grant-funded at this time, it is hoped that produce prescriptions will eventually be included as a health insurance benefit by both public and private third-party payers.

Psychographic information: In communications, knowledge of particular audiences' values, attitudes, beliefs, challenges, and concerns. Knowing and understanding one's audience are essential in crafting nutrition messaging that will resonate with the target audience.

Puberty: The period during which a person develops from a child into an adult; includes the development of secondary sexual characteristics and attainment of adult stature with the closure of the skeletal epiphyses in late puberty. Puberty also includes substantial neurologic development, which encompasses growth in intellectual, emotional, decision-making, and social capabilities.

Public Health Emergency Preparedness and Planning Model: In 2018, the CDC Center for Emergency Preparedness and Response (CDC-CEPR) published national standards for emergency response capabilities for state, local, tribal, and territorial public health agencies, and the materials were updated in 2021. The standards and accompanying guidance provide a framework for assessing, planning, and implementing specific public health functions during emergency situations. The standards are designed to promote effective emergency preparedness and response.

Public health nutrition (PHN): The branch of public health that seeks to protect and improve community health through nutrition policy recommendations, nutrition education and outreach, and research focused on the prevention, detection, and management of nutrition-related diseases.

Public health: "The science and art of preventing disease, prolonging life, and promoting health through the organized efforts and informed choices of society, organizations, public and private communities, and individuals." (Adapted from: Winslow C. The untilled fields of public health. Science, *New Series*. 1920;51(1306):23–33. https://doi.org/10.1126/science.51.1306.23)

Racism: A societal system, consisting of structures, policies, practices, and norms, that assigns value and determines opportunity based on racial hierarchies, which negatively affects the mental and physical health of millions of people.

Registered dietitian nutritionist (RDN): A U.S.-based credential for nutrition professionals. RDNs complete coursework in basic, social, and nutritional sciences and at least 1,000 hours of practical experience before completing a national exam. After initial exam-based credentialing, RDNs must complete 75 hours of continuing professional education every 5 years.

Relaxin: The hormone that promotes softening and stretching of the pelvic muscles and ligaments throughout pregnancy, and especially during the third trimester, to promote and prepare for a safe delivery.

Resilience: The process and outcome of successfully adapting to difficult or challenging life experiences, especially by demonstrating flexibility and the ability to change and adjust. It is often described as the ability to "bounce back." As humans age, their ability to bounce back from physical insults such as illness and injury decreases, and the body loses reserve capacity to deal with physical stress. Older adults who age successfully eventually lose physical resilience, but often have great reserves of mental and emotional resilience that they apply to dealing with the challenges and inevitable losses of aging.

Responsive feeding: Recognizing and responding to the child's hunger and fullness cues.

Return on investment (ROI): A ratio expressed as the (current value of investment – cost of the investment)/cost of investment. So, if a person purchased a property at a cost of $50,000 and sold it several years later for $75,000, the ROI would becalculated as follows: (75,000 – 50,000)/50,000 = 0.50, or 50% ROI. Investments in health, such as following a nutritious diet and engaging in regular exercise, may not be as tangible or easy to measure, but have multiplier implications on all tiers of economic factors—household, firms, government, and the rest of the world.

Risk factors (modifiable and nonmodifiable): Interactions between contextual environment factors (nonmodifiable, such as age, gender and genetics) and an individual's lifestyle behaviors (modifiable, such as diet, physical activity, tobacco use) that increase the likelihood of developing a chronic disease.

Rooting: A feeding reflex in infants to turn their head to the side and open their mouth when one cheek is touched.

Sarcopenia: Gradual loss of muscle mass, strength, and function. It is associated with many poor outcomes and is often a precursor to malnutrition and frailty.

Satiety: A feeling of fullness upon eating that reduces the subsequent desire to eat more. In a general sense, satiety is one-half of the appetite mechanism, with the other half being hunger.

School-age child: Child between the ages of 5 and 12 years.

Screen time: Time spent in any activity done while watching a screen, including computer use, TV watching, and video gaming

Secondary prevention: Identification (screening) of persons to detect chronic disease early; the main focus of interventions is at-risk populations.

Sedentary behavior: Any waking behavior that is completed in a sitting or reclining posture.

Self-efficacy: An individual's belief in their own abilities to reach a goal.

Senescence: The aging process that takes place over a lifetime, and results in the gradual loss of physiologic capabilities including healing and protective processes that ultimately leads to death. There is great variation among individuals in the rate and process of senescence.

Sensitive period of childhood development: A time when brain and body alignment are optimal for a particular developmental task; however, the time period during which the task can be accomplished remains somewhat malleable.

Severe obesity: BMI ≥120% of the 95th percentile

Short Form Cultural Intelligence Assessment (SFCIA): An assessment that consists of 10 statements about one's experience when interacting with people from other cultures. The result of over a decade of academic research, the SFCIA was developed and validated in response to the need for an easy-to-administer assessment of individual differences in cultural intelligence. Each statement is rated using a Likert-type scale.

Shoulder dystocia: A complication of vaginal birth that is considered an obstetric emergency. It occurs when the infant's head is delivered but the shoulder becomes obstructed at the mother's pubic bone, and requires additional interventions for delivery to be completed. The major risk factor for shoulder dystocia is fetal macrosomia.

Six domains of emergency preparedness: (1) Community resilience; (2) incident management; (3) information management; (4) countermeasures and mitigation; (5) surge management; and (6) biosurveillance. This plan was defined by the CDC Center for Preparedness and Response.

Small for gestational age (SGA): A birth weight below the 10th percentile for gestational age. Infants with SGA status are at higher risk of death during the *neonatal period,* about 22% of infant deaths worldwide during the neonatal period associated with SGA status. Inadequate weight gain during pregnancy increases the risk of SGA birth.

Social determinants of health (SDOH): SDOH are factors that affect health, function, and quality-of-life and can be grouped into five major domains, including economic stability, education access and quality, healthcare access and quality, neighborhood and built environment and social and community context. Socioeconomic and environmental factors are powerful determinants of health and are largely outside the control of individuals and groups.

Social-ecological model (SEM): A public health framework that is used to describe the importance of public policy, community, institutional, interpersonal, and individual drivers of health outcomes.

Social media: A collective term for websites and applications that focus on communication, community-based input, interaction, content-sharing, and collaboration. Facility in the use of social media is increasingly becoming an essential skill for nutrition communicators.

Social vulnerability: Referring to community resilience in the face of external stressors on human health.

Social vulnerability index (SVI): A tool based on 16 factors recorded in Census tract data and grouped into four thematic domains: (1) socioeconomic status; (2) household composition and disability; (3) minority status and language; and (4) housing type and transportation. The tool is designed to identify communities which may need support prior to, during, and after disasters.

Socioeconomic status (SES): The term used to characterize social position and social class. Research has shown that a higher SES is associated with better health outcomes due to completion of higher levels of education, higher incomes, more autonomy at work, more access to grocery stores, health resources, knowledge, skills, and the capacity to act on health recommendations. Four major factors related to SES that influence health outcomes are education, income, occupation, and occupational settings.

Special healthcare needs: Increased risk for chronic physical, developmental, behavioral, or emotional conditions; require greater health and related services.

Stadiometer: A piece of equipment for measuring height; usually consists of a vertical measuring stick and a horizontal stick that can be moved up or down to rest on the top of the head.

Standard drink: The amount of a particular kind of alcoholic beverage that is likely to contain about 14 g of pure alcohol, or 12 oz beer, 5 oz wine, or 1.5 oz (1 shot) spirits/hard liquor.

Strengths-based assessment: An approach to emergency planning that focuses first on community strengths, existing social networks, resources, and community assets in order to leverage existing resources to promote community resilience and recovery in the face of emergencies. An assessment of strengths can help communities enhance existing resources, prioritize areas for improvement, and deploy resources for optimal impact.

Structural inequities: Systemic disadvantages of one group that coexists with others related to societal structures and disparities.

Stunting: Impaired growth and development that children experience from poor nutrition, repeated infection, and inadequate psychosocial stimulation; too short for age.

Subclinical iron deficiency: Insufficient iron level for red blood cell production, but not yet detectable by low hemoglobin levels.

Successful aging: See *Healthy aging*.

Suckling: The earliest feeding reflex of moving the tongue forward and backward.

*Supplemental Nutrition Assistance Program (SNAP):*The largest antihunger program in the United States; it provides food support to low-wage workers and people living with disabilities, among others.

Surge management: The implementation of strategies to optimize and increase the capacity of essential organizations during emergency situations. In disasters, facilities such as hospitals and shelters may become overwhelmed by demand for services. Roles for public health nutrition professionals in surge management may include providing food to first responders and other emergency response personnel and collaborating with community healthcare facilities in regard to deployment of emergency food supplies.

Surveillance: The collection of health data in a systematic way, continuously over time. Surveillance data is regularly analyzed and interpreted to determine needed actions and to inform policy development.

Systems thinking: Holistically considering the connections among a set of factors and how they contribute to potential outcomes.

Tanner stages: In clinical settings, the progress of puberty is often assessed by the use of Tanner stages. The Tanner stages were developed as the result of longitudinal observation studies conducted in England from the 1940s to the 1960s by Drs. J.M. Tanner and W.A. Marshall, with their classic studies published in 1969 and 1970. Also known as *sexual maturity* ratings (SMR), the Tanner stages provide medical providers with a five-stage reference standard for documenting the development of external genitalia throughout puberty for females and males.

Temperament: How a child reacts to the world; temperament can include different emotions and behaviors.

Ten Essential Public Health Services Framework: A framework that defines and describes the public health activities in which all communities should participate. It was originally released in 1994 and updated in 2020 by the Public Health National Center for Innovations and the de Beaumont Foundation.

Ten Tasks of Adolescent Development: The areas in which teens transition from childhood into adulthood. Based on the work of Dr. A. Rae Simpson, the *Ten Tasks of Adolescent Development* are housed at the Raising Teens website, Massachusetts Institute of Technology MIT Work-Life Center. Along with the *Ten Tasks,* the website provides links to resources and suggestions for supporting each area of development.

Tertiary prevention: Treatment or management strategies to prevent secondary disease complications by slowing disease progression, improving disease management, and delaying disease complications. Ultimately, tertiary prevention strategies are intended to promote the highest possible quality of life for persons with chronic diseases.

The Law of Unintended Consequences: Actions—however well-intentioned—may have results, either positive or negative, that are different from, or in addition to, expected outcomes.

Theory of Change (TOC): A method used to explain how an intervention is expected to lead to the desired change and guide policy making by using evidence gathered in the TOC process.

Time preference: The extent to which people value current consumption over future consumption.

Toddler: Child between the ages of 1 and 3 years.

Trimester: A 3-month period during pregnancy. Healthcare professionals usually describe the 9 months of pregnancy as occurring in three consecutive 3-month periods called the first, second, and third trimesters. During the first trimester, initial differentiation and development of virtually all body systems and tissues takes place. During the second trimester, growth and development of organs, body systems, and other physical characteristics continue at a rapid pace. During the third trimester of pregnancy, the fetus continues to grow larger, accumulate fat, and gain weight.

U.S. Department of Agriculture (USDA): A federal agency that implements policies related to food quality, nutrition, farming, and other agriculture-related issues. USDA comprises 29 agencies, including the Food and Nutrition Service and the Center for Nutrition Policy and Promotion, and is responsible for several nutrition programs including SNAP and WIC .

Upstream factors. Risk factors from social and environmental factors that affect an individual's behaviors. Examples of upstream factors include social determinants of health such as income level, education level, access to healthcare, access to healthful food, exposure to violence, and the like. Policies directed at upstream factors may substantially and positively impact downstream factors, that is, individual health behaviors.

Upstream, Midstream, Downstream Model: In 2019, the de Beaumont Foundation proposed a model for strategies and tactics to impact social determinants of health at clinical, individual, and community levels, called downstream, midstream, and upstream domains, respectively. If one thinks of health as a river or stream, it follows that the source of the river—the upstream component—will have a major impact on downstream results. According to the model, clinical health encounters are downstream from social determinants of health that affect individuals, and individual impacts are downstream from societal conditions that affect social determinants of health. Thus, the greatest health and nutrition impacts will result from strategies and tactics that impact upstream factors in ways that promote health for everyone.

Very low birth weight: Birth weight <1,500 g (<3 lb 5 oz).

Vitamin K deficiency bleeding (VKDB): Unstoppable bleeding in infants due to lack of *vita*min K for blood clotting.

Wasting: Impaired growth and development that children experience from poor nutrition, repeated infection, and inadequate psychosocial stimulation; too thin for age.

Water security: The ability to reliably access sufficient water for all household uses.

Weaning: Process of changing an infant's diet from breast milk or formula to other foods and fluids.

Weight stigma: Negative attitudes and beliefs that devalue people based on their weight status that may include bias, discrimination, stereotyping, and social exclusion.

WHO Decade of Healthy Ageing Report (DHAR): A report that describes three determinants of healthy aging: functional ability, intrinsic capacity, and environments; published in 2016. The WHO Decade of Healthy Ageing is currently ongoing from 2020 to 2030.

Xerostomia: Dry mouth, or lack of saliva flow, often caused by polypharmacy or other diseases or dysfunctions of oral tissues. Xerostomia is associated with dental problems and subsequent poor food intake.

Youth: The period from 15 to 24 years of age, encompassing the first years of early adulthood.

Young-old: Ages 65 to 74, within the three stratifications of age.

Zygote: The fertilized egg after conception occurs; it travels through a fallopian tube into the uterus where it implants into the uterine wall.

INDEX

Note: Page numbers in *italics* denote tables and figures.

www.ingramcontent.com/pod-product-compliance
Lightning Source LLC
LaVergne TN
LVHW082025200926
848481LV00010B/2923